✓ £34.99

The Library
The Learning Centre
Huddersfield Royal Infirmary
Occupation Road
Huddersfield HD3 3EA
Tel: 01484 342581

due for return on or before the last date shown below.

- 4 APR 2012
2 4 OCT 2012

2 2 FEB 2013

2 8 MAR 2013

D0279125

Property of

OXFORD MEDICAL PUBLICATIONS

Handbook of
Surgical Consent

This book is

Handbook of
Surgical
Consent

Edited by

Rajesh Nair

MBBS MRCS
Specialist Trainee in Urology
South Thames Rotation
London Deanery

David J Holroyd

MSc(Res) MB ChB BSc MedSci(Hons) MRCS
EPSRC Clinical Research Fellow
Transplantation Research Group
Nuffield Department of Surgical Sciences
University of Oxford

OXFORD
UNIVERSITY PRESS

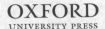

OXFORD
UNIVERSITY PRESS

Great Clarendon Street, Oxford OX2 6DP

Oxford University Press is a department of the University of Oxford.
It furthers the University's objective of excellence in research, scholarship,
and education by publishing worldwide in

Oxford New York

Auckland Cape Town Dar es Salaam Hong Kong Karachi
Kuala Lumpur Madrid Melbourne Mexico City Nairobi
New Delhi Shanghai Taipei Toronto

With offices in

Argentina Austria Brazil Chile Czech Republic France Greece
Guatemala Hungary Italy Japan Poland Portugal Singapore
South Korea Switzerland Thailand Turkey Ukraine Vietnam

Oxford is a registered trade mark of Oxford University Press
in the UK and in certain other countries

Published in the United States
by Oxford University Press Inc., New York

© Oxford University Press, 2012

The moral rights of the author have been asserted
Database right Oxford University Press (maker)

First published 2012

All rights reserved. No part of this publication may be reproduced,
stored in a retrieval system, or transmitted, in any form or by any means,
without the prior permission in writing of Oxford University Press,
or as expressly permitted by law, or under terms agreed with the appropriate
reprographics rights organization. Enquiries concerning reproduction
outside the scope of the above should be sent to the Rights Department,
Oxford University Press, at the address above

You must not circulate this book in any other binding or cover
and you must impose this same condition on any acquirer

British Library Cataloguing in Publication Data
Data available

Library of Congress Cataloguing-in-Publication-Data
Data available

Typeset by Cenveo, Bangalore, India
Printed in Great Britain
on acid-free paper by
Ashford Colour Press Ltd, Gosport, Hampshire

ISBN 978–0–19–959558–7

10 9 8 7 6 5 4 3 2 1

Dedication

To our families and friends, without your support
and understanding this work would
not have been completed.

To our colleagues, without whom this work
would not have begun.

Oxford University Press makes no representation, express or implied, that the drug dosages in this book are correct. Readers must therefore always check the product information and clinical procedures with the most up-to-date published product information and data sheets provided by the manufacturers and the most recent codes of conduct and safety regulations. The authors and publishers do not accept responsibility or legal liability for any errors in the text or for the misuse or misapplication of material in this work. Except where otherwise stated, drug dosages and recommendations are for the non-pregnant adult who is not breastfeeding.

Preface

Patients have the ethical and legal right to decide whether to undergo medical or surgical intervention. Before this can occur, they need to be provided with sufficient information so that they can make an appropriately informed decision about their care. The amount of information given will vary from patient to patient depending on individual circumstances. Valid consent to treatment is vital in all forms of healthcare and extends from simple examination to disclosing confidential information to undertaking major surgery.

The Department of Health has highlighted, for consent to be *valid*, the patient must be fully informed of the risks, benefits, and alternatives to the procedure in question. This is particularly applicable to invasive investigations and surgical procedures. All significant risks should be disclosed and this will vary from patient to patient (significance depends on individual circumstances). Many complaints and medicolegal cases involve inadequate disclosure of the potential risks and benefits of the procedure in question. The information included in this book is not exhaustive: it is neither practical nor possible to list every possible risk for every procedure. Similarly, every possible risk cannot be disclosed during consent.

Also, the consent process cannot be reduced to information contained within a book—it is far more than that. Consent needs to be tailored to each patient as, while a given benefit or risk may not be significant for one patient, it may be greatly significant to another, depending on the circumstances that the patient finds themselves in. Thus, the information in this book is intended to be used as a *basis* for consent and should be individualized accordingly for the patient concerned.

Several published audits have demonstrated that there is great variability in the quality of consent for surgical procedures. This is at all levels: from foundation year trainees through to consultants. Improving the consent process can only be beneficial to both the patient and the clinician.

Gaining informed consent for individual procedures is a structured process that is often not included in formal medical education. All too often it is the junior surgical trainee who is requested to consent patients for surgery, but who although 'trained' to undertake consent is unable to perform the procedure as they do not fully understand all of the significant risks of the procedure. This is poor practice (put yourself in the patient's shoes!). The person taking consent should ideally be the person about to undertake the procedure, as per the Department of Health, General Medical Council, and the Royal Colleges' guidelines. If this is not possible, consent must be taken, at the very least, by someone who is capable of performing the procedure or someone who has sufficient knowledge of the procedure, techniques, benefits, alternatives, and risks.

Although aimed at surgical trainees, this handbook offers all healthcare professionals general guidance in the principles of consent, followed by procedure-specific information regarding risks and benefits. The aim of this book is not to 'teach' consent to junior trainees and is not intended to reduce the need for the person undertaking consent to be able to perform the procedure. Rather, it is intended to be an adjunct to surgical training as a pocket reference for the clinician to help improve the quality and content of verbal and written consent in surgical practice. Thus, we hope this book will help medical staff to discuss surgical treatments with patients, particularly with disclosure, improve understanding of the principles of consent and encourage good consent practice.

RN
DH
March 2011

Acknowledgements

We are indebted to all those who have helped us produce this book, especially to all our contributors and their consultant supervisors for their expertise and timely submissions. We are grateful to the staff at Oxford University Press who have been both professional and a pleasure to work with. Particular mention goes to Elizabeth Reeve, Anna Winstanley, Andrew Sandland, Michael Hawkes, and Kate Smith at OUP, and Lotika Singha for copy-editing. A special mention goes to the consultant staff at Chase Farm Hospital, where the idea for this book was conceived, and to Mr Robert Wheeler, whose expertise in medical law has been invaluable in the production of this book.

Contents

Contents

Contributors

Adebayo Alli
BA(Hons) BM BCh
Ear, nose, and throat surgery
CT2 in ENT Surgery
Northwick Park and St Mark's
Hospital
London

Aiden Armstrong
MD FRCSI FRCS(Gen)(Glas)
FEBSQ(Coloproc)
Colorectal surgery
Consultant Colorectal Surgeon
Belfast City Hospital
Belfast

Nadeem Ashraf
FRCS(Gen)
Vascular surgery
Specialist Registrar in General
Surgery
Basildon University Hospital
Basildon, Essex

Atul Bagul
MD FRCS
Transplantation surgery
NIHR ACL and SpR in
Transplant Surgery
University Hospitals of Leicester
Leicester

Catherine C L Bryant
MB ChB MRCS
*Upper gastrointestinal and
bariatric surgery*
Clinical Research Fellow in Surgery
Barts and the Royal London
Queen Mary's School of
Medicine and Dentistry
London

Bernie Chang
BSc MB ChB FRCSEd FRCOphth
Ophthalmic surgery
Consultant Ophthalmologist
Leeds Teaching Hospitals NHS Trust
Leeds

Asif Chaudry
MA BM BCh FRCS(Gen)
*Upper gastrointestinal and
bariatric surgery*
SpR in General Surgery
Barts and the Royal London
NHS Trust
London

Daniel D'Aquino
MBBS MSc BA(Hons) MRCS
Neurosurgery
ST2 in Neurosurgery
Queen's Medical Centre
Nottingham

Jessica Farren
BA(Hons) MBBS
*Obstetrics and gynaecological
surgery*
Specialist Trainee in Obstetrics
and Gynaecology
London Deanery

Daren L Francis
MD FRCS(Gen Surg)
*General surgical procedures
and Laparoscopic surgery*
Consultant Colorectal,
Laparoscopic, and General Surgeon
Barnet and Chase Farm
NHS Trust, Middlesex

Thomas W Hester
BSc(Hons) MBBS MRCS
Orthopaedic surgery
ST3 in Orthopaedic Surgery
Southeast Thames Rotation
London Deanery

Richard E Hill
MB ChB BSc(Hons) MRCS
*General paediatric surgery and
Neonatal surgery*
Senior Clinical Fellow in
Paediatric Surgery
King's College Hospital NHS Trust
London

Arvind Singh
MBBS DLO FRCS(Orl-HNS)
Ear, nose, and throat surgery
Consultant Otolaryngologist
Northwick Park and St Mark's
Hospitals
Middlesex

Richard P Stevenson
MB ChB MRCS
Colorectal surgery
Clinical Research Fellow
Beatson Institute for Cancer
Research
University of Glasgow
Glasgow

Ajay Sud
MBBS MRPharmS MRCS
Breast surgery and *Vascular surgery*
Core Surgical Trainee
London Deanery

Natalie Suff
MB BCh(Hons) BSc(Hons)
Obstetrics and gynaecological surgery
Academic Clinical Fellow in
Obstetrics and Gynaecology
London Deanery

Guy M Webster
MB ChB FRCS(Urol) FEBU
Urological surgery
Consultant Urological Surgeon
Barnet and Chase Farm NHS
Trust, Middlesex

Robert A Wheeler
MB LLB(Hons) FRCS FRCPCH
General principles of consent,
General paediatric surgery, and
Neonatal surgery
Consultant Paediatric and
Neonatal Surgeon
Wessex Regional Centre for
Paediatric Surgery
Southampton University Hospitals
NHS Trust

Barrie White
BSc MBBS FRCP FRCS(SN)
Neurosurgery
Consultant in General and
Spinal Neurosurgery
Queen's Medical Centre,
Nottingham

Symbols and abbreviations

✍	Web reference
📖	Cross-reference
▶▶	Note (important)
2°	Secondary
↓	Decrease
ACS	acute coronary syndrome
AD	advanced decision
AF	atrial fibrillation
AFP	A-fetoprotein
APACHE	acute physiology and chronic health evaluation
AR	aortic regurgitation
ARDS	adult respiratory distress syndrome
AS	aortic stenosis
ASA	American Society of Anesthesiologists
BAUS	British Association of Urological Surgeons
BCC	basal cell carcinoma
BCG	bacille Calmette Guérin
BIPP	bismuth iodoform paraffin paste
BSO	bilateral salpingo-oophorectomy
BTS	British Thoracic Society
BWS	Beckwith–Wiedemann syndrome
BXO	balanitis xerotica obliterans
CABG	coronary artery bypass graft
CAT	combined approach tympanoplasty
CBD	common bile duct
CBDE	common bile duct exploration
CDH	congenital diaphragmatic hernia
CFA	common femoral artery
CHA	Canadian Heart Association
CIN	cervical intra-epithelial neoplasia
CIS	carcinoma in situ
CMV	cytomegalovirus
CPAP	continuous positive airway pressure
CT	computed tomography
CTG	cardiotocography
CVA	cerebrovascular accident/incident

CVC	central venous catheter
CVP	central venous pressure
CVS	chorionic villus sampling
DALK	deep anterior lamellar keratoplasty
DBD	donation after brain death
DCD	donation after cardiac death
DIEP	deep inferior epigastric perforator
DLCO	carbon monoxide diffusion capacity
DLEK	deep lamellar endothelial keratoplasty
DSAEK	Descemet's stripping automated endothelial keratoplasty
DSEK	Descemet's stripping endothelial keratoplasty
DVT	deep vein thrombosis
dwMRI	diffusion weighted magnetic resonance imaging
EAC	external auditory canal
EACTS	European Association for Cardio-Thoracic Surgery
EAU	European Association of Urology
ECG	electrocardiogram
ECMO	extra-corporeal membrane oxygenation
ECP	endoscopic cyclophotocoagulation
ECV	external cephalic version
EF	ejection fraction
ERCP	endoscopic retrograde cholangio-pancreatography
ERM	epiretinal membranes
ERPC	evacuation of retained products of conception
ESC	European Society of Cardiology
ESWL	extracorporeal shock wave lithotripsy
EVLT	endovenous laser therapy
FAP	familial adenomatous polyposis
FBC	full blood count
FDG-PET	$[^{18}F]$2-fluoro-2-deoxy-D-glucose positron emission tomography
FESS	functional endoscopic sinus surgery
FETO	fetal endoscopic tracheal occlusion
FFP	fresh frozen plasma
FNAC	fine needle aspiration cytology
FROA	flow-rate (urine) on arrival (outpatient)
FTSG	full thickness skin graft
GnRH	gonadotropin-releasing hormone
GTN	glyceryl trinitrate
HCG	β-human chorionic gonadotrophin

HDU	high dependency unit
HFOV	high frequency oscillatory ventilation
HIV	human immunodeficiency virus
HNPCC	hereditary non-polyposis colorectal cancer
HoLEP	holmium laser enucleation of prostate (gland)
HPT	hyperparathyroidism
HTA	Human Tissue Act
HTLV	human T-lymphotropic virus
ICSI	intracytoplasmic sperm injection
ILM	internal limiting
IMA	internal mammary artery
IMCA	independent mental capacity advocate
INR	international normalized ratio
ISC	intermittent self-catheterization
ITU	intensive treatment/care unit
IUD	intrauterine device
IV	intravenous
IVC	inferior vena cava
IVF	*in vitro* fertilization
IVU	intravenous urogram
KUB	kidney–ureter–bladder
LAD	left anterior descending (artery)
LARC	long-acting reversible contraception
LD	latissimus dorsi
LDH	lactate dehydrogenase
LLETZ	large loop excision of the transformation zone
LOS	lower oesophageal sphincter
LPA	lasting power of attorney
LPS	levator palpebrae superioris
LSV	long saphenous vein
LUTS	lower urinary tract symptoms
LV	left ventricle
LVESD	left ventricular end-systolic dimension
MALT	mucosa-associated lymphoid tissue
MEN	multiple endocrine neoplasia
MIBG	metaiodobenzylguanidine scan
MODS	multiple organ dysfunction syndrome
MR	mitral regurgitation
MRM	modified radical mastoidectomy
MVR	mitral valve replacement

NAC	nipple–areolar complex
NACSDR	6th National Adult Cardiac Surgical Database Report of the Society for Cardiothoracic Surgery in Great Britain & Ireland
NEC	necrotizing enterocolitis
NICE	National Institute of Health and Clinical Excellence
NYHA	New York Heart Association
OAB	overactive bladder
OASIS	obstetric anal sphincter injuries
OGD	oesophago-gastro-duodenoscopy
OMC	osteomeatal complex
OPSI	overwhelming post-splenectomy infections
OSA	obstructive sleep apnoea
PAP	pulmonary artery pressure
PCA	patient-controlled analgesia
PCI	percutaneous coronary intervention
PCNL	percutaneous nephrolithotomy
PEG	percutaneous endoscopic gastrostomy
PFA	profunda femoris artery
PFS	preformed silastic silo
PNALD	parenteral nutrition-associated liver disease
POIC	progesterone-only injectable contraceptive
POSSUM	Physiologic and Operative Severity Score for the enumeration of Mortality and Morbidity
PPV	patent processus vaginalis
PSA	prostate specific antigen
PTH	parathyroid hormone
PTLD	post-transplant lymphoproliferative disorders
PVP	photo-selective vaporization of the *prostate*
RFA	radiofrequency ablation
ROM	range of motion
RT-PCR	reverse transcriptase polymerase chain reaction
RV	residual volume
SAPS	Simplified Acute Physiological Score
SCC	squamous cell carcinoma
SCTS	Society for Cardiothoracic Surgeons
SFA	superficial femoral artery
SIRS	systemic inflammatory response syndrome
SLNB	sentinel lymph node biopsy
SPK	simultaneous pancreas-kidney (transplant)
STEMI	ST-segment elevation myocardial infarction

STSG	split-thickness skin graft
SVG	saphenous vein graft
TCC	transitional cell carcinoma
THR	total hip replacement
TIA	transient ischaemic attack
TOE	transoesophageal echocardiogram
TOF	tracheo-oesophageal fistula
TOP	tracheo-oesophageal puncture
TPN	total parenteral nutrition
TR	tricuspid regurgitation
TRAM	transverse rectus abdominis myocutaneous (flap)
TURBT	transurethral resection of bladder tumour
TURP	transurethral resection of prostate (gland)
TV	tricuspid valve
U&E	urea and electrolytes
UDT	undescended testes
VATS	video-assisted thoracoscopic surgery
VEGF	vascular endothelial growth factor
WLE	wide local excision
WHO	World Health Organization

General principles of consent

Quick reference guide to consent

The aim of this short section is to provide answers to some of the common questions and issues involved in consenting. Each of the issues listed in Box 1.1 is covered in greater depth within the main body of the chapter.

Box 1.1 Key principles of consent

- The patient must be competent
- There must be sufficient disclosure of information
- The information disclosed must be understood, processed, and evaluated in terms of the patient's own beliefs and values
- Consent must be voluntary

What procedures/treatments?

- Consent is required for *all* examinations, investigations, and procedures, except in some emergencies
- This may range from simple verbal consent for examination to written consent
- Consent is also required for the disclosure of confidential information to other parties and this must not be forgotten

What type of consent and how should it be documented?

There is generally no legal requirement for the specific procedures that require *written* consent (exceptions are those procedures listed in the Human Fertilization and Embryology Act 1990).

- However, in practice and in keeping with the Department of Health, Royal Colleges', and trusts' guidelines, written consent should be gained for surgical procedures
- The consent form simply documents that a discussion has taken place about the procedure or investigation
- Good oral consent is valid consent, but it is difficult to prove it occurred in retrospect
- Documentation needs to be made in the clinical records when the complete details of a discussion that has occurred cannot be fully documented on a consent form, or when oral consent has been given

Who should gain consent?

- Ideally, the person who will perform the procedure should gain consent
- Failing that, a clinician who can undertake the procedure him/herself, or a clinician who is fully familiar with the procedure, its alternatives, benefits, and risks, and has received appropriate training

What information should be disclosed?

- The following information should be discussed:
  - The diagnosis, including uncertainties
  - The purpose of the treatment or investigation
  - What the treatment or investigation involves
  - Alternatives, including the option not to treat

- Prognosis
- The likely benefits of the investigation or procedure and the probability of success
- Significant risks, complications or side effects
- The clinician responsible
- The patient's right to change their mind
- All significant risks should be disclosed
- There is no numerical cut-off regarding risk—clinical judgement needs to be used to determine whether a risk is significant or not
- The 'reasonable patient standard' is used, meaning any risk that a reasonable patient would find significant should be disclosed
- Significance may vary from patient to patient

How long is consent valid for?
- Consent is a process rather than a single event
- If consent is gained in advance, it should be confirmed immediately prior to undertaking the investigation or procedure
- Patients have the right to withdraw consent, or change their mind at any stage, and this should be explained to the patient

Assessing competence
- All people over the age of 16 are legally presumed to have the capacity to consent, unless there is evidence to the contrary
- Where there is doubt, it is important to assess competence fully: e.g. not all patients with a mental disability lack competence to consent
- To demonstrate capacity, a patient needs to:
  - Understand the nature of the proposed treatment, why it is being proposed and what it involves
  - Understand the relative benefits and risks of the treatment
  - Understand the potential consequences of not receiving the treatment
  - Retain and weigh up the information in order to come to a decision regarding treatment

Adults who lack capacity to consent
- Incapacity may be temporary, e.g. due to medications, drugs, pain, sedation, shock
- Relatives cannot provide consent on an incompetent person's behalf (even if they have power of attorney). However, in Scotland, an appointed proxy decision maker may provide consent
- In emergency situations, treatment should be provided in the patient's best interests, unless there is a valid advanced decision (AD)
- If there is sufficient time, advice should be sought from the trust's legal team as an independent mental capacity advocate (IMCA) may be required to help assess and determine the patient's best interests
- For less-urgent treatment, the case should be referred to the local clinical ethics committee and the Court of Protection for it to decide whether a proposed treatment is legal

Advanced decisions

- Patients may draw up an AD to refuse treatment that may be proscribed
- Patients may also appoint a lasting power of attorney, who may refuse consent on the patient's behalf, although they are constrained by the wording of the legal document
- The AD needs to be applicable to the clinical circumstances
- If there is clear refusal of treatment by an AD, which is applicable to the clinical situation faced, and the AD was made when the patient was competent and fully informed, the AD should be respected
- If there is doubt over the validity of an AD, or it is not relevant to the clinical situation, it should be presumed that the patient wishes to live

Children and adolescents

- Young people under the age of 16 must *demonstrate* competence (Gillick competence), i.e. they are presumed to lack competence to consent
- If a person under 16 can demonstrate that they are competent, i.e. they have sufficient understanding of the treatment proposed and that they can weigh up and retain this information, they may provide consent independently
- Gillick competence does not extend in the same way to the refusal of treatment
- Children aged 16 and 17 are presumed to be competent to consent. However, this does not extend to consent for involvement in research
- If a child under the age of 16 is not competent to give valid consent, somebody with parental responsibility may give consent to treatment
- Not all parents have parental responsibility:
  - The mother automatically has parental responsibility
  - Both parents have parental responsibility if they were married at the time of the child's conception, birth, or at some point after the child's birth
  - Neither parent loses parental responsibility on divorce
  - The father also has parental responsibility if the child was born after 2003 and the father is named on the birth certificate
  - The father may also apply through the courts to be granted parental responsibility, or apply to have the birth certificate changed

Emergencies

- Valid consent is required if the patient is competent to consent
- In an emergency, if consent cannot be obtained, clinicians should provide treatment that is in the patient's best interests
- The treatment should be limited to that required to save life or treat the immediate emergency situation
- Treatment to treat non-emergency pathology should wait until the patient has regained capacity
- If there is *clear* evidence of a *valid* AD that is applicable to the clinical situation, this must be respected. However, if this is not the case, it should be presumed that the patient wishes to live

- In the case of children under 16, if the patient lacks the capacity to consent, someone with parental responsibility should provide consent. If urgent treatment is required, the child lacks capacity and nobody with parental responsibility is available, treatment should be provided in the child's best interests

Research

- Separate consent is required for research
- Consent for research should be written consent
- When consenting for research purposes, information must be provided in the fullest possible form, including the aims, methods, risks, and benefits of the research, along with the parts that are experimental and, as such, subject to unpredictable outcomes
- If randomization is involved, this should also be disclosed, including the potential of being allocated to a non-treatment group
- Adequate time must be allocated to allow the patient to reflect
- Obtaining tissues or organs for research purposes also requires consent and is subject to the Human Tissue Act 2004
- Adults who lack capacity can be involved in research, although the local ethics committee should be consulted and the research is likely to be 'therapeutic' in nature
- When involving children in research, someone with parental responsibility should be consulted, even if the child is competent to make the decision him/herself

Teaching

- Consent should be sought from patients before engaging them in any teaching activities
- Patients should be able to decline, if they so wish, without pressure
- Anaesthetized patients have the same right to give or withhold consent, and specific consent for teaching purposes should be gained prior to administration of an anaesthetic
- Consent is required for photography/video recordings and their use for teaching purposes. Patients may withdraw their consent at any point and the material should be destroyed if this occurs

A guide to consent forms

Which consent form?

 See Appendices 1–4 for exemplar forms used in the National Health Service (NHS).
- Consent form 1 (Appendix 1)—Used for patients able to consent for themselves
- Consent form 2 (Appendix 2)—Used for those with parental responsibility consenting on behalf of a child
- Consent form 3 (Appendix 3)—Used for procedures performed with no impairment of consciousness (both adults and children)
- Consent form 4 (Appendix 4)—Used for adults without capacity to consent for themselves

What information?
- Consent forms 1 and 2 (consent form 3 is a shortened version):
  - Patient identifiable details
  - Name of responsible healthcare professional, contact details
  - Intended procedure
  - Intended benefits of the procedure
  - Significant risks, complications
  - Any additional procedures
  - Consent for possible blood transfusions
  - Type of anaesthesia/sedation
  - Signature and details of clinician gaining consent
  - Signature and details of interpreter, if applicable
  - Patient's name, signature and date
  - Confirmation of consent—if first-stage consent taken at an earlier encounter
- Consent form 4:
  - Patient identifiable details
  - Name of responsible healthcare professional, contact details
  - Intended procedure
  - Assessment of the patient's capacity—why the patient is unable to consent on his/her own behalf; how this judgement has been made
  - Why it is believed that performing the proposed procedure is in the patient's best interests
  - Why the treatment cannot wait until the patient regains capacity
  - Documentation of family members consulted. However, they do not have a right to consent on behalf of the patient: the final decision lies with the clinician responsible for the patient
  - Any concerns
  - Signature and details of the clinician proposing treatment
  - Signature and details of a clinician giving a second opinion
- Additional information should be documented in the notes, e.g. where an extensive discussion/disclosure has taken place

Introduction to the consent 'process'

Consent is essential to the fundamental principle of autonomy. It does not only apply to interventions and surgical procedures; a patient's consent is necessary prior to commencing any examination and is also required to share confidential information. Guidance in *Good Medical Practice*,[1] published by the General Medical Council (GMC), requires doctors to be satisfied that they have consent (Box 1.2) from a patient or other valid authority prior to commencing an examination, investigation, or treatment. Similar consent is also required before involving a patient in research or teaching. This chapter covers general issues on consent, including current guidance and legal aspects, but is aimed to be a practical guide.

Box 1.2 The elements of informed consent

- The patient must be competent
- There must be sufficient disclosure of information
- The information disclosed must be understood, processed, and evaluated in terms of the patient's own beliefs and values
- Consent must be voluntary

Many of the procedural aspects of consent stem from guidance issued by the GMC, Department of Health, and the Royal Colleges, rather than from legal obligation.[1–3] It should also be noted that there is no legal obligation to obtain written consent for any procedure, bar a few exceptions detailed in the Human Fertilization and Embryology Act 1990 or the Mental Capacity Act 2005.[4] Verbal consent can be good consent. Rather, it is more important to gain *valid* consent.

►►**Consent is a process, not a one-off event**

Ideally, consent should not be a singular event and should not be obtained only immediately prior to a planned intervention. By doing so, it does not allow a patient sufficient time to retain, process, and weigh up information in order to provide 'informed' consent. Patients need sufficient time and information to make informed decisions and therefore consent should be a gradual 'process', where possible. In practice, this usually means that the consent 'process' usually starts in the outpatient department and continues right up to the preoperative period. A signature on a consent form is not sufficient in itself; indeed it does not constitute consent or evidence of adequate consent. Unfortunately, consent within the NHS all too often seems to focus on the completion of the consent form.

As with any patient interaction, a discussion regarding consent needs to be conducted in an appropriate location, with sufficient privacy to maintain patient dignity and confidentiality.

The various components of the consent 'process' are covered in detail in the individual sections within this chapter. Assessment of capacity commences at the first encounter with the patient. If there are any concerns or doubts, a more formal assessment may need to be made. The path that subsequent discussions and decisions will need to take will depend on the outcome of this and should be adjusted accordingly.

As with all patient encounters, good communication is key to making the consent 'process' effective. A partnership between the patient and the doctor needs to be established whereby each has a role in making decisions about treatment or care and a level of trust is developed. An effective partnership involves:
- Listening to and respecting the views and decisions of the patient
- Discussing what the diagnosis, treatment and prognosis involves
- Disclosing relevant information that a patient needs to make informed decisions
- Listening and responding to questions and concerns
- Maximizing the patient's opportunities and the ability to make decisions for themselves

If the patient does not share a common language, then it should be arranged for a translator to be present. In practice, the consent process should be a series of discussions between the clinician and the patient, whereby information is shared, questions regarding the possible treatment options are raised and answered, and a decision as to the best treatment option for that patient is made in partnership. In emergency situations, obviously this may not be possible. In general, the following information should be discussed/disclosed during the consent process for a particular treatment or intervention:
- The diagnosis and prognosis, including any uncertainties and options for further investigations/treatment
- Options for managing the condition, including the option not to treat, and the relative benefits and risks of each
- The purpose of any investigation or treatment, and what it will involve
- A summary of the main details of the investigation or procedure
  - This needs to be presented in language that the patient can understand
  - Visual aids or information sheets/leaflets may help with this process
- The likely postoperative course
- The potential benefits and risks of the investigation/treatment/procedure
- The likelihood of success for each treatment option
- If the benefits/risks are affected by the specific organization or doctor chosen to provide care
- Whether a proposed investigation or treatment is part of a research programme or, if it is an innovative treatment, designed for a specific patient's benefit
- The people responsible for the patient's healthcare
- The extent that any students may be involved
- The patient's right to refuse to be involved in teaching or research
- The right to a second opinion
- Any conflicts of interest
- Any costs involved (i.e. private practice)
- A reminder that the patient can change their mind at any time
- Any questions should be answered honestly and accurately

It is impossible and impractical to inform patients of all known risks for a given procedure. Different risks are of different importance to different individuals and the consent 'process' needs to reflect this. Therefore, disclosure must be adapted to each individual process and disclosure for a given procedure may vary substantially between patients, depending on their values, needs, and situations. However, what is certain is that patients should be told of significant risks even if the likelihood of them occurring is small.

Finally, in many cases, once an informed decision has been made, adequate documentation of consent should follow, including documentation on what information was disclosed. However, not all consent needs to be written: implied or verbal consent may be adequate in many cases. All of the principles mentioned here are discussed in greater depth within this chapter.

References

1. General Medical Council. *Consent: Patients and Doctors Making Decisions Together.* London: GMC, 2008.
2. Department of Health. *Reference Guide to Consent for Examination or Treatment*, 2nd edn. London: DH, 2009.
3. Royal College of Surgeons of England. *Good Surgical Practice*. London: Royal College of Surgeons of England, 2008.
4. Mental Capacity Act 2005.

Seeking consent from a person who is fully aware of the clinical risks and benefits should concentrate the mind of both surgeon and patient. If the process has failed to dispel doubts in either mind that intervention is the right thing to do, abandon the procedure, reconsider the situation, and do something different.

References

1. Bolam v. Friern Barnet Hospital Management Committee. [1957] 1 WLR 582.
2. Pearce v. United Bristol Healthcare NHS Trust. [1999] 48 BMLR 118.

How should consent be recorded, and for what procedures?

Consent is necessary for any intervention, but the form of consent, and its mode of recording, can differ widely. Individual hospital trusts often have their own view of what type of procedures merit written consent and it is prudent to adhere to local rules. However, from a broader perspective, there is no doubt that oral consent is good consent. There is no national legal requirement to obtain written consent for surgery, although there is a statutory requirement for written consent for fertility treatment.[1]

But the reality remains; that the existence of oral consent is very hard to prove in retrospect, and this difficulty is proportionate to the time that has elapsed since the intervention in question took place. For this reason, the Department of Health advocates written consent for all forms of surgery.[2] However, as will be seen later in this section, neither the form of the written consent, nor the definition of 'surgery', is stated. Thus a practical approach to the problem is proposed.

You require permission to touch patients. Patients with capacity are entitled to refuse your touch if they wish, although this is almost never problematic. They want to be cured; you need to touch them for this to occur, so there is a tacit understanding that touching will need to ensue. Nevertheless, permission to touch should never be taken for granted. If you want to examine the patient, simply let them know what you want to do, and ask if that is alright. They will almost inevitably agree that it is and you can proceed in a dignified manner. It is no more difficult than that. If the patient refuses, try to ascertain why they do not want to be touched, and find a solution. But do not imagine that your professional position confers authority to force the patient to be examined. Quite the contrary; you have a fiduciary duty to respect the patient's wishes, while working out how you are going to fulfil your other duty of providing good clinical care. This is a clinical challenge, and if you feel unable to deal with it effectively, seek help from your seniors, or an experienced nurse.

Patients who lack capacity may be unable to consent for a relatively complex procedure, such as an operation. However, you are not entitled to assume that they are indifferent to whether they are indifferent to being touched, examined, or bled, and so you should presume that their permission is required for these things, as with a person with normal capacity. If truly incapacitated for all intents and purposes, patients still must be afforded politeness and dignity. It can only be hoped that someone will remember this if we ourselves end up in this unenviable situation.

Once you accept that consent is required for any and every time you want to touch the patient, and that obtaining this consent is an elementary process, it can be seen that most of our clinical activities can be easily performed on the basis of the form of verbal consent that is based on the concept sometimes described as 'good manners'. This would certainly include physical examination, measuring blood pressure, venesection, inserting intravenous cannulae and urinary catheterization. None of these activities are usually controversial, and oral consent is entirely appropriate. However, there may be particular circumstances when you start to feel anxious about the situation. Perhaps you encounter the rare clinical circumstance of a woman with urinary retention, who needs to have a catheter. She is very reluctant to have one passed, but eventually agrees, though still reluctant.

It is purely a clinical judgement whether you feel that consent needs to be recorded more formally. This has little to do with the law. Oral consent is good consent, but it may be difficult, months later, confidently to recall that you obtained consent orally, and what you disclosed in obtaining it. If in doubt, make a note in the case notes: That you have discussed catheterization, that you noted her reluctance, but that you advised the necessity for urinary drainage, while acknowledging some risk of ascending infection; but balancing this against the risks of retention. This is powerful evidence of consent. Far more so than some incompletely filled-in 'consent form', which may well be mislaid. Such interventions as thoracocentesis and chest drain insertions on the ward, diagnostic lumbar punctures and many other everyday procedures may often have a patient's consent recorded in this way.

Which interventions are 'so serious' that formal consent form must be completed? This will usually have been decided for you, codified by the local trust's consent policy. Commonly, any surgical or interventional radiology procedure will require a consent form, as will any procedure that requires local or general anaesthesia. If in doubt, it is prudent to use a form, but ensure that it is properly filled in. The disclosure that leads to valid consent is infinitely more important than the signature.

Indeed, failure to ensure that the patient has capacity, inadequate disclosure of information, or failing to ensure that the patient provides consent voluntarily are all errors that invalidate the consent, irrespective of a signature: 'Consent expressed "in form only" is no consent at all'.[3]

For this reason, providing evidence by a handwritten entry in the case notes becomes potent evidence of a diligent approach to consent. This is also a prudent move when you have completed a consent form with a patient, but still remain anxious that the form does not wholeheartedly reflect the conversation, or the inherent uncertainties of the procedure. For example, you may have spent an hour with some parents, weighing up the risks and benefits of excising their infant's thoracic neuroblastoma. The Department of Health form gives precious little space for a full account of your deliberations, or a relevant diagram, which better describes the surgical dilemma. Putting your thoughts on paper will allow you to state your position, beyond doubt.

Oral consent is valid, but writing provides a record. Get consent for any intervention, but take a proportionate approach as to what form of documentation is necessary.

References

1. Human Fertilization and Embryology Act 1990, Sch. 3.
2. Department of Health. *Reference Guide to Consent for Examination or Treatment*. 2nd edn. London: DH, 2009.
3. *Chatterton v. Gerson*. [1981] 1 All ER 257 at 265.

Implied, presumed, or inferred consent

Paradoxically, in a society where autonomy is given priority, there are observable trends towards reducing the requirements for explicitly expressed consent. Recently, there was an attempt to implement an 'opt out' system to increase the supply of donated organs. This system avoided the need for expressed consent,[1] replacing it with implied or presumed 'consent'. For this reason, among others, the project stalled. However, the willingness at government level even to consider compromising the principle of explicit consent is instructive.

By asserting that a patient has consented to an intervention, we are referring to the state of the patient's mind. Properly informed, the patient has made a voluntary decision, agreeing to the intervention. Usually, the patient then expresses their state of mind either orally or in writing. The caveat that a signature is not necessarily adequate evidence of consent is, in part, based on the anxiety that the signed form may not be indicative of what the patient truly thinks, i.e. his/her state of mind. But the expressed consent usually suffices, since there is no practicable alternative.

There are circumstances when it is possible to imply that a person has acquiesced to a situation, for example it might have been in the era of routine non-inactivated polio vaccination: the unaccompanied non-English-speaking parent who brings his child for polio vaccination sits in silence with the child on his knee, holding open the baby's mouth for oral vaccination. Once inoculated, the child and father leave. A reasonable observer viewing this would acknowledge that the father acquiesced to the procedure, satisfying the legal test for implied consent.[2]

However, the father's 'consent' is based on fiction. The observer cannot assume that the father's action is based on an informed decision. The father, who is not vaccinated, now risks contracting polio, infected by the live inoculum that his child excretes. It seems unlikely that he would have consented to this outcome.

Implied (or presumed) consent is a term for a legal device that allows an intervention to be performed without expressed consent to be recognized as legal. It requires that a reasonable observer would conclude, on the basis of the patient's conduct, that there was acquiescence to the intervention. It has the effect of preventing a person subsequently deny that he/she consented, even though they did not do so. This stops patients who choose not to express their consent from subsequently complaining that they have not consented to the intervention.

In the generality of routine medical practice, the device of implied consent facilitates practice. The GMC recognizes that for routine investigations, implied consent suffices.[3] However, it qualifies this, ensuring that the practitioner 'is satisfied that the patient understands' what is proposed. This describes inferred, not implied, consent where the reasonable observer is not only satisfied that acquiescence has occurred, but also deduces that the patient's state of mind is that of consent.

The distinction between implied and inferred is not mere pedantry. The state of a patient's mind, in terms of their attitude to consent, is deduced (inferred)[4] by courts when deciding whether contested consent was valid. This is completely different from merely relying on a patient's conduct to license an intervention, irrespective of the presence of consent. Implied consent is an unfortunate term, since it indicates that there is consent, where none may exist. The false belief that it represents valid consent leads those who need to legitimize their unconsented activity to select implied consent as the appropriate licence.

Furness' pithy description[5] of implied consent—'provide an information sheet and invite objections' is accurate. 'Implied consent' should be abandoned. We should understand that in circumstances when we claim that the patient gave his/her 'implied consent', in reality what we were hoping for was acquiescence, not consent.

In general terms, it is always better simply to ask the competent patient whether they mind us commencing our intervention, whatever that may be. They almost invariably agree, and you carry on. What could be easier?

References

1. Wheeler RA. Presumed or implied, it's not consent. *Clin Risk* 2010;**16**:1–2.
2. Hurwitz B. Negligence in general practice. In: Powers M, Barton A, Harris N, eds. *Clinical Negligence*, 4th edn. West Sussex: Haywards Heath, Tottel Publishing, 2008.
3. General Medical Council. *Consent: Patients and Doctors Making Decisions Together*. London: GMC, 2008.
4. Grubb A. *Principles of Medical Law*, 2nd edn. Oxford: Oxford University Press, 2004.
5. Furness P. Consent to using human tissue. *BMJ* 2003;**327**:759–60.

The consequences of proceeding with invalid consent

In many senses, the most significant problem arising from failing to ensure that valid consent is in place is that it may interfere with your good relationship with the patient. This benefits no one. Furthermore, formal retribution may flow, either from your employer, the patient, or regulatory authorities.

Local disciplinary activities

It is likely that the organization for which you work will have a consent policy in place. Failure to conform with this puts you at risk of conflict with your employer, and disciplinary measures may be taken against you.

Clinical negligence

There is a duty to provide care of a reasonable standard. This includes ensuring that valid consent is in place before surgery, and failure to provide consent at this standard has led to a series of court actions. In one of the more recent,[1] a surgeon was found to have provided inadequate information before spinal surgery. For this reason, his care was held to be below the reasonable standard. The case is notable for unlinking the necessary causative link between the substandard care and the harm caused. Unusually, Ms Chester did not assert that she would never, at some later stage, have undergone surgery. This assertion would often prove fatal to a consent case (since most claimants rely on the fact that adequate disclosure would have prevented them from running the risk). However, the Court of Appeal found in her favour. It could be argued that this is a measure of the importance with which the courts regard disclosure for consent, waiving the usually invariable rule that a causative link must exist, before a claim in negligence can succeed.

Involvement in civil litigation is a stressful experience. It could be costly, and does not enhance your reputation.

General Medical Council

A patient who feels that he or she has suffered an unwanted touch without providing valid consent is entitled to refer the case to the GMC.

The GMC is unequivocal in its insistence that consent is always required,[2] and will act against doctors who are proved to have defied this requirement.

Civil and criminal charges

Treatment without consent may amount to the civil wrong of battery, or the crime of assault. Individual citizens could use the civil courts to assert their right to veto care proposed by doctors, and the state is free to pursue crimes through the criminal courts. However, these are rare occurrences since such civil and criminal actions have a very limited role to play in healthcare law.[3] In part, this is because the standard of proof required to prove a crime is higher than that to prove a civil wrong, and because the claimant stands to gain far more from a successful clinical negligence action than from actions in battery or crime.

The decision of the English judiciary to use the clinical negligence as the principal legal framework for consent means that damage to your relationship with the patient, local disciplinary measures, clinical negligence actions, and the attention of the GMC remain the principal consequences of proceeding with invalid consent.

References

1. *Chester v. Afshar.* [2002] EWCA Civ 724.
2. General Medical Council. *Consent: Patients and Doctors Making Decisions Together*. London: GMC, 2008.
3. Montgomery J. *Health Care Law*. Oxford: Oxford University Press, 2003, p.228.

What should be disclosed, and by whom?

The summary answer to this question is easy. When taking consent, any matter that a reasonable person would consider significant, when deciding whether they wish to agree to treatment, should be disclosed to them. Additionally, the disclosure should be provided by a clinician capable of performing the intervention.

Getting to this point is more complex.

The particular patient standard

The legal history of disclosure extends over 50 years. It started as something of a shock to the medical profession, that any form of explanation to the patient was required. This pendulum rather rapidly swung in the opposite direction, to a point where North American courts were suggesting that the standard for valid consent was based on what the particular patient in question wished to know. This was the originally conceived doctrine of 'informed consent'. This proved impractical.

Consider the disappointed patient, suing a doctor on the grounds that he has been given insufficient information about his procedure and that if he had known the information, he would have refused to proceed. Even with a wide-ranging and comprehensive disclosure of preoperative information by the defendant doctor, a particular nugget of information will go unmentioned. This, the litigant patient asserts (in retrospect), was crucial for him to know, and will establish his claim, however rare and obtuse that piece of information might have been. Such a doctrine left a door open to unfair claims, and has not been wholeheartedly supported in English law.

The professional standard

The next attempt at setting a standard for disclosure was to suggest that it should be provided by expert medical evidence, the so-called 'professional' standard, akin to the standard setting in other aspects of clinical care. Although this was accepted for some years, it has fallen into disrepute. Courts became increasingly anxious that doctors were 'protecting their own', and acting in a paternalistic manner by, in effect, telling the patient what they should be worried about, rather than asking the patient what worried them.

The reasonable patient standard

Subsequently, courts felt able to put themselves in the position of the claimant patient asking themselves whether, in the circumstances of the case, they would regard the disclosure as adequate. The courts do not feel the need to ask an expert doctor's view on this matter. They consider themselves, as reasoning citizens, amply equipped to set the standard. Thus the stage is set for the 'reasonable patient'. This patient is a fictional creation of the court, imbued with all of the characteristics of the claimant patient, but whose sense of reasonableness is provided by the court:

'If there is a significant risk which would affect the judgement of a reasonable patient, then in the normal course it is the responsibility of a doctor to inform the patient of that significant risk, if the information is needed so that the patient can determine what course he or she should adopt.'[1]

This leaves open to question what a 'significant risk' entails. However, if you apply your personal criteria to the phrase, you are likely to consider that most of the unintended harms that flow from surgery could be construed as 'significant'. The great difficulty is that there exists a gap between what you, as an experienced clinician, and what an average patient might foresee as the result of surgery.

On how many citizens whom you might encounter walking down your local high street will it dawn that surgery on a painful back might result in faecal incontinence? Or that it is foreseeable that an inguinal hernia repair could result in the loss of a testis? Or that a hysterectomy could lead to urinary ascites? Or that operation on one eye could lead to contralateral blindness? While commonplace knowledge for surgeons, these potentials for disaster are not widely known by those who have not had a medical education, and that is why they should be disclosed, when obtaining consent. In addition to this gap in surgical knowledge is the reverse; the recognition that the patient is intimately acquainted with their own circumstances, of which you know little, or nothing.

Financial considerations; perhaps the imminent maturation of an insurance policy; family matters, such as forthcoming wedding; employment; perhaps starting a manual job; and countless other considerations will go into the melting pot when a patient decides whether or not to have surgery. The fact that they may die, or be made impotent, or paraplegic, may have almost boundless implications as to these future activities and since they do not have any awareness of these risks, why would they ask about them?

To address this gap created by a combination of the professional knowledge of the doctor and the personal circumstances, the GMC makes it clear that the duty to disclose is onerous:[2]

'You must tell patients if an investigation or treatment might result in a serious adverse outcome, even if the likelihood is very small.'

The risk may be tiny, but of great importance when deciding whether or not to have surgery, which may be elective.

Statistics are a valuable form of description when articulating risk to patients. In a recent case, the court confirmed the importance of comparative statistics when describing alternative procedures that a patient might want to consider in deciding which intervention she should consent for. Faced with a choice between a catheter cerebral angiography and a magnetic resonance angiogram, the patient was not informed of the comparative risks of stroke.[3] The court held that the patient, as a result, could not provide properly informed consent.

The numerical threshold of risk

The most commonly asked question relating to disclosure refers to the importance, or otherwise, of the numerical threshold for risk; how common does a risk have to be before we disclose it to the patient?

When describing the risk of a clinical intervention to a patient, there is a common and mistaken supposition by doctors that there exists a numerical threshold of improbability beyond which there is no need to disclose.

Where should the line be drawn?

Doctors are comfortable with ubiquitous numerical thresholds to guide their interventions, and depend on plasma levels, and physiological or radiological measurements to carry a patient across a threshold from non-treatment to treatment. However, the numerical risk of most complications of therapy is usually low, and may not be caught by a realistic threshold. Is it right that such a threshold should (inadvertently) conceal relevant matters from the putative patient's consideration?

Courts have briefly explored the notion of a numerical threshold. In 1980, a Canadian court[4] held that a 10% risk should automatically be disclosed when obtaining consent; in this case, to disclose the possibility of a stroke following surgery. This built on the American concept of a material risk, where a reasonable person in the patient's position is likely to attach significance to the risk.

Since then, courts have steadily distanced themselves from a numerical threshold. Three years later, an American case[5] determined that a 200/1 complication rate would not equate to a material risk. A 'landmark' English consent case[6] held that Mrs Sidaway, who had spinal cord damage after surgery, failed to prove that a prudent patient would regard a <1% complication rate as constituting a significant risk.

In 1997, it was held that there was no certainty that an unqualified duty to disclose a risk of around 1% existed, in the context of a family which was not told that permanent neurological damage could result from cardiac transplantation surgery.[7] An Australian case[8] held that the failure to warn of the 14000/1 risk of blindness following ophthalmic surgery fell below the reasonable standard of care. From the legal perspective, this was the death knell of the numerical threshold. To disclose all risks of this frequency would be impractical. The court was demanding that significant risks should be disclosed, irrespective of the likelihood of occurrence. The UK courts followed this lead in 1995,[9] holding that failure to disclose the risk of spontaneous vasectomy reversal (1/2300) equated to substandard care.

The explicit switch from a quantitative to a qualitative approach came in a maternity case,[10] when a patient lost her baby. She had reluctantly agreed to the deferral of her delivery, in the absence of full disclosure of the possible consequences of so doing. Lord Woolf, giving the leading judgement, held that it was not necessarily inappropriate to fail to disclose a risk in the order of 0.1–0.2%; but that the correct standard was to disclose 'a(ny) significant risk which would affect the judgement of the reasonable patient',[10] as described previously.

In a subsequent case,[11] where it was held that there was a failure to warn parents of the risk of fetal abnormality of a pregnancy that coincided with maternal chickenpox, the threshold that the disclosure had to satisfy was that of the patient's determination of a risk, albeit insubstantial; the court accepted Lord Woolf's dictum proscribing the use of a numerical threshold.

Legal scholars support this trend, warning against reducing the meaning of 'substantial' or 'grave' (or 'significant') to quantifiable (numerical) risks,[15] since such reduction misses the central point; that only the patient can judge what risk is material to them, irrespective of its frequency of occurrence.

The concept of a numerical threshold for disclosing risk is therefore outdated from the legal point of view. There is no reference whatsoever to a threshold either from the GMC[12] or the Department of Health,[17] other than to give information about all significant adverse outcomes.

The commonest question asked by doctors, when discussing the law of consent, is where to draw the line between matters that must be disclosed, and those that require no mention. Invariably, they demand a numerical threshold, and are disappointed when this is not forthcoming. Although it is understandable that doctors continue to use this artificial threshold, it is submitted that they should follow the lead of the courts, because a better formula that identifies what needs to be disclosed has been provided for our use. It is better because it provides an assurance that patients will not be 'ambushed' by a serious complication that the doctor could foresee, but of which the patient remained oblivious until it was too late for him/her to avoid it.

Who should disclose the information?

There is no clear rule. However, since it is very clear that every significant risk should be disclosed, there is no doubt that the person best placed to disclose is a person who is familiar with the procedure, since he or she has performed it many times. Some surgeons prefer to delegate this duty to trainees or nurses who are unable to perform the intervention, but who are armed with an information sheet, and have been 'trained' in consenting patients. One wonders whether they would wish their own families treated in this way. It is recommended that consent, and the disclosure that makes it valid, should be taken by the person who is about to perform, or at least who is capable of performing, the procedure.

References

1. *Pearce v. United Bristol Healthcare Trust. Butterworths Med Law Rep* 1999;**48**:118.
2. General Medical Council. *Consent: Patients and Doctors Making Decisions Together.* London: GMC, 2008, para32.
3. *Birch v. University College London Hospital NHSFT.* [2008] EWHC 2237.
4. *Reibl v. Hughes. DLR Canada* 1980;**114**:11.
5. *F v. R. South Austr Supreme Court* 1983;**33**:189.
6. *Sidaway v. Board of Governors of the Bethlem Royal Hospital. All Engl Rep, House of Lords* 1985;**1**:643.
7. *Poynter v. Hillingdon Health Authority. Butterworths Med Law Rep* 1997;**37**:192.
8. *Rogers v. Whittaker. CLR HC Austr* 1993;**175**:479.
9. *Newell v. Goldenberg. Med Law Rep* 1995;**6**:371.
10. *Pearce v. United Bristol Healthcare Trust. Butterworths Med Law Rep* 1999;**48**:118.
11. *Wyatt v. Curtis. Engl Wales Court of Appeal* 2003:1779.
12. Kennedy I. *Treat Me Right.* Oxford: Clarendon Press, 1991, p.200.
13. General Medical Council. *Consent: Patients and Doctors Making Decisions Together.* London: GMC, 2008.
14. Department of Health. *Reference Guide to Consent for Examination or Treatment,* 2nd edn. London: DH, 2009.

Testing capacity in adults

Adults are presumed to have the capacity to provide consent for interventions. If they are unconscious, it will be self evident that the patient lacks capacity. Your immediate reaction will be to treat the patient on the basis of necessity, saving their lives, or preventing permanent irremediable harm (provided there is no valid advance decision to refuse such treatment).

If the patient is conscious, there may still be clinical grounds to suspect that their capacity is impaired, rendering them incompetent to provide consent.

Your next clinical decision will be whether the patient's capacity is only temporarily impaired. The apparent lack of capacity may be caused by confusion, fear, fatigue, or medication.[1] The passage of a few hours may allow the patient to become competent, so can the intended intervention be delayed this long? If this is not possible, you will need to assess their capacity to provide consent for the intervention that you propose.

- The test now used is directly derived from the Mental Capacity Act 2005, drafted broadly on the basis of the common law[2]
- The test is based on the negative, reminding us once more of the presumption that an adult is competent

'A person is unable to make a decision if they cannot do one or more of the following things:
- Understand the information given to them that is relevant to the decision
- Retain that information long enough to be able to make the decision
- Use or weigh up the information as part of the decision-making process
- Communicate their decision—this could be by talking or using sign-language and includes simple muscle movements such as blinking an eye or squeezing a hand'[3]

Practically, you will use the disclosure appropriate to the proposed intervention to test the patient's competence. This ensures that the patient's capacity for making this specific decision is tested. Testing in this way will therefore confirm the patient's capacity for making only this particular decision; no others.

It must be emphasized that measurement of the patient's competence by comparing the reasonableness of his/her decision with your own view of the situation is inappropriate. Patients are entitled to make unwise or irrational decisions, and the fact that they choose to do so is not an indicator of their incompetence. It is only when their understanding, retention, or use of the information (or communication of the decision) is at fault that their capacity may be impaired. Thus, a man who believes that his foot is gangrenous, and understands the consequences of non-treatment, yet chooses this course, may be competent to do so. Contrast this with a man who believes (incorrectly) that his gangrene is merely a curious and superficial fungus, which he could wipe off if he chose to do so. This person is likely to be incompetent, because he does not understand the information given to him that is relevant to the decision.

References

1. Department of Health. *Reference Guide to Consent for Examination or Treatment.* London: DH, 2009, p.10.
2. *Bolam v. Friern.* Barnet Hospital Management Committee. [1957] 1 WLR 582.
3. Department of Health. *Reference Guide to Consent for Examination or Treatment.* London: DH, 2009, p.9.

Adults without the capacity to provide their consent for treatment

The starting point for treating any patient is that you have a duty to save life, or prevent permanent irremediable harm. If no consent is available, and there are no visible provisions made by the patient to refuse treatment, then in an emergency, save the patient's life and limb, without hesitation. You are doing this without consent, and relying on the principle of necessity. Those that survive will be unlikely to complain.

However, there is a presumption that adults have capacity, and are therefore competent; either to provide their consent, or refuse to give it. (▶▶For the purposes of this section, 'competence' and 'capacity' should be treated as synonyms.) In some clinical situations, it will be self-evident that the patient is incompetent; for instance, if unconscious. In others, the patient will be conscious, but so obtunded by their disease or medication that their capacity is in doubt. Further to complicate the problem, some patients will be only temporarily incapacitated, while others will be incompetent for all of the foreseeable future.

Whichever of these groups your patient is in, it must be remembered that at some time in the past, they probably did have capacity. At some stage, they might have made an advance decision (AD) that could still influence their present circumstances. In particular, they may have decided to refuse treatment. This they may have done either by providing a document laying out the treatment they do not want, or by appointing a person to act on their behalf. This advance decision making has been recognized by the common law for some years, but was recently codified in the Mental Capacity Act 2005.

The effect of the Act is clearly laid out in the Department of Health's guidance,[1] which is by far the best and most concise advice on the subject available to doctors in England and Wales. However, if you wish further to investigate the workings of the Act, the Code of Practice is recommended. It is exhaustive, and addresses most potential clinical applications when dealing with patients without capacity.[2]

In summary, patients with capacity may influence their treatment by anticipating a time when they may be incompetent but want to refuse treatment in advance of this time. It should be noted that there is no power to insist on treatment; the patient's rights extend only to refusal. The patient may draw up a written and witnessed document[3] (an AD[4]); if valid, this prevents clinicians administering treatments that the patient proscribes. Older incarnations of the AD include 'living wills' and 'advanced directives'. These were less formalized, and thus, less enforceable, but still have validity under the common law.

However, despite the formality of ADs to refuse treatment, there is ample scope for finding them invalid. Patients who remain competent through the early stages of what will predictably become a drawn out and onerous illness may well be able to foresee, with some accuracy, their own terminal event. Consider a patient with advanced coronary artery disease who wishes to avoid tracheal intubation, should he require it. An appropriately drafted AD could ensure that his views are well known. However, if the same patient has an anaphylactic response to flu vaccination, manifesting as laryngospasm, clinicians are unlikely to regard the AD as valid in the circumstances, and would rightly intubate (if the AD refused intubation without specifying the underlying clinical indication).

Immediately, it can be seen that to draft an AD so that it will operate only in the circumstances anticipated by the patient is difficult. When in doubt, clinicians will avoid the AD, and presume the patient wishes to live. For this reason, the application of ADs in clinical practice may be limited.

Alternatively, the patient, when competent, may have appointed a person to hold a lasting power of attorney (LPA).[5] This person may be thus authorized to refuse clinical treatment on the behalf of the (now incompetent) patient.[6] The legal instrument may contain an express provision to the effect that the person who is instructed to hold the LPA can consent to or refuse life-sustaining treatment on the patient's behalf. If this is the case, then the patient has truly been able to influence their own fate, at a time when they would be otherwise powerless to do so.

The great advantage of the LPA is that it empowers a proxy decision maker, who may be able to put the patient's point of view in clinical situations that the patient may not have been able to anticipate, and almost certainly would have failed to include in an AD. The person who holds the LPA will still be entirely restricted by the words of the legal instrument; but plainly, this form of advanced decision making is more likely to result in a patient's wishes being complied with. However, to be a holder (donee) of an LPA is an onerous duty, and it is still rare to meet a patient who has made such a provision.

In the absence of advance provisions by the patient, the surgeon may be left with a patient who lacks capacity, but requires treatment. All treatment in these circumstances must accord with the patient's best interests.

In most clinical circumstances, it is possible to gather sufficient information about the patient to determine whether the proposed treatment is in his or her best interests. This information may come from previous conversations with the patient, or discussions with the family, or accompanying friends or associates. Provided that the planned intervention is unequivocally agreed during these discussions as being consistent with the patient's best interests, you should proceed. However, if there is any element of disagreement, either between clinicians or with those accompanying the patient, this should be resolved, if possible, before the treatment proceeds.

Such disagreements are unusual, and merit further exploration. If the intervention is so urgent that it is necessary to save life or prevent serious irremediable harm, the time available for this exploration is obviously limited. In these circumstances, you should try to consult with a colleague, if only to reassure yourself that you are acting reasonably. Provided this is the case, you should proceed. Thus if disagreement is raised over the emergency drainage of a pharyngeal abscess that is threatening the airway, the consultation will be hurried and limited.

If you have sufficient time for a formal second opinion, the views of the local clinical ethics committee, or a review from outside the hospital, so much the better. The need for this more wide-ranging review is proportional to the severity of the intervention over which there is dispute, and inversely proportional to the time available. For example, consider a young man with severe learning difficulties who needs an appendicectomy in the next 12h, whose the parents propose antibiotic treatment as an alternative therapy. Thorough discussions can ensue in the intervening hours, but there is a relatively narrow timeframe available to reach an agreement on treatment. Contrast this with a dispute as to whether a percutaneous endoscopic gastrostomy (PEG) is appropriate in a demented patient as an elective procedure. In the latter situation, the conflicting views should be resolved, and there is time to do so. Although rare, such disputes sometimes need the assistance of a court to achieve resolution. Once other channels are exhausted, referral to the Court of Protection for a declaration as to whether a proposed treatment is lawful is entirely appropriate, and envisaged under the Act.[7]

Although understandably reluctant to involve the court, surgeons should recognize that it is precisely for these purposes that our judicial structure has been created, and they should make use of it, when required. In a recent example, the case of a 55-year-old woman who lacked the capacity to consent for the surgery necessary to cure her uterine cancer was taken to the Court of Protection. It was held that such treatment was lawful; as were measures to get her into hospital for the surgery, and to keep her in hospital postoperatively until it was safe to discharge her.[8] This judgment was of great assistance, removing the (additional) anxiety of acting unlawfully from a situation that already posed a significant clinical challenge.

However, there are also situations in which the legal situation becomes complex. In another recent case, there was a dispute as to whether a patient was being lawfully kept in hospital under the Mental Capacity Act 2005, or the Mental Health Act 1983.[9] Although this does matter, it had little bearing on surgical practice; save to remind us all that if in doubt, a court should be consulted, in a similar way to our consultation with colleagues when facing a clinical dilemma.

It is not unusual to encounter a patient who lacks capacity, and who has no appropriate person with whom you can consult in determining what would be in the patient's best interests. In this situation, as before, if emergency treatment is necessary to save life or prevent permanent harm, then you must proceed. However, if the clinical situation permits, you need to seek advice from the hospital, because there may be a requirement to instruct an independent mental capacity advocate (IMCA).[10]

The IMCA will interview the patient, and others, to ascertain as best they can what the patient's wishes and feelings would be likely to be, if she had capacity. Essentially, the IMCA formulates the information that you will then use to determine whether the proposed intervention is in the patient's best interests. This process is important for supporting an 'unbefriended' incompetent patient during decisions over serious medical treatment, accommodation, and other welfare matters.

In patients who anticipate will regain their competence in the foreseeable future, you are effectively 'playing for time'. It is plainly better to await their return to competence before undertaking major interventions. This will put the patient in the position where he or she can decide whether to proceed, given the risks and benefits that are disclosed to them. But in the meantime, you may need to intervene to save their life, or prevent serious harm. Whether you are proceeding on the basis of necessity, or have has the benefit of discussions with friends and relatives to ensure that you are acting in a manner that is consistent with the patient's best interests, avoid giving treatment that is not absolutely necessary.

Consent in emergencies is dealt in detail elsewhere. But in principle, only take interventional steps that are proportionate to the clinical emergency that you are facing. Furthermore, if there are several clinical options open to you then employ the technique that is least restrictive to the patient's subsequent decision making.

References

1. Department of Health. *Reference Guide to Consent for Examination or Treatment*, 2nd edn. London: DH, 2009.
2. Mental Capacity Act 2005, Code of Practice, 2007. London: TSO.
3. Mental Capacity Act 2005, s.25.
4. Mental Capacity Act 2005, s.24(1).
5. Mental Capacity Act 2005, s.9.
6. Mental Capacity Act 2005, s.11(8)(a).
7. Mental Capacity Act 2005, ss.15 and 16.
8. *DH NHS Foundation Trust v. PS (Official Solicitor)*. [2010] Med LR 320 [Court of Prot].
9. *GJ v. The Foundation Trust*. [2010] Med LR 167 [Court of Prot].
10. Mental Capacity Act 2005, ss.35 and 36.

Treating children

From the legal perspective, a child is someone who has not yet reached 18 years of age. Legal synonyms include 'minor' and 'infant'. The latter is instructive since it is derived from the Latin: infants, unable to speak. This reflects the legal rules that prevent children from speaking for themselves in court, although this impediment has been at least partly addressed over the past two decades. Nevertheless, it begs a fundamental question, as to whether children can provide their own consent, or whether they depend on their parents to provide it for them.

People under 18 years can be considered in three broad groups.

Children under the age of 16 who lack capacity

This is the simplest group. Although presumed to lack capacity, some will be able to demonstrate their competence to provide independent consent for treatment (see 'Children under 16 who can demonstrate their capacity', p.29).

For those who cannot, a person with parental responsibility has the right to provide consent where necessary. The child's mother (the woman who gave birth to the baby, rather than the person who provided the egg from which he or she was conceived, if different) has parental responsibility automatically. The child's father gains parental responsibility automatically if married at the time of the birth registration. Since 2003, unmarried fathers also get parental responsibility automatically, when they register the birth. Alternatively, parental responsibility can be acquired by the unmarried father; either with the agreement of the child's mother, or by application to a court.

Parental responsibility is passed to adoptive parents on legal adoption. It may be shared with guardians appointed by parents, with local authorities, and is linked to various legal orders. For a full account, see Bainham.[1]

The person with parental responsibility who provides consent for a child's surgery must act in the child's best interests in so doing. These are usually self-evident, and the agreement between parents and surgeon is reached after full disclosure of the relevant information. This agreement is not invariable. In a case[2] concerning a child (T) with biliary atresia, the clinicians wished to perform a liver transplantation and considered the prospects of success to be good. The parents refused their consent on the grounds that the surgery was not in the child's best interests. The Court of Appeal held that the assessment of the child's best interests went wider than the narrower medical best interests, and that T's connection with his family held great weight in this regard. Accordingly, the court refused to enforce the hospital's request that the mother would bring T in for surgery. The judgment could be criticized, in failing to differentiate between the interests of the child and those of his mother. However, the case provides an example of the balancing act performed by courts.

Children under 16 who can demonstrate their capacity

Depending on their maturity and the intervention that is proposed, children from a young age may be able to provide independent consent. A 4-year-old may be able to consent to a blood pressure measurement; a 6-year-old to a venepuncture; a 10-year-old to the removal of an early stage appendicitis. This is not suggesting that parents should be excluded from this process; such an exclusion would be quite wrong. It is for the family, as a whole, to decide what part the child's potential capacity should play in the consenting process. But the involvement of children in this process will strengthen the therapeutic relationship, and is to be encouraged.

A child's previous experience is of great importance. It is submitted that following the very recent diagnosis of leukaemia, a 15-year old, who has been healthy up to this point, will be so horrified by the dissolution of his comfortable and well-organized life as to be incoherent and entirely incapable of consenting for the necessary tunnelled central venous catheter (CVC). Contrast this child with a 10-year-old on the same ward with relapsed leukaemia. He has already undergone three line insertions and two removals. He knows (effectively) everything there is to know about CVC placement, complications, and disadvantages. Now facing his fourth insertion, he will likely be competent to provide independent consent.

Therefore, it is important objectively to determine whether a child of 15 years or younger has capacity to provide independent consent for the proposed intervention.

For this assessment, the Gillick test is used, derived from a landmark case where it was established that a child with capacity to provide consent should be allowed to do so, independently of her parents. The test requires that a child has sufficient understanding and intelligence to enable them to understand fully what is involved in a proposed intervention.[3] Thus, if a child can understand:

- That a choice exists
- The nature and purpose of the procedure
- The risks and side effects
- The alternatives to the procedure; and is able:
  - To retain the information long enough
  - To weigh the information
  - To arrive at a decision
  - And to be free from undue pressure

he or she would be deemed competent for the proposed intervention. It will be seen that competence rests on intelligence, maturity, and experience, not on age.

During the Gillick case, an additional set of guidelines were suggested by Lord Fraser, specifically for doctors who assist with reproductive decision making by children under 16. It should be noted that these guidelines do not replace the Gillick test, nor are they synonymous with it.[4]

Gillick provides a high threshold for consent, consistent with public policy. It would be highly undesirable to allow incompetent children to provide consent for interventions that they could not fully understand. The fact that a child has to 'prove' their competence places a barrier to *children* that is never experienced by adults, whose capacity is presumed. One can only speculate how many adults would 'pass' the test in *Gillick*.

The Gillick-competent child does not enjoy an equal right to refuse treatment. Only those cases in which the refusal of life-saving treatments in these children is at issue have reached the court. But given this opportunity, courts have resolutely denied the (otherwise) competent minor the right to choose death. A 15-year-old girl[5] refusing her consent for a life-saving heart transplant had her refusal overridden by the courts. M's reason was that she 'would rather die than have the transplant and have someone else's heart. I would feel different with someone else's heart—that's a good enough reason not to have a heart transplant, even if it saved my life . . .'. The court authorized the operation, as being in her best interests.

In another case,[6] a 14-year-old girl with serious scalding required a blood transfusion. She was a Jehovah's Witness, and refused the treatment. The court found that even if she had been Gillick competent, her grave condition would have led the court to authorize the transfusion. As it was, the girl was unaware of the manner of death from anaemia, and was basing her views on those of her congregation, rather than on her own experiences. For these reasons, she was judged incompetent to make this decision for herself.

It must be remembered that the vast majority of Gillick-competent children who refuse treatment are refusing relatively trivial procedures. You would be entitled to rely upon their parent's consent if necessary, but it is a matter for clinical judgement whether the procedure could be deferred, to allow the child further time to consider, and be reconciled with what is likely to be an inevitable outcome. The problem of refusal in Gillick-competent children is dealt with in the same way as for the 16 and 17 years age group.

People of 16 and 17 years of age

People of 16 and 17 years of age are presumed to have the capacity to provide consent for surgical, medical, and dental treatment. This was made possible by a law enacted in 1969,[7] which recognized that the decisions that teenagers were taking, irrespective of the law, contrasted sharply with the age of majority (21 years) at the time. The new law reduced the age of majority to 18 years, and introduced the presumption of capacity for 16- and 17-year-olds.

What the new law did not do was extend this right to consent for research, or interventions that do not potentially provide direct health benefit to the individual concerned. However, if competent along 'Gillick' lines, a young person may be able to provide consent for these activities.

Young people of 16 and 17 are thus able to provide consent for treatment in absence of their parents. However, the parental right to provide consent for treatment lasts until the end of childhood. This has the effect of providing a 'safety net'; allowing a 16/17-year-old the opportunity of consent for herself; or deferring to her parents, if he or she sees fit. Once a child reaches adulthood on his or her 18th birthday, their parents' right disappears. For the rest of his or her life, they alone can provide consent, either directly, in person; or in some circumstances, by a proxy method.

If parents and a child of this age disagree, it is wise to exercise caution. If a 16- or 17-year-old wishes to exercise his right to consent, and his parents oppose the decision, then you would be entitled to rely on this consent. However, it would be important to understand the basis for their disagreement. For instance, if you suspected that the young person was not competent, you should challenge the presumption. This can simply be done by establishing whether he understands the relevant information, can retain the information, believe it, weigh it up, and communicate his decision. If the child can, then he or she has capacity. However, it is still wise to tease out where the problem lies, since this is a most unusual situation, and it would be in the young person's best interests to resolve the issue before surgery, if that is feasible.

The problem, reversed, is of a young person who refuses treatment, but who is accompanied by a parent who provides consent. Valid parental consent will make the procedure 'legal', but as with the situation of consent withdrawal, you will have to make a clinical judgement as to whether proceeding with the treatment against the young person's wishes is both practicable, and in their best interests.

In summary, it is recommended that an elective procedure should be abandoned until the dispute is resolved. If emergency treatment is required, but could be administered in a different way, which is still consistent with the patient's best interests, the alternative should be explored. If their life or limb is threatened, and there is no choice but to provide a definitive operation, then reluctantly, you may feel the need to restrain and proceed. A supracondylar fracture of the humerus that has resulted in an ischaemic hand could be an example of this situation. It should be noted that in reality, the amount of resistance that a child of any age puts up is usually inversely proportional to their malaise and discomfort. In the gravely ill, refusal is rare.

There are those who are gravely ill in need of urgent rather than emergency treatment. If a 16- or 17-year-old in this category refuses treatment for the preservation of their life, such as the transfusion of blood,[8] or feeding[9] (in anorexia), courts invariably choose to override the child's autonomy, and provide an order which allows lawful provision of the treatment against the child's wishes. This either upholds the parental wishes for treatment, or overrides parental refusal. These cases are rare, but the timescale within which the decision needs to be made allows sufficient time for the court to be contacted, providing the surgeon with the necessary authority.

References

1. Bainham A. *Children: The Modern Law'* 2005 Family Law. Bristol: Jordan Publishing.
2. *Re T.* Wardship. Medical treatment. [1997] 1 FLR 502.
3. *Gillick* v. *West Norfolk & Wisbech AHA.* AHA [1986] AC 112.
4. Wheeler RA. Gillick or Fraser? A plea for consistency over competence in children. *BMJ* 2006;**332**:807.
5. *Re M.* Medical treatment: consent. [1999] 2 FLR 1097.
6. *Re L.* Medical treatment: Gillick competency. [1998] 2 FLR 810.
7. Family Law Reform Act 1969, s.8.
8. Re P. Medical treatment: best interests. [2004] 2 All ER 1117.
9. Re W. A minor—medical treatment: court's jurisdiction. [1992] 3 WLR 758.

Treatment in emergencies

It is commonplace to encounter patients who require emergency surgical treatment. This may range from cleaning an abrasion to repairing a dissecting aneurysm. As already noted, patients may have provided advance refusals of treatment, either as ADs or via an LPA. However, in the emergency situation, these advance indications may be either inapplicable or unobtainable. While the surgeon should take reasonable steps to ascertain details of advance refusals, the patient's clinical condition must take priority. It would be wrong to allow an irrevocable clinical situation to develop while simply awaiting confirmation of a legal instrument.

In adult patients with capacity, (or children accompanied by someone with parental responsibility) following appropriate disclosure, the consent will be forthcoming, and the treatment administered. In the rare situation where an adult patient appears to have capacity, but refuses treatment, their capacity should be assessed. This is because the injury, or its effects, may have rendered them temporarily incompetent to make decisions for themselves. If it is clear that their competence is unaffected by their injury, the consequences of non-treatment should be made clear to them. Any alternatives to the treatment initially proposed should also be discussed, in an effort to minimize the harm that may flow from an insufficient intervention.

However, if the competent adult patient steadfastly refuses treatment in an emergency, in the face of full disclosure of the risk he or she is taking, the refusal must be complied with. Equally, a patient's advance decision refusing treatment should be respected, but may be rendered invalid by the clinical circumstances.

In adult patients who temporarily lack capacity but require emergency treatment, the treatment may be provided without their consent. Nobody can give proxy consent; but the patient may be lawfully treated without consent, on the grounds of necessity.

This doctrine enables the surgeon to save the patient's life, and to prevent the occurrence of serious or irremediable harm. In this way, it is accepted that acting without consent may be justified by the clinical result, if this is the only way of achieving it; despite not strictly adhering to the law of consent. This is not a rare event; it is happening on a daily basis, throughout the country, and is entirely acceptable practice. Without this doctrine, surgical practice would be paralysed; unable to operate without consent, and yet unable to obtain consent. It would become impossible to deal with spontaneous neurosurgical, cardiac, and vascular catastrophes, let alone the patient with high velocity trauma. The use of this doctrine should cause you no anxiety; but it is important to distinguish this from operating with consent.

But there are limits to the scope of the unconsented treatment. You may be confronted by a patient who has suffered a traumatic duodenal laceration that can only be treated by open operation; the trauma has temporarily rendered the patient incompetent to provide consent. It is your duty to treat the laceration, and perform peritoneal toilet. But do not be tempted to remove the stone-laden gallbladder at the same time. Cholecystectomy does not fall within the clinical remit of saving life or preventing irremediable harm in this circumstance, and can wait until the patient has recovered his capacity sufficient to decide for himself. Thus in Murray v McMurchy,[1] the surgeon who ligated the patient's fallopian tubes at the time of her Caesarean section without her prior consent was found to have acted inappropriately. There was no immediate danger posed by leaving her tubes intact; it was simply convenient to ligate them while she was unconscious.

In practical terms, the surgeon operating in an emergency situation who encounters unanticipated pathology needs to question whether it is reasonable to postpone treatment of this pathology. The great benefit of postponement will be that it gives an opportunity to consult the patient, and allow them to provide consent once in full possession of the pertinent facts. But will the postponement confer such a clinical disadvantage as to outweigh the benefits of consent?

In a case where a patient[2] was found to have provided consent to the urgent replacement of her leaking breast prosthesis and capsulotomy, the surgeon encountered widespread silicone deposits within both the breast tissue and pectoralis major. The court found that the resulting subcutaneous mastectomy and excision of the majority of the pectoralis major was a reasonable surgical response to the pathology. But it was not performed with consent. The implication may be drawn that the surgeon could not rely on the defence of necessity. The operation could have been abandoned, the skin closed and the necessity for radical excision discussed with patient, before this irrevocable step was taken.

In summary, emergency surgical treatment may be provided to patients who are temporarily unable to provide consent. This is lawful, providing the treatment is confined to meeting the emergency and needs to be carried out at once, before the patient is likely to be in a position to make the decision for him or herself.

References

1. *Murray* v. *McMurchy.* [1949] 2 DLR 442.
2. *Williamson* v. *East London & City Health Authority.* [1998] Lloyd's Rep Med 6.

Patients who request a form of treatment with which you are unwilling to comply

The consent of a competent patient is crucial in making a procedure lawful. However, the patient's influence does not extend to enabling them either to insist on a particular treatment, or to impose a restriction on the surgeon that is clinically unacceptable.

The former situation is more common, and easier to deal with. Surgeons cannot be required to provide treatment that is contrary to their professional judgement.[1] So, if you wish to manage a patient's appendix abscess initially with antibiotics, while they demand that you go for immediate drainage, your position is quite clear. They cannot use their wish for drainage as some form of battering ram. If you believe that non-operative management is correct and appropriate, this should be explained to the patient, along with your reasoning.

It is always prudent to check your reasoning, and any available evidence, before having this conversation. Your aim is to share the advantages and risks of the alternative treatments in their entirety with the patient, putting them in the position where they can appreciate as fully as you can why the suggested approach may be superior. If the patient remains unconvinced, wavering, it is prudent to offer them a second opinion.

If you reach an impasse, finding yourself unable to accede to the patient's request, there is arguably a duty to refer the patient to another colleague. This is analogous to the principle that if you are unwilling to perform an abortion,[2] you should nevertheless refer the patient to a surgeon who might be prepared to do so.[3]

Do not let yourself be talked into performing surgery that you believe is inappropriate. If you believe that a non-therapeutic circumcision in a child who is incompetent to provide consent is inconsistent with his best interests, you are perfectly entitled to decline, and refer the patient on to a colleague, who may feel differently. The same would apply, at the other end of the spectrum of magnitude, to patients with body dysmorphic disorder who want their healthy limbs removed.

Jehovah's witnesses

Patients who wish to impose conditions on their treatment are less common, but Jehovah's Witnesses are one recognizable group, refusing to accept the administration of blood products. These patients, if competent adults, may refuse blood even though the consequences may include their death, serious irremediable harm, or death of their unborn child. They must be offered any alternatives to blood products that may be acceptable to them, and that are available. Their refusal must be carefully documented. But unpalatable as it may seem, they may not be given blood products without their consent.

Children of Jehovah's Witnesses are an entirely different matter. If it is necessary to provide blood or its products to a person who is under 18 years, and no alternative therapy is available, simple legal mechanisms are in place to facilitate this. There are provisions under the Children Act 1989, enabling a clinician to obtain a Specific Issue Order[4] from the court, which permits the lawful administration of blood in these circumstances,[5] despite opposition from either parents or child. The great advantage of this system is that the Order simply passes a singular matter, in this case, administration of blood, to the control of the clinicians. All other aspects of parental responsibility are left with the parents, avoiding them being left with the impression that all aspects of the child's welfare has been taken out of their hands.

If faced with a child who needed a blood transfusion as an emergency, despite parental opposition, and there really is no time to seek court approval, then the transfusion must be provided; but this situation will be rare, since the order can (and should) be obtained over the telephone in these circumstances, whatever the hour.

Perhaps the most difficult situation is the incompetent patient who is alleged to be a Jehovah's Witness, but cannot assert this for him or herself. In the absence of other information, we must always make the presumption that the incompetent patient would wish to live. In *Re T*, an adult Jehovah's Witness,[6] when competent, signed a form refusing blood. Later, when she was unconscious, and deteriorating after a complex caesarean section, a court order was obtained authorizing her doctors to give her a blood transfusion. This appears to contradict a direct instruction from a competent adult. The court was able to do this by 'finessing' her competence, reasoning that at the time of signing the form, she had deteriorated, and was not competent, after all. The form was thus invalid, the court made a presumption in favour of life and authorized a transfusion.

So what do we do with the incompetent patient, in dire need of blood, who arrives in the emergency department with his newly diagnosed and freely bleeding oesophageal varices? His friends and family assert his adherence to Jehovah's teaching, and insist that he (would) refuse the administration of blood products? Since he is incompetent, should we follow *Re T*, and presume in the favour of life, irrespective of the testimony of his family? The first step (once someone else takes over the resuscitation, and agrees that there is no feasible alternative other than blood products) is to find some evidence backing up this claim.

As was seen previously, competent citizens can make advance arrangements to influence treatment that they might receive when later they lack capacity to choose for themselves. These arrangements may be written, in the form of an AD, or entrusted to another person, who is the 'donee' of an LPA. By either of these mechanisms, it is theoretically possible that Jehovah's Witness might be able to avoid receiving blood, even if this were to result in their death. But it should be noted that in any circumstance where a patient is making an advance refusal of life-saving treatment, written evidence, as strictly prescribed by the Mental Capacity Act 2005, must be presented.

If such written (and witnessed) materials are available, do the clinical situations they envisage correspond with the present circumstances? If they do, and you are absolutely sure they do, you may be present at one of the rare occasions when an advance refusal of treatment could produce its author's desired effect. Clearly, you should discuss your decision with the most senior colleague you can contact. However, since (in 2010) this is still an untested legal principle, you are also strongly advised to call the Court of Protection to seek its assurance that withholding transfusion is the correct thing to do. This is because the confusion caused by Re T has yet to be resolved.[7]

If the patient comes with no evidence of an advance refusal, either as an AD or in the form of an LPA, it is submitted that whatever the family tell you, you should presume that the patient would rather live than die, and thus if you have no alternative, you should administer blood. Again, discussions with colleagues and the Court of Protection are necessary. But the decision, in a grave emergency, to administer blood is a great deal easier than the one to withhold it, since the consequences of the latter are irreversible.

References

1. Re B. A minor—wardship: medical treatment. [1981] 1 WLR 1421, 4.17.
2. Abortion Act 1967, s.4(1).
3. Barr v Matthews. (1999) 52 BMLR 217, 227.
4. Children Act, 1989, s.8(1).
5. Re P. Medical treatment: best interests. [2003] EWHC 2327 (Fam).
6. Re T. Adult refusal of medical treatment. [1992] 4 All ER 649.
7. Mason JK, Laurie GT. Mason and McCall Smith's Law and Medical Ethics. Oxford: Oxford University Press, 2010, section 4.56.

Situations where a simple consent may be insufficient

In the vast majority of surgical procedures, a single consent is sufficient to authorize a procedure as legitimate. However, some procedures may be considered by society as controversial; and society's anxieties are sometimes reflected by Parliament and the courts; in legislation, or the common law.

Prohibited interventions, not in the patient's best interests

Some interventions are therefore prohibited, irrespective of whether consent is available. This is because the performance of these activities has been judged as never being consistent with the person's best interests. Thus, female genital mutilation for no therapeutic purpose is proscribed by statute,[1] as is the tattooing of children,[2] and the ritual incision of a person's face.[3] In the same way, amputation of a child's foot, to facilitate the process of begging for money, is illegal.[4]

Interventions that may be in the patient's best interests, but require the sanction of a court

Other interventions may be in the person's best interests, but are so controversial that the sanction of a court is required before the procedure can take place. This would include the non-therapeutic sterilization[5] of a child, or of an adult who lacked capacity. The courts have already held that sterilization for the purposes of eugenics will not be sanctioned.[6]

Similarly, prior sanction is required for the donation of regenerative tissue, such as bone marrow[7] by a child or incompetent adult. In *Re Y*, the court left open the question as to whether blood or other regenerative tissue fluids would be considered in the same way. Whether a court would ever sanction the donation by a child or incompetent adult of non-regenerative tissue, such as a kidney, is 'open to considerable doubt'.[8]

No sanction required, but a clinical decision

Some interventions that may be in a patient's best interests require no such prior sanction. However, it will always be a matter of clinical judgement as to whether the activity is consistent with best interests or not, and it is this element of the clinical 'transaction' which is prone to scrutiny.

The performance of cosmetic surgery and piercing of children illustrates this well. A court[9] has accepted that 'parents (are) plainly able to consent to plastic surgery to correct serious disfigurement for purely cosmetic purposes even though not "therapeutic" within the accepted meaning of that word'. However, it qualified this by noting that 'there may well be some limitations upon the power to consent to cosmetic surgery on a child, depending upon its purpose'.

A further example is that of elective amputation of a healthy limb, on the basis of a *body dysmorphic disorder*.[10] Although the possibility that such an amputation could be in the best *interests of a patient if it was to* benefit their mental health is acknowledged,[11] this is clearly an onerous clinical decision.

Finally, and far more common, is non-therapeutic circumcision. This, in children, requires the consent of both parents.[12]

References

1. Female Genital Mutilation Act 2003.
2. The Tattooing of Minors Act 1969.
3. *R v. Adesanya. The Times* 16 July 1974;17.
4. *Secretary Department of Health and Community Services v. JWB and SMB.* [1990] 14 Fam LR. 427 448.
5. *Re F.* Mental patient: sterilization. [1990] 2 AC 1.
6. *Re E.* A minor—wardship: sterilization. [1988] AC 199.
7. *Re Y.* Mental patient: bone marrow donation. [1997] Fam 110, 116.
8. Grubb A, Laing J, McHale J. *Principles of Medical Law* . Oxford: Oxford University Press, 2010, 10.193.
9. *Secretary, Department of Health and Community Services v. JWB and SMB.* CLR 1992;**175**:218.
10. Elliott T. Body dysmorphic disorder, radical surgery and the limits of consent. *Med Law Rev* 2009;**17**:149–82.
11. Grubb A, Laing J, McHale J. *Principles of Medical Law.* Oxford: Oxford University Press, 2010, 8.34.
12. Wheeler RA. Consent for non-therapeutic male circumcision. *Arch Dis Child* 2008;**93**:825–6.

Withdrawal of consent

A patient with capacity (or a person providing consent on behalf of a patient) may withdraw consent at any stage.[1] In practical terms, the withdrawal needs to be made without ambiguity. What happens next is largely dependent on whether the patient is about to undergo a procedure under general or local anaesthesia.

Procedures under general anaesthesia

Withdrawal of consent is seen in starkest relief when it occurs in the anaesthetic room, before a general anaesthetic is administered.

If a competent patient indicates that they have changed their mind, the clinical situation must be reviewed. The patient should be moved out of the anaesthetic room and taken to a quiet location in the theatre complex. Here, their capacity can be assessed. It should be noted that a patient who was competent to consent for surgery might have been rendered incompetent by premedication.

However, if the patient still has capacity, and despite being aware of the consequences of not receiving the intervention still refuses to proceed, their withdrawal must be honoured, and the procedure cancelled. Alternatives to the original procedure should be offered; perhaps a lesser procedure, or conservative management may be agreed upon.

In adult patients who lack capacity, their withdrawal of consent is invalid, but may still cause significant difficulties. The patient who has been rendered incompetent by the premedication may put up stiff resistance to the induction of anaesthesia. This provides a clinical rather than legal problem. Assuming the procedure is in the patient's best interests, it may be clinically proportionate to restrain the patient and carry on. Alternatively, if the theatre staff demurs to restraining the patient, or the patient's resistance is violent, it may be necessary to postpone the operation. Later options include rearranging the procedure after planned sedation, which can itself be agreed after a discussion with the patient, once capacity is regained.

In children whose parents withdraw consent in the anaesthetic room, the procedure should be cancelled and completely re-discussed. The rare exception would be an emergency procedure is required to save life or limb, in the next few minutes. In this situation, the best interests of the child will overcome the parents' lack of consent, and the procedure should be performed on this basis.

The reality of the clinical situation is that few patients requiring life-saving surgery in this context will have the capacity to withdraw their consent. If the intervention can be postponed without putting the patient's life or limb at risk, it should be, since the withdrawal of a competent patient must be respected. There are no 'withdrawal' cases in English common law, indicating that clinical pragmatism is very likely to be successful.

Procedures under local anaesthesia

Procedures under local anaesthesia pose a particular problem.

Patients who are initially competent, once mid-way through a procedure under local anaesthesia, sometimes indicate their refusal to carry on. In a Canadian case,[2] a woman undergoing a cerebral angiogram (awake) withdrew her consent when she had a painful reaction to the intravenous contrast. The court accepted that a patient had a right to withdraw consent in these circumstances, but pointed out that the physiological effects of the intervention may render the patient incapable of so doing, since an incompetent patient is unable to withdraw consent. For this reason, it is most important that the capacity of the patient is checked when they withdraw treatment. Simple questioning of the patient about why they want you to stop, what the effects of 'stopping now' will be, and the long-term outcome of terminating the operation, will reveal whether they have capacity or not.

As a general rule, if a competent patient indicates unambiguously that they have withdrawn their consent midway through a procedure under local anaesthesia, you should continue the procedure only until you have ensured that the clinical situation is safe; and then stop what you are doing. The whole situation should be reassessed, including the feasibility of converting to general anaesthesia, since many withdrawals are prompted by intolerable pain.

The same approach should be adopted for the incompetent child, accompanied by their parent.

If a patient lacking capacity is being correctly treated under local anaesthesia, they are being subjected to the procedure on the basis that it is consistent with their best interests. If they are clearly in pain, and distressed, you should stop as soon as clinical safety is achieved, and find an alternative humane approach. However, if they are simply objecting, and not distressed, it is a clinical decision as to whether the procedure should continue. If the patient needs to be restrained to complete the procedure, and thus prevent harm, that is lawful. In this situation, restraint may be used[3] to ensure the procedure is safe, although it must be proportionate to the likelihood of the patient otherwise suffering harm.

References

1. Department of Health. *Reference Guide to Consent for Examination or Treatment,* 2nd edn. London, DH, 2009.
2. *Ciarlariello v. Keller.* Med Law Rev 1994;2:115.
3. Mental Capacity Act 2005, s.6.

Consent for research and teaching

Consent for research

It is common, especially in university or teaching hospitals, for doctors and other health professionals to recruit patients to ongoing research programmes. This may range from recruiting a patient for a multicentre randomized controlled study, which could significantly affect their treatment pathway, to requesting a patient's consent to use tissues or specimens for research that have been acquired as part of routine practice, or specifically for research purposes.

As with all consent, it is only valid and acceptable if the participant is competent, has agreed without coercion and the relevant information has been disclosed. An open discussion between the patient and the health professional is vital to clarifying objectives and understanding. It is important that the following information is disclosed and should preferably be provided in writing, as well as verbally:[1]

- The aims of the research; what it is hoped to achieve
- Confirmation of approval by a research ethics committee
- An outline of the methods involved
- The legal rights of participants
- The reason the patient has been asked to participate
- Potential benefits and risks
- If the research involves randomization, the process and reasons for it should be disclosed to the patient. If the research study is double-blinded, then it should be discussed that neither the research team nor the patient will know whether he or she is receiving the treatment or is in the control group
- An explanation of which parts of the treatment are experimental and not fully tested
- In case of an adverse event, details of what the patient should do should be provided
- Advice that a patient may withdraw from the study at any time without penalty and it will not affect the relationship with their care provider, or future treatment
- Details of how and what personal information will be stored, shared, and published
- Confidentiality and the possibility of access to confidential notes by third parties (e.g. regulatory authorities, ethics committees, auditors)
- What information will be given to the patient about the outcomes of the research
- Any details of financial compensation
  - Expenses
  - Compensation in the event of any research-related injury or harm

Adequate time must be given for reflection prior to the patient giving consent. In practice, this usually means that the consent 'process' should take place over a *period of time, meeting* with the patient on more than one occasion.

Any research that involves potentially vulnerable people, namely children and adults who are unable to consent for themselves, but also vulnerable adults who have capacity to consent, requires special safeguards.

Adults who lack capacity

There is no legislation in England, Wales, and Northern Ireland detailing the circumstances under which research that involves adults who lack capacity to consent may be undertaken. However, research that could be undertaken equally well by recruiting adults with capacity should always be done this way, rather that involving patients with incapacity. In essence, that means that the only areas of research that should involve patients with incapacity are those that involve the conditions or illnesses that are linked to the incapacity itself.

Thus, in a surgical setting, it is fairly rare that you will need to involve adult patients who lack capacity, except for perhaps some areas of research in neurosurgery or critical care. If research is to be conducted in this group of patients, it must be demonstrated that:

- There could be a direct benefit to the patient's health
- It will significantly improve the scientific understanding of the adult's incapacity, leading to a direct benefit to them or others with the same incapacity
- The research is ethical and will not lead to harm
- The patient does not express any physical or verbal objections
- The right to withdraw from the research is respected at all times. Implied refusal may be in the form of signs of pain, distress, or physical/verbal indication of refusal

If there has been any expression of a patient's wishes about participation in research in an AD, then this should be taken into account. Any refusal to participate in a research project or trial in a statement made when an adult was competent is legally binding and must be respected.

Children and young people

Involving children and young people in research is important in advancing knowledge of conditions affecting children only and validating the benefits of treatment shown to be beneficial in adults However, the child without competency is vulnerable in that they cannot make informed choices about their treatment, including the potential risks and benefits of research, their best interests, and express their own needs. Similar to vulnerable adults, children or young people should only be involved in research when research on adults is unable to provide the same benefits. Before embarking on research involving children, the necessary approval must have been granted by the relevant research ethics committee and advice may have been sought from a Royal College, the Medical Research Council or other professional or research body.

If the child is not competent to consent for themselves, they should not participate in research unless someone with parental responsibility has given valid consent following disclosure. Even when a minor is competent to consent to participate in therapeutic research, then current guidance advises that the approval of someone with parental responsibility should also be sought before proceeding, in most cases. If a child or young person objects either verbally or physically, then they should not be involved in research in general, even if an adult with parental responsibility consents.

Emergencies

In some emergency situations, consent cannot be obtained. Treatment in these circumstances can be given only if it is limited to what is necessary to preserve life or avoid significant deterioration in the patient's condition. For more details, 📖 see 'Treatment in emergencies', p.33.

Emergency treatment may, in some circumstances, include treatment that is part of a research project. In this case, the risks of the treatment that is being researched should not be known to or be believed to exceed the risks of the standard treatment. If possible, the situation should be discussed with the next-of-kin or relatives.

If the patient regains capacity during the course of the treatment, they should be informed about the research as soon as is practically possible and their consent to continue with the research should be obtained.

Consent for obtaining tissue, organs, or body fluids[4]

Following the controversies in Bristol, Liverpool, and several other locations in the UK, where it was found patients' organs or tissues had been removed and retained without the consent of the patient, family, or parents, there was a major change in law, which led to the creation of the Human Tissue Act (HTA) 2004.[2] Scotland has separate legislation in the form of the Human Tissue (Scotland) Act 2006, although this is very similar to the HTA (2004) in practical terms.

The HTA (2004) only applies to some specific activities, for both living and deceased persons. The use of tissue, organs, and body fluids for the diagnosis and treatment of the patient from whom the samples are derived from, are not governed by the HTA (2004) and are instead covered by common law. However, tissues being used for the diagnosis and treatment of another person are covered by the HTA (2004), for example the use of tissue or blood for a predictive genetic test that would mainly benefit a relative of the patient from whom the tissue was obtained. The activities covered by the HTA (2004) are:

• Anatomical examination
• Research
• Transplantation
• Determining cause of death
• Establishing the efficacy of a treatment or drug post-mortem
• Public display

For deceased persons, there are some additional activities that are covered by the HTA (2004):

• Clinical audit
• Health-related training/education
• Public health monitoring
• Performance assessment and quality assurance

Thus, if a tissue sample is taken from a living patient for use in health-related training, then the HTA (2004) is not applicable. For example, if a sample of tissue is taken from a living person for teaching purposes, the consent is provided for this in the usual way. This need not be written consent. However, should the patient die, then the HTA (2004) would then apply to the tissue sample. Although the HTA (2004) does not stipulate that written consent is required in every case, it is necessary for anatomical specimens and specimens for public display. Wherever possible, written consent should also be given for any post-mortem activities. This is one reason that there is a section on the Department of Health consent forms for patients to consent to the use of their tissues for diagnostic, teaching, and audit purposes. The use of tissue or organs for research is, however, covered by the HTA (2004), whether the patient is alive or deceased.

Tissue samples, organs and body fluids are frequently collected as part of routine practice and can be a valuable research resource. Whether they are collected routinely, or specifically for research purposes, appropriate consent/authorization must be sought and granted by the patient or volunteers. In the case of samples collected as part of a routine treatment or operation, the wish to use the samples for research must be specifically disclosed, and specific consent for this purpose must be granted.

If tissue, organ, or fluid samples obtained from a routine surgical procedure are going to be retained for research purposes, separate consent should be obtained for the procedure and the research. It is important that the following information is discussed during disclosure:
- The amount and nature of the tissue/organs/fluid that will be collected
- The intended use for the material
  - Details of a specific project
  - For retention for use in future research projects
- The right to decline or to withdraw consent for use of the material in research projects at any time
- Arrangements for the disposal of the material, once the research has concluded
- Details of what information will be used or stored (e.g. access to medical records for research purposes)
- What information will be given to the patient or volunteer about the outcomes of the research

If the person is not competent to give consent, the HTA (2004) stipulates the doctor should refer to the Mental Capacity Act 2005.[3] The consent for the activity that would fall under the HTA (2004) in a competent patient is then included in the consent under which the tissue sample will be obtained under the Mental Capacity Act 2005. This Act describes the process of consent and the recording of consent for an incompetent patient under these circumstances.

Post-mortems
There are three situations in which post-mortems are undertaken:
- First, in the case where a coroner has instructed a post-mortem to take place, such as to determine the cause of death in a sudden, unexpected death then, by law, the post-mortem has to take place whether the next-of-kin is in agreement or not
- The second situation is where the hospital would like to conduct a post-mortem, usually to provide further information about a death, the underlying conditions and to further medical research. Post-mortems are an important part of medical research because they can provide information about medical conditions that cannot be gained in any other way. If a hospital is requesting a post-mortem, written consent

must be gained from the deceased patient's next-of-kin or nominated representative. If the pathologist wishes to take tissues or organs for further research or study, this can only be done with the written consent of the next-of-kin
- The third situation is where the next-of-kin or family request a post-mortem to gain information on the deceased patient's cause of death

Specific consent forms for post-mortem examinations, based on the model consent form, are available from the Human Tissue Authority

Consent for teaching and education

It is necessary, as well as polite, to seek patients' consent for students or other observers to be present during a consultation, examination, investigation or procedure. The doctor responsible should explain that a medical student or observer would like to sit in on the consultation, including the reasons why, and request the patient's consent for this to happen. Patients should feel able to refuse and should be reassured that their decision will not affect their treatment in any way. Ideally, this discussion should occur in the absence of the observer and he or she should be invited to observe the consultation or procedure once consent has been given by the patient for this to happen. In the case of most consultations, examinations, and investigations, verbal consent is all that is required.

In the case of anaesthetized patients, they have the same right to give or refuse consent as any other patients. The presence of medical students/ observers should be discussed during the consent process prior to the procedure and the patient's consent/refusal documented in the clinical notes or on the standard consent form that is being used for the procedure.

Likewise, consent is also required for the use of photography or video recording for educational or teaching purposes. In the case of children, permission should be sought from someone with parental responsibility if the child is unable to consent for him/herself. However, once the child reaches an age where he/she is competent to consent independently, then permission should be sought for continued use of the material for educational purposes and withdrawn if consent is denied. Also, it should be made clear that patients have the right to change their mind at any point and if this happens, the material should be withdrawn and erased.

Consent should also be sought from a patient if clinicians are wishing to use data that could potentially identify an individual in a publication, e.g. a case report. The immediate identifiable data will have been removed from this (i.e. name, date of birth), however, it is often easy to identify patients from the literature if their history is known. Many journals demand for evidence of consent to be included at the time of submission, usually in the form of a signed consent form. However, if this is not the case, it is still prudent and correct to seek the patient's consent and for this to be documented in their clinical records.

References

1. *General Medical Council. Research: The Roles and Responsibilities of Doctors.* London: GMC, 2002.
2. Human Tissue Act 2004, s.53. Available at: ℘ www.legislation.gov.uk/ukpga/*2004/30/contents* (accessed 4 May 2011).
3. Mental Capacity Act 2005. Available at: ℘ www.legislation.gov.uk/ukpga/2005/9/contents (accessed 4 May 2011).
4. Lucassen A, Wheeler R. Legal implications of tissue. *Ann R Coll Surg Engl* 2010;**92**:189–92.

Other elements of good surgical practice

Surgical site marking

The surgeon undertaking a procedure is responsible for ensuring the surgical site is marked. This is vital, especially when performing a side-specific operation, e.g. nephrectomy, and is a constituent of the World Health Organization (WHO) Surgical Safety Checklist and detailed within the Royal College of Surgeons of England's *Good Surgical Practice* guideline.[1] Documentation within the patient's clinical records and consent form should also reflect the intended side and the side should be documented in *full* on the consent form. Prior to this, the intended side should be confirmed by reviewing the clinical notes and radiology and it should be verified with the patient. Following this, the side should be marked in indelible ink and the side should be double-checked against the consent form prior to commencing the procedure.

Anaesthetic consent

It is the responsibility of the anaesthetist to discuss the aspects of consent relating to the anaesthesia. In practice, this is likely to include a discussion regarding the transition into the anaesthetic room, the application of monitoring equipment, insertion of lines, method of induction, method of airway management, recovery, and the immediate postoperative period. The benefits and risks of anaesthesia will also be disclosed. There is commonly some overlap in content with the surgical consent, such as the intention to insert lines or a catheter and the plans for postoperative care, especially if it is likely that the patient will return to a high-dependency or intensive care setting.[2]

References

1. Royal College of Surgeons of England. *Good Surgical Practice*. London: Royal College of Surgeons of England, 2008.
2. Royal College of Anaesthetists. *Information and Consent for Anaesthesia*. London: Royal College of Anaesthetists, 1999.

Further reading

General Medical Council. *Research: The Roles and Responsibilities of Doctors*. London: GMC, 2002.

General Medical Council. *Consent: Patients and Doctors Making Decisions Together*. London: GMC, 2008.

Mental Capacity Act 2005.

Royal College of Surgeons of England. *Good Surgical Practice*. London: Royal College of Surgeons of England, 2008.

Department of Health guidance for clinicians

Department of Health. *Good Practice in Consent Implementation Guide: Consent to Examination or Treatment*. London: DH, 2001.

Department of Health. *Seeking Consent: Working with Children*. London: DH, 2001.

Department of Health. *Seeking Consent: Working with Older People*. London: DH, 2001.

Department of Health. *Seeking Consent: Working with People with Learning Disabilities*. London: DH, 2001.

Department of Health. *Reference Guide to Consent for Examination or Treatment*, 2nd edn. London: DH, 2009.

Department of Health guidance for patients

Department of Health. *Consent—A Guide for Children and Young People*. London: DH, 2001.

Department of Health. *Consent—What You Have the Right to Expect: A Guide for Adults*. London: DH, 2001.

Department of Health. *Consent—What You Have the Right to Expect: A Guide for Parents*. London: DH, 2001.

General surgical procedures

Abdominal paracentesis

Description

This is an aseptic procedure in which a needle or catheter is inserted into the peritoneal cavity to obtain ascitic fluid for diagnostic or therapeutic purposes. It is performed 2cm below the umbilicus or 5cm superior and medial to the anterior superior iliac spine on either side. Ideally the procedure should be performed under radiological guidance.[1] One must be aware of coagulopathies, an acutely peritonitic abdomen, distended bowel, organomegaly, an abdominal wall with scars from previous surgery, pregnancy, and abdominal wall sepsis (cellulitis, fasciitis) before performing this procedure, to reduce the risk of complications.[2]

Additional procedures that may become necessary

- Ultrasound guidance
- Catheterization—to empty urinary bladder
- Insertion of paracentesis/ascitic drain

Benefits

- Minimally invasive
- *Diagnostic*: new-onset ascites enabling biochemical analysis (transudate versus exudate), microbiology (culture and sensitivities) and cytological evaluation
- *Therapeutic*: drainage of tense ascites to relieve pressure on diaphragm causing respiratory distress

Alternative procedures/conservative measures

- *Conservative/medical*: no fluid is aspirated and the patient is treated on the assumption that the fluid is a transudate or exudate
- *Surgical*: laparoscopy or open surgery with aspiration of fluid under direct vision

Serious/frequently occurring risks[2]

- Intraperitoneal bleeding, especially in patients with cirrhotic ascites and coagulopathy
- Visceral perforation leading to peritonitis
- Introduction of infection resulting in peritonitis
- Failure to aspirate fluid
- Acute fluid loss and hypotension due to fluid shifts from therapeutic drainage
- Persistent fluid leak from puncture site
- Dilutional hyponatraemia, hypoalbuminaemia

Blood transfusion necessary

- None/group and save
- Occasionally request for Human Albumin Solution (HUS) if anticipated *ascitic drainage is high*

Type of anaesthesia/sedation
- Local or no anaesthetic infiltration if simple diagnostic tap

Follow-up/need for further procedure
- May need repeated drainage for recurrent tense ascites
- Rapid fluid shifts may require albumin/blood product/fluid replacement
- Further medical or surgical treatment may be required following initial diagnostic paracentesis

References
1. Nazeer SR, Dewbre H, Miller AH. Ultrasound-assisted paracentesis performed by emergency physicians vs the traditional technique: a prospective randomized study. *Am J Emerg Med* 2005;**23**(3):363–7.
2. Wong CL, Holroyd-Leduc J, Thorpe KE, Straus SE. Does this patient have bacterial peritonitis or portal hypertension? How do I perform a paracentesis and analyze the results? *JAMA* 2008;**299**(10):1166–78.

Arterial cannulation

Description

A needle or cannula is inserted into the radial artery (Fig. 2.1; although any peripheral artery can be used, e.g. ulnar, brachial, femoral) in order to obtain arterial blood sampling for biochemical gas analysis or to allow continuous blood pressure monitoring. The latter is used in an intraoperative or high-dependency setting.

If the radial artery is used, Allen's test should be performed to ensure adequate collateral blood supply to the hand prior to cannulation.

Additional procedures that may become necessary

- Non-invasive blood pressure monitoring

Benefits

- Arterial blood gas sampling
- Invasive, real-time blood pressure monitoring
- Guidance of fluid and inotrope management

Alternative procedures/conservative measures

- Mixed venous saturations and blood gas analysis
- Peripheral pure venous blood gas analysis
- Central venous line to aid fluid management

Serious/frequently occurring risks

- Bruising or bleeding leading to haematoma/false aneurysm formation
- Infection
- Blockage of cannula requiring reinsertion
- Thrombosis of artery/distal embolic phenomenon leading to end vessel ischaemia/infarction
- Prolonged arterial spasm resulting in ischaemia or infarction especially if end-organ collateral arterial arcades are inadequate

Blood transfusion necessary

- None

Type of anaesthesia/sedation

- Local anaesthesia/no anaesthesia required

Follow-up/need for further procedure

- Ensure arterial lines are dressed, observed, handled, changed, or replaced according to local infection control policy

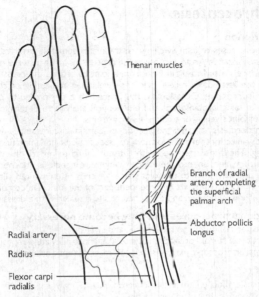

Fig. 2.1 Anatomy of the radial artery for cannulation.

Reproduced with permission from Ramrakha PS and Hill J. *Oxford Handbook of Cardiology*. 2006. Oxford: Oxford University Press, p.211, Figure 5.2.

Arthrocentesis

Description

Common causes of joint swelling are trauma, rheumatoid arthritis, gout and osteoarthritis. Arthrocentesis is the process by which a sterile needle and syringe is used to drain fluid from a joint to reduce the pressure of fluid in an attempt to relieve pain and swelling in an acutely or chronically inflamed joint. Occasionally, this procedure is performed to obtain a sample for microbiological and biochemical analysis to determine the cause of joint swelling or exclude septic arthritis.

Arthrocentesis can be therapeutic in certain circumstances where steroids injections are performed to reduce joint inflammation and swelling. The skin is sterilized with antiseptic fluid to reduce the risk of introducing infection into the joint. A wide-bore needle is attached to a syringe and inserted into the joint space, which is often marked clinically as the most fluctuant part or dependent part of the joint. On completion the needle is withdrawn and the puncture site is sealed with a dressing.

Additional procedures that may become necessary

- Repeated aspirations to reduce pain and swelling
- Injection of steroid or synthetic synovial agent to alleviate symptoms
- Formal arthroscopic joint washout—in cases of septic arthritis

Benefits

- *Diagnostic:* biochemical analysis, microbiological analysis with microscopy, culture and sensitivities
- *Therapeutic:* steroid joint injections

Alternative procedures/conservative measures

- None

Serious/frequently occurring risks

- Usually a straightforward procedure with minimal risks
- Bleeding within the joint during aspiration, leading to bruising or more swelling. In rare circumstances, in particular in patients with coagulopathies, evacuation of a haemarthrosis may need to be performed
- Repeated injections can lead to loss of skin pigmentation around the needle entry site
- Infection within the joint cavity leading to septic arthritis
- Occasionally, repeated injections with corticosteroids given too frequently may lead to systemic side effects of steroid use including weight gain, skin bruising, and osteoporosis

Blood transfusion necessary

- None/group and save

Type of anaesthesia/sedation

- None/local anaesthesia

Follow-up/need for further procedure

- Follow-up review in outpatient clinic
- Microbiology review may necessitate antibiotics/arthroscopic washout in septic arthritis

Blood transfusions

There has been considerable debate in UK concerning consent pertaining to the transfusion of blood products, with concerns that the practice of obtaining consent for blood transfusion is inconsistent and that the relevant benefits, risks, and alternatives may not be being disclosed to patients in many cases. The issue has been recently highlighted by the recent stakeholder consultation, initiated by the UK's Independent Advisory Committee on the Safety of Blood, Tissue and Organs.[1]

As with any examination, investigation, or treatment, the relevant information should be disclosed to the patient and the patient should consent to treatment with this information in hand, before commencing the intervention. Indeed, the Royal College of Surgeons of England issued a position statement in October 2010 stating that patients should be fully aware of the likelihood of blood/blood product transfusion, along with the indications, benefits, risks and alternatives before their operation.[2] This discussion should begin in the outpatient department and continue as part of the immediate preoperative discussion, especially if a patient is to undergo a procedure where there is a high likelihood for the need for blood transfusion.

It is the responsibility of the operating surgeon, as with consent for the operative procedure itself, to ensure that consent for perioperative blood transfusion is discussed and the outcome documented. Regarding the issue over whether consent for blood/blood product transfusion should be documented separately, the Royal College of Surgeons of England believes that best practice should be applied by using the existing national consent form and that a separate consent form is unnecessary. However, it is the clinician's responsibility to ensure that the national consent form is used properly, including disclosure of the likelihood of the need for a blood transfusion for a given procedure, and the relative benefits and risks of this.

Blood transfusions are administered more often than is necessary, as highlighted by the Chief Medical Officer, which exposes patients to needless risk and wastes valuable blood products. Therefore, it is good practice to ensure that blood products are administered only when appropriate (see the British Committee for Standards in Haematology (BCSH) guidelines[3] on transfusion of red cells and separate guidance on fresh frozen plasma (FFP), cryoprecipitate, and platelets).

Blood products include:
- Packed red cells
- Fresh frozen plasma (FFP)
- Platelets
- Cryoprecipitate
- Clotting factor concentrates, e.g. prothrombin complex (Octaplex®)

Jehovah's Witnesses

In the case of patients who do not agree to allogeneic blood transfusion, such as Jehovah's Witnesses, it is imperative to discuss the alternatives to and consequences of refusing a blood transfusion. In some cases, patients may agree to specific blood products and it is important that this is carefully documented, with the exact products they are willing to receive.

Both the Royal College of Surgeons of England and the Association of Anaesthetists of Great Britain and Ireland have produced guidelines on the management of patients who are Jehovah's Witnesses.[2,4] For major operations where there is a likelihood of significant blood loss, planning needs to commence at an early stage.

A number of techniques can be employed to replace allogeneic blood transfusion. However, some patients may not find these techniques acceptable either, so it is important to discuss and document what is acceptable to them as an individual. Patients may already be in possession of an AD that may specify the blood products that they do not wish to receive. There are a number of other products that Jehovah's Witnesses may also find unacceptable, e.g. human albumin solution, immunoglobulins.

Benefits
As with all treatments, the rationale behind the need for a blood product transfusion should be discussed with the patient, e.g. acute blood loss, symptomatic anaemia.

Alternative treatments
- Investigate and treat cause of anaemia preoperatively, e.g. iron deficiency
- Preoperative erythropoietin over several weeks to increase haematocrit
- Autologous blood salvage (intraoperative blood salvage)
  - Lost blood is collected, the red cells filtered, washed, stored, and subsequently autotransfused
- Autotransfusion
  - Venesection is performed on the patient in the weeks prior to surgery and blood is stored for subsequent use
  - This is no longer routinely practised

Serious/frequently occurring risks
Acute transfusion reactions
- Incorrect blood—this is a major risk associated with blood transfusions, although this risk is not disclosed to the patient
- Febrile non-haemolytic transfusion reaction
  - Affect 1–2% of recipients
  - Increased risk with multi-transfused or parous patients
- Mild allergic reaction—urticaria
- Haemolytic transfusion reaction
  - Usually related to ABO incompatibility
  - Almost always an administrative error leading to the transfusion of incorrect blood components
- Volume overload
- Anaphylaxis
- Infections
- Every blood donation is screened for hepatitis B surface antigen, hepatitis C antibody and RNA, human immunodeficiency virus (HIV) I+II, human T-lymphotropic virus (HTLV)-1 and *Treponema pallidum*
- Bacterial infection—highest with platelet transfusions

- Viral infections
  - Hepatitis B—1:850 000
  - Hepatitis C—1:51 000 000
  - HIV—1:6 000 000
  - Variant *Creutzfeldt–Jacob* disease—extremely rare, in the event of enquiry by patient. Only three possible transmissions by blood transfusion have been reported
- Transfusion-related acute lung injury
  - Rare—approximately 20 cases per year
  - May be fatal
- Delayed reactions

Delayed haemolytic transfusion reaction
- >24h after transfusion
- Occurs in patients who have been immunized to a red cell antigen by a previous transfusion or pregnancy
- Transfusion-associated graft versus host disease
  - Rare
  - Usually occurs in immunocompromised patients, or those who receive a transfusion from a 1st or 2nd degree relative
- Post-transfusion purpura
  - Typically at 5–9 days post transfusion of red cells or platelets
  - Thrombocytopenia, leading to bleeding
  - Rare, especially since exclusion of all previously transfused donors

References

1. Advisory Committee on the Safety of Blood, Tissue and Organs, Department of Health. *Patient consent for blood transfusion: a SaBTO consultation.* London: Department of Health, 2010. Available at: ℜ www.dh.gov.uk/en/Publicationsandstatistics/Publications/PublicationsPolicyAndGuidance/DH_113481?ssSourceSiteId=ab (accessed 6 May 2011).
2. Royal College of Surgeons of England. *Code of Practice for the Management of Jehovah's Witnesses.* London: Royal College of Surgeons of England, 2002.
3. British Committee for Standards in Haematology. *Guidelines on the Clinical Use of Red Cell Transfusion, for the Use of Platelet Transfusions and on the Use of Fresh Frozen Plasma, Cryoprecipitate and Cryosupernatant.* Available at: ℜ www.bcshguidelines.com (accessed 6 May 2011).
4. Association of Anaesthetists of Great Britain and Ireland. *Management of Anaesthesia for Jehovah's Witnesses,* 2nd edn. London: Association of Anaesthetists of Great Britain and Ireland, 2005.

Central venous cannulation

Description

This is an invasive procedure where a central vein is cannulated. Its role extends beyond central vascular access and measurement of central venous pressure to guide fluid management.

Current guidelines stipulate that central venous cannulation should be performed under sonographic guidance. This is usually carried out in the operating theatre, intensive care unit or the radiology department under sterile conditions with adequate monitoring.

Commonly the internal jugular vein in the neck is used, but occasionally the subclavian vein is used (Figs. 2.2, 2.3). Rarely, in an emergency or when access to the neck is poor, the femoral vein is used for vascular access. The patient needs to be supine with head turned to the opposite side and with a 15° head down tilt. Following ultrasound identification of the vein, a needle is inserted to enable passage of a guide-wire and then cannula (Seldinger technique). The central venous line is then fixed in place with sutures and dressing.

Additional procedures that may become necessary

- Ultrasound guidance
- Chest radiograph—to ensure adequate position of central venous line and exclude a silent pneumothorax

Benefits

- Vascular access
- Administration of total parenteral nutrition
- Infusion of toxic drugs
- Measurement of central venous pressure
- Cardiac catheterization
- Renal dialysis/filtration
- Pulmonary artery catheterization
- A means to perform transvenous cardiac pacing

Alternative procedures/conservative measures

- None/use of peripheral veins and arterial cannulation to aid fluid management, trans-oesophageal Doppler ultrasound

Serious/frequently occurring risks

- Catheter infection leading to systemic sepsis and need for line removal
- Arterial puncture
  - Rarely, can lead to stroke
- Pneumothorax, haemothorax
- Multiple unsuccessful attempts
- Haematoma formation
- Malposition of catheter
- Dysrhythmias
- Arteriovenous fistula formation
- Tamponace

The risk of complications increases, depending upon:
- Difficult anatomy: obesity, short neck, scarring due to surgery or radiation
- Repeated catheterization: increased risk of thrombus formation
- Coagulopathies
- Patients on mechanical ventilation

Blood transfusion necessary
- None/group and save

Type of anaesthesia/sedation
- Local anaesthesia
- General anaesthesia for fluid balance management pre/during major surgery

Follow-up/need for further procedure
- Chest radiography is performed to confirm correct placement and level of CVC and to identify a pneumothorax/haemothorax/mediastinal haemorrhage leading to widening
- Daily line care/checks
- Central line removal and reinsertion—also refer to local trust infection control policy

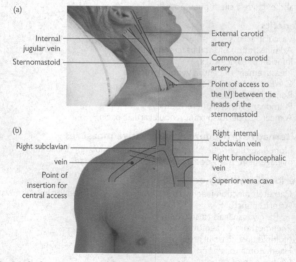

(a)

Internal jugular vein

Sternomastoid

External carotid artery

Common carotid artery

Point of access to the IVJ between the heads of the sternomastoid

(b)

Right subclavian vein

Point of insertion for central access

Right internal subclavian vein

Right branchiocephalic vein

Superior vena cava

Fig. 2.2 Surface anatomy showing internal jugular (IJV) and subclavian veins.

Reproduced with permission from Thomas J and Monaghan T. *Oxford Handbook of Clinical Examination and Practical Skills.* 2007. Oxford: Oxford University Press, p.573, Figure 17.6.

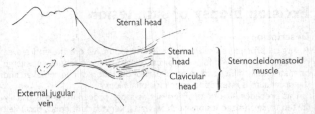

(a) Surface anatomy of external and internal jugular veins

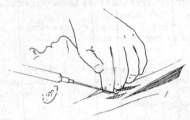

(b) Anterior approach: the chin is in the midline and the skin puncture is over the sternal head of SCM muscle

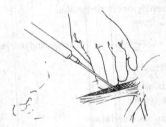

(c) Central approach: the chin is turned away and the skin puncture is between the two heads of SCM muscle

Fig. 2.3 Technique for catheterization of the internal jugular and subclavian veins.

Reproduced with permission from Ramrakha PS and Hill J. *Oxford Handbook of Cardiology*. 2006. Oxford: Oxford University Press, p.681, Figure 18.2.

Excision biopsy of skin lesion

Description

A surgical procedure used to remove skin lesions where the entire area of concern is removed for histological review. Often if the lesion is large or anatomically difficult to access, a part of the lesion can be removed and the procedure is referred to as an incisional biopsy.

This procedure is often carried out as a day procedure and is usually limited to small-sized lesions such as warts, keratoacanthomas, basal cell carcinomas and skin naevi.

Additional procedures that may become necessary

- Completion excision of lesion
- Regional lymph node biopsies/lymph node clearance
- V-Y flap to close the skin defect

Benefits

- Often a local anaesthesia or day-case procedure
- The entire lesion is excised with a macroscopically normal circumferential margin; the procedure is usually therapeutic so that no further procedure is required

Alternative procedures/conservative measures

- None

Serious/frequently occurring risks

- Bleeding and bruising
- Wound infection
- Skin necrosis leading to wound disruption and delayed healing
- Seroma
- Local pain and scarring

Blood transfusion necessary

- None/group and save

Type of anaesthesia/sedation

- Local anaesthesia/general anaesthesia

Follow-up/need for further procedure

Histology is reviewed and for most benign lesions no follow-up is required, with copy of the biopsy result sent to the patient's general practitioner and a letter to the patient. However, in cases of malignant lesions, clinic follow-up should be arranged to discuss results and any additional treatment if required. Rarely if the lesion is malignant and there is involvement of the excised margin, further excision or regional lymph node sampling/clearance may be required. Advice is given regarding the removal of skin sutures if non-dissolvable material is used.

Excision of soft tissue mass/lump (lipoma/sebaceous cyst)

Description

This is a surgical procedure to remove fatty lumps or cysts from skin or adipose tissue deep to it. Excision is commonly performed for alleviating symptoms, which include pain, cosmesis, recurrent cyst infection, impaired limb function, and patient anxiety. In certain circumstances, lipomas may be intramuscular in nature and, therefore, more extensive excision may be necessary.

Additional procedures that may become necessary

- Occasionally a drain left in situ—for larger lipoma excisions to reduce the risk of seroma formation

Benefits

- Symptom relief
- Cosmesis
- To obtain tissue diagnosis in suspicious atypical lesions

Alternative procedures/conservative measures

- For long-standing benign asymptomatic lesions, conservative treatment with observation alone is possible
- Disadvantage: larger lipomas have a theoretical risk of becoming malignant in nature over time

Serious/frequently occurring risks

- Seroma—needing drainage/aspiration
- Bruising of skin
- Wound infection
- Scar
- Keloid (higher preponderance in African Caribbean patients)
- Recurrence (especially of sebaceous cyst or lipoma if excision is incomplete)

Blood transfusion necessary

- None/group and save

Type of anaesthesia/sedation

- Local anaesthesia for smaller superficial lesions
- General anaesthesia for larger, deeper lesions

Follow-up/need for further procedure

- None or routine/urgent review in outpatient clinic with histology results

Femoral hernia repair

Description

A hernia is caused by the abnormal protrusion of a viscus (in the case of groin hernias, an intra-abdominal organ) through a weakness in the containing wall. This weakness may be inherent, as in the case of inguinal, femoral, and umbilical hernias. Femoral hernias occur just below the inguinal ligament, when abdominal contents pass through a naturally occurring defect known as the femoral canal (Fig. 2.4). Femoral hernias are relatively uncommon, accounting for only 3% of all hernias and occur more commonly in women and in adults more than children.

Surgery is performed to relieve discomfort and to prevent complications including incarceration and strangulation. Surgery involves exploration of the groin, reduction of the hernia contents, and repair the defect with sutures or mesh.

Additional procedures that may become necessary

- Bowel resection
- Laparotomy
- Postoperative surgical drain insertion

Benefits

- Reduce the risk of future surgical emergency (incarceration, bowel obstruction)
- To treat the complications of an incarcerated or obstructed hernia

Alternative procedures/conservative measures

- *Conservative* management: includes not operating on hernia until it becomes symptomatic
- *Disadvantage:* risk of incarceration and obstruction leading to gangrenous and perforated bowel

Serious/frequently occurring risks[1]

- Bruising
- Vascular injury (femoral vessels)
- Wound infection (<1% in elective cases)
- Mesh infection (may require removal of mesh)
- Sensory changes over skin at hernia site or genitalia
- Recurrence after surgical repair is <1% (depending on surgical technique and experience)
- In event of needing bowel resection there is a 1–3% risk of anastomotic leak
- Female patients are at risk of injury to the ovarian and uterine neurovascular bundles

Blood transfusion necessary

- *None/group and save*

Type of anaesthesia/sedation
- Local/regional (spinal)/general anaesthesia

Follow-up/need for further procedure
- None/outpatient follow-up if concerns

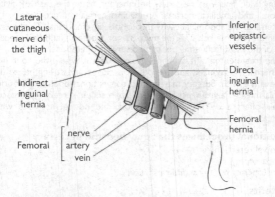

Fig. 2.4 Groin anatomy showing anatomy of femoral and inguinal hernias.

Reproduced with permission from Longmore M, Wilkinson IB, Davidson EH et al. Oxford Handbook of Clinical Medicine. 8th edition. 2010. Oxford: Oxford University Press, p.617.

Reference
1. Prather C. Inflammatory and anatomic diseases of the intestine, peritoneum, mesentery, and omentum. In: Goldman L, Ausiello D, eds. Cecil Medicine, 23rd edn. Philadelphia, PA: WB Saunders/Elsevier, 2007.

Inguinal hernia repair

Description

A hernia is caused by the abnormal protrusion of a viscus (in the case of groin hernias, an intra-abdominal organ) through a weakness in the containing wall. This weakness may be inherent, as in the case of inguinal, femoral, and umbilical hernias. An inguinal hernia is a protrusion of the contents of the abdominal cavity through the inguinal canal. They are very common (lifetime risk 27% for men, 3% for women[1]), and their repair is one of the most frequently performed surgical operations.

The treatment in a fit patient is usually surgical, where the contents of the hernia are reduced and the defect is closed and strengthened using a mesh (Fig. 2.5). Surgery may involve conventional open exploration of hernia through a groin incision, or by laparoscopic surgery. Laparoscopic repair offers a quicker return to work and normal activities with a decreased pain.

Additional procedures that may become necessary

- Bowel resection
- Laparotomy
- Postoperative surgical drain insertion

Benefits

- Reduce the risk of future surgical emergency (incarceration, bowel obstruction)
- To treat the complications of an incarcerated or obstructed hernia

Several prospective randomized trials comparing open versus laparoscopic repair have reported reduced postoperative pain, earlier return to work, and fewer complications and decreased recurrence rate via a laparoscopic approach.

Alternative procedures/conservative measures

The discomfort from direct and indirect inguinal hernias may be reduced by a truss hernia support. This can be useful while the patient is waiting for an operation of if the patient is unfit for surgery.

- *Disadvantage*: a truss hernia support is not curative as the underlying mechanical muscle wall defect is not addressed

Serious/frequently occurring risks

Conventional open repair[2]

- Recurrence of the hernia—about 0.5% or 1 in 200 (first time repairs)
- Wound infection—less than 0.5% or 1 in 200
- Bleeding (fully controlled)—less than 1% or 1 in 100
- Swelling and bruising (temporary)—about 5% or 1 in 20
- Injury to bladder or bowel—extremely rare (less than 1 in 400)
- *Actual or perceived change in testicular size/function[3]*
  - 0.5% for primary repairs (*1 in 200, usually in large scrotal or neglected hernias*)
  - 1–5% for recurrent repairs
- Injury to the vas deferens—~0.3% or less

- Infertility, directly caused by inguinal hernia surgery is *extremely rare*. This would occur only if both sides (left and right) were repaired and both vas deferens or testicular injury occurred
- Numbness and/or chronic incisional pain—1–2%; generally mild, non-debilitating and self-limiting. In about 1 in 800 cases the chronic pain may require nerve blockade to relieve symptoms[3]
- Retention of urine necessitating bladder catheterization

Laparoscopic repair

The complication of laparoscopic hernia repair can be summarized as follows:[2]

- Immediate
  - Visceral injury—less than 0.1%; as with any laparoscopic procedure (📖 see Chapter 10, p.279)
  - Vascular injury—inferior epigastric vessels (0.5–1%) and femoral vessels (<0.1%)
  - Injury to vas/spermatic vessels—spermatic cord vessels (0.5–1%) causing testicular atrophy or scrotal haematoma
- Late
  - Nerve entrapment—the lateral cutaneous nerve of thigh (2%), causing paraesthesia of upper aspect of thigh, and the femoral branch of genitofemoral nerve (~1%) are the two nerves most vulnerable to trauma caused by indiscriminate placement of staplers lateral to the spermatic cord on the iliopubic tract
  - Bowel—adhesions to mesh and migration of mesh are extremely rare (<0.1%)
  - Recurrence rates for a totally extraperitoneal repair are approximately 0.3–1% and for a transabdominal pre-peritoneal repair are approximately 0.4–1%. Immediate recurrence within 6 weeks is usually due to technical failure

Blood transfusion necessary

- None/group and save

Type of anaesthesia/sedation

- General/regional (spinal/epidural)/local anaesthesia

Follow-up/need for further procedure

- None or review in outpatient clinic if concerns

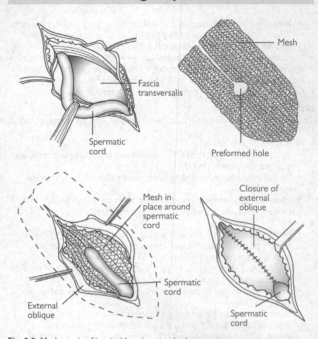

Fig. 2.5 Mesh repair of inguinal hernia—standard steps.

Reproduced with permission from McLatchie GR and Leaper DJ. *Oxford Specialist Handbook of Operative Surgery* 2nd edition. 2006. Oxford: Oxford University Press, p.369, Figure 11.1.

References

1. Rutkow IM. Demographic and socioeconomic aspects of hernia repair in the United States in 2003. *Surg Clin North Am* 2003;**83**(5):1045–51, v–vi.
2. Fitzgibbons RJ Jr, Greenberg AG. *Nyhus and Condon's Hernia*, 5th edn. Philadelphia: Lippincott William & Wilkins, 2002.
3. Wantz GE. Testicular atrophy and chronic residual neuralgia as risks of inguinal hernioplasty. *Surg Clin North Am* 1993;**73**:571–81.

Hernia repair—umbilical/paraumbilical/epigastric/incisional

Description
Umbilical/paraumbilical
This is a weakness or defect in the anterior abdominal wall, which may be congenital or acquired. It results in the protrusion of intra-abdominal contents, which are at risk of strangulation or obstructing, or is simply painful. The hernia is usually repaired via a transverse incision over the hernial protrusion, and may require a mesh cover if the defect is larger than 3cm or is recurrent in nature.

Epigastric hernia
This hernia develops due to a weakness in the midline linea alba where the fibres of the rectus sheath decussate. It is usually repaired by primary closure of the defect, and does not routinely require a mesh unless the neck of the hernia is large.

Incisional hernia
This is an iatrogenic hernia resulting from previous incisions over the anterior abdominal wall. Incisional hernia formation is due to poor abdominal wall structure, infection, or failure in surgical technique. The rate of incisional hernia occurrence has been reported as high as 13%.[1]

Both laparoscopic and open surgical repair have been used for incisional hernias. The use of mesh is dependent on the surgeon, however, it is now commonly used.

Additional procedures that may become necessary
- More than one repair—since recurrence rates are high, especially for incisional hernia
- Postoperative surgical drain insertion

Benefits
- Relief of local symptoms of pain, discomfort, and cosmetic improvement
- Reduction in the risk of future surgical emergency (incarceration, bowel obstruction)
- To treat the complications of an incarcerated or obstructed hernia

Alternative procedures/conservative measures
The discomfort from direct and indirect inguinal hernia may be improved by a truss hernia support. This can be useful while the patient is waiting for an operation or if the patient is unfit for surgery.
- Disadvantage: a truss hernia support is not curative as the underlying mechanical muscle wall defect is not addressed. Its use, however, is not routinely recommended due to poor long-term efficacy and risk of strangulation of bowel

Serious/frequently occurring risks

- The risk of complications has been shown to be about 13%[2,3]
- The risk of recurrence and repeated surgery is as high as 20–52%,[2–4] particularly with open procedures in obese patients
- Laparoscopy with mesh has shown rates of recurrence as low as 3.4%, with fewer complications[2]

Postoperative complications include:
- Seroma, sometimes requiring aspiration
- Postoperative bleeding, though seldom enough to require repeat surgery
- Prolonged pain, treated with pain medication or anti-inflammatory drugs
- Intestinal injury due to adhesions with the sac
- Nerve injury
- Surgical wound infection
- Infected mesh with chronic sinus, requiring removal of mesh
- Urinary retention in immediate postoperative period
- Respiratory distress due to loss of domain from large hernia repair

Blood transfusion necessary

- None/group and save/cross-match 2–4 units blood

Type of anaesthesia/sedation

- Local/regional (spinal/epidural)/general anaesthesia

Follow-up/need for further procedure

- None or review in outpatient clinic as required

References

1. Fitzgibbons RJ Jr, Greenberg AG. *Nyhus and Condon's Hernia*, 5th edn. Philadelphia: Lippincott William & Wilkins, 2002.
2. Goodney PP, Birkmeyer CM, Birkmeyer JD. Short-term outcomes of laparoscopic and open ventral hernia repair. *Arch Surg* 2002;**137**:1161–5.
3. Luijendijk RW, Hop WCJ, Van Den Tol MP, et al. A comparison of suture repair with mesh repair for incisional hernia. *N Engl J Med* 2000;**343**:392–8.
4. Mathes SJ, Steinwald PM, Foster RD, et al. Complex abdominal wall reconstruction: A comparison of flap and mesh closure. *Ann Surg* 2000;**232**:586–96.

Incision and drainage of abscess

Description

An abscess is a collection of pus that has accumulated in a cavity as a result of an infective process. It is a part of the host defence response to prevent the spread of sepsis systemically. Abscesses tend to present with local symptoms of pain, swelling, redness, and limitation of movement. Systemic symptoms, which include pyrexia, are not uncommon. The most common organisms involved are *Staphylococcus aureus* and *Streptococcus*. Surgical treatment is with incision and drainage of the sepsis, and those with weakened immune systems, e.g. patients on steroids or chemotherapy and patients with diabetes, renal failure on dialysis, or HIV develop abscesses frequently and need to have treatment instituted urgently.

Additional procedures that may become necessary

- Multiple incision and drainages for recurrent abscesses
- Debridement of necrotic tissue
- Packing abscess cavity and changing packs under anaesthesia for large abscess cavities

Benefits

- Resolution of sepsis
- Drainage of pus for microbiological culture and sensitivities

Alternative procedures/conservative measures

- Needle aspiration (breast/facial abscesses)
  - *Disadvantage:* recurrence rates higher and multiple drainage procedures may be required
- Ultrasound or computed tomography (CT)-guided drainage of abscess
- Laparoscopic washout
  - *Disadvantage:* general anaesthesia required and invasive procedure
  - *Advantage:* debridement or washout can be performed with irrigation of pelvic or intra-abdominal abscess cavities

Serious/frequently occurring risks

- Bleeding from injury to underlying vessels, especially in the neck, axilla, and groin
- Unsightly scar in event of large abscess requiring debridement of skin
- Prolonged period of wound healing, especially if there is underlying osteomyelitis
- Recurrence of abscess
- Fistula formation in the perianal region (incidence 15–25%)
- Development of chronic sinus in presence of infected underlying foreign body, e.g. infected mesh, bony prosthesis, or vascular prosthetic graft

Blood transfusion necessary

- None/group and save

Type of anaesthesia/sedation
- Local/regional (spinal/epidural)/general anaesthesia

Follow-up/need for further procedure
- None or review in outpatient clinic as required, especially in circumstances where perianal fistulation has taken place
- Often dressing change and packing by a district nurse is required until the abscess cavity has healed to completion

Intercostal drain insertion

Description

A drain is inserted percutaneously into the pleural cavity through an intercostal space for the purpose of drainage (Fig. 2.6). This could be therapeutic in nature or diagnostic to obtain pleural fluid for biochemical, cytological, or microbiological analysis. Intercostal drain insertion can be performed by blunt dissection (surgical drain, Fig. 2.7) or via Seldinger's technique for smaller drains. Ultrasound guidance may be used to guide placement, especially for basal drains.

Indications for insertion[1]

- Pneumothorax
  - In any ventilated patient with chest trauma
  - Post needle thoracocentesis in a tension pneumothorax
  - Persistent or recurrent pneumothorax
  - Large secondary spontaneous pneumothorax
- Malignant pleural effusions
- Empyema and complicated para-pneumonic pleural effusions
- Traumatic haemopneumothorax
- Postoperative—for example, thoracotomy, oesophagectomy, cardiac surgery, and nephrectomy

Additional procedures that may become necessary

- Massive haemothorax may necessitate thoracotomy to control bleeding

Benefits

- Diagnostic (microbiological/biochemical/cytological)
- Therapeutic (drainage)

Alternative procedures/conservative measures

- Aspiration (pleural fluid aspiration, aspiration of small spontaneous primary pneumothoraces)
- Conservative/medical management of pleural effusions
- In certain transudates, fluid management with fluid restriction and diuretics can decrease the volume of pleural fluid in an overall oedematous patient

Serious/frequently occurring risks[2,3]

- Insertional complications—23%
  - Bleeding from intercostal vessels
  - Perforation of underlying lung causing a broncho-pleural fistula
  - Diaphragm/abdominal cavity penetration (placed too low)
  - Stomach/colon injury (diaphragmatic hernia not recognized)
  - Blockage of drain by blood clot or debris
  - Injury to liver on right side and spleen on left side during drain insertion
- Positional complications—73%
  - Tube placed subcutaneously (not in thoracic cavity)
  - Dislodgement—drain falls out
  - Infection
  - Iatrogenic pneumothorax on removal of chest drain

Blood transfusion necessary

- None

Type of anaesthesia/sedation

- Local anaesthesia is infiltrated into the site of insertion to raise a dermal bleb before deeper infiltration of the intercostal muscles and pleural surface
- Sedation in the form of midazolam 1–5mg may be used in the anxious patient (be wary of respiratory compromise in such patients!)

Follow-up/need for further procedure

- Depends on underlying pathology

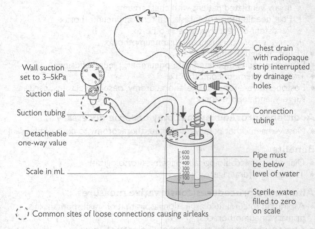

Wall suction set to 3–5kPa

Suction dial

Suction tubing

Detacheable one-way value

Scale in mL

Chest drain with radiopaque strip interrupted by drainage holes

Connection tubing

Pipe must be below level of water

Sterile water filled to zero on scale

Common sites of loose connections causing airleaks

Fig. 2.6 Intercostal chest drain insertion—site and position.

Reproduced with permission from O'Connor IF and Urdang M. *Oxford Handbook of Surgical Cross-Cover*, 2008. Oxford: Oxford University Press, p.203, Figure 5.5.

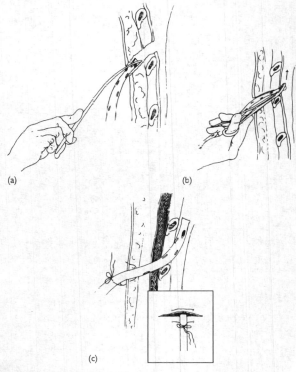

Fig. 2.7 Insertion of chest drain.

Reproduced with permission from Ramrakha PS, Moore KP, and Sam A. *Oxford Handbook of Acute Medicine* 3rd edition. 2010. Oxford: Oxford University Press, p.789, Figure 15.13.

References

1. Laws D. BTS Guidelines for the insertion of a chest drain. *Thorax* 2003;**58**(Suppl II):ii53–ii9.
2. Bailey RC. Complications of tube thoracostomy in trauma. *J Accid Emerg Med* 2000;**17**:111–14.
3. Maritz DF. Complications of tube thoracostomy for chest trauma. *S Afr Med J* 2009;e(2):114–17.

Colorectal surgery

General issues in consent for colorectal procedures

Introduction

- The procedure-specific complications will be detailed in each section.
- For any colorectal procedure it is important to mention the following general consent issues:
  - Scarring
  - Possibility of administration of antibiotics
  - Allergic reactions
  - Possibility of administration of blood products (consequently transfusion reactions and transmission of infectious diseases)
  - Thromboembolism (deep vein thrombosis (DVT), pulmonary embolism)
  - Wound infection and/or dehiscence
  - Peritoneal sepsis
  - Risks related to anaesthesia
  - Urinary retention
  - Urinary tract infection
  - Lower respiratory tract infection
  - Myocardial infarction
  - Death
- It should also be documented that should any unforeseen pathologies be identified then additional procedures (in particular hysterectomy and bilateral salpingo-oophorectomy (BSO) should they be involved in a malignant process) should be authorized if deemed in the best interest of the patient
- Where appropriate, it is prudent to discuss the disposal of tissues
- For laparoscopic procedures it is important to mention the following: perforation of bowel (following port-site insertion), port-site haematoma, port-site hernia and the potential for the operation to be converted to an open procedure

Risk predictors

When discussing a proposed operation with a patient, it is important to mention all significant potential complications, their evidence-based rates where appropriate, the expected recovery, and perceived benefits of surgery. While studies and departmental audits can indicate likely complication rates for a particular procedure, the morbidity and mortality is more difficult to predict.

- Risk predictor scoring systems have been in use since the American Society of Anesthesiologists (ASA) scoring system was introduced in 1963. This is a simple and effective scoring system, which classifies the physical status of a patient
- In 1981 the Acute Physiology and Chronic Health Evaluation (APACHE) scoring system was introduced to classify the severity of a disease based on a number of different physiological parameters. There have since been two updated versions: APACHE II in 1985 and APACHE III in 1991. The APACHE system is used predominantly in the

intensive care setting and calculates the mortality risk for a group of patients within a specific disease category
- The Simplified Acute Physiological Score (SAPS) is a derivation of the APACHE system that uses fewer of the physiological parameters and is used to calculate the predicted hospital mortality

In 1991, Copeland et al.[1] introduced the Physiologic and Operative Severity Score for the enumeration of Mortality and Morbidity (POSSUM) score.[1] It was initially developed in the context of the general surgical population and has since been modified for use in gastrointestinal/colorectal, vascular, head and neck, and orthopaedic patients. ▶▶ It has been shown to over-predict mortality, in particular for patients in the lowest risk category.[2] It utilizes 12 physiological parameters and six operative variables to give a percentage estimation of mortality risk[2]

- Physiological
  - Age
  - Cardiac signs
  - Respiratory
  - Systolic blood pressure
  - Pulse
  - Glasgow Coma Scale
  - Haemoglobin
  - White cell count
  - Urea
  - Sodium
  - Potassium
  - Electrocardiogram (ECG)
- Operative
  - Operative severity
  - Multiple procedures
  - Total blood loss
  - Peritoneal soiling
  - Malignancy
  - Mode of surgery

For the purpose of this chapter we will consider the colorectal (CR) POSSUM score which involves the following parameters:
- Physiological
  - Age
  - Cardiac
  - Systolic blood pressure
  - Pulse rate
  - Haemoglobin
  - Urea
- Operative parameters (if calculating risk preoperatively)
  - Operation type
  - Peritoneal contamination
  - Malignancy status
  - National Confidential Enquiry into Patient Outcome and Death (NCEPOD) classification

When consenting a patient for a colorectal operation (suitable operations for which this would be relevant are indicated in later sections) a colorectal

(CR) POSSUM score should be calculated in order to predict mortality risk from a particular procedure. These details can then be conveyed to the patient when consenting for procedural risks.[3] This is in order to more accurately estimate the mortality risk involved.

References

1. Copeland GP, Jones D, Walters M. POSSUM: a scoring system for surgical audit. *Br J Surg* 1991;**78**(3):355–60.
2. Prytherch DR, Whiteley MS, Higgins B, *et al*. POSSUM and Portsmouth POSSUM for predicting mortality. Physiological and operative severity score for the enumeration of mortality and morbidity. *Br J Surg* 1998;**85**(9):1217–20.
3. Smith JJ, Tekkis PP. Risk prediction in surgery. Available at: ℘ www.riskprediction.org.uk (accessed 5 May 2011).

Anal fissure (botulinum toxin injection, lateral internal sphincterotomy, advancement flap)

Description

An anal fissure is a breach in the skin in the anal canal, which can be acute (within 6 weeks' duration) or chronic in nature. Classically patients experience painful defecation and bright per rectal bleeding. Surgical or chemical sphincterotomy is generally reserved for symptomatic chronic anal fissures. For difficult or recurrent anal fissures (particularly in patients without sphincter hypertonia), excision of the fissure with anal advancement flap may be an option.[1]

- *Lateral internal sphincterotomy*: this can be performed as a day case either under local or general anaesthesia. A small incision is made in order to access the internal sphincter followed by a small incision in the sphincter in order to relieve the spasm associated with the fissure itself
- *Intra-anal botulinum toxin*: the toxin is injected in either three or four positions between the internal and external anal sphincter causing paralysis. This in turn prevents the anal spasm associated with the fissure, encouraging fissure healing
- *Anal advancement flap*: the fissure is excised and adjacent healthy tissue is used as a flap to cover the excised area[2]

Additional procedures that may become necessary

- Anal fissure excision or curettage

Benefits

- *Diagnostic*: examination under anaesthesia will aid in confirming the diagnosis of an anal fissure, in particular those cases who cannot be examined in clinic or in the emergency department due to pain
- *Therapeutic*: relief of pain, allows painless defecation, and decrease constipation rates due to painful infrequent defecation cycles

Alternative procedures/conservative measures

- *Conservative*: dietary advice, stool softeners and the use of topical analgesic agents
- *Medical*: topical glyceryl trinitrate (GTN) ointment, topical diltiazem (calcium channel blocker)

Serious/frequently occurring risks

- *Anal sphincter surgery*: bleeding, infection, faecal incontinence, recurrence, acute urinary retention (in patients with pre-existing obstructive lower urinary tract symptoms)
- *Lateral internal sphincterotomy*: haematoma—2.5%, haemorrhage—2.5%, incontinence at 2 months—7.5%, incontinence at 3 years—5%, overall recurrence—7.5%

- *Intra-anal botulinum toxin injection*: haematoma—2.5%, incontinence at 2 months—5%, incontinence at 3 years—0%, overall recurrence—55%
- *Anal advancement flap*: the American Society of Colon and Rectal Surgeons' guidelines have suggested this as an acceptable alternative to lateral internal sphincterotomy, however, there is a lack of prospective, randomized studies in the literature at the present time

Blood transfusion necessary
- None/group and save

Type of anaesthesia/sedation
- Regional/general anaesthesia (this can be a particularly painful procedure when curetting the base of a chronic ulcer and may require forewarning the anaesthetist to deepen the anaesthesia at this point)

Follow-up/need for further procedure
- On discharge patients must be reminded of the need for regular sit baths, high-fibre diet, high fluid intake (assuming no contraindications) and the use of bulk-forming agents and/or stool softeners
- Routine outpatient review if required

References
1. Orsay C, Rakinic J, Perry B, et al. Practice parameters for the management of anal fissures (Revised). *Dis Colon Rectum* 2004;**47**:2003–7.
2. Arroyo A, Pérez F, Serrano P, et al. Surgical versus chemical (botulinum toxin) sphincterotomy for chronic anal fissure: Long-term results of a prospective randomized clinical and manometric study. *Am J Surg* 2005;**189**(4):429–34.

Anal sphincter repair

Description

Faecal incontinence is the loss of voluntary control of stool or bowel movements. Incontinence of flatus implies the loss of control of flatulence whilst maintaining faecal control.[1] There are a number of different causes of faecal incontinence, which are beyond the scope of this handbook (□ see *Oxford Specialist Handbook of Colorectal Surgery*).

If surgery is considered, sphincteroplasty is the mainstay. When explaining to the patient it is often helpful to describe the two anal sphincters (internal and external) as complete circles like doughnuts, which encircle the anal canal. If a defect or tear exists in one or both of these circles, sphincteroplasty is possible. This involves cutting the sphincter, overlapping the two ends, and then securing them in place with sutures. This aims to restore the circle and improve control. This is performed under regional or general anaesthesia with the patient positioned in the lithotomy or jack-knife position.

Preoperatively, the surgeon may recommend either endo-anal ultrasound or MRI in order to fully understand the anatomy of the sphincter complex. Indications for surgery include:[2]

- Perineal trauma/iatrogenic injury following anorectal surgery
- Obstetric anal sphincter injuries (OASIS), which are symptomatic (incontinence, perineal pain, and dyspareunia). These include only grade 3 and 4 perineal tears (classification based on the Royal College of Obstetricians and Gynaecologists guideline[3])

It is the external anal sphincter which is repaired using, in general, two recognized sphincteroplasty techniques: first, an end-to-end (approximation) or second, an overlap repair.

If recognized at the time of injury and repaired within 24h, this is termed a primary repair. If left and repaired subsequently (recommended minimum of 3 months) this is termed a secondary repair. Most obstetricians perform primary end-to-end repair, whereas colorectal surgeons would opt for the overlap technique.

Additional procedures that may become necessary

- Defunctioning colostomy
- Further trauma surgery—if other organs injured in the presence of traumatic sphincter injury

Benefits

- *Therapeutic*: restore continence or reduce the risk of further incontinence

Alternative procedures/conservative measures

- *Conservative*: dietary lifestyle change, the use of bulk-forming agents, pelvic floor exercises, and biofeedback training

Serious/frequently occurring risks

- Bleeding, infection, difficulty voiding with acute retention of urine, faecal impaction, dyspareunia, perineal pain, failure of procedure, deterioration from preoperative continence level, deterioration in continence with time, the possibility of requiring a further operation
- *Sphincteroplasty*:[4]
  - Short-term results: 60–88% patients achieved an excellent or good outcome which was defined as perfect continence or incontinence of flatus with minor staining, 15–20% experienced no change or deterioration in symptoms
  - Long-term results: 15% patients required further surgery for incontinence, 0% were continent of both stool and flatus, 10.5% were totally continent for stool, 15.8% had no faecal urgency, 52.6% wore a pad for incontinence
- Overlapping sphincteroplasty: overall 16.5% complication rate (1.3% mortality, temporary difficulty in voiding, excessive bleeding, abscess formation, haematoma, faecal impaction[5])

Blood transfusion necessary

- None/group and save

Type of anaesthesia/sedation

- Regional/general anaesthesia

Follow-up/need for further procedure

- Routine outpatient review
- Continue conservative measures including dietary lifestyle change, use of bulk-forming agents, pelvic floor exercises, and biofeedback training

References

1. Bartolo DCC, Paterson HM. Anal incontinence. *Best Pract Res Clin Gastroenterol* 2009;**23**(4):505–15.
2. Madoff RD, Parker SC, Varma MG, *et al.* Faecal incontinence in adults. *Lancet* 2004;**364**(9434):621–32.
3. Royal College of Obstetricians and Gynaecologists. The management of third- and fourth-degree perineal tears. London: Royal College of Obstetricians and Gynaecologists, 2007 (Green-top guideline; no. 29).
4. Malouf AJ, Norton CS, Engel AF, *et al.* Long-term results of overlapping anterior anal-sphincter repair for obstetric trauma. *Lancet* 2000;**355**(9200):260–5.
5. Fang DT, Nivatvongs S, Vermeulen FD, *et al.* Overlapping sphincteroplasty for acquired anal incontinence. *Dis Colon Rectum* 1984;**27**(11):720–2.

Anorectal abscesses (incision and drainage)

Description

An anorectal abscess (Fig. 3.1) is a collection of pus formed adjacent to the anus commonly as a result of an infection originating in the crypts of Morgagni.[1] Without intervention in the form of incision and drainage, the abscess will progress, expand in size, and act as an underlying source of sepsis and necrotizing infection.[2] Once the abscess has formed, antibiotics are unable to penetrate and are ineffective when used alone. The abscess cavity is generally incised and drained under general anaesthesia, although, if small, it can be treated under local anaesthesia.

It is recommended that an anal speculum or proctoscope should be used to visualize the rectum prior to incision in order to detect the presence of a fistula-in-ano. An incision is made over the most fluctuant point, loculations are broken down, and the abscess cavity is thoroughly irrigated with either saline or hydrogen peroxide. It is important to inform the patient that the wound will most likely be left open, packed on a daily basis, and heal through secondary intention.

Additional procedures that may become necessary

- Examination of rectum under anaesthesia
- Some surgeons advocate immediate management, should a fistula-in-ano be found at the time of incision and drainage

Benefits

- *Diagnostic*: assess the size and extent of abscess and whether there is communication with the rectal mucosa in the form of a fistula-in-ano
- *Therapeutic*: resolve sepsis, prevent fistula formation

Alternative procedures/conservative measures

- *Medical*: antibiotic therapy is often used in conjunction with incision and drainage, and may help with systemic sepsis. The abscess cavity does, however, need to be drained surgically or allowed to discharge spontaneously to allow for evacuation of pus from a septic focus[3]

Serious/frequently occurring risks

- Bleeding, infection, damage to sphincter mechanism, potential for faecal incontinence, fistula-in-ano formation, recurrence, urinary retention
- Even with incision and drainage: up to 60% may develop a fistula-in-ano later in life and up to 35% present at the time of incision and drainage (there is some variation in the literature regarding the incidence of fistula-in-ano)[4]

Blood transfusion necessary

- None/group and save

Type of anaesthesia/sedation

- General anaesthesia/regional anaesthesia (spinal/epidural)

Follow-up/need for further procedure
- Regular dressing changes and packing of wound
- Occasionally a course of oral or intravenous antibiotics will be given
- Follow-up is necessary in cases where fistulas have been identified with subsequent examination under anaesthesia and fistula surgery

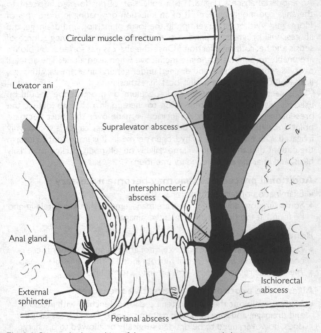

Fig. 3.1 Sites and relationships of the commonest anorectal abscesses.

Reproduced with permission from MacKay GJ, Dorrance HR, Molloy RG, et al. Oxford Specialist Handbook of Colorectal Surgery. 2010. Oxford: Oxford University Press, p.275, Figure 6.6.

References
1. Marcus RH, Stine RJ, Cohen MA. Perirectal abscess. Ann Emerg Med 1995;**25**(5):597–603.
2. Lichtenstein D, Stavorovsky M, Irge D. Fournier's gangrene complicating perianal abscess: Report of two cases. Dis Colon Rectum 1977;**21**(5):377–9.
3. Scoma JA, Salvati EP, Rubin RJ. Incidence of fistulas subsequent to anal abscesses. Dis Colon Rectum 1974;**17**(3):357–9.
4. Ramanujam PS, Prasad ML, Abcarian H, et al. Perianal abscesses an fistulas: A study of 1023 patients Dis Colon Rectum 1984;**27**(9):593–7.

Appendicectomy

Description

Appendicectomy is the surgical removal of the vermiform appendix either due to clinically or radiologically suspected appendicitis or alternative pathology (i.e. tumour, mucocoele etc). The operation is performed (Fig. 3.2) under general anaesthesia with the patient in the supine position. Both open and laparoscopic appendicectomy are acceptable, local practice may influence the surgeon's decision.

- Open: a gridiron or Lanz incision is made in the right iliac fossa. The layers are divided and the peritoneum is opened. The peritoneal cavity is entered and the appendix is identified, ligated, and excised. If the appendix has perforated, a washout is performed. The peritoneum is closed and the layers are closed with absorbable sutures
- Laparoscopic:[1] in general, three or four small port incisions are be made in the abdominal wall, the ports and camera are inserted following the introduction of a pneumoperitoneum. The appendix is identified, ligated, and removed. The port sites are subsequently closed

Recent Cochrane review recommends that all patients undergoing appendicectomy should be prophylactically administered antibiotics. If the appendix has perforated antibiotics may need to be continued over a number of days (either intravenously or oral).

If an intra-abdominal mass is found (commonly following a perforated appendix) the decision may be made to manage this with antibiotics. Some surgeons may elect to subsequently perform an interval appendicectomy.

If the appendix is found to be macroscopically normal and the operation is performed open it is best practice to perform the appendicectomy for two reasons: the first is that the appendix may be microscopically inflamed, the second being if a patient is noted to have either a gridiron or Lanz incision it is assumed (rightly or wrongly) that they have previously undergone appendicectomy.

If the operation is performed laparoscopically and the appendix is noted to be normal, the decision to perform the appendicectomy is less clear. If, for example in a young female blood is noted in the pelvis (commonly from a ruptured ovarian cyst) the diagnosis is clear and an appendicectomy would confer additional unnecessary risks. If no other obvious cause is found an appendicectomy may be indicated as a proportion will be histologically inflamed.

Once the operation has been performed, the appendix will be sent to the histopathology lab for examination. Possible aetiologies of the appendicitis include faecaliths, intestinal parasites, carcinoid appendix, caecal tumour, and inflammatory bowel disease.

Additional procedures that may become necessary

- Conversion to open procedure (from laparoscopic) or laparotomy
- Need for alternative procedure (i.e. right hemicolectomy, Meckel's diverticulectomy) if alternative diagnosis encountered
- Excision of appendix despite macroscopically normal appearance

Benefits
- *Diagnostic*: to identify the cause of pain/sepsis/symptoms
- *Therapeutic*: remove a diseased appendix and source of sepsis

Alternative procedures/conservative measures
- *Medical*: intravenous followed by oral antibiotic therapy (a comparison of 252 men with suspected appendicitis, randomized to antibiotic therapy or early surgery showed 86% improved with antibiotics of which 14% required surgery within 24h)[2]

Serious/frequently occurring risks
- Bleeding, infection[3] (including intra-abdominal abscess, wound infection and urinary infection), perforation of bowel, stump leak/blow out with resultant peritonitis, colo-cutaneous faecal fistula, subfertility (a potentially rare complication following pelvic abscess)
- Open versus laparoscopic appendicectomy: wound infections are half as likely following open appendicectomy. Intra-abdominal abscess formation is three-fold higher following laparoscopic appendicectomy[4]
- ▶▶ <1% risk of pulmonary complications, urinary tract complications, venous thrombosis/pulmonary embolism, post-procedure haemorrhage

Blood transfusion necessary
- Group and save

Type of anaesthesia/sedation
- Regional (spinal/epidural)/general anaesthesia

Follow-up/need for further procedure
- No routine outpatient follow-up required unless histopathological examination of appendix alters management plan

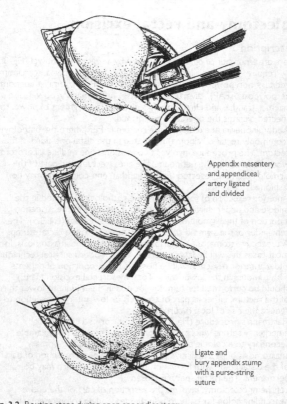

Appendix mesentery
and appendiceal
artery ligated
and divided

Ligate and
bury appendix stump
with a purse-string
suture

Fig. 3.2 Routine steps during open appendicectomy.

Reproduced with permission from McLatchie GR and Leaper DJ. *Oxford Specialist Handbook of Operative Surgery* 2nd edition. 2006. Oxford: Oxford University Press, p.247, Figure 7.19.

References

1. Sauerland S, Lefering R, Neugebauer EAM. Laparoscopic versus open surgery for suspected appendicitis. *Cochrane Database Syst Rev* 2004 4:CD001546.
2. Styrud J, Eriksson S, Nilsson I, et al. Appendicectomy versus antibiotic treatment in acute appendicitis: a prospective multicenter randomized controlled trial. *World J Surg* 2006;**33**(6):1033–7.
3. Andersen BR, Kallehave FL, Andersen HK. Antibiotics versus placebo for prevention of postoperative infection after appendicectomy. *Cochrane Database Syst Rev* 2005;**3**:CD001439.
4. Nguyen NT, Zainabadi K, Mavandadi S, et al. Trends in utilization and outcomes of laparoscopic versus open appendectomy. *Am J Surg* 2004;**188**(6):813–20.

Colectomy and rectal excision

Description

There are a number of different reasons why a segment of bowel (Fig. 3.3) may require resection. Indications include benign polyps, carcinoma, hereditary non-polyposis colorectal cancer (HNPCC), familial adenomatous polyposis (FAP), diverticular disease, inflammatory bowel disease, ischaemia, trauma, and Hirschsprung's disease. The segment of bowel that is affected dictates the operation performed.[1]

- Abdominoperineal excision of the rectum (APER): here the pathology (commonly rectal carcinoma) is situated in the distal one-third of the rectum. The procedure involves two incisions: one midline laparotomy wound and one in the perineum. The anus, rectum, and part of the sigmoid colon are resected (Fig. 3.4) and an end-colostomy may be fashioned
- Anterior resection of rectum: here the pathology is situated in the middle and upper thirds of the rectum. This involves the resection of a portion of the sigmoid colon and part of the rectum (Fig. 3.5). The remainder of the sigmoid colon is anastomosed to the rectal stump. A protective stoma can be performed to protect the anastomosis. In most cases this will be later reversed. With modern surgical techniques a low anterior resection will be possible in a proportion of patients with tumours in the lower third. Total mesorectal excision (TME) should be performed for tumours located in the middle to lower third of the rectum, either as part of an APER or low anterior resection to reduce the risk of local recurrence
- Hartmann's procedure (Fig. 3.6): this is performed either in the emergency setting where gross contamination exists (for example secondary to a colonic perforation) thereby precluding primary anastomosis or as a palliative procedure. It involves resection of part of the distal colon with formation of a colostomy, which may be permanent. The rectal stump is closed
- Left hemi-colectomy: involves the resection of part or the entire descending colon for pathology in the descending colon or splenic flexure. If it is extended, part of the transverse colon is also resected beyond the middle colic vessels. An anastomosis is made between the proximal colon and the distal colon. A defunctioning ileostomy or colostomy may be performed which the surgeon will decide in the postoperative period whether or not to reverse
- Transverse colectomy: a rarely performed procedure for pathology in the transverse colon
- Right hemi-colectomy: the caecum and ascending colon are resected. If it is extended, part of the transverse colon is also resected beyond the middle colic vessels. An anastomosis is made between the proximal segment of bowel and the transverse colon. It is performed for pathology in the caecum, ascending colon, or hepatic flexure
- Total colectomy: this procedure involves resection of the entire colon with formation either of an ileorectal anastomosis or an end-ileostomy and mucous fistula. If the rectum is also excised it is termed

a proctocolectomy. Indications include pancolitis refractory to medical therapy, patients with known HNPCC or FAP. An end-ileostomy may be fashioned. Alternatively, an ileoanal pouch or ileorectal anastomosis may be performed
- Ileocaecal resection: for pathology in the terminal ileum and caecum. It is commonly performed for Crohn's disease or occasionally an appendiceal mass. Here, the terminal ileum and caecum are resected. The ileum is then anastomosed with the ascending colon

The operations listed can all be performed either open or laparoscopically. Preoperatively the patient may be asked to undergo bowel preparation.[2] If the colectomy is planned open this will be performed under general anaesthesia with the patient in the supine or lithotomy position. A midline laparotomy wound will be made, the segment of bowel identified and resected.

Depending on the operation, an anastomosis of healthy bowel will be made or alternatively an end-ileostomy or colostomy will be performed. Should the surgeon wish to protect the anastomosis they may elect to fashion a defunctioning stoma. This may be temporary and is potentially reversible—the decision for this will be made in the postoperative period once the patient has recovered from the initial operation.

Additional procedures that may become necessary
- Extension of resection margins to include extended colectomy, sub-total colectomy or pan-proctocolectomy depending on intraoperative findings
- Excision of gynaecological or urological organs
- Formation of defunctioning stoma

Benefits
- *Diagnostic*: to provide histopathological diagnosis of underlying pathology with or without local staging
- *Therapeutic*: to remove underlying pathology/disease process of bowel and restore function or reduce the risk of future complications

Alternative procedures/conservative measures
- *Malignancy*: should a patient be deemed fit for surgery and it thought possible to achieve an R0 resection, surgery should be advised. If there is evidence of metastatic disease then alternative treatments such as chemo-radiotherapy should be discussed. If a tumour is likely to obstruct then options other than surgery include the use of colonic stents or diverting stomas. The appropriateness of this will be somewhat dependant on the patient's life expectancy and multidisciplinary team discussion
- *HNPCC/FAP*: should the patient be in a high-risk category for future development of colonic carcinoma, alternatives to surgery include surveillance colonoscopies at regular intervals. It is important to inform the patient of the possibility of an interval cancer developing between consecutive colonoscopies. For most FAP patients with polyps total proctocolectomy is advised

- *Diverticular disease*: dietary advice can be given for symptomatic disease. In acute diverticulitis perforates this may be treated initially with antibiotics or, alternatively if an abscess cavity develops, this may be radiologically drained. It is important to inform the patient that the disease process may persist or recur despite these measures at which point surgery may be the only option
- *Inflammatory bowel disease*: medical therapy (steroids, immunosuppressants and 5-aminosalycilic acid (5-ASA) drugs) is generally advocated as first-line treatment for acute exacerbations. If unresponsive or there is risk of imminent perforation or indeed perforation of bowel, surgery would be advocated
- *Ischaemia*: antibiotics, adequate oxygenation, intravenous fluids and bowel rest may resolve the acute event. If the bowel is non-viable and the patient is fit for surgery, resection of the affected bowel with stoma formation is advocated

Serious/frequently occurring risks

- Bleeding, infection (including intra-abdominal sepsis in the presence or absence of an anastomosis and wound infection), perforation of bowel, anastomotic leak, ileus, possibility of blood transfusion, irresectability of tumour and recurrence, incisional or parastomal hernia, mortality (guidelines recommend operative mortality should be <20% for emergency surgery and <7% for elective surgery for colorectal cancer[1]), possibility of splenectomy (for left-sided colectomies), damage to or resection of female organs (e.g. hysterectomy, BSO) or resection of a segment of bladder, ureteric injury
- *Pelvic surgery*: urinary and sexual dysfunction (impotence and retrograde ejaculation), faecal urgency, increased frequency of defecation[3]
- *Anastomotic leak*: anterior resection (leak rate varies from 6% to 7.4%), other colonic anastomosis (leak rate varies from 2.6% to 4.1%). ▶▶Anastomotic leak is associated with fivefold increased 30-day mortality[4]

Blood transfusion necessary

- Group and save/cross-match 2–6 units

Type of anaesthesia/sedation

- General anaesthesia (often with a regional block for postoperative pain control)

Follow-up/need for further procedure

Follow-up is often required depending on the underlying pathology. This may necessitate further imaging to identify local and systemic recurrence or a review of postoperative symptoms.

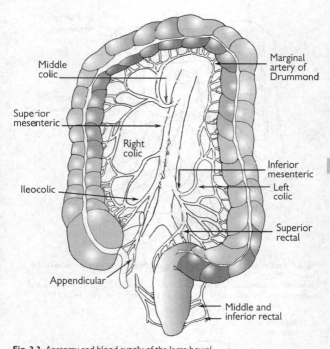

Fig. 3.3 Anatomy and blood supply of the large bowel.
Reproduced with permission from MacKay GJ, Dorrance HR, Molloy RG, et al. *Oxford Specialist Handbook of Colorectal Surgery*. 2010. Oxford: Oxford University Press, p.23, Figure 1.11.

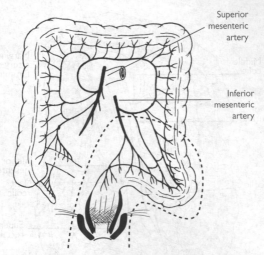

Fig. 3.4 Section of bowel removed during an abdominoperineal excision of the rectum (APER).

Reproduced with permission from McLatchie GR and Leaper DJ. *Oxford Specialist Handbook of Operative Surgery* 2nd edition. 2006. Oxford: Oxford University Press, p.295, Figure 7.53.

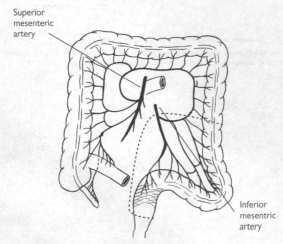

Fig. 3.5 Section of bowel removed during an anterior resection.

Reproduced with permission from McLatchie GR and Leaper DJ. *Oxford Specialist Handbook of Operative Surgery* 2nd edition. 2006. Oxford: Oxford University Press, p.287, Figure 7.49.

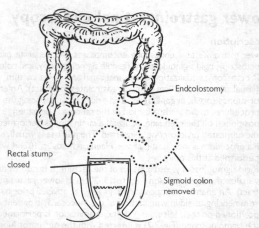

Fig. 3.6 Hartmann's procedure.

Reproduced with permission from McLatchie GR and Leaper DJ. *Oxford Specialist Handbook of Operative Surgery* 2nd edition. 2006. Oxford: Oxford University Press, p.301, Figure 7.55.

References

1. The Association of Coloproctology of Great Britain and Ireland. *Guidelines for the Management of Colorectal Cancer*, 3rd edn. London: The Association of Coloproctology of Great Britain and Ireland, 2007.
2. Guenaga KKFG, Matos D, Wille-Jergensen P. Mechanical bowel preparation for elective colorectal surgery. *Cochrane Database Syst Rev* 2009;**1**:CD001544.
3. Jayne DG, Brown JM, Thorpe H, et al. Bladder and sexual function following resection for rectal cancer in a randomized clinical trial of laparoscopic versus open technique. *Br J Surg* 2005;**92**(9):1124–32.
4. Matos D, Atallah ÁN, Castro AA, et al. Stapled versus handsewn methods for colorectal anastomosis surgery. *Cochrane Database Syst Rev* 2001;**3**:CD003144.

Lower gastrointestinal endoscopy

Description

Lower gastrointestinal endoscopy encompasses four separate procedures: proctoscopy, rigid sigmoidoscopy, flexible sigmoidoscopy, and colonoscopy.

- Proctoscopy: visualization of the anal canal and lower rectum (visualization up to 10cm of lower gastrointestinal tract). An enema or suppository is, in general, advised prior to commencing the listed procedures to aid in visualization of the mucosa. The patient is positioned on their left side. A digital examination is performed before the lubricated proctoscope is inserted. The mucosa is visualized and if a procedure is indicated (☐ see 'Haemorrhoids', p.102) it will be performed at this point

- Rigid sigmoidoscopy: visualization of the rectum (it is rare to directly visualize the sigmoid colon—up to 15–20cm of lower gastrointestinal tract). An enema or suppository is, in general, advised prior to commencing to aid in visualization of the mucosa. The patient is positioned on their left side. A digital examination is performed before the sigmoidoscope (Fig. 3.7) is inserted with the obturator lubricated. Once inside the rectum the obturator is removed and the bellows are used to insufflate air and dilate the rectum. The sigmoidoscope is advanced to approximately 15cm while negotiating the valves of Houston. Patients may experience discomfort and the sensation of the need to pass flatus

- Flexible sigmoidoscopy: visualization of the rectum, sigmoid colon, and up to two-thirds of the transverse colon (in the majority of cases the descending colon is not seen). An enema will be administered prior to commencement. The patient is positioned on their left side with both knees brought forward. A digital examination is performed before the sigmoidoscope is inserted. The flexible sigmoidoscope is inserted into the rectum and advanced to the splenic flexure. Air will be insufflated during the procedure in order to view the mucosa adequately and aid advancement. The images are transmitted onto a screen, which the operator will observe. Should there be an abnormal area a biopsy can be taken which will be sent to pathology. The patient may experience an uncomfortable sensation and abdominal cramps as a result of the insufflated air. The procedure should last less than 10min

- Colonoscopy: here the entire lower gastrointestinal tract can be visualized up to and including the caecum. Skilled endoscopists are able to cannulate the ileocaecal valve to visualize the terminal ileum. In the 2–3 days leading up to the procedure the patient is advised to maintain a low fibre, clear fluid-only diet. The day before, a laxative preparation is taken with large quantities of clear fluid. This will enable the colon to be free of solid matter. The patient is positioned on their left side with their left leg. A sedative can be administered to relax the patient. A digital examination is performed before the colonoscope (Fig. 3.8) is inserted. The colonoscope is inserted into the rectum and advanced to the terminal ileum. Air will be insufflated during the procedure in order to view the mucosa adequately and aid advancement. The images are transmitted onto a screen, which the operator will observe. Should there be an abnormal area a biopsy can be taken which will be sent to pathology. Should a tumour be noted, ndia ink can be injected at the site to aid location during surgery. The patient may experience an uncomfortable sensation and abdominal cramps as a result of the insufflated air. The procedure will last 15–20min

Through these techniques, both visualization and biopsy of lesions are possible. Therapeutic procedures are also possible for certain conditions.

Additional procedures that may become necessary

Biopsy, polypectomy, decompression of volvulus, injection of India ink at tumour site (for intraoperative identification), colonic stenting for obstructing/potentially obstructing colonic tumours, argon laser coagulation, treatment of haemorrhoids, insertion of flatus tube, insertion of percutaneous endoscopic colostomy (PEC).

Benefits

- *Diagnostic*: investigate change in bowel habit, investigate lower gastrointestinal bleeding for surveillance (previous h story of colonic polyps or cancer, ulcerative colitis, strong family history of colonic cancer), investigation of colorectal neoplasia, investigation of symptoms suggestive of anorectal pathology[1]
- *Therapeutic*: permits biopsy of lesions, polypectomy, decompression of volvulus, injection of ink at tumour site (for intraoperative identification), colonic stenting for obstructing/potentially obstructing colonic tumours, argon laser coagulation for the management of colorectal disease (palliative therapy for obstructing or bleeding, malignancies, anastomotic strictures, ablation of colonic mucosal lesions, radiation proctitis), treatment of haemorrhoids (band ligation, injection of oily phenol), insertion of flatus tube, insertion of PEC for the management of recurrent sigmoid volvulus or acute colonic pseudo-obstruction

Alternative procedures/conservative measures

- *Radiological*: CT colonogram/pneumocolon, barium/Gastrografin enema, capsule endoscopy (poor sensitivity for lower gastrointestinal lesions)
- *Surgical*: open or laparoscopic surgical procedure for biopsy or tissue diagnosis or colostomy formation

Serious/frequently occurring risks

- Bleeding, infection (local/systemic), post-procedure pain, bloating, perforation, respiratory compromise, abdominal distension, flatulence
- Flexible sigmoidoscopy: UK multicentre randomized trial of 40 322 patients undergoing flexible sigmoidoscopy shows approximate risk of perforation at 1 in 40 000)
- Caution is advised in neutropenic patients owing to the potential of bacteraemia. Antibiotics may be considered in this scenario and for patients with prosthetic heart valves
- In a UK multicentre randomized trial of 2377 patients undergoing colonoscopy there were four perforations (approximate risk of

1 in 500), all following snare polypectomy. Nine patients were admitted with bleeding
- For the insertion of colonic stents, a review of 27 studies performed between 2000 and 2006 concluded that the perforation rate was 2.5%, distal migration of stents 4.4%, rectal tenesmus 2.2%, occlusion 0.8% and recto-vaginal fistula 0.8%[2]
- There are limited data available with reference to argon laser coagulation, however, perforation is a recognized complication[3]
- With regard to PEC, the most common complications reported in the published literature are granular formation and infection. Other reported complications included pain, colonic leakage, and tube erosion.[4] Unpublished data from a multicentre UK audit showed a 12% (13/105) infection rate following the procedure. Two deaths were also reported in patients with recurrent sigmoid volvulus due to late tube dislodgement. There were seven other cases of reported tube dislodgement following the procedure as well as four cases of migration (Simson, unpublished data, 2005)

Blood transfusion necessary
- None/group and save

Type of anaesthesia/sedation
- Local/general anaesthesia (particularly for children)

Follow-up/need for further procedure
- Dependent on the underlying indication, findings and therapeutic intervention during lower gastrointestinal endoscopy

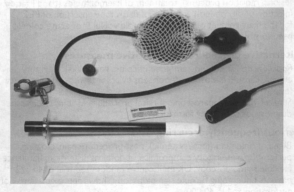

Fig. 3.7 Rigid sigmoidoscope.

Reproduced with permission from MacKay GJ, Dorrance HR, Molloy RG, et al. Oxford Specialist Handbook of Colorectal Surgery. 2010. Oxford: Oxford University Press, p.67, Figure 2.24a.

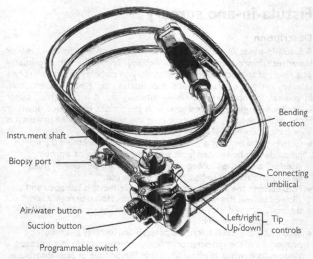

Bending section

Instrument shaft

Biopsy port

Connecting umbilical

Air/water button

Suction button

Left/right | Tip
Up/down | controls

Programmable switch

Fig. 3.8 Colonoscope.

Reproduced with permission from MacKay G., Dorrance HR, Molloy RG, et al. *Oxford Specialist Handbook of Colorectal Surgery*. 2010. Oxford: Oxford University Press, p.61, Figure 2.20.

References

1. Ransohoff DF. Lessons from the UK sigmoidoscopy screening trial. *Lancet* 2002;**359**(9314):1266–7.
2. Dionigi G, Villa F, Rovera F, et al. Colonic stenting for malignant disease: Review of literature. *Surg Oncol* 2007;**16**(Suppl):153–5.
3. Manner H, Plum N, Pech O, et al. Colon explosion during argon plasma coagulation, *Gastrointest Endosc* 2008;**67**(7):1123–7.
4. National Institute for Health and Clinical Excellence. Percutaneous endoscopic colostomy. London: NICE, 2006. Available at: ℜ www.nice.org.uk/guidance/IPG161.

Fistula-in-ano surgery

Description

A fistula-in-ano is an abnormal communication between the anal canal or lower rectum and the perianal skin (Fig. 3.9). They either result primarily as a result of anorectal sepsis or secondary to pathology such as Crohn's disease, malignancy, hidradenitis suppurativa, or, rarely, tuberculosis. In general, for operations involving fistula-in-ano, it is performed either under local or general anaesthesia with the patient either face down or in the supine position. When explaining the procedure to the patient it is important to cover the following points:

- Conventional fistulotomy: the tract must first be identified (hydrogen peroxide may be injected from the external opening or a probe inserted) and is then subsequently 'laid-open' (or de-roofed) using cautery and allowed to heal from the inside out
- Fistulectomy: the entire fistulous tract is excised. It is left open and allowed to heal through secondary intention, closed primarily with sutures, or closed with an advancement flap. The rectal side of the tract is closed internally
- Seton suture: if the fistulous tract is high and involves a significant proportion of the sphincter complex, the surgeon may elect to pass a seton suture (which is essentially a thin Silastic tube or non-absorbable suture) through the tract and the two ends tied together outside the body. There are two types of seton available, the first being a cutting seton which is gradually tightened every 2 weeks (over an approximate 6–8-week period). This allows fibrosis to occur and the tract to gradually heal or becomes low enough to be 'laid-open'. The second is a draining seton which is inserted in the presence of sepsis (if, for example a fistula is noted during incision and drainage of an anorectal abscess). This can be left indefinitely until the abscess has drained and then definitive treatment considered
- Marsupialization fistulotomy: a conventional fistulotomy is performed and the wound edges are marsupialized to the fistulous tract with absorbable sutures
- If the fistula is deemed to be 'high' (i.e. includes a substantial amount of the sphincter complex), fistulotomy is relatively contraindicated, given the high incidence of incontinence
- Parks is the recognized classification system and defines four different types of fistula-in-ano: intersphincteric, trans-sphincteric, suprasphincteric and extrasphincteric (Fig. 3.9)[1]

Additional procedures that may become necessary

- Incision and drainage of perianal/anorectal abscess
- Packing of wound
- Biopsies of fistula tract/rectal mucosa

Benefits

- *Diagnostic*: confirm cause of underlying fistula tract (i.e. Crohn's disease)
- *Therapeutic*: allow for fistula healing, reduce symptoms (pain/bleeding/mucopurulent discharge/incontinence)

Alternative procedures/conservative measures
- Radiofrequency ablation, anal fistula plug, fibrin glue
- It should be emphasized, however, that these treatments are associated with a high fistula recurrence rate

Serious/frequently occurring risks[1]
- Postoperative pain, bleeding, incontinence, recurrence, delayed healing, need for multiple procedures
- *Conventional fistulotomy*: recurrence rates range from 1.9% to 12.5% with an incontinence rate ranging from 4.2% to 12.8%
- *Fistulectomy*: fewer studies are available to contrast fistulectomy, however, one study demonstrated a recurrence rate of 9.5% with an incontinence rate of 14.3%
- *Seton suture*: regarding conventional seton suture placement, the recurrence rate is 6.2% with an incontinence rate of 12.5%
- *Marsupialization fistulotomy*: recurrence rate of 4.5% with incontinence rate of 6%

Blood transfusion necessary
- None/group and save

Type of anaesthesia/sedation
- Local/regional/general anaesthesia

Follow-up/need for further procedure
- Dressing change/pack changes if abscess drained
- Routine outpatient review with histopathology results and review of symptoms
- Review in outpatient clinic if seton is of cutting type and has to be tightened

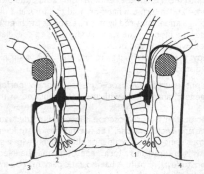

Fig. 3.9 Parks' classification of fistula-in-ano: 1: extrasphincteric; 2: intersphincteric; 3:trans-sphincteric; 4: suprasphincteric.
Reproduced with permission from McLatchie GR and Leaper DJ. *Oxford Specialist Handbook of Operative Surgery* 2nd edition. 2006. Oxford: Oxford University Press, p.235, Figure 7.9.

References
1. Jacob TJ, Perakath B, Keighley MR. Surgical intervention for anorectal fistula. *Cochrane Database Syst Rev* 2010;5:CD006319.
2. Parks AG, Gordon PH, Hardcastle JD. A classification of fistula-in-ano. *Br J Surg* ;**63**(1) 1–12.

Haemorrhoids

Description

Haemorrhoids are enlarged vascular cushions around the anus and can be classified into internal (proximal to the dentate line) and external. Internal haemorrhoids can be further subdivided into grades 1–4.

Traditionally, treatment of haemorrhoids has fallen into two categories: *non-surgical* techniques such as rubber band ligation, sclerotherapy, infrared coagulation, and cryotherapy; and *surgical* procedures such as haemorrhoidectomy and stapled haemorrhoidopexy.

Non-surgical treatments should be advocated in the first instance for 1st and 2nd degree haemorrhoids with surgical procedures reserved for:
- 3rd and 4th degree haemorrhoids
- Those that have failed to respond to non-surgical measures
- Significant external component
- Extensive thrombosis (may best be managed conservatively)
- Associated fissure-in-ano

Non-surgical procedures can generally be performed in the outpatient clinic. If the haemorrhoids are above the dentate line no anaesthesia is required. The patient will be positioned in the left lateral position and a proctoscope or rigid sigmoidoscope will be inserted into the rectum in order to adequately visualize the mucosa.
- Rubber band ligation: a small elastic band will be placed just above the haemorrhoid. This cuts the blood supply and as a consequence the haemorrhoid will undergo necrosis and fall off within a few days. The area will then heal naturally
- Sclerotherapy: a solution of 5% oily phenol (in a solution of almond oil) is injected into the base of the haemorrhoid causing the blood supply to thrombose and in turn the haemorrhoid to shrink and disappear
- Infra-red coagulation: infra-red light is directed at the haemorrhoid which causes the blood in the surrounding veins to coagulate, the haemorrhoid will shrink and eventually disappear
- Cryotherapy: the haemorrhoid is frozen, causing it to shrink and eventually disappear

For *surgical* procedures, the procedure is generally performed under regional or general anaesthesia with the patient placed in the lithotomy position.
- Haemorrhoidectomy: a proctoscope is inserted to adequately visualize the ano-rectal mucosa. The haemorrhoids are identified and excised either using cautery/scalpel or alternatively with a staple gun. Haemostasis is ensured and a local anaesthetic may be injected to minimize postoperative pain. A haemostatic pack may be inserted in the rectum to aid haemostasis and this will pass within a day or two. If the Milligan–Morgan technique is used the mucocutaneous defect is left open. Alternatively, *if the Hil–Ferguson technique is* adopted the mucocutaneous defect is closed
- Stapled haemorrhoidopexy: a circular anal dilator is inserted and the prolapsed mucous membrane falls within the device. A purse-string suture anoscope is then inserted and rotated allowing a purse-string suture to be stitched into the anal circumference. A circular stapler is

then introduced and traction applied to the purse-string. This pulls the prolapsed mucous membrane into the stapler and the device is fired excising a circumferential layer of mucosa. Meticulous haemostasis is then achieved

Patients should also be advised about conservative measures such as dietary modification, topical ointments and retraining in toilet habit (i.e. the avoidance of straining).

Additional procedures that may become necessary
- Nil

Benefits
- *Therapeutic*: reduce the symptoms associated with haemorrhoids and prevent complications associated with large haemorrhoids (e.g. thrombosis/ulceration)

Alternative procedures/conservative measures
- *Conservative*: dietary modification, topical ointments, retraining in toilet habit (i.e. the avoidance of straining)

Serious/frequently occurring risks
- Bleeding, infection, post-procedural pain, prostatitis (following injection sclerotherapy), anaphylaxis (the 5% oily phenol is in a solution of almond oil, therefore, it is important to ascertain if the patient has a nut allergy), recurrence[1]
- *Rubber band ligation*: overall success between 69% and 94%. Overall complication rate less than 2% (vasovagal syncope, anal pain, minor bleeding, chronic ulcer formation, priapism, difficulty in urination, thrombosis of external haemorrhoids)[2]
- *Haemorrhoidectomy*:
  - Early: urinary retention (20.1%), bleeding (secondary (7–10 days post-procedure) or (reactionary 2.4–3%), subcutaneous abscess (0.5%)
  - Late: anal fissure (1.2–6%), anal stenosis (1%), incontinence (0.4%), fistula (0.5%[1])
- *Stapled haemorrhoidopexy*: postoperative bleeding (1.5–9%), urinary retention (<5%), external haemorrhoidal thrombosis (1.2–4.7%), pelvic sepsis, rectovaginal fistula, rectal perforation, and anal stenosis are well-recognized complications of stapled haemorrhoidopexy and should be included in the consent process. Temporary faecal incontinence and faecal urgency have been documented, although these resolved in all cases by 3 months[3]

Blood transfusion necessary
- None/group and save

Type of anaesthesia/sedation
- Local/regional/general anaesthesia

Follow-up/need for further procedure
- Routine outpatient review if required

- Patients must be discharged on laxatives and analgesia, and given appropriate advice regarding diet and toilet habits

References

1. Jayaraman S, Colquhoun PH, Malthaner RA. Stapled hemorrhoidopexy is associated with a higher long-term recurrence rate of internal hemorrhoids compared with conventional excisional hemorrhoid surgery. *Dis Colon Rectum* 2007;**50**(9):1297–305.

2. Shanmugam V, Campbell KL, Loudon MA, *et al.* Rubber band ligation versus excisional haemorrhoidectomy for haemorrhoids. *Cochrane Database Syst Rev* 2005;**1**:CD005034.

3. Lehur PA, Gravie JF, Meurette G. Circular stapled anopexy for haemorrhoidal disease: results. *Colorectal Dis* 2001;**3**(6):374–9.

Percutaneous caecostomy

Description

This is largely performed as a palliative procedure in patients with significant comorbidities unable to receive more aggressive surgery. It is not the optimal treatment modality, however, given the limited options as a result of the condition of the patient, it may be considered necessary. Primary indications include distal colonic obstruction colonic pseudo-obstruction, caecal perforation, caecal volvulus, and to divert the stream in order to protect a distal anastomosis.

There are a number of techniques for the insertion of a caecostomy tube. The basic principle is to inflate the caecum with air (through a catheter inserted per rectum) and then, under fluoroscopic guidance, a small incision is made in the right lower quadrant of the abdomen. Access is gained to the caecum via a needle, a tract is then formed using a dilator. Contrast is used to confirm correct position and a catheter is then inserted and sutured in place.

Additional procedures that may become necessary

- Surgical fashioning of a caecostomy/appendicostomy
- Blind percutaneous caecostomy formation

Benefits

- *Therapeutic*: Percutaneous caecostomy is a palliative procedure and is only performed when other surgical alternatives are deemed unsuitable

Alternative procedures/conservative measures

- *Surgical*: blind percutaneous caecostomy, open surgery to fashion caecostomy/appendicostomy/loop colostomy/trephine

Serious/frequently occurring risks

- Bleeding, infection (intra-abdominal and wound), pericatheter leak tube occlusion, skin excoriation, premature tube dislodgement, colo-cutaneous fistula, ventral hernia
- Up to 45% patients experience minor complications including: pericatheter leak, superficial wound infection, tube occlusion, skin excoriation, premature tube dislodgement, colo-cutaneous fistula, ventral hernia[1]

Blood transfusion necessary

- None/group and save

Type of anaesthesia/sedation

- Local anaesthesia/sedation

Follow-up/need for further procedure

- Patients will need regular caecostomy care involving cleaning, skin care, and flushing of port on a regular basis
- Complications with caecostomy may necessitate removal or replacement

Reference

1. Benacci JC, Wolff BG. Cecostomy—therapeutic indications and results. *Dis Colon Rectum* 1995;**38**(5):530–4.

Perianal skin tag excision

Description

Perianal skin tags are a common problem and may represent underlying or coexistent pathology. They are commonly the result of a previous anorectal insult for example haemorrhoids. A sentinel tag is one that is situated at the inferior border of an infection, injury, or chronic anal fissure. The excision will either be performed under local or general anaesthesia with the patient either positioned on their side or in the lithotomy position. The excision will result in an irregular anal verge and this should be emphasized to patients who request excision for cosmetic reasons. An examination of the surrounding area will be performed for coexistent pathology, the lesion will be excised either with a scalpel or electrocautery and the tag sent for histological analysis.

Additional procedures that may become necessary

- Curettage of chronic anal fissure/intra-anal botulinum toxin/advancement flap
- Biopsy of anorectal mucosa

Benefits

- *Diagnostic*: to obtain a histological diagnosis of the lesion in question
- *Therapeutic*: symptomatic benefit for perianal skin tag (pruritis/bleeding/pain), interference with perianal hygiene, cosmesis

Alternative procedures/conservative measures

- *Conservative*: manage symptoms with good perianal hygiene, moisturizing cream, antipruritic agents

Serious/frequently occurring risks

- Bleeding, infection, postoperative pain, recurrence, prolonged healing time which may take several weeks, irregular anal verge, poor cosmetic result

Blood transfusion necessary

- None/group and save

Type of anaesthesia/sedation

- Local/regional/general anaesthesia

Follow-up/need for further procedure

- Maintain good perianal hygiene, change dressings regularly, laxatives, and diet to ensure soft stool during wound healing
- No outpatient follow-up necessary

Pilonidal sinus

Description

A pilonidal sinus is a small tract present in or near the natal cleft at the top of the buttocks. They commonly form around a dilated hair follicle into which hairs, desquamated skin, and other debris become entrapped leading to secondary infection (the pit is the primary cause). The operation is performed under local or general anaesthesia and the patient is positioned either face down or in the lateral position. An incision is made either in the midline or off midline, the sinus tracts are obliterated, and then irrigated. The wound is either closed with sutures or left open to close by secondary intention.

There are two traditional methods for excising the pilonidal sinuses and two for closing the wound. Regarding the excision the first is a midline approach, the second off-midline. When closing the wound following the excision of pilonidal sinuses one method is to leave the wound open (therefore allowing healing through secondary intention), the second method is for primary closure.[1] Risks involved have been structured around the categories mentioned here, however, within these categories there are a number of different surgical procedures for which individual risks have not been given (e.g. the use of classic and modified rhomboid flaps, V-Y advancement flap, Bascom procedure, Karydakis procedure, marsupialization, and z-plasty).

- Rhomboid flap: the sinus tracts are excised and a rhomboid flap is transposed to cover the defect
- V-Y advancement flap: in this technique a V incision is made, this is then approached to cover the defective as a Y shape
- Bascom procedure: lateral (or off-line) incision to access the pilonidal cavity followed by curettage. The midline pits are then excised separately. The midline incisions are closed, the lateral incision is left open
- Karydakis procedure: midline elliptical incision of the sinus down to the sacrum. A flap is then created by undercutting the midline side of the wound and advanced across the wound to the opposite side and sutured in place. The skin is then closed
- Marsupialization: the sinus is incised, the borders are raised and stitched to form a pouch. This gradually closes and may need to be packed until this has happened

Additional procedures that may become necessary

- Drainage of underlying sepsis
- Laying open of sinus tract
- Insertion of surgical drain

Benefits

- *Diagnostic*: assess extent of injury
- *Therapeutic*: to resolve a symptomatic or recurrent pilonidal sinus

Alternative procedures/conservative measures

- *Conservative*: meticulous hygiene although resolution of the sinus is unlikely

Serious/frequently occurring risks

- Bleeding, infection, pain, scar, prolonged healing, wound dehiscence, need for regular dressing changes, large cavity/dimple/scar, recurrence (open wound 5.3%, closed wound 8.7%)
- *Midline procedures*: surgical site infection (12.4%), recurrence rate (9.4%), variable healing time (*midline open* wound is 41–91 days, *midline closed* wound is 10–27 days)
- *Off-midline procedures*: surgical site infection (3.6–9.3%), recurrence rate (1.5–2.4%), variable healing time (*off-midline open wound is* 41–120 days, *off-midline closed* wound is 15–23 days)[2]

Blood transfusion necessary

- None/group and save

Type of anaesthesia/sedation

- Regional/general/local anaesthesia

Follow-up/need for further procedure

- Regular follow-up is required to monitor progress

References

1. Petersen S, Koch R, Stelzner S, *et al*. Primary closure techniques in chronic pilonidal sinus: a survey of the results of different surgical approaches. *Dis Colon Rectum* 2002;**45**(11):1458–67.
2. AL-Khamis A, McCallum I, King PM, *et al*. Healing by primary versus secondary intention after surgical treatment for pilonidal sinus. *Cochrane Database Syst Rev* 2010;**1**:CD006213.

Rectal prolapse surgery

Description

This is a full thickness prolapse of the rectum through the anal canal. There are two approaches to the repair of a rectal prolapse; either a trans-abdominal or perineal. The trans-abdominal approach can be further subdivided into the traditional open and the newer laparoscopic method. Generally, younger patients may benefit from a trans-abdominal approach, given the lower risks of recurrence, whereas older patients may be more suitable for a perineal approach, given the higher morbidity associated with the trans-abdominal approach.[1]

The perineal approach encompasses several recognized techniques:

- Perineal recto-sigmoidectomy (Altemeier's procedure): indicated in patients with external full thickness prolapse. It is performed under regional or general anaesthesia, the patient is placed in the lithotomy or prone position. The rectum is withdrawn as fully as possible and an incision is made 1.5cm proximal to the dentate line and is continued through the full thickness of the bowel wall and extended circumferentially. The peritoneum is entered, the sigmoid colon is pulled down and the transection line determined. In general, 15–30cm of bowel is resected and a colo-anal anastomosis is performed
- Delorme's procedure (Fig. 3.10): indicated in full thickness rectal prolapse. It is performed under regional or general anaesthesia, the patient is placed in the lithotomy or prone position. The basic principle is that only the mucosa (inner lining) of the prolapsed rectum is resected and the lining above is sutured back down to the anal canal. The outer wall of the rectum is plicated to strengthen the repair. The prolapse is then reduced, the stitches tied and a circular doughnut of tissue is left just inside the rectum

The trans-abdominal approach encompasses several recognized techniques:

- Trans-abdominal Marlex rectopexy (Ripstein's procedure): is indicated in patients with rectal prolapse without constipation and a redundant sigmoid colon. It is performed under general anaesthesia with the patient in the supine position. A midline incision is made and the abdominal cavity is entered. The rectum is mobilized down to the coccyx posteriorly often with division of the upper portion of the lateral ligament and the anterior cul-de-sac. The rectum is retracted and placed under tension. A non-absorbable Marlex mesh is then fixed to the presacral fascia and wrapped round and sutured to the anterior wall of the rectum to keep it in position
- Trans-abdominal suture rectopexy: indicated in patients with rectal prolapse without constipation and a redundant sigmoid colon. Essentially the same as the Marlex rectopexy, with the exception that the rectum is sutured in place to the presacral fascia as opposed to the use of the mesh

Anterior resection

Some authors have advocated resection for patients with constipation, however, evidence is lacking. It is performed under general anaesthesia with the patient in the supine position. A midline incision is made and the abdominal cavity is entered. The rectum is mobilized to the level of the lateral ligaments and the redundant sigmoid colon is resected. An anastomosis is then performed between the cut end of the colon and the proximal end of the rectum. The colon is maintained under tension in order to prevent the prolapse recurring.

Trans-abdominal rectopexy with sigmoid resection (Frykman–Goldberg operation)

Advocated by some for patients with a significant degree of associated constipation. It is performed under general anaesthesia with the patient in the supine position. A midline incision is made and the abdominal cavity is entered. The rectum is mobilized to the coccyx posteriorly and the cul-de-sac anteriorly. A section of the sigmoid colon is resected with the cut end of the colon being subsequently anastomosed with the proximal end of the rectum. The presacral fascia is then sutured either to the lateral ligament or to the rectal fascia itself thus maintaining the rectum under tensions and preventing subsequent prolapse.

Orr–Loygue rectopexy

More commonly performed in mainland Europe in patients with full thickness rectal prolapsed. It is performed under general anaesthesia with the patient in the supine position. A midline incision is made and the abdominal cavity is entered. Essentially the same as the traditional abdominal rectopexy, the difference being that the dissection is limited to the anterior and posterior rectal wall.

Additional procedures that may become necessary

- Abdominal or perineal drain insertion
- Defunctioning colostomy/ileostomy when redundant bowel is resected and anastomosed

Benefits

- *Therapeutic*: symptomatic rectal prolapse (incontinence, bowel habit disturbances, rectal bleeding)

Alternative procedures/conservative measures

- *Conservative*: treatment involves advice regarding safe reduction of the prolapse itself and advice regarding bowel habit

Serious/frequently occurring risks

- Bleeding, infection, recurrence (full thickness and mucosal), incontinence, constipation, anastomotic dehiscence, incisional hernia and pelvic sepsis
- *Perineal rectosigmoidectomy (Altemeier's procedure)*: 8.6% major complications, pelvic haematomas, anastomotic dehiscence, sigmoid perforation, pararectal abscess, late anal strictures, 14% minor complications, 18% recurrence rate at 41 months[2]
- *Delorme's procedure: urinary retention 12%, Clostridium difficile colitis 4%*, myocardial infarction 1.3%, 4% suture line bleeding, 3% anastomotic disruption, 1.3% anastomotic stricture, 6.6% faecal incontinence postoperatively (includes patients who were continent and incontinent

prior to procedure), 7% postoperative constipation, 14.5% recurrence rate at 60 months[3]

- *Trans-abdominal suture rectopexy*: complication rates ranging from 9.4% to 20%, recurrence rate of 2–3.1%, postoperative incontinence of 16–26%, postoperative constipation of 31–71%[4]
- *Trans-abdominal Marlex rectopexy (Ripstein procedure)*: complication rates ranging from 2.3% to 28%, recurrence rate of 2–14%, post-operative incontinence of 28–50%, post-operative constipation of 17–43%[5]
- *Trans-abdominal rectopexy with sigmoid resection (Frykman–Goldberg operation)*: 6.3% full thickness recurrence, 8.5% mucosal prolapsed, 6.3% constipation (in patients who had not pre-operatively experienced this), 12.8% patients experienced diminished continence postoperatively, 8.5% developed significant diarrhoea[6]
- *Anterior resection*: 15% morbidity, 7% recurrence at 5.5 years, 7.3% incisional hernia, 4.9% small bowel obstruction, 2.4% stroke[7]
- *Orr–Loygue rectopexy*: prolapse recurrence 4.11% (mean follow-up 27.5 months) pelvic abscess 0%, 62.5% patients who were preoperatively incontinent of faeces were 'totally cured'
- Common: bleeding; swelling; pain; scar; prolonged wound healing, infection

Blood transfusion necessary

- Group and save/cross-match 2–6 units

Type of anaesthesia/sedation

- Regional/general anaesthesia

Follow-up/need for further procedure

- Monitor patient in hospital until patient passes urine and faeces prior to discharge
- Symptomatic review in outpatient clinic

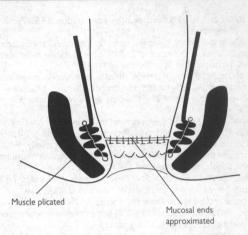

Muscle plicated

Mucosal ends
approximated

Fig. 3.10 Delorme's procedure.
Reproduced with permission from McLatchie GR and Leaper DJ. *Oxford Specialist Handbook of Operative Surgery* 2nd edition. 2006. Oxford: Oxford University Press. p.241, Figure 7.14.

References

1. Tjandra JJ, Clunie GJA, Kaye AH, *et al. Textbook of Surgery*. Oxford: Wiley-Blackwell. 2006, p.247.
2. Altomare DF, Binda G, Ganio E, *et al.* Long-term outcome of Altemeier's procedure for rectal prolapse. *Dis Colon Rectum* 2009;**52**(4):698–703.
3. Lieberth M, Kondylis LA, Reilly JC, *et al.* The Delorme repair for full-thickness rectal prolapse: a retrospective review. *Am J Surg* 2009;**197**(3):418–23.
4. Blatchford GJ, Perry RE, Thorson AG, *et al.* Rectopexy without resection for rectal prolapse. *Am J Surg* 1989;**158**(6):574–6.
5. Novell JR, Osborne MJ, Winslet MC. Prospective randomized trial of Ivalon sponge versus sutured rectopexy for full-thickness rectal prolapse. *Br J Surg* 1994;**81**(6):904–6.
6. Madoff RD, Williams JG, Wong WD, *et al.* Long-term functional results of colon resection and rectopexy for overt rectal prolapse. *Am J Gastroenterol* 1992;**87**(1):101–4.
7. Cirocco WC, Brown AC. Anterior resection for the treatment of rectal prolapse: a 20-year experience. *Am Surg* 1993;**59**(4):265–9.

Rectocele repair

Description

A rectocele is the result of a defect in the rectovaginal septum (a tough fibrous layer), which separates the vagina (anteriorly) from the rectum (posteriorly). This defect results in the protrusion of the rectum into the vagina and the resultant symptoms.

The primary indication for repair of a rectocele is obstructive defecation with objective evidence of faecal trapping demonstrated through a defecating proctogram. Other indications include a subjective sensation of 'pressure' in the vagina and a feeling of incomplete evacuation post-defecation. This may progress to difficult or painful defecation or sexual intercourse, constipation, incontinence, vaginal bleeding, and even prolapse of the bulge through the opening of the vagina.

Various approaches are employed in the repair of a rectocele including posterior colporrhaphy, trans-anal and trans-perineally. For the purpose of this colorectal chapter we will consider the trans-anal and trans-perineal approach.

- Trans-anal rectocele repair: the procedure is performed under regional or general anaesthesia with the patient positioned either in the jack-knife position or supine. An incision is generally made just proximal to the dentate line, the redundant rectal mucosa is either removed or plicated and the rectal submucosa and mucosa are closed in separate layers
- Trans-perineal rectocele repair: this approach is also performed under general anaesthesia with the patient positioned either in the jack-knife position or supine. The recto-vaginal septum is repaired through an incision in the perineum and a decision whether or not to use a prosthetic mesh is made

Additional procedures that may become necessary

- Cystocoele repair
- Suprapubic catheter insertion
- Pelvic floor reconstruction
- Defunctioning colostomy/ileostomy

Benefits

- *Therapeutic*: symptomatic improvement from rectocoele (e.g. constipation, incontinence, painful vaginal bulge, painful intercourse, vaginal bleeding)

Alternative procedures/conservative measures

- *Conservative*: pelvic floor strengthening exercises should be advised
- Biofeedback devices
- Vaginal pessaries
- Transvaginal/transcutaneous electrical stimulation to allow muscle contraction

Serious/frequently occurring risks

- *Trans-anal rectocele repair*: bleeding, infection 3.3%, incomplete evacuation, faecal impaction, faecal incontinence, recto-vaginal fistula, dyspareunia, sexual dysfunction, failure of procedure, recurrence 40%–66% reported an excellent/good/fair result[1,2]
- *Trans-perineal rectocoele repair*: anatomical cure 89.2%, bleeding 3.6%, infection 4.8%, incomplete evacuation, faecal impaction, faecal incontinence, recto-vaginal fistula, dyspareunia, sexual dysfunction, failure of procedure, recurrence, if a mesh is used there is potential for mesh erosion and infection[3]

Blood transfusion necessary

- Group and save

Type of anaesthesia/sedation

- General anaesthesia

Follow-up/need for further procedure

- Monitor patient in hospital until patient passes urine and faeces prior to discharge
- Symptomatic review in outpatient clinic

References

1. Heriot AG, Maxwell P, Kumar D. Functional and physiological outcome following transanal repair of rectocele, *Gastroenterology* 2000;**118**(4):A126.
2. Nieminen K, Hiltunen KM, Laitinen J, *et al.* Transanal or vaginal approach to rectocele repair: a prospective, randomized pilot study. *Dis Colon Rectum* 2004;**47**(10):1636–42.
3. Leventoğlu S, Menteş BB, Akin M, *et al.* Transperineal rectocele repair with polyglycolic acid mesh: a case series. *Dis Colon Rectum* 2007;**50**(12):2085–92.

Restorative proctocolectomy (ileo-anal pouch)

Description

Restorative proctocolectomy (Fig. 3.11) is a procedure designed to use loops of small bowel as a reservoir for faeces prior to defecation. The ileo-anal pouch is indicated in patients with ulcerative colitis (resistant to medical therapy), FAP, HNPCC, and has been performed in some patients with constipation.[1]

The operation is performed under general anaesthesia with the patient positioned in the lithotomy position. If performed open, a midline laparotomy incision is made, the layers divided and the abdomen entered. The colon and rectum are excised, a mucosectomy may be performed, the small intestine is mobilized and the pouch is formed (either fully stapled or hand-sewn). A pouch-anal anastomosis is fashioned and the decision is then made whether or not to form an ileostomy.

The procedure can be performed either laparoscopically or as an open procedure. It can be performed as one operation or divided into two or three procedures.

Additional procedures that may become necessary

- Defunctioning ileostomy
- Failure to create pouch and alternative procedure performed (end-ileostomy, total colectomy with ileorectal anastomosis)

Benefits

- *Therapeutic*: avoid an end-stoma, allow for an element of continence, avoid social stigmas associated with stoma formation, allow for defecation through anus

Alternative procedures/conservative measures

- *Surgical*: total colectomy with ileorectal anastomosis, total colectomy and end-ileostomy formation

Serious/frequently occurring risks[2]

- Bleeding, infection (including intra-abdominal abscess, wound, urinary tract pelvic sepsis 4.7%, peritoneal abscess 1%), perforation of bowel, sexual and urinary dysfunction infertility, anastomotic dehiscence and leak, anastomotic stricture 21.3%, pouchitis 15–50% (ulcerative colitis patients only), staple line ulcer 13.5%, pouchitis 5.4%, bowel obstruction 7.1%, alteration in bowel habit, incontinence, entero-cutaneous fistula, incisional hernia 4%, anal fistula 4%, the need for a temporary defunctioning ileostomy
- Regarding mucosectomy (excision of the rectal mucosa prior to ileo-anal anastomosis), one review article concluded that whereas performing mucosectomy results in both lower rates of inflammation and dysplasia in patients with ulcerative colitis and lower rates of cuff polyposis in FAP patients, it also leads to worse functional outcomes[3]

Blood transfusion necessary

- Group and save/cross-match 4–6 units

Type of anaesthesia/sedation

- General anaesthesia with regional epidural block for postoperative analgesia

Follow-up/need for further procedure

- Monitor patient in hospital until patient passes urine and faeces prior to discharge
- Symptomatic review in outpatient clinic
- Patients will often require follow-up pouchoscopy with rigid/flexible sigmoidoscopy, especially if symptomatic to ensure no evidence of pouchitis or recurrence of pathology in pouch[4]

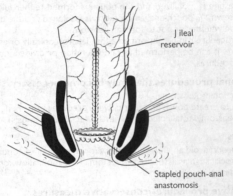

J ileal reservoir

Stapled pouch-anal anastomosis

Fig. 3.11 Restorative proctocolectomy with ileoanal pouch.

Reproduced with permission from McLatchie GR and Leaper DJ. *Oxford Specialist Handbook of Operative Surgery* 2nd edition. 2006. Oxford: Oxford University Press, p.299, Figure 7.54.

References

1. Stewart J, Kumar D, Keighley MR. Results of anal or low rectal anastomosis and pouch construction for megarectum and megacolon. *Br J Surg* 1994;**81**(7):1051–3.
2. Arai K, Koganei K, Kimura H, *et al.* Incidence and outcome of complications following restorative proctocolectomy. *Am J Surg* 2005;**190**(1):39–42.
3. Chambers WM, McC Mortensen NJ. Should ileal pouch-anal anastomosis include mucosectomy?. *Colorectal Dis* 2007;**9**(5):384–92.
4. Pardi DS, D'Haens G, Shen B, *et al.* Clinical guidelines for the management of pouchitis. *Inflamm Bowel Dis* 2009;**15**:1424–31.

Small bowel resection

Description

Small bowel resection is performed under general anaesthesia with the patient in the supine position. The procedure is performed either open or laparoscopically for the following conditions:

- Small bowel tumour (benign/malignant)
- Crohn's disease resistant to medical treatment
- Small bowel ischaemia (i.e. superior mesenteric artery infarction)
- Radiation or Crohn's disease induced stricture

Open: a midline laparotomy or other appropriate incision is made, the layers are divided and the abdomen is entered. The diseased segment of bowel is identified and resected. The two healthy ends are then either anastomosed (using hand sewn or stapled technique) or alternatively a stoma is brought to the skin surface.

Laparoscopic: 3–5 small incisions are made on the abdomen in order that the camera and instruments can be inserted. The diseased segment of bowel is identified and resected. The two healthy ends are then either anastomosed (using hand-sewn or stapled technique) or, alternatively, a stoma is brought to the skin surface.

As the length of the small bowel varies from person to person, the length of small bowel resected is not as important as the amount left behind. The British Society of Gastroenterology suggests that if there is <200cm small bowel, nutritional or fluid supplements are likely to be needed. If it is anticipated that there will be <150cm of small bowel remaining it is important to discuss the possibility of the long-term need of total parenteral nutrition.[1]

Following distal ileal resection patients are more prone to the formation of gallstones. As a consequence of dehydration and abnormal oxalate metabolism, certain patients following small bowel resection will also be more prone to developing kidney stones.

Additional procedures that may become necessary

- End-ileostomy/loop ileostomy/defunctioning stoma/abdominal drain insertion

Benefits

- *Diagnostic*: to obtain tissue for histopathological diagnosis
- *Therapeutic*: remove diseased segment of small bowel

Alternative procedures/conservative measures

- *Medical*: for Crohn's disease, medical therapy and immunotherapy can be used to decrease the inflammatory process and reduce the risk of stricture formation and fistulation
- *Surgical*: for small bowel structuring disease in patients where length of bowel will need to be conserved, stricturoplasty can be considered as an alternative to small bowel resection

Serious/frequently occurring risks

- Bleeding, infection (including intra-abdominal abscess, wound and urinary infection), perforation of bowel, anastomotic dehiscence or leak (1.1%), small bowel syndrome, intestinal failure, entero-cutaneous fistula, incisional hernia, alteration of bowel habit, mortality rate (1.7%)[2]

Blood transfusion necessary

- Group and save/cross-match (depending on starting haemoglobin)

Type of anaesthesia/sedation

- Regional/general anaesthesia

Follow-up/need for further procedure

- Routine outpatient review if required

References

1. Nightingale J, Woodward JM. *Guidelines for Management of Patients with a Short Bowel*, 2006 (on behalf of the Small Bowel and Nutrition Committee of the British Society of Gastroenterology). Available at: ℜ www.bsg.org.uk/images/stories/docs/clinical/guidelines/sbn/short_bowel.pdf (accessed 5 May 2011).
2. Pickleman J, Watson W, Cunningham J, *et al.* The failed gastrointestinal anastomosis: an inevitable catastrophe? *J Am Coll Surg* 1999;**188**(5):473–82.

Small bowel strictureplasty

Description

Obstructing small bowel fibrotic strictures are commonly secondary to Crohn's disease or tuberculosis. Strictures up to 25cm are amenable to strictureplasty. Heineke–Mikulicz technique is preferred for strictures smaller than 10cm with the Finney technique reserved for segments over 10cm.

- *Heineke–Mikulicz:*[1] the operation is performed under general anaesthesia with the patient placed in the supine position. A midline laparotomy incision is made, the layers are divided, and the abdomen entered (Fig. 3.12). The small bowel is carefully examined to identify the previously imaged strictures and ensure none are missed. Non-traumatic bowel clamps are secured at either end of the stricture. A longitudinal incision is made over the entire length of the stricture, and stay sutures are placed to retract and aid in the transverse closure.
- *Finney:* the operation is performed under general anaesthesia with the patient placed in the supine position. A midline laparotomy incision is made, the layers are divided and the abdomen entered. The small bowel is carefully examined to identify the previously imaged strictures and ensure none are missed. The segment of bowel containing the stricture is brought together in a side-to-s de U-shaped configuration with stay sutures placed to maintain this (Fig. 3.13). The enterotomy over the stricture is closed, suturing the opposed surfaces of the bowel together.

Additional procedures that may become necessary

- Small bowel resection and anastomosis
- Defunctioning small bowel stoma

Benefits

- *Diagnostic:* identify the underlying cause of structuring disease, histopathological analysis of underlying stricture (Crohn's disease)
- *Therapeutic:* to relieve symptoms, signs and complications of small bowel obstruction

Alternative procedures/conservative measures

- *Conservative:* high fluid intake, low-residue diet, low-volume frequent meals
- *Surgical:* small bowel resection

Serious/frequently occurring risks

- Bleeding, infection (including intra-abdominal abscess and wound infection), perforation of bowel, enterocutaneous fistula, incisional hernia, alteration of bowel habit, new disease at site of strictureplasty or at alternative small bowel segments
- One long-term study of 314 patients undergoing Heineke–Mikulicz (88%) and Finney (11%) strictureplasties (1% not clearly defined) demonstrated the following: overall morbidity 18%, septic complications 5%, intra-abdominal abscess 2%, anastomotic leak or enterocutaneous fistula 2%, wound infection 1%, reoperation in postoperative period 1%, prolonged ileus 4%, mechanical small bowel obstruction 1%, luminal bleeding requiring transfusion 7%, at a mean period of 7.7 years 37% had undergone a reoperation (92% as a result of obstruction)[2]

Blood transfusion necessary

- Group and save/cross-match (dependent on preoperative haemoglobin)

Type of anaesthesia/sedation

- General anaesthesia

Follow-up/need for further procedure

- Dependent on underlying cause of stricture formation and post operative course

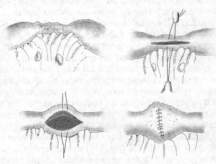

Fig. 3.12 Heineke-Mikulicz strictureplasty. Short (<10cm) strictures are opened longitudinally and closed transversely.

Reproduced with permission from MacKay GJ, Dorrance HR, Molloy RG, *et al. Oxford Specialist Handbook of Colorectal Surgery.* 2010. Oxford: Oxford University Press, p.141, Figure 4.15.

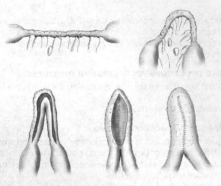

Fig. 3.13 Finney strictureplasty for longer (>10cm) strictures.

Reproduced with permission from MacKay GJ, Dorrance HR, Molloy RG, *et al. Oxford Specialist Handbook of Colorectal Surgery.* 2010. Oxford: Oxford University Press, p.142, Figure 4.16.

References

1. Brown CJ. Heineke-Mikulicz and Finney strictureplasty in Crohn's disease. *Oper Tech Gen Surg* 2007;**9**(1):3–7.
2. Dietz DW, Laureti S, Strong SA, *et al.* Safety and longterm efficacy of strictureplasty in 314 patients with obstructing small bowel Crohn's Disease. *J Am Coll Surg* 2001;**192**(3):330–7.

Stoma (formation/reversal)

Description

The formation of a stoma will likely form only part of an operation. It is advisable that a specialist stoma nurse discuss with the patient preoperatively (when possible) the implications involved and also to aid in the siting. The important points when informing a patient of a potential stoma are:

- *Permanent* or *temporary*: if it is anticipated to be temporary it is important to stress that it may be permanent depending on intra- and postoperative events
- *Site*: an ileostomy is commonly sited in the right iliac fossa (Fig. 3.14) with a colostomy commonly sited in the right iliac fossa (Fig. 3.15)
- *Single-* versus *double-barrelled*
- Possibility of a *mucous fistula*

Ileostomy

- *End*—formed following the complete removal of the colon including the rectum (Fig. 3.16). A mucous fistula may be fashioned in addition, termed a double-barrelled stoma
- *Loop*—formed in order to defunction either a distal obstructing colonic lesion or in order to protect a distal anastomosis

Colostomy

- *End*—formed in order to defunction a distal segment of bowel (Fig. 3.17). Commonly performed following an anterior resection, APER, or as part of a Hartmann's operation. May be indicated in a distal colonic fistula. A mucous fistula may be fashioned in addition to this procedure
- *Loop*—formed in order to defunction either a distal obstructing colonic lesion, a distal anastomosis or complex pelvic disease

Reversal of ileostomy or colostomy: is performed in order to restore the integrity of the intestinal tract. If performed open, involves either a circumferential incision around the stoma or possibly through the previous laparotomy incision. Reversal of loop ileostomies or colostomies can generally be performed through the circumferential incision around the stoma whereas reversal of end-ileostomies or colostomies usually involves opening the old scar in order to safely access the bowel. The anastomosis is performed and the wound is closed.

The formation of a stoma and indeed the reversal may also be performed either *open* or *laparoscopically*.

Additional procedures that may become necessary

- Stoma formation can be both the primary procedure or part of a larger sequence of events as a temporary stoma (defunctioning)

Benefits

- *Therapeutic*: Diversion stoma—divert faeces away from a segment of bowel that has been removed or away from the perineum in trauma or pathology (i.e. necrotizing fasciitis). Defunctioning stoma—to allow a segment of bowel, distal pathology, or anastomosis to heal

- *Therapeutic*: to relieve symptoms, signs and complications of small or large bowel obstruction

Alternative procedures/conservative measures

The patient should be advised of the indications and reasons for stoma formation. If it feasible to avoid the formation of a stoma (which may result in the increased risk of an anastomotic leak) and the patient is advised of these risks then the operating surgeon may opt to forego the stoma. This should be appropriately documented on the consent form.

Serious/frequently occurring risks

- *Formation of a stoma*: overall complication rates ranging from 13.1% to 69.4%; bleeding, infection (including intra-abdominal abscess, wound and urinary infection), vascular compromise (ischaemia and infarction of the stoma 2.3–17%), retraction, prolapsed, peristomal skin irritation (3–42%), peristomal infection/abscess/fistula formation (2–14.8%), stenosis, alteration of bowel habit, parastomal hernia (early and late presentation 4.6–13%)[1]
- *Reversal of stoma*: Bleeding, infection (intra-abdominal abscess, urinary and wound infection), perforation of bowel, anastomotic leak, enterocutaneous fistula, ileus, stricture at the anastomotic site, reoperation

Blood transfusion necessary

- Group and save/cross-match blood (dependent on preoperative haemoglobin and nature of the primary procedure being performed)

Type of anaesthesia/sedation

- General anaesthesia

Follow-up/need for further procedure

- Dependent on underlying reason for stoma formation and postoperative course of patient

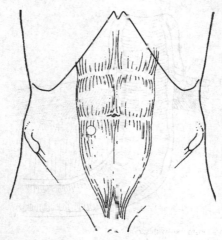

Fig. 3.14 Usual site of ileostomy.

Reproduced with permission from McLatchie GR and Leaper DJ. *Oxford Specialist Handbook of Operative Surgery* 2nd edition. 2006. Oxford: Oxford University Press, p.255, Figure 7.24.

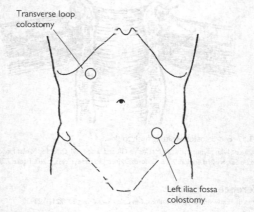

Fig. 3.15 Sites of colostomy.

Reproduced with permission from McLatchie GR and Leaper DJ. *Oxford Specialist Handbook of Operative Surgery* 2nd edition. 2006. Oxford: Oxford University Press. p.263, Figure 7.28.

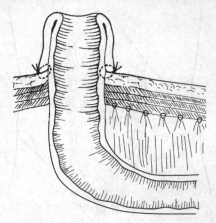

Fig. 3.16 End-ileostomy—with spout.

Reproduced with permission from McLatchie GR and Leaper DJ. *Oxford Specialist Handbook of Operative Surgery* 2nd edition. 2006. Oxford: Oxford University Press, p.255, Figure 7.25.

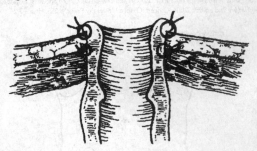

Fig. 3.17 End-colostomy, sitting flush to skin.

Reproduced with permission from McLatchie GR and Leaper DJ. *Oxford Specialist Handbook of Operative Surgery* 2nd edition. 2006. Oxford: Oxford University Press, p.263, Figure 7.29.

Reference

1. Kann BR. Early stomal complications. *Clin Colon Rectal Surg* 2008;**21**(1):23–30.

Vascular surgery

Abdominal aortic aneurysm— endovascular aneurysm repair

Description

The abdominal aorta is considered to be aneurysmal when there is focal abnormal dilatation of the aorta to over 1.5 times its expected diameter. Complications from aneurysms relate to the size. The '5,10,20' rule suggest that there is a 5% annual risk of rupture for a 5cm aneurysm, 10% for a 6cm aneurysm, and 20% for a 7cm aneurysm. Other complications include thrombosis, embolism, pressure effects, and rarely fistulae between the aorta and bowel, inferior vena cava, or ureter.

Aneurysms should therefore be repaired once they have reached a critical size if the patient is a suitable candidate. Open and endovascular techniques may be employed. Not all aneurysms are morphologically suitable for endovascular stent grafting. Calcification, excessive angulation, thrombus at landing zones and quality of access vessels are important considerations. Patients should also be compliant with long-term surveillance.

Operative technique

Endovascular repair is performed in the operating room with image intensifier or in a dedicated interventional angiography suite. Percutaneous or open access to the femoral artery is obtained on both sides. An angiogram is performed to confirm the site of the renal and internal iliac arteries. The main body of the stent graft is deployed below the lowest renal artery (Fig. 4.1) and positioned to allow easy cannulation of the contra-lateral limb. Ballooning may be required and a completion angiogram must be performed to ensure patency of critical side branches, rule out endoleaks, assess limb patency and ensure access vessel integrity.

Additional procedures that may become necessary

- Internal iliac artery embolization if the distal landing zone is in the external iliac artery
- Pre-dilatation or a conduit if access vessels are smaller than the delivery system
- Brachial access to cannulate contralateral limb by snaring
- Balloon dilatation/extension cuffs/stents to contain endoleaks
- Aorto-uni-iliac stent graft, iliac occlusion on contralateral side and femoro-femoral crossover graft
- Conversion to open if arterial dissection, avulsion, or rupture
- Embolectomy

Benefits

- Fewer postoperative complications, less operative blood loss, and shorter stay than open repair
- Reduced physiological insult as aortic cross clamping is not necessary

Alternatives procedures/conservative measures

- Non-operative management in high-risk patients or those not expected to survive at least 2 years
- Open aneurysm repair

Serious/frequently occurring risks
- Risk to life and limbs
- *Early*: groin or wound complications (bleeding, haematoma, or pseudoaneurysm), injury to access vessels, dissection, distal embolization, malposition, graft limb dislocation, occlusion of essential branch vessels, postimplantation syncrome
- *Late*: endoleak, graft migration, late rupture, failure of device integrity, limb occlusion, graft infection, structural failure

Blood transfusion necessary
- Group and save

Type of anaesthesia/sedation
- General, regional, or local anaesthesia

Follow-up/need for further procedure
- Patients need to be followed up for life with surveillance duplex scans or CT scans to detect endoleaks, device failure, migration and limb occlusion

Further reading
National Institute for Health and Clinical Excellence. *Endovascular Stent—Grafts for the Treatment of Abdominal Aortic Aneurysms*. Technology appraisal TA167. London: NICE, 2009.
Patient information—endovascular abdominal aortic aneurysm repair. Available at: ℬ www.circulationfoundation.org.uk and ℬ www.nhs.uk (accessed 17 May 2011).

Abdominal aortic aneurysm—open repair

Description

The risk of aneurysm rupture can be prevented by open surgical repair in patients who are fit enough to undergo major surgical intervention. The cardiopulmonary reserve of the patients is assessed when the aneurysm crosses the threshold for intervention, which is accepted as greater than 5.5cm for infrarenal aortic aneurysms. Patients whose aneurysms expand over 1cm in a year and those who are symptomatic may also be considered for intervention. Once ruptured, the mortality is over 90% despite intervention.

Operative technique (Figs. 4.1 and 4.2)

The aorta is approached through a transperitoneal or retroperitoneal approach and the aorta and iliac vessels are controlled. After systemic heparinization, the aorta above and iliac vessels below the aneurysm are crossclamped. The aneurysm is opened, atheroma removed and back bleeding controlled before inlay grafting with a suitably sized graft. The sac is used to cover the graft after ensuring that there are no bleeding or ischaemic complications.

Additional procedures that may become necessary

- Embolectomy if acute limb ischaemia noted following surgery
- Reimplantation of inferior mesenteric artery if visceral collateral flow is insufficient
- Aorto-iliac or bifemoral graft if iliacs are also aneurysmal
- Axillo-bifemoral if infrarenal aorta not suitable for grafting

Benefits

- Life saving after rupture
- Reduce risk of rupture in elective cases

Alternatives procedures/conservative measures

- Non-operative management in high-risk patients or those not expected to survive at least 2 years
- Endovascular abdominal aortic aneurysm repair

Serious/frequently occurring risks

- Risk to life and limbs
- Elective perioperative mortality is around 5%
- Emergency surgery carries mortality of over 50%
- *Early*: bleeding, ischaemia (organ failure, gut ischaemia, rarely spinal cord ischaemia), nerve injury resulting in sexual dysfunction
- *Late*: graft infection, aorto-enteric fistula

Blood transfusion *necessary*

- *Cross*-match 6 units for elective cases; 10 units for rupture
- Intraoperative blood salvage may be used as adjunct to reduce transfusion requirements

Type of anaesthesia/sedation

- General anaesthesia combined with epidural in elective situation
- Combined spinal and epidural anaesthesia in selected high-risk patients

Follow-up/need for further procedure

- May need further surgery if patient develops aneurysmal dilatation in juxta-anastomotic aorta or graft infection

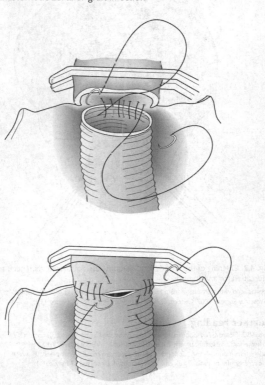

Fig. 4.1 Open aortic aneurysm repair: aortic stent graft.

Reproduced with permission from Hands L, Murphy N, Sharp M, et al. *Oxford Specialist Handbook of Vascular Surgery*. 2007. Oxford: Oxford University Press. p.243, Figure 13.3.

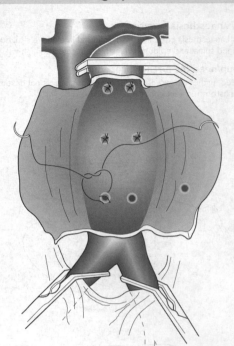

Fig. 4.2 Opening of the aortic sac to demonstrate aortic aneurysm neck and aortic bifurcation for anastomosis.

Reproduced with permission from Hands L, Murphy M, Sharp M, et al. *Oxford Specialist Handbook of Vascular Surgery.* 2007. Oxford: Oxford University Press, p.241, Figure 13.1.

Further reading

Rubin BG, Sicard GA. Abdominal aortic aneurysms. In: Cronenwett JL, Johnston KW, eds. *Rutherford's Vascular Surgery*, 7th edn. Philadelphia: WB Saunders, 2010, pp1949–72.

Patient information—open abdominal aortic aneurysm repair. Available at: ℛ www.circulationfoundation.org.uk and ℛ www.nhs.uk (accessed 17 May 2011).

Amputations

Description

Amputations of the lower limb are performed for peripheral vascular disease, trauma, tumours, and infection. The level of the amputation is influenced by the viability of soft tissues, functional requirement, cosmesis, and comfort. In lower limb amputations, the level of amputation in relation to the knee influences postoperative mobility, with half as many patients with below-knee amputations being able to walk with a prosthesis as compared with those with above-knee amputations.

Lower limb amputations are the most common amputation performed for vascular disease as the upper limb has an excellent collateral circulation. Lower limb amputations include digital, trans-metatarsal (Fig. 4.3), Syme's, guillotine, through-knee (Fig. 4.4), below-knee (Fig. 4.5), above-knee (Fig. 4.6), and hind quarter amputations. For major limb amputations, blood loss can be reduced with the application of a tourniquet.

Careful selection of level of amputation, and good surgical technique and postoperative care are essential to ensure a successful outcome. The more common digital, below-knee, and above-knee amputations are described as follows.

Operative technique

Digital lower limb amputations are usually performed for sepsis and therefore the wound should not be closed. The side should be marked preoperatively. A racquet incision is made around the digit, taking care not to encroach on the neurovascular bundle of the adjacent toes. The bone is divided with bone cutters ensuring removal of the articular surface. Haemostasis and saline lavage are performed. A non-adherent dressing is then applied.

Below-knee amputations may be performed using the skew or long posterior flap. In the skew flap incisions are made such that two equal flaps are skewed off of the midline and centred along the saphenous veins. In the long posterior flap, perforating branches from the gastrocnemius muscles help supply the overlying skin. In both cases, the incision are taken down to the tibia and fibula, dividing and ligating the major neurovascular bundles. The tibia and fibula are divided ensuring that the bone edges are even. Haemostasis and saline lavage is performed before the wound is closed in layers.

Above-knee amputations are performed using a slightly unequal anterior and posterior flaps so that the suture line is not over the end of the stump. Muscle is divided down to bone, dividing and ligating major neurovascular bundles. The femur is divided ensuring that the bone edge is even. Haemostasis and saline lavage is performed before the wound is closed in layers.

Additional procedures that may become necessary

- Debridement of further tissue if sepsis and ischaemia are present
- Stump revision or a more proximal amputation if the stump fails to heal

Benefits

- Treatment of infection
- Removal of a painful or useless limb

Alternatives procedures/conservative measures
- If gangrene is dry, digits may auto-amputate
- Opiate analgesia to control pain
- Long-term antibiotics to treat osteomyelitis
- Palliation should be considered when a non-viable limb occurs in patient with significant comorbidity

Serious/frequently occurring risks
- Bleeding, wound infection, osteomyelitis or gangrene necessitating further surgery, DVT and pulmonary embolism, myocardial infarction, falls, phantom limb pain

Blood transfusion necessary
- Group and save

Type of anaesthesia/sedation
- General or regional anaesthesia
- Epidural anaesthesia before surgery may help reduce the likelihood of phantom limb pain
- Local anaesthesia using blocks may be sufficient for digital amputations

Follow-up/need for further procedure
- Stump revision or a more proximal amputation may become necessary if the patient develops stump complications
- Referral for further rehabilitation and limb fitting should be considered

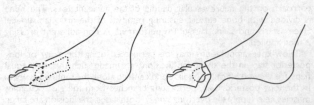

Fig. 4.3 Trans-metatarsal amputation.

Reproduced with permission from Hands L, Murphy M, Sharp M, *et al. Oxford Specialist Handbook of Vascular Surgery*. 2007. Oxford: Oxford University Press, p.345, Figure 15.4.

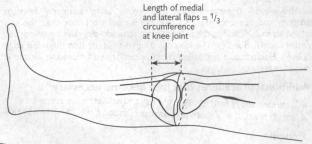

Length of medial and lateral flaps = $1/3$ circumference at knee joint

Fig. 4.4 Through-knee amputation.

Reproduced with permission from Hands L, Murphy M, Sharp M, *et al. Oxford Specialist Handbook of Vascular Surgery*. 2007. Oxford: Oxford University Press, p.341, Figure 15.3.

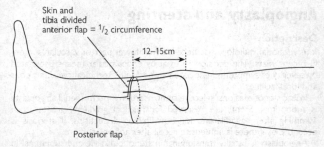

Skin and
tibia divided
anterior flap = $^1/_2$ circumference

12–15cm

Posterior flap

Fig. 4.5 Below-knee amputation.

Reproduced with permission from Hands L, Murphy M, Sharp M, et al. *Oxford Specialist Handbook of Vascular Surgery*. 2007. Oxford: Oxford University Press, p.337, Figure 15.2.

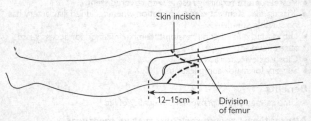

Skin incision

12–15cm

Division
of femur

Fig. 4.6 Above-knee amputation.

Reproduced with permission from Hands L, Murphy M, Sharp M, et al. *Oxford Specialist Handbook of Vascular Surgery*. 2007. Oxford: Oxford University Press, p.335, Figure 15.1.

Futher reading

Dormandy J. Heeck L, Vig S. Major amputations: clinical patterns and predictors. *Semin Vasc Surg* 1999;**12**(2):154–61.

Datta D, Atkinson G. Amputation, rehabilitation and prosthetic developments. In: Beard JD, Gains PA (eds). *Essential Vascular Surgery* 4th edition. London: WB Saunders, 2009, pp. 97–109.

Patient information—leg amputation. Available at: ℘ www.circulationfoundation.org.uk (accessed 17 May 2011).

Angioplasty and stenting

Description

Interventional radiology has become an integral part of vascular surgery in recent years. The decision to treat by endovascular means is dictated by severity of symptoms, associated comorbidity, technical considerations and local facilities.

In iliac stenotic lesions, selective stent insertion is performed if angioplasty is suboptimal. Stents are reserved for residual gradients greater than 10mmHg after vasodilators, for flow-limiting dissections, if stenosis is eccentric or if there is immediate recoil after angioplasty.

Angioplasty is usually transluminal in stenotic disease and subintimal in infrainguinal occlusions.

Additional procedures that may become necessary

- Vessel rupture requiring rescue with covered stent
- 'Kissing' iliac stents at aortic bifurcation when occluded iliac artery has no suitable stump
- Ultrasound-guided compression/thrombin injection for access vessel false aneurysm
- Closure device for arterial seal
- Surgery for major complications

Benefits

- Limb salvage and improvement in quality of life

Alternatives procedures/conservative measures

- Best medical treatment with optimization of risk factors
- Supervised exercise programme
- Surgical intervention

Serious/frequently occurring risks

- Complications related to access: groin or retroperitoneal haematoma, dissection, false aneurysm
- Complications related to angioplasty: vessel rupture, need for conversion to open surgery, distal emboli, and trash foot
- Complications related to stent: stent infection (rare), migration or failure to deploy
- Contrast-induced nephropathy

Blood transfusion necessary

- Group and save

Type of anaesthesia/sedation

- Local anaesthesia

Follow-up/need for further procedure

- *Patient advised to take* bedrest for 4–6h to ensure adequate haemostasis at the puncture site

Further reading

Norgren L, Hiatt WR, Dormandy JA, et al. Inter-Society Consensus for the Management of
  Peripheral Arterial Disease (TASC II). *J Vasc Surg* 2007;**45**(Suppl S):S5–67.
Faries P, Morrissey NJ, Teodorescu V, et al. Recent advances in peripheral angioplasty and
  stenting. *Angiology* 2002;**53**(6):617–26.
Patient information—Angioplasty and stent. Available at: ℞ www.circulationfoundation.org.uk
  (accessed 17 May 2011).

Arteriovenous fistula formation

Description

Arteriovenous fistulas are fashioned to provide a high-flow vessel that is easily accessible for haemodialysis in patients with chronic renal failure. Superficial veins from the upper limb such as the cephalic and basilic vein can be anastomosed to adjacent arteries. The fistula must then mature over the following 4–6 weeks before it can be used for dialysis.

Operative technique

Venous anatomy may be determined preoperatively using duplex ultrasound. The site should be marked preoperatively. An appropriate incision is made that allows access to both the vein and artery. The vein is dissected and mobilized towards the artery. The vessels are anastomosed with non-absorbable sutures.

Additional procedures that may become necessary

It may be impossible to form a fistula due to the unsuitability of the vein. A synthetic graft could be an alternative conduit in this situation.

Benefits

- Provides access for haemodialysis

Alternatives procedures/conservative measures

- Central venous catheters may be used
- Synthetic grafts are an alternative when no suitable vein is available
- Peritoneal dialysis may also be considered
- Renal transplant
- Patients not suitable for dialysis or renal transplant may be managed with best medical therapy

Serious/frequently occurring risks

- Bleeding, thrombosis, infection, steal syndrome, aneurysm formation, venous hypertension

Blood transfusion necessary

- None

Type of anaesthesia/sedation

- General, regional and local anaesthesia

Follow-up/need for further procedure

- Fistula may fail due to technical complications and if detected early may be salvaged by prompt surgical intervention
- Exclude long-term complications that may require ligation of fistula, such as aneurysm formation or steal syndrome

Further reading

Murphy GJ, White SA, Nicholson ML. Vascular access for haemodialysis. Br J Surg 2000;**87**(10):1300–15.

Shenoy S. Innovative surgical approaches to maximize arteriovenous fistula creation. Semin Vasc Surg 2007;**20**(3):141–7.

Patient information—arteriovenous fistula first. Available at: ℘ www.fistulafirst.org (accessed 17 May 2011).

Bypass surgery—infrainguinal

Description

Atherosclerotic and diabetic arterial disease account for most cases of symptomatic occlusive disease in the ageing population. The decision to intervene is based on the extent of patient's disability, associated comorbidities and the nature of the stenotic disease.

The indications for infrainguinal bypass surgery include critical limb ischaemia and short distance claudication. The occluded segment can be recanalized by subintimal balloon angioplasty or surgically bypassed. The surgical options include femoropopliteal or femorodistal bypass (Fig. 4.7) with native vein grafts as reversed or *in situ* grafts or using prosthetic grafts.

Femoropopliteal bypass is performed from the femoral artery to the above- or below-knee popliteal artery. Femorodistal bypass is usually undertaken for limb salvage in critical limb ischaemia. The inflow is established from femoral artery to the tibial vessel, which has the best run-off. When the graft is on to lower-third peroneal artery, excision of a segment of fibula may be required to access the vessel.

Additional procedures that may become necessary

- Procedures to improve inflow, such as proximal angioplasty, stenting and crossover bypass graft (Fig. 4.8)
- Vein harvest from another extremity
- Debridement of infected tissue
- Free tissue transfer combined with revascularization
- Lumbar sympathectomy
- For below-knee femoropopliteal bypass, vein patch, collar or boot to reduce neointimal hyperplasia

Benefits

- Improve quality of life
- Prevent limb and life loss

Alternatives procedures/conservative measures

- Best medical treatment with statins, antiplatelets, and exercise with optimization of all vascular risk factors
- Interventional radiology
- Spinal cord stimulator
- Intermittent pneumatic compression of the calf and foot
- Palliation in extreme cases where patients are too high risk for any intervention

Serious/frequently occurring risks

- Infection, bleeding, thromboembolism, graft failure secondary to technical problems, compartment syndrome, progression of disease

Blood transfusion necessary

- Group and save

Type of anaesthesia/sedation
- General/regional anaesthesia

Follow-up/need for further procedure
- Graft surveillance
- Further surgery in the case of graft complications
- Major limb amputation

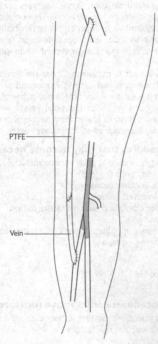

Fig. 4.7 Femorodistal bypass graft with PTFE/vein.

Reproduced with permission from Hands L, Murphy M, Sharp M, et al. *Oxford Specialist Handbook of Vascular Surgery.* 2007. Oxford: Oxford University Press, p.307, Figure 14.6.

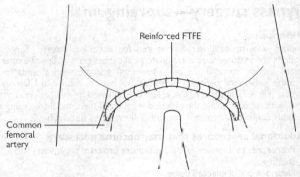

Fig. 4.8 Femoro-femoral crossover bypass graft.

Reproduced with permission from Hands L, Murphy M, Sharp M, et al. Oxford Specialist Handbook of Vascular Surgery. 2007. Oxford. Oxford University Press, p.421, Figure 19.3.

Further reading

Adam AJ, Beard JD, Cleveland T, et al. BASIL trial participants. Bypass versus angioplasty in severe ischaemia of the leg (BASIL): multicentre, randomized controlled trial. Lancet 2005;**366**:1925–34.
Scottish Intercollegiate Guideline Network. Diagnosis and Management of Peripheral Arterial Disease. Clinical guideline no. 89 . London: Scottish Intercollegiate Guideline Network, 2006.
Patient information—femoropopliteal and femoro-distal bypass. Available at: ℘ www. circulationfoundation.org.uk (accessed 17 May 2011).

Bypass surgery—suprainguinal

Description
Suprainguinal procedures are required for aortoiliac disease. Surgical options are anatomical or extra-anatomical bypass grafting. Specific operations include aortoiliac or aorto-bifemoral grafting, surgical endarterectomy, iliofemoral bypass, femoro-femoral bypass, and axillo-bifemoral bypass (Fig. 4.9). In general, the inflow is established from a proximal site to a distal vessel beyond the diseased segment of the arterial tree using a suitable conduit. Outcome is primarily influenced by distal run-off.

Additional procedures that may become necessary
- Procedures to improve inflow procedures proximal angioplasty and stenting
- Debridement of infected tissue
- Free tissue transfer combined with revascularization
- Lumbar sympathectomy

Benefits
- Improve quality of life
- Prevent limb and life loss

Alternatives procedures/conservative measures
- Best medical treatment with statins, antiplatelets, and exercise, with optimization of all vascular risk factors
- Interventional radiology
- Spinal cord stimulator
- Intermittent pneumatic compression of the calf and foot
- Palliation in extreme cases where patients are too high risk for any intervention
- Major limb amputation
- Laparoscopic aortoiliac reconstruction

Serious/frequently occurring risks
- Bleeding, infection, thromboembolism, false aneurysm at anastomotic sites, graft stenosis, graft occlusion, graft infection, injury to ureters, bladder and iliofemoral veins, sexual dysfunction, myocardial infarction, limb loss, and death

Blood transfusion necessary
- Group and save
- Cross-match necessary for aortic and iliac surgery

Type of anaesthesia/sedation
- General or regional anaesthesia

Follow-up/need for further procedure
- Graft surveillance
- Further surgery in the case of graft complications
- Major limb amputation

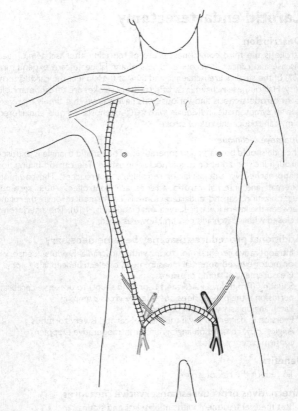

Fig. 4.9 Axillo-bifemoral bypass graft.

Reproduced with permission from Hands L, Murphy M, Sharp M, et al. Oxford Specialist Handbook of Vascular Surgery. 2007. Oxford: Oxford University Press, p.417, Figure 19.1.

Further reading

Adam AJ, Beard JD, Cleveland T. et al. BASIL trial participants. Bypass versus angioplasty in severe ischaemia of the leg (BASIL): multicentre, randomized controlled trial. Lancet 2005;**366**:1925–34.

Scottish Intercollegiate Guideline Network. Diagnosis and Management of Peripheral Arterial Disease. Clinical guideline no. 89. Edinburgh: Scottish Intercollegiate Guideline Network, 2006.

Patient information—aorto/axillo-bifemoral surgery. Available at: ℘ www.circulationfoundation.org.uk (accessed 17 May 2011).

Carotid endarterectomy

Description

Stroke is the third commonest cause of mortality after ischaemic heart disease and cancer. It accounts for 5% of annual healthcare expenditure. 80% of the strokes are ischaemic and 80% of these affect the carotid territory. Half of these ischaemic carotid territory strokes are thromboembolic from carotid stenosis and various trials have shown that timely intervention in symptomatic individuals with >70% stenosis, carotid endarterectomy can reduce the risk of stroke.

Operative technique

The side should be marked preoperatively. The carotid triangle is exposed through incision anterior to sternocleidomastoid. The carotid bifurcation is approached via antejugular or retrojugular approaches. The common, external, and internal carotid arteries are controlled. After systemic heparinization, carotid endarterectomy is performed through the plane between the internal elastic lamina and plaque (Fig. 4.10). The arteriotomy is closed with a patch and cerebral flow restored.

Additional procedures that may become necessary

- Intraoperative cerebral monitoring with transcranial Doppler, sensory or motor evoked potential measurement, or electroencephalography
- Measurement of stump pressures
- Shunting (Pruitt–Inahara (Fig. 4.11) or Javid shunt) to preserve cerebral perfusion if the patient does not tolerate cross-clamping
- Patch angioplasty with vein or Dacron
- Eversion endarterectomy if the internal carotid is very tortuous
- Angioscopy, completion angiogram, or intraoperative Doppler to confirm patency of flow

Benefits

- To reduce the risk of stroke

Alternatives procedures/conservative measures

- Best medical treatment with antiplatelets and statins
- Carotid stenting, particularly in restenosis and in hostile necks after previous radiotherapy

Serious/frequently occurring risks

- *Early*: infection, bleeding, thromboembolism, stroke, myocardial infarction, death, reperfusion injury, cranial nerve injury (recurrent laryngeal, vagus, hypoglossal, glossopharyngeal, accessory and marginal mandibular nerve), Horner's syndrome, great auricular nerve injury
- *Late*: patch infection, restenosis

Blood transfusion necessary

- Group and save

Type of anaesthesia/sedation

- General or local anaesthesia (cervical plexus block)

Follow-up/need for further procedure

- Patients may develop restenosis over time, however, this may be asymptomatic and not require further treatment
- Symptomatic restenosis may be treated with surgery or stenting

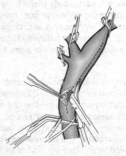

Fig. 4.10 Arteriotomy during carotid endarterectomy.

Reproduced with permission from Hands L, Murphy M, Sharp M, et al. Oxford Specialist Handbook of Vascular Surgery. 2007. Oxford: Oxford University Press, p.359, Figure 16.3.

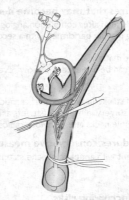

Fig. 4.11 Insertion of a Pruitt-Inahura shunt during carotid endarterectomy.

Reproduced with permission from Hands L, Murphy M, Sharp M, et al. Oxford Specialist Handbook of Vascular Surgery. 2007. Oxford: Oxford University Press, p.359, Figure 16.4.

Further reading

Chaturvedi S, Bruno A, Feasby T, et al. Carotid endarterectomy-an evidence-based review: report of the Therapeutics and Technology Assessment Subcommittee of the American Academy of Neurology. Neurology 2005;65(6):794–801.

Rothwell PM, Eliasziw M, Gutnikov SA. For the carotid endarterectomy trialists collaboration. analysis of pooled data from the randomized controlled trials of endarterectomy for symptomatic carotid stenosis. Lancet 2003;361:107–16.

Patient information—carotid endarterectomy Available at: ℘ www.nhs.uk, ℘ www.cks.nhs.uk and ℘ www.circulationfoundation.org.uk (accessed 17 May 2011).

Carotid stenting

Description

Carotid stenting is accepted as an alternative in patients who have symptomatic carotid stenosis. It is particularly useful in patients with a surgically hostile neck and in symptomatic restenosis after previous endarterectomy. Dual antiplatelet treatment with aspirin and clopidogrel is commenced 1 week prior to stenting. Anatomical suitability is confirmed by 'overview' imaging of the arterial anatomy from arch of aorta to the circle of Willis.

Technique

Access is obtained through femoral or upper limb vessels with systemic heparinization. The common carotid artery is catheterized and a stiff wire is placed in the external carotid artery. A guiding catheter is passed over the stiff wire and calibrated angiography performed to assess size of internal and common carotid artery. The carotid sinus baroreceptor is blocked with atropine or glycopyrrolate. The internal carotid stenosis is crossed with a protection device with filter or occlusion balloon. The stenosis is pre-dilated to 3mm before stent delivery and the stent is balloon dilated. Completion angiography is performed and arterial access closed with closure device.

Additional procedures that may become necessary

- If plaque protrusion is seen after completion angiography, re-ballooning or double-scaffolding may be performed with a second stent inside the first
- Aspiration of embolic material
- Cerebral protection can be achieved with flow reversal

Benefits

- To reduce the risk of stroke in symptomatic carotid stenosis
- Useful alternative to surgery in high-risk patients and those with restenosis, and in hostile necks after previous radiotherapy

Alternatives procedures/conservative measures

- Best medical treatment with antiplatelets and statins in asymptomatic patients
- Surgery

Serious/frequently occurring risks

- Access-related—bleeding, dissection, pseudoaneurysm
- Procedure-related—stroke from embolism, vessel spasm, perforation, haemodynamic instability, bradycardia, hyperperfusion, intracranial haemorrhage, headache

Blood transfusion necessary

- Group and save

Type of anaesthesia/sedation

- Local anaesthesia

Follow-up/need for further procedure

- Dual antiplatelet therapy with aspirin and clopidogrel for 28 days

Further reading

Mas JL, Chazellier G, Beyssen B, et al. Endarterectomy versus stenting in patients with symptomatic severe carotid stenosis. *N Engl J Med* 2006;**355**(16):1660–71.

National Institute for Health and Clinical Excellence. *Carotid Artery Stent Placement for Carotid Stenosis.* Interventional Procedure Guidance IPG 191. London: NICE, 2006.

Patient information—carotid endarterectomy—alternatives. Available at: ℘ www.nhs.uk (accessed 17 May 2011).

Common femoral endarterectomy

Description

The common femoral artery (CFA) commences at the mid-inguinal point and soon after bifurcates into the profunda femoris artery (PFA) and the superficial femoral artery (SFA). Atherosclerotic disease is common at this point as it is subject to increased wall shear stress. Unlike the iliac artery and SFA, the CFA is not amenable to angioplasty and stenting as it crosses the hip joint and is subject to the stress of hip flexion. CFA endarterectomy is therefore the procedure of choice to manage disease here. The clinical manifestation of CFA disease ranges from thigh and calf claudication through to critical limb ischaemia if there is associated distal disease.

Operative technique

The side should be marked preoperatively. A longitudinal skin incision is made and the CFA, PFA, and SFA are dissected and isolated. These vessels are controlled and vascular clamps applied after heparinization. A longitudinal arteriotomy is made and extended with Potts scissors. A Watson–Cheyne dissector is used to develop the plane between the internal elastic lamina and the plaque. This is removed avoiding raising flaps that may result in dissection. The vessel is flushed with heparinized saline before being closed with a prosthetic/vein patch.

Additional procedures that may become necessary

- Further bypass graft—to improve limb perfusion
- Profundaplasty to improve inflow to profunda

Benefits

- Limb salvage
- Improvement in symptoms

Alternatives procedures/conservative measures

- Lifestyle changes such as losing weight and stopping smoking
- Supervised exercise programme
- Secondary prevention and drugs to improve perfusion such as cilostazol
- Opiate analgesia

Serious/frequently occurring risks

- Bleeding, embolization, arterial dissection, lymph leak, pseudoaneurysm

Blood transfusion necessary

- Group and save

Type of anaesthesia/sedation

- General, regional or local anaesthesia

Follow-up/need for further procedure

- Further procedure may be required if the patient develops complications or there is disease progression

Further reading

Ballotta E, Gruppo M, Mazzala F, et al. Common femoral artery endarterectomy for occlusive disease: an 8-year single-center prospective study. *Surgery* 2010;**147**(2):268–74.

Kang JL, Patel VI, Conrad MF, et al. Common femoral artery occlusive disease: contemporary results following surgical endarterectomy. *J Vasc Surg* 2008;**48**(4):872–7.

Embolectomy

Description

Embolectomy is performed for acute limb ischaemia occurring secondary to an embolism. This is most commonly a thromboembolism arising from the diseased heart or from atherosclerotic or aneurysmal disease. It is important to differentiate embolism from *in situ* thrombosis as the management of these conditions is very different. Occasionally, however, both conditions may coexist.

Embolectomy should be performed when the embolism is significant and results in a threatened limb. This is determined by the size and site of the embolus as well as the state of the collateral circulation. Prompt treatment of the threatened limb can result in limb salvage. Embolectomy should not be performed when the limb is non-viable. In this situation a decision must be made as to whether the patient is a candidate for major limb amputation or palliation as acute limb ischaemia often arises in elderly patients with significant comorbidity and may herald the end of life.

Embolectomy is most often performed for lower limb ischaemia as the upper limb has an excellent collateral circulation.

Operative technique

The side should be marked preoperatively and both limbs should be prepared in case a crossover graft is required. An oblique or longitudinal incision is made at the mid-inguinal point and dissection performed down to the CFA. The CFA and bifurcation should be controlled. A transverse or longitudinal arteriotomy is made proximal to the bifurcation and a Fogarty balloon catheter is passed proximally (Fig. 4.12) and withdrawn to clear thrombus and establish good inflow. Heparinized saline is flushed into the vessel before the application of a vascular clamp. The balloon catheter is passed distally down the profunda and superficial femoral vessels, and the balloon gradually inflated as it is withdrawn, avoiding excess tension, which may lead to intimal damage. Once adequate back bleeding is obtained, heparinized saline is flushed down both vessels before applying a vascular clamp. The arteriotomy is then closed using a polypropylene suture. Completion angiography may be performed.

Embolectomy of the upper limb is performed in a similar fashion although a lazy S skin incision is utilized to prevent flexion contracture at the elbow.

Additional procedures that may become necessary

- Systemic anticoagulation
- Systemic or intra-arterial catheter delivered thrombolysis
- Angioplasty
- Distal bypass
- Crossover graft if inadequate inflow
- Fasciotomies to prevent or treat compartment syndrome
- *Amputation if failure*

Benefits
- Limb salvage
- Improving limb function and limiting the extent of amputation should it become necessary

Alternatives procedures/conservative measures
- Peripheral intra-arterial thrombolysis
- Percutaneous thrombectomy devices, including clot aspiration devices
- Anticoagulation
- Primary amputation
- Palliation

Serious/frequently occurring risks
- Bleeding, failure, recurrent embolism, thrombosis, nerve damage, limb loss, lymphatic leak, compartment syndrome, reperfusion injury resulting in organ failure and death, pseudoaneurysm

Blood transfusion necessary
- Group and save

Type of anaesthesia/sedation
- Local, regional or general anaesthesia
- If local anaesthesia is used, it is important to have an anaesthetist available to provide analgesia and sedation or administer a general anaesthetic if the patient cannot tolerate the procedure or a more extensive procedure becomes necessary

Follow-up/need for further procedure
- Anticoagulation
- Frequent neurovascular limb observations are essential
- Investigation to identify and treat underlying cause of embolus

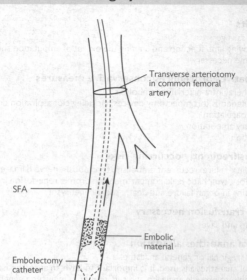

Fig. 4.12 Femoral embolectomy. SFA, superficial femoral artery.

Reproduced with permission from Hands L, Murphy M, Sharp M, *et al. Oxford Specialist Handbook of Vascular Surgery.* 2007. Oxford: Oxford University Press, p.319, Figure 14.10.

Further reading

O'Connell JB, Quiñones-Baldrich WJ. Proper evaluation and management of acute embolic versus thrombotic limb ischemia. *Semin Vasc Surg* 2009;**22**(1):10–16.

Fasciotomy

Description

Fasciotomy is used to relieve elevated compartment pressures and improve limb perfusion. It is most commonly performed for the prevention or treatment of acute compartment syndrome. This can occur secondary to revascularization of the acutely ischaemic limb or as a result of tissue swelling following vascular, soft tissue, or bony injury.

Once established the cardinal symptom of acute compartment syndrome is of pain that is out of proportion to the extent of the injury. Signs include a tense, tender muscle compartment with severe pain on passive muscle stretching. The absence of pulses is not a reliable sign of acute compartment syndrome. The diagnosis is primarily clinical and requires prompt management of the underlying condition and fasciotomy to prevent limb dysfunction and loss. Compartment pressure measurement may be useful in patients who are unable to be assessed clinically.

Acute compartment syndrome most commonly occurs in the lower leg but can also occur in the thigh and upper limb. There are four compartments in the lower leg, the anterior, peroneal, superficial posterior, and deep posterior compartments.

Operative technique

Subcutaneous fasciotomies are inadequate. Lower limb fasciotomy requires a four-compartment release to be effective. This requires two incisions (Fig. 4.13). The posteromedial incision is made along the length of the lower leg two finger-breadths posterior to the tibia. It is important to avoid damaging the long saphenous vein. The anterolateral incision is made along the length of the lower leg two finger-breadths lateral to the anterior border of the tibia. This incision avoids the peroneal nerve and allows access to the anterior and peroneal compartments, which must be individually incised along their length. The skin incisions are left open but various techniques may be employed to facilitate later closure.

Additional procedures that may become necessary

- Vascular repair and external fixation in trauma cases
- Skin grafting to close the fasciotomy wounds at a later stage
- Debridement of non-viable tissue
- Primary amputation if limb is not salvageable
- The application of a vacuum dressing to subsequently close the wound

Benefits

- Life saving
- Limb salvage
- Prevent limb dysfunction

Alternatives procedures/conservative measures

- Consider primary amputation in clinically non-viable limb
- Circumferential casts in long bone fractures should be split immediately

Serious/frequently occurring risks

- Limb loss, reperfusion injury leading to organ failure (sometimes death), bleeding, nerve and muscle injury resulting in impaired function, infection, problems with wound healing

Blood transfusion necessary

- Group and save

Type of anaesthesia/sedation

- General or regional anaesthesia

Follow-up/need for further procedure

- Frequent neurovascular limb observations are essential
- Delayed primary closure usually at 3 to 5 days
- Fasciotomy wounds which are not amenable to delayed primary closure may require skin grafting
- Appropriate rehabilitation programme

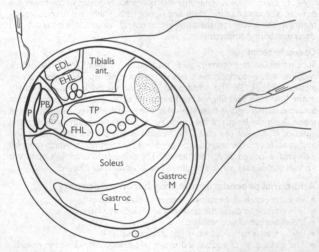

Fig. 4.13 Lower limb fasciotomy, compartments, and incisions. P, peroneus longus; PB, peroneus brevis; EDL, extensor digitalis longus; EHL, extensor hallucis longus; TP, tibialis posterior; FHL, flexor hallucis longus; gatroc, gastrocnemius; L, lateralis; M, medialis.

Reproduced with permission from Hands L, Murphy M, Sharp M, et al. *Oxford Specialist Handbook of Vascular Surgery*. 2007. Oxford: Oxford University Press, p.325, Figure 14.12.

Further reading

Ernst CB. Fasciotomy—in perspective. *J Vasc Surg* 1989;**9**(6):829–30.

Pearse MF, Harry L, Nanchahal J. Acute compartment syndrome of the leg. *BMJ* 2002;**325**(7364):557–8.

Popliteal aneurysm repair

Description

Popliteal artery aneurysms are common, comprising 80% of all peripheral aneurysms. The popliteal artery is considered aneurysmal if its diameter exceed 2cm. Popliteal aneurysms may be bilateral and are associated with abdominal aortic aneurysms in 50% of cases.

Symptoms include compression of adjacent structures, rupture and limb ischaemia secondary to emboli or thrombosis. Once detected a decision must be made as to whether repair of the popliteal aneurysms is justified. This depends on aneurysm size, comorbidity and whether the patient is symptomatic.

Definitive management is surgical and involves ligating proximal and distal to the aneurysm and restoring cistal flow with a femoropopliteal bypass.

Operative technique

The side is marked preoperatively and the aneurysm is approached either from a posterior or medial approach. The popliteal artery is controlled and after heparinization the aneurysm is excluded and bypassed. An alternative form of repair is with an inlay graft as an end-to-end anastomosis.

Additional procedures that may become necessary

- Thrombolysis if run off is poor or if distal embolization occurs
- Amputation

Benefits

- Prevention of limb loss

Alternatives procedures/conservative measures

- If patient is high surgical risk and has limited lifespan, the aneurysm may be managed conservatively
- Endovascular repair with stent grafts
- Intra-arterial thrombolysis for acute aneurysm thrombosis

Serious/frequently occurring risks

- Bleeding, thromboembolism, limb loss, nerve injury, compartment syndrome, graft stenosis, critical limb ischaemia following graft failure, graft infection

Blood transfusion necessary

- Group and save

Type of anaesthesia/sedation

- General or regional anaesthesia

Follow-up/need for further procedure

- Consider graft surveillance
- Angioplasty or graft revision may be required for stenosis
- Contralateral procedure may be required

Further reading

Hamish M, Lockwood A, Cosgrove C, *et al.* Management of popliteal artery aneurysms. *ANZ J Surg* 2006;**76**(10):912–15.

Mousa AY, Beauford RB, Henderson P, *et al.* Update on the diagnosis and management of popliteal aneurysm and literature review. *Vascular* 2006;**14**(2):103–8.

Sympathectomy

Description

The sympathetic nervous system is part of the autonomic nervous system and has a thoraco-lumbar outflow from T1 to L2. The sympathetic nerves synapse within ganglia and contribute to the supply of smooth muscle, cardiac muscle, and glands. The effects of sympathetic stimulation therefore include vasoconstriction of cutaneous blood vessels, tachycardia, and sweating.

Sympathectomy is the disruption of the sympathetic outflow and has been primarily performed to reduce sweating of the axilla and hands and to help heal painful cutaneous ulcers in patients with inoperable arterial disease.

Operative technique

Open techniques for sympathectomy have been replaced by minimal access and radiological methods. Thoracic sympathectomy is usually performed with video-assisted thoracoscopy and involves dividing the sympathetic chain below the stellate ganglion. Lumbar sympathectomy may be surgical or chemical. The latter is performed under radiological guidance and involves the injection of phenol into the sympathetic chain.

Additional procedures that may become necessary

• Chest drain insertion for pneumothorax

Benefits

• Treatment of hyperhidrosis
• Prevention of the vasoconstrictive skin changes associated with Raynaud's disease
• Pain relief and healing of ischaemic foot ulcers and areas of cutaneous gangrene in patients with inoperable arterial disease

Alternatives procedures/conservative measures

• Hyperhidrosis may be treated with anticholinergic drugs and injection of botulinum toxin
• Raynaud's disease may be managed by stopping smoking, avoiding the cold, using heated gloves, calcium channel antagonists and the infusion of prostacyclin analogues
• Arterial ulcers may be treated with opiate analgesia
• Spinal cord stimulators may also be used in patients with intractable pain
• If refractory to treatment, amputation may be required

Serious/frequently occurring risks

• *Thoracic sympathectomy*: bleeding, infection, pneumothorax, lung injury, Horner's syndrome failure, compensatory hyperhidrosis, hypotension
• *Lumbar sympathectomy*: inadvertent injection into soft tissue, vessels or nerves, failure, post-sympathectomy neuralgia, sexual dysfunction

Blood transfusion necessary

- Group and save for thoracoscopic sympathectomy

Type of anaesthesia/sedation

- General anaesthesia for open or thoracoscopic sympathectomy
- Local anaesthesia for chemical lumbar sympathectomy

Follow-up/need for further procedure

- In the case of lumbar sympathectomy for rest pain or non-healing painful ulcers amputation may be required

Further reading

Gordon A, Zechmeister K, Collin J. The role of sympathectomy in current surgical practice. *Eur J Vasc Surg* 1994;**8**(2):129–37.

Malmivaara A, Kuukasjarvi P, Autti-Ramo I, *et al.* Effectiveness and safety of endoscopic thoracic sympathectomy for excessive sweating and facial blushing: a systematic review. *Int J Technol Assess Health Care* 2007;**23**(1):54–62.

Patient information—thoracoscopic sympathectomy. Available at: Ⓜ www.circulationfoundation. org.uk (accessed 17 May 2011).

Thoracic outlet decompression

Description

Thoracic outlet syndrome describes a collection of symptoms caused by the compression of the subclavian vessels and roots of the brachial plexus at the thoracic outlet (Fig. 4.14). This may lead to neurological symptoms such as pain and weakness and less commonly symptoms from vascular compression. The aetiology includes trauma, loss of muscle tone, hypertrophy of the scalene muscles, congenital fibromuscular bands, and accessory cervical ribs.

There is controversy about the best form of treatment for this diverse group of conditions. The surgical management of this condition is surgical decompression. This usually involves the resection of the first rib and any constricting lesion via a transaxillary or combined supraclavicular and infraclavicular approach. The type of approach used depends on whether the symptoms are primarily neurological or vascular.

Operative technique

The transaxillary approach involves placing the patient in the lateral position with the arm elevated. An incision is made at the level of the third rib and dissection extended towards the apex of the axilla. Upon reaching the first rib, the scalenus medius, scalerus anterior, and subclavius muscles are divided at their origins. The rib is then removed and any remaining fibrous bands around the nerves or vessels divided.

The combined infraclavicular and supraclavicular approach involves an S-shaped incision over the clavicle and division of the pectoralis major and minor and subclavius muscles. The scalenus anterior and medius are approached from above the clavicle and also divided. The subclavian vessels are freed and the first rib divided and disarticulated. Any accessory cervical rib can also be removed using this approach. If there is significant arterial disease, resection and primary anastomosis or an interposition graft using vein or synthetic graft may be performed.

Additional procedures that may become necessary

- Embolectomy
- Insertion of chest drain

Benefits

- Relief of symptoms
- Decreased risk of embolization

Alternatives procedures/conservative measures

- Avoid heavy lifting and working with arms above shoulder level
- Physiotherapy

Serious/frequently occurring risks

- Nerve injury—brachial plexus or phrenic nerve
- Subclavian vein or artery injury
- Bleeding and haematoma
- Pneumothorax

Blood transfusion necessary
- Group and save

Type of anaesthesia/sedation
- General anaesthesia

Follow-up/need for further procedure
- Physiotherapy

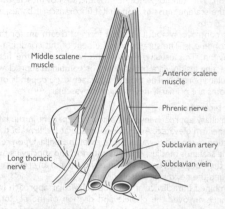

Middle scalene muscle

Anterior scalene muscle

Phrenic nerve

Subclavian artery

Subclavian vein

Long thoracic nerve

Fig. 4.14 Structures impinged on with thoracic outlet syndrome.

Reproduced with permission from Hands L, Murphy M, Sharp M, *et al. Oxford Specialist Handbook of Vascular Surgery*. 2007. Oxford: Oxford University Press, p.373, Figure 16.7.

Further reading

Povlsen B, Belzberg A, Hansson T, *et al.* Treatment for thoracic outlet syndrome. *Cochrane Database Syst Rev* 2010;**1**:CD007218.

Patient information—thoracic outlet syndrome. Available at: ℰ www.tos-syndrome.com (accessed 17 May 2011).

Thrombolysis

Description

Thrombolysis has become an important adjunct or alternative to surgery in both arterial and venous disease. Thrombus dissolution can be achieved by systemic or catheter-directed thrombolysis. The common use of thrombolysis on the venous side is for extensive proximal iliofemoral vein thrombosis and in subclavian vein thrombosis. Systemic thrombolysis is used in pulmonary embolism and for non-haemorrhagic stroke.

Thrombolysis is used mostly for infrainguinal graft occlusion within 2 weeks of occlusion where the limb is viable. The absolute contraindication to thrombolysis is active internal bleeding.

The technique of catheter-directed thrombolysis involves placing a catheter intravascularly close to or within the thrombus. The risk of pericatheter thrombosis is reduced by infusing low-dose heparin into the side-arm of the sheath.

Additional procedures that may become necessary

- Mechanical thrombectomy
- Angioplasty of underlying stenosis
- Arterial stenting
- Aspiration thromboembolectomy
- Fasciotomy

Benefits

- Thrombolysis avoids the need for difficult redo surgery and helps to clear run-off vessels more effectively
- On completion of treatment, it may unmask the underlying cause for thrombosis, which may also be treated by endovascular means

Alternatives procedures/conservative measures

- Systemic anticoagulation
- Surgical thromboembolectomy or bypass

Serious/frequently occurring risks

- Allergic reaction, bleeding (puncture site, intra-abdominal, retroperitoneal), stroke, death, distal embolization, pericatheter thrombosis, reperfusion injury, contrast-induced nephropathy

Blood transfusion necessary

- Group and save

Type of anaesthesia/sedation

- Local anaesthesia for access

Follow-up/need for further procedure

- Neurological observations during thrombolysis and CT scan of the head if any focal neurological deficit is noted
- Imaging to monitor thrombus dissolution
- Heparin post-lysis for 48h
- Long-term anticoagulation or dual antiplatelet treatment

Further reading

Earnshaw JJ, Whitman B, Foy C. National Audit of Thrombolysis for Acute Leg Ischemia (NATALI): clinical factors associated with early outcome. *J Vasc Surg* 2004;**39**(5):1018–25.

Working Party on Thrombolysis in the Management of Limb Ischemia. Thrombolysis in the management of lower limb peripheral arterial occlusion—a consensus document. *Am J Cardiol* 1998;**81**(2):207–18.

Varicose vein surgery—long saphenous vein

Description

Varicose veins are defined as abnormally dilated, superficial, tortuous veins. Varicose veins may arise due to intrinsic vein wall or valve weakness. Other causes include extrinsic compression of pelvic veins and DVT leading to valve damage. Varicose veins primarily affect the lower limb and the majority arise from the long saphenous system. Fig. 4.15 shows normal venous anatomy of the leg.

Clinical assessment includes history of previous DVT, previous vein surgery, or limb trauma. Limbs should be examined for unusual distribution of the varicosities and signs of venous hypertension such as oedema, lipodermatosclerosis, and pigmentation. In all cases of redo surgery, duplex scan is mandatory.

If patients are symptomatic or have complications of bleeding, ulceration, or recurrent superficial thrombophlebitis, they may be considered for surgical management.

Operative technique

Troublesome varicosities should be marked preoperatively with the patient standing. Exposure of the long saphenous vein is gained through a groin incision located just inferomedial to the femoral pulse. The saphenofemoral junction (SFJ) and tributaries draining into the long saphenous vein are identified prior to their division and ligation. The long saphenous vein is then stripped with the endoluminal stripper (Fig. 4.16), from the groin to just below the knee. Finally small stab incisions are made over the varicosities and they are avulsed.

A third of patients after varicose vein surgery develop recurrent disease. Surgery for recurrence is complex with greater risk of complications. The operation requires dissection of the femoral vein and division and ligation of any tributaries that may have been missed at initial surgery.

Additional procedures that may become necessary

- A more proximal incision to deliver the stripper if unable to strip the vein to below the knee

Benefits

- Symptom relief

Alternatives procedures/conservative measures

- Conservative measures, which include lifestyle alterations (losing weight and avoiding prolonged standing)
- Compression hosiery, class II graduated compression stockings
- Endovenous laser therapy or radiofrequency ablation (RFA)
- Injection and foam sclerotherapy

Serious/frequently occurring risks

- Bruising, bleeding, wound infection, scars, residual or recurrent varicosities, phlebitis, limb swelling, saphenous nerve damage (paraesthesia to medial calf and ankle), DVT/pulmonary embolism, skin tattooing, lymph leak, common femoral vein or artery damage

Blood transfusion necessary

- Not required

Type of anaesthesia/sedation

- General anaesthesia with local anaesthesia
- Regional anaesthesia

Follow-up/need for further procedure

- Class II compression stockings to be worn for at least 4–6 weeks after surgery
- May require injection sclerotherapy for residual varicosities

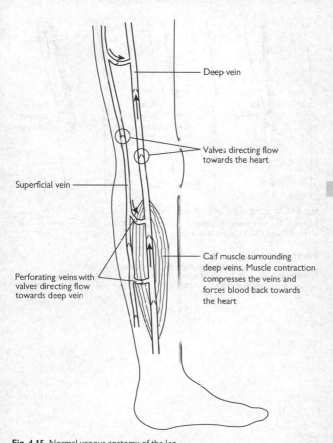

Fig. 4.15 Normal venous anatomy of the leg.

Reproduced with permission from Hands L, Murphy M, Sharp M, et al. *Oxford Specialist Handbook of Vascular Surgery*. 2007. Oxford: Oxford University Press, p.17, Figure 1.5.

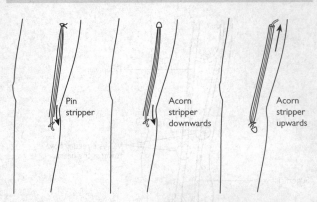

Fig. 4.16 Stripping of the long saphenous vein.

Reproduced with permission from Hands L, Murphy M, Sharp M, *et al. Oxford Specialist Handbook of Vascular Surgery*. 2007. Oxford: Oxford University Press, p.451, Figure 21.2.

Further reading

Campbell B. Varicose veins and their management. *BMJ* 2006;**333**(7562):287–92.
Patient information—varicose veins. Available at: ℘ www.cks.nhs.uk, ℘ www.nhs.uk and ℘ www.circulationfoundation.org.uk (accessed 17 May 2011).

Varicose vein surgery—short saphenous vein

Description

Varicose veins in the short saphenous distribution are less common than those associated with the long saphenous vein (Fig. 4.15). A combination of disease arising from the two systems may exist and failure to identify concomitant short saphenous vein disease may be a cause of treatment failure. Clinical assessment reveals the distribution of varicosities be in the posterolateral region of the lower leg. Hand-held Doppler assessment with the calf-squeeze test helps to support the diagnosis. All patients should undergo preoperative venous duplex to confirm the diagnosis and identify the site of the variable sapheno–popliteal junction (SPJ).

Operative technique

Preoperative identification and marking of the SPJ is essential. Troublesome varicosities should be also be marked with the patient standing. The short saphenous vein is exposed with a horizontal skin incision at the level of the SPJ with the patient lying prone. Careful dissection is performed to the SPJ making sure that the sural nerve is preserved. The short saphenous vein and any tributaries are divided and ligated. Finally small stab incisions are made over the varicosities and they are avulsed.

Additional procedures that may become necessary

- None

Benefits

- Symptom relief

Alternatives procedures/conservative measures

- Conservative measures, which include lifestyle alterations (losing weight and avoiding prolonged standing)
- Compression hosiery, class II graduated compression stockings
- Endovenous laser therapy or RFA
- Injection and foam sclerotherapy

Serious/frequently occurring risks

- Bruising, bleeding, wound infection, scars, residual or recurrent varicosities, phlebitis, limb swelling, sural nerve damage (paraesthesia, numbness to outer calf and outer foot), DVT/pulmonary embolism, skin tattooing, lymph leak, popliteal vein bulge

Blood transfusion necessary

- Not required

Type of anaesthesia/sedation

- General anaesthesia with local anaesthesia
- Regional anaesthesia

Follow-up/need for further procedure

- Class II compression stockings to be worn for at least 4–6 weeks after surgery
- May require injection sclerotherapy for residual varicosities

Further reading

Leopardi D, Hoggan BL, Fitridge RA, *et al*. Systematic review of treatments for varicose veins. *Ann Vasc Surg* 2009;**23**(2):264–76.

Perkins JM. Standard varicose vein surgery. *Phlebology* 2009;**24**(Suppl 1):34–41.

Patient information—varicose veins. Available at: ℘ www.cks.nhs.uk, ℘ www.nhs.uk and ℘ www.circulationfoundation.org.uk (accessed 17 May 2011).

Varicose veins—endovenous therapy

Description

Endovenous therapy allows for the treatment of varicose veins without requiring a groin incision. It includes endovenous laser therapy (EVLT), RFA, and foam sclerotherapy.

EVLT and RFA utilize energy from laser and radiofrequency sources respectively to ablate the saphenous vein trunks. This action is analogous to the effect of the stripper in open surgery. Although no treatment is given to the groin tributaries, recent studies have shown no significant difference in rates of recurrence. Multiple stab avulsions may still be necessary to remove the varicosities.

Operative technique

RFA or EVLT for varicose veins arising from the long saphenous vein involves marking the varicosities with the patient standing. The patient is placed in the reversed Trendelenburg position and an ultrasound probe allows the abnormally dilated long saphenous or anterior thigh vein to be followed down the leg. The vein is cannulated and catheter passed to a point distal to the SFJ. The distance is noted and the patient is placed head down. Tumescence is infiltrated around the vein along the length of the catheter. The position of the catheter is re-checked before either radiofrequency or laser energy is used to disrupt the vein as the catheter is withdrawn. The procedure for the short saphenous vein is similar with the short saphenous vein being cannulated in the lower leg and short saphenous vein being disrupted to a point distal to the SPJ. Finally small stab incisions are made over the varicosities and they are avulsed.

Foam sclerotherapy involves mixing air and sclerosant to form a foam that is then injected under ultrasound guidance into the superficial main trunk veins. This procedure can be performed without anaesthesia.

Additional procedures that may become necessary

- An incision to cannulate the vein if unable to do so percutaneously

Benefits

- Symptom relief
- Avoids groin incision and associated complications

Alternatives procedures/conservative measures

- Open varicose vein surgery
- Conservative measures, which include lifestyle alterations (losing weight and avoiding prolonged standing)
- Compression hosiery, class II graduated compression stockings
- Injection sclerotherapy

Serious/frequently occurring risks

- Bruising, bleeding, residual or recurrent varicosities, phlebitis, limb swelling, saphenous or sural nerve damage, DVT/pulmonary embolism, skin burns, skin tattooing, common femoral vein damage, allergic reaction, failure to cannulate or to advance catheter

Blood transfusion necessary

- Not required

Type of anaesthesia/sedation

- Local or general anaesthesia

Follow-up/need for further procedure

- Class II compression stockings to be worn for at least 4–6 weeks after surgery
- May require injection sclerotherapy for residual varicosities

Further reading

Mundy L, Merlin TL, Fitridge RA, et al. Systematic review of endovenous laser treatment for varicose veins. Br J Surg 2005;**92**(10):1189–94.

National Institute for Clinical Excellence. Radiofrequency Ablation of Varicose Veins. Interventional procedure guidance IPG8. London: NICE, 2003.

Patient information—endovenous therapy. Available at: ℬ www.cks.nhs.uk, ℬ www. circulationfoundation.org.uk and ℬ www.nhs.uk (accessed 17 May 2011).

Endocrine surgery

Adrenalectomy

Description

The adrenal glands are paired retroperitoneal organs situated superior to the kidneys. They consist of two functional units, the adrenal cortex (secreting glucocorticoids (cortisol), mineralocorticoids (aldosterone), and sex hormones) and the adrenal medulla (secreting catecholamines, e.g. noradrenaline, adrenaline, and dopamine).

Adrenal masses can be classified into functioning and non-functioning tumours. In over 5% of routine cross-sectional imaging, an incidental adrenal mass (incidentaloma) may be found. Benign adrenal adenomas represent the commonest adrenal tumours (>60%). Adrenocortical carcinoma is rare and carries a dismal prognosis. Metastases to the adrenal gland from melanoma, lung, breast, and renal carcinoma can be found in up to 73% of cases. Indications for surgery are listed as follows.

Non-functioning tumours

- Incidentaloma >4cm or increasing in size
- Symptomatic adrenal cyst/angiolipoma
- Solitary adrenal metastasis
- Adrenocortical carcinoma

Functioning tumours

- Phaeochromocytoma
- Conn's syndrome (adenoma)
- Cushing's syndrome
- Unsuccessful hypophysectomy for Cushing's disease
- Bilateral adrenal hyperplasia
- Feminizing/virilizing tumours
- Adrenocortical carcinoma
  Preoperative work-up for these patients include:
- Metaiodobenzylguanidine (MIBG) scintigraphy and [^{18}F]2-fluoro-2-deoxy-D-glucose positron emission tomography (FDG-PET) may be used selectively
- Assessment of hormonal function
- Lateralization of abnormal function—angiography and adrenal vein sampling may be used to accurately determine laterality of disease in Conn's syndrome
- Preoperative control of hormonal dysfunction is mandatory (e.g. α-adrenergic blockade in phaeochromocytoma, control of blood pressure and hypokalaemia in Conn's syndrome)

Cross-sectional imaging

CT and MRI are the gold standard and allow for assessment of size and further characterization of the mass. Size is the strongest predictor of malignancy (prevalence of adrenocortical cancer: 2% with lesions <4cm, 6% with lesions 4.1–6cm, 25% with lesions >6cm)[1]

Operative procedure

Laparoscopic adrenalectomy represents the standard of care for resection of benign functioning or non-functioning adrenal tumours. More recently, the retroperitoneoscopic adrenalectomy is gaining wider acceptance. There is currently little evidence to support the oncological safety of laparoscopic techniques in management of adrenocortical cancer and thus an open adrenalectomy is recommended.

Approach to the adrenal glands requires clear appreciation of anatomy and the relationship of the glands to other retroperitoneal organs. The laparoscopic transperitoneal adrenalectomy is carried out with the patient in the lateral decubitus position. A four-port technique is commonly used for approach to the right adrenal gland with the most medial port being used for insertion of a liver retractor.

The right adrenal gland is exposed by rotating the liver medially by dividing the triangular ligament. On the left, a three-port technique is used. Exposure of the left adrenal gland requires division of the lienophrenic ligament and medial rotation of the spleen. It is of paramount importance to ensure minimal traction on the liver or the spleen to prevent problematic haemorrhage from capsular tears.

The right adrenal vein has a short drainage course into the inferior vena cava. In up to 20% of cases, the adrenal vein may drain into an accessory right hepatic vein. Incision of the peritoneal layer over the right adrenal gland is followed by dissection along the course of the retrohepatic inferior vena cava to its confluence with the adrenal vein. The adrenal vein is skeletonized and ligated. Blood supply to the adrenal gland is segmental and individual feeding arteries need to be accurately controlled.

Exposure of the left adrenal gland follows the same principles. Care is required to preserve the left renal vein, particularly if an accessory adrenal vein drains into it. Dissection of the adrenal gland is carried out within the peri-adrenal fat with careful attention to haemostasis and minimal manipulation of the gland. On the left, the tail of the pancreas is in close proximity to the gland and needs to be avoided. Where tumour infiltration into the surrounding tissues is encountered, conversion from a laparoscopic to open technique may be required with view to en-bloc resection of involved organs.

Close postoperative monitoring is specifically required following resection of phaeochromocytomas as large fluctuations in blood pressure are anticipated. Peri- and postoperative glucocorticoid and mineralocorticoid supplementation is initiated as required.

Additional procedures that may become necessary

- Abdominal drain insertion
- Chest drain insertion
- Nephrectomy

Benefits
- *Diagnostic:* to provide a histological diagnosis for underlying adrenal tumour development
- *Therapeutic:* treatment of symptomatic adrenal pathology, remove tumour from adrenal gland whether primary or secondary, restore hormonal equilibrium after surgery with medication as required

Alternative procedures/conservative measures
- *Medical:* conservative watchful waiting with serial radiological follow-up, analgesia, hormonal and steroid therapy as necessary
- *Surgical:* open, laparoscopic, RFA (currently in research phase)

Serious/frequently occurring risks
- Intra-/postoperative haemorrhage from adrenal vein stump, accessory adrenal veins or accessory hepatic veins
- Inadvertent injury to adjacent organ; liver capsule or parenchymal injury, splenic injury requiring splenectomy, bowel injury (especially splenic flexure during left adrenalectomy), damage to the tail of the pancreas, injury to bowel during laparoscopic port insertion
- Pleural effusion/lower lobe pneumonia
- DVT/pulmonary embolism
- Pneumothorax
- Postoperative adrenal insufficiency (addisonian crisis)
- Death (2009 national crude mortality rate 0.6%)[2]

Blood transfusion necessary
- Group and save

Type of anaesthesia/sedation
- General anaesthesia with appropriate invasive and non-invasive monitoring (central venous pressure (CVP)/arterial line)

Follow-up/need for further procedure
- Routine postoperative surgical follow-up to ensure satisfactory healing
- Endocrinological follow-up for clinical and biochemical confirmation of cure (e.g. reduction in antihypertensive requirements and potassium supplementation in Conn's syndrome)
- Short Synacthen test—indicated following unilateral adrenalectomy in Cushing's syndrome as predictor of return of contralateral adrenal function

References
1. Zeiger MA, Thompson GB, Duh QY, *et al.*; American Association of Clinical Endocrinologists; American Association of Endocrine Surgeons. American Association of Clinical Endocrinologists and American Association of Endocrine Surgeons Medical Guidelines for the Management of Adrenal Incidentalomas: executive summary of recommendations. *Endocr Pract* 2009;**15**:450–3.
2. *British Association of Endocrine and Thyroid Surgeons. Third National Audit Report.* Oxfordshire: Dendrite Clinical Systems, 2009.

Parathyroidectomy

Description

Hyperparathyroidism (HPT) is a condition of abnormal excessive parathyroid hormone (PTH) production and a resultant calcium and phosphate disturbance. It is broadly categorized into primary, secondary (e.g. chronic kidney disease), and tertiary. Primary HPT is the commonest metabolic condition requiring surgical intervention. Commonly, it is as a result of a single hyperfunctioning adenoma (80%) and less frequently due to multiple gland hyperplasia (~15%). Parathyroid carcinoma is a rare cause (<1%).

Indications for surgery

- Symptomatic primary HPT ± evidence of end-organ damage (e.g. nephrolithiasis, osteopaenia/porosis)
- Asymptomatic primary HPT (meeting National Institutes of Health (NIH) criteria: age <50 years, osteitis fibrosa cystica, nephrocalcinosis, serum $[Ca^{2+}]$ >1mg/dl above normal range, urinary calcium excretion >400mg/day, reduced bone mineral density >2SD matched controls, surveillance not possible or undesirable)[1]
- Hypercalcaemic crisis (Ca >3.5mmol/L)
- Parathyroid carcinoma
- Renal HPT (current practice follows evidence-based guidelines, e.g. Kidney Disease Outcomes Quality Initiative (KDOQI))[2]

Preoperative work-up

- Unequivocal biochemical diagnosis is mandatory (exclude other causes, e.g. familial hypocalciuric hypercalcaemia)[3]
- Assessment of severity of HPT and evidence of end-organ damage
- Imaging: extensive attempts should be made to localize the abnormal glands with concordance between two imaging modalities.[4] The commonest imaging techniques uses are ultrasound and sestamibi-scintigraphy. Other techniques are selectively used (e.g. CT, MRI, PET, selective venous sampling). Localization is seldom indicated in primary surgery for renal HPT. Localization studies do not impact cure rates but influence the choice for targeted approach to parathyroidectomy
- Preoperative vocal cord check (mandatory)[5]

Operative procedure

The surgical management of HPT requires a thorough understanding of the anatomy and embryology of the parathyroid glands. The surgical approach (bilateral cervical exploration versus focused approach) may be dictated by the localization studies and the underlying pathology. Accurate localization allows for the use of focused and minimally invasive techniques.

The open/bilateral cervical exploration remains the gold standard approach. An open parathyroidectomy is performed through a 4–5cm midline cervical incision with dissection through layers as for a thyroidectomy. The superior glands are constant in position and lie in a more posterior plane to the thyroid gland and intimately related to the recurrent laryngeal nerve, which lies in a medial plane at the level of the larynx. The position of the inferior glands is more variable, and they are often found within the thyrothymic ligament. However they can occur anywhere along the line of decent of the gland from foramen caecum to the mediastinum.

The aim of parathyroidectomy is to remove the pathological gland(s). In multiple gland disease two, three, three-and-half or all four glands may be excised. In rare occurrence of ectopic parathyroid glands, exploration of paraoesophageal space, the carotid sheath and the anterior mediastinum (via a sternotomy) may be required. More recently, rapid intraoperative PTH analysis has been used to aid intraoperative validation of cure.

Additional procedures that may become necessary
- Drain insertion
- Multiple parathyroidectomy
- Rarely thyroid lobectomy for an intra-thyroidal gland

Benefits
- *Diagnostic:* provide histological diagnosis for underlying parathyroid abnormality
- *Therapeutic:* prevention of complications of symptomatic HPT and prevent associated end-organ damage, treatment of parathyroid carcinoma

Alternative procedures/conservative measures
- *Medical:* conservative watchful waiting with serial radiological follow-up, analgesia, biochemical and electrolyte correction with calcium binding agents as necessary, and calcimimetics e.g. Cinacalcet

Serious/frequently occurring risks
- Early postoperative haemorrhage requiring reoperation (0.6–0.8%)[5]
- Injury to the recurrent laryngeal nerve (primary surgery = 0.8%, redo surgery 2%)[4]
- Failure to cure (overall ~5%[5]—rates are marginally higher in un-localized disease and multiple endocrine neoplasia (MEN) 1)
- Postoperative hypocalcaemia
- Complication rates are higher in reoperative cases

Blood transfusion necessary
- None/group and save

Type of anaesthesia/sedation
- Local/regional anaesthesia may be feasible in minimally invasive/focused approach
- General anaesthesia required for cervical exploration

Follow-up/need for further procedure
- Interval follow-up to ensure normalization of calcium and PTH
- Postoperative vocal cord check (recommended)[3]

References

1. National Institutes of Health. *Diagnosis and Management of Asymptomatic Primary Hyperparathyroidism*. NIH Consensus Statement 1990;8(7):1–18.
2. National Kidney Foundation. KDOQI clinical practice guidelines: bone metabolism and disease in chronic kidney disease. *Am J Kidney Dis* 2003;42(Suppl 4):S1–S201.
3. British Association of Endocrine and Thyroid Surgeons. *Pre and Post Operative Laryngoscopy in Thyroid and Parathyroid Surgery*. British Association of Endocrine and Thyroid Surgeons Consensus 2010.
4. British Association of Endocrine Surgeons. *Guidelines for the Surgical Management of Endocrine Disease and Training Requirements for Endocrine Surgery*. Available at: ⅋ www.baets.org.uk/Pages/BAE_S%20Guidelines.pdf (accessed 25 May 2011).
5. British Association of Endocrine and Thyroid Surgeons. *Third National Audit Report*. Oxford-shire: Dendrite Clinical Systems, 2009.

Thyroidectomy

Description
Thyroid surgery involves a variety of operations including:
- Total thyroidectomy
- Hemithyroidectomy (excision of one thyroid lobe and the isthmus)
- Isthmusectomy (resection of the isthmus only)
- Subtotal thyroidectomy (seldom practised due to high recurrence/reoperation rate)

Indications for surgery
- Goitre/nodule with local compressive symptoms
- Graves' thyrotoxicosis refractory/unsuitable to medical treatment
- Thyroid cancer
- Diagnostic procedure for a cytologically indeterminate lesion
- Improving cosmesis in a large goitre

Preoperative work-up
- Assessment of thyroid function—thyroidectomy is contraindicated in uncontrolled thyrotoxicosis
- Cytological assessment of a solitary nodule (fine needle aspiration cytology (FNAC))
- Imaging—assessment of functionality with I^{123} scintigraphy, ultrasound and cross-sectional imaging with CT (for assessment of retrosternal/mediastinal extension and airway compromise)
- Preoperative vocal cord check (mandatory)[1]

Operative procedure
The patient is prepared supine with next extension (Fig. 5.1). A transverse (Kocker's) skin crease incision is made 1–2cm below the cricoid cartilage (Fig. 5.2). Platysmal flaps are raised with preservation of the anterior jugular veins. The strap muscles are separated along their midline raphe and the plane between the thyroid gland and the strap muscles created. Ligation of the middle thyroid vein confers further mobility to the gland.

The upper pole of the thyroid gland is isolated by ligation and division of the superior thyroidal vessels. Care is taken to preserve the external branch of the superior laryngeal nerve in the avascular space between the upper pole and the cricothyroid muscle. The superior parathyroid gland and the recurrent laryngeal nerve (RLN) are identified and preserved. The branches of the inferior thyroidal artery and veins are ligated in the per-capsular plane of the thyroid. Inferiorly, the thyroid gland is dissected from the thyrothymic ligament, while identifying and preserving the inferior parathyroid glands.

Dissection at Berry's ligament requires special care due to the close proximity of RLN entering the larynx. Meticulous attention to haemostasis is mandatory. Occult venous bleeding can be identified by placing the patient head down and increasing venous pressure with the Valsalva manoeuvre. Closure is carried out with approximation of the strap muscles, platysma, and the skin.

In a hemithyroidectomy, the dissection is completed at the level of the isthmus with excision of the pyramidal lobe (present in ~80%). A total thyroidectomy involves the dissection of the contralateral lobe following the principles already outlined. In the presence of a retrosternal goitre, a sternotomy is occasionally required (<10% of cases).

Additional procedures that may become necessary

- Drain insertion
- Parathyroid autotransplantation

Benefits

- *Diagnostic:* obtain a histopathological diagnosis of underlying thyroid pathology
- *Therapeutic:* treatment of symptomatic thyroid pathology, remove tumour of thyroid gland whether primary or secondary, restore hormonal equilibrium with surgery and postoperative thyroid hormone replacement as required

Alternative procedures/conservative measures

- Selective cervical lymphadenectomy (levels III–VI) is recommended for locoregional control in clinically apparent lymph node metastases. In medullary thyroid cancer bilateral cervical lymphadenectomy is recommended
- The role of prophylactic central compartment (level VI) lymphadenectomy in management of papillary thyroid cancer is contentious and currently recommended in patients with clinically uninvolved central compartment nodes and more advanced tumours (stages T3 and T4)[3]
- Radio-iodine thyroid ablation
- Chemical (drug induced) thyroid suppression

Serious/frequently occurring risks

- Early postoperative haemorrhage requiring reintervention (maximal risk in the first 6–12h, overall rate 0.9%)[2]
- Voice change (overall 4.9%)[2]
- Injury to the RLN (overall 2.5%)[2]
- Hypocalcaemia (may be temporary or permanent; overall rate 11%, long-term 7%)[2]
- Mortality (0.24%)[2]
- Risk of RLN palsy and postoperative hypocalcaemia is greater following lateral cervical lymphadenectomy
- Complication rates are higher in reoperative cases. Individual surgeon complication rates vary and may depend on caseload

Blood transfusion necessary

- None/group and save

Type of anaesthesia/sedation

- General anaesthesia

Follow-up/need for further procedure

- Check for calcium and PTH homeostasis following a total thyroidectomy
- Thyroid function test (thyroxine replacement is titrated against clinical and biochemical response)
- Post-operative vocal cord check (recommended)[1]

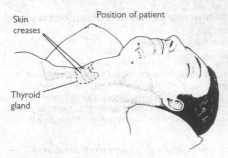

Fig. 5.1 Patient positioning for thyroidectomy.

Reproduced with permission from McLatchie GR and Leaper DJ. *Oxford Specialist Handbook of Operative Surgery* 2nd edition. 2006. Oxford: Oxford University Press, p.647, Figure 15.3a.

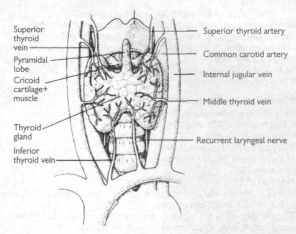

Fig. 5.2 Gross anatomy and vascular supply to the thyroid gland.

Reproduced with permission from McLatchie GR and Leaper DJ. *Oxford Specialist Handbook of Operative Surgery* 2nd edition. 2006. Oxford: Oxford University Press, p.177, Figure 5.8.

References

1. Palazzo F. *Pre and Post Operative Laryngoscopy in Thyroid and Parathyroid Surgery*. British Association of Endocrine and Thyroid Surgeons Consensus 2010. Available at: ℰ www.baets. org.uk/Pages/Vocal_cord_check_consenus_document_2010_final.pdf (accessed 17 May 2011).
2. British Association of Endocrine and Thyroid Surgeons. *Third National Audit Report*. Oxfordshire: Dendrite Clinical Systems, 2009.
3. *Revised American Thyroid Association (ATA) Guidelines for Patients With Thyroid Nodules and Differentiated Thyroid Cancer*. American Thyroid Association, 2009.

Breast surgery

Axillary lymph node dissection

Description

Axillary nodal status is the single most important prognostic indicator of systemic relapse in breast cancer. This is routinely assessed with a pre-operative ultrasound scan and FNA analysis of any pathological nodes. Axillary lymph node dissection (ALND) remains the gold standard of managing clinically positive axillary lymph nodes or following a positive sentinel lymph node biopsy.[1]

Anatomically, the axilla can be divided into three zones (Fig. 6.1):

• Level I nodes: inferior to pectoralis minor
• Level II nodes: posterior to pectoralis minor
• Level III nodes: superior to pectoralis minor

Routine practice involves the dissection of lymph nodes up to level II, where level III clearance may be selectively carried out in the presence of extensive level II lymph node metastases.

Procedure

Access to the axilla is best achieved via a 5–8cm horizontal or vertical incision. When performing a mastectomy, the axillary contents are reached via the same mastectomy wound as a continuation of the axillary tail of the breast.

Dissection involves incising the clavipectoral fascia to gain access to the axillary contents. Lateral border of pectoralis major is identified and the plane between the lateral chest wall and the axilla is created. On the posterior aspect of this space, the long thoracic nerve (nerve to serratus anterior) is identified and preserved. The dissection is continued cranially to the apex of the axilla where the axillary vein forms the superior boundary of level I nodes. Care must be taken to avoid avulsion of branches of the lateral thoracic vein from the main axillary vein trunk as troublesome bleeding will be encountered.

At this point, the thoracodorsal pedicle is identified and preserved. All axillary tissue is swept caudally off the axillary vein and laterally to the medial border of the latissimus dorsi (LD) muscle, which forms the lateral border of the axilla. Access to level III nodes can be aided by abduction and flexion of the shoulder, which relaxes the fibres of pectoralis major and minor. Where possible, axillary contents are dissected off en bloc. The intercostobrachial nerve traverses the middle of the axilla. Attempt should be made to preserve this nerve unless heavy involvement with nodal metastases may require it to be sacrificed.

Good haemostasis is ensured and routine use of a closed suction drain is common practice. Wound closure is carried out in layers using absorbable sutures.

Serious/frequently occurring risks[2]

• Wound infection
• Bleeding and haematoma formation
• Lymphoedema (rates of up to 20%)
• Venous thrombosis (axillary vein)
• Sensory loss medial aspect of upper arm (intercostobrachial nerve palsy; >50%)

- Arm stiffness (20–30%)
- Chronic pain
- Winging of the scapula (long thoracic nerve palsy—rare)
- Arm weakness (thoracodorsal nerve or long thoracic nerve injury—rare)

Blood transfusion necessary

- None (but group and save recommended)

Type of anaesthesia/sedation

- General anaesthesia
- Infiltration of local anaesthesia into the wound for postoperative analgesia

Follow-up/need for further procedure

- Routine postoperative wound check
- Review of histology and decision for adjuvant treatments
- Aspiration of seroma or haematoma if symptomatic

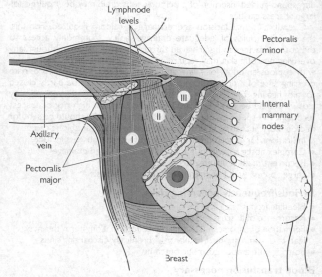

Fig. 6.1 Breast and axillary anatomy.

Reproduced with permission from Chaudry MA and Winslet MC. *Oxford Specialist Handbook of Surgical Oncology*. 2009. Oxford: Oxford University Press, p.115, Figure 2.6.

References

1. National Institute for Health and Clinical Excellence. *NICE Guidance: Early and Locally Advanced Breast Cancer*. London: NICE, 2009.
2. Mansel RE Fallowfield L, Kissin M, et al. Randomized multicenter trial of sentinel node biopsy versus standard axillary treatment in operable breast cancer: the ALMANAC Trial. *J Natl Cancer Inst* 2006;**98**(9):599–609.

Management of breast abscess

Description
Breast abscesses can be broadly divided into lactational and non-lactational causes. An abscess can complicate up to 10% of lactational mastitis and may affect up to 2.5% of breastfeeding mothers. The commonest cause of non-lactational breast abscess is periductal mastitis. Smoking is the strongest risk factor for this. An abscess may also arise from infective exacerbation of skin lesions (e.g. sebaceous cysts or hidradenitis suppurativa). Presentation of mastitis or a breast abscess in postmenopausal women should raise the suspicion of an inflammatory carcinoma and when tolerated, routine triple assessment should be completed.

The principal pathway of managing breast abscesses is by non-operative means. Serial ultrasound guided aspiration (± washout) of the abscess cavity is augmented with an appropriate antibiotic cover.[1] This commonly achieves a successful resolution of the abscess with superior cosmetic outcomes compared with incision and drainage. Occasionally, an ultrasound-guided insertion of a percutaneous drain may be required for large abscess cavities.

Overall, a formal incision and drainage is seldom required. For this, the core principles of 'adequate drainage' apply. Commonly access to the abscess cavity can be achieved through a small incision, although any overlying necrotic skin may require an excision. The cavity is washed out with copious amounts of saline and gently packed with an appropriate dressing. Use of a drain is rarely required. Wounds can be partly closed to aid healing by secondary intention. Attempt at delayed primary closure should be carefully considered as it carries a high risk of abscess recurrence. A specimen of pus or tissue from the cavity should be sent for microbiological analysis in order to direct appropriate antibiotic cover.

Indications for an incision and drainage of a breast abscess include:
- Complex abscess cavity not amenable to ultrasound drainage
- Recurrent/multiloculated abscess cavity
- Large abscess with significant overlying skin necrosis

Serious/frequently occurring risks
- Bleeding from the cavity
- Recurrence of abscess requiring further drainage
- Formation of chronic, multiloculated collection. Long-term this may lead to a mammary duct fistula or a chronically discharging sinus
- Scarring with a poor cosmetic outcome

Blood transfusion necessary
- None

Type of anaesthesia/sedation
- Image-guided aspiration/drainage carried out under local anaesthesia
- Surgical drainage carried out under general anaesthesia

Follow-up/need for further procedure

- Daily wound irrigation, packing of cavity to allows healing by secondary intention
- A delayed primary closure can be considered if wound remains clean and dry to aid faster healing of skin
- Where a non-infective aetiology is suspected (e.g. inflammatory carcinoma or underlying ductal carcinoma *in situ* (DCIS) with comedo necrosis), definitive triple assessment is mandatory

Reference

1. Dixon JM. Outpatient treatment of non-lactational breast abscess. *Br J Surg* 1992;**79**(1):5.

Reduction mammoplasty

Description

Reduction mammoplasty is a common cosmetic procedure used to reduce the size and alter the shape of the breast.

The indications for a reduction mammoplasty include:

- Symptomatic gigantomastia (e.g. resulting in chronic shoulder, neck and back pain, persistent intertrigo, shoulder grooving/ulceration from bra straps)
- Virginal breast hypertrophy (have high rate of recurrence following surgery)
- Gynaecomastia
- Patient preference/to improve cosmesis
- As part of contralateral symmetrization after breast reconstruction

Recently, mammoplasty techniques have been amalgamated with oncological breast surgery as part of oncoplastic breast surgery. This has broadened the application of breast-conserving surgery, allowing for wide excisions of the tumour, while maintaining the optimal breast shape.

Procedure

To date several different mammoplasty techniques have been described. Common to all is the reduction in breast volume that is achieved by excision of skin, fat, and glandular tissue, with subsequent repositioning of the nipple–areolar complex (NAC).

Some of the commonly utilized techniques include:

- *The Wise pattern mammoplasty* (Fig. 6.2)—this remains the most popular technique allowing for safe excision of large volumes of glandular tissue. Maintaining an adequate dermoglandular pedicle (commonly inferior or superomedial pedicle) preserves the blood supply to the NAC. The resultant scar has an inverted 'T' shape
- *(Lejour)[1] vertical mammoplasty*—this technique is a modification of the technique described by Lassus[2] and further popularized by Hall-Findlay,[3] excises the bulk of breast tissue directly inferior to the NAC. The breast envelope is reapproximated, leaving a vertical scar only
- *The 'Round-block' (Benelli)[4] technique*—this technique involves a periareolar incision and excision of a 'donut' of breast tissue. Reapproximation of the periareolar incision allows for a more discrete scar. The procedure can be combined with an augmentation mammoplasty to correct any ptosis. Limitations remain in the amount of glandular tissue that may be excised

The choice of the techniques is dependent on patient as well as surgeon factors. The breast tissue is commonly excised using sharp dissection (with a knife) or with the use of diathermy. Excessive bleeding can be minimized by infiltration of breast tissue with a diluted adrenaline solution (typically 1:1000 solution). Care is required to preserve an adequate width of the dermoglandular pedicle in order to preserve nipple–areolar viability. Careful haemostasis is of paramount importance. The routine use of suction drains have not been show to alter outcomes.

Serious/frequently occurring risks
- Early bleeding/haematoma formation requiring re-exploration (~5%)
- Wound infection
- Wound dehiscence (specially the T-junction scar in a Wise pattern mastectomy)
- Change in sensation of nipple (30–40%)
- Nipple loss (1–5%)
- Scarring (including widened/hypertrophic or keloid scars)
- Poor cosmesis
- Inability to breastfeed

Blood transfusion necessary
- None (group and save sufficient)

Type of anaesthesia/sedation
- General anaesthesia
- Local anaesthetic infiltration for postoperative analgesia

Follow-up/need for further procedure
- Routine postoperative review to ensure satisfactory wound healing and cosmetic outcome
- Following oncoplastic surgery, review of final histological results and plans for adjuvant therapies required

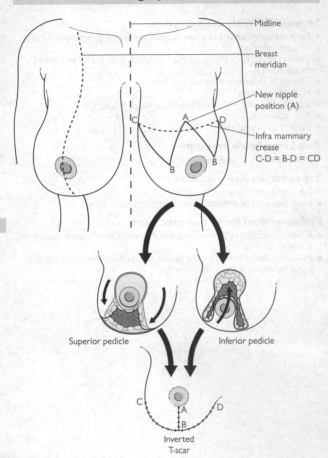

Fig. 6.2 Reduction mammoplasty (Wise pattern).

Reproduced with permission from Chaudry MA and Winslet MC. *Oxford Specialist Handbook of Surgical Oncology*. 2009. Oxford: Oxford University Press, p.133, Figure 2.13.

References

1. Lejour M. Verical mammoplasty and liposuction of the breast. *Plast Reconstr Surg.* 1994;**94**(1):100–14.
2. Lassus C. A technique for breast reduction. *Int Surg* 1970;**55**(1):69–72.
3. Hall-Findlay EJ. A simplified vertical reduction mammoplasty: shortening the learning curve. *Plast Reconstr Surg* 1999;**104**(3):748–59.
4. Benelli L. A new periareolar mammoplasty: the 'round block' technique. *Aesthetic Plast Surg* 1990;**14**(2):93–100.

Implant-based breast reconstruction

Description

Implant-based breast reconstructions are a frequently performed technique and according to recent national data, account for 37% of all immediate and 16% of delayed reconstructions following a mastectomy.[1]

The key advantages of implant reconstructions are the relatively short operative time and quicker postoperative recovery. However, unlike autologous reconstructions, the cosmetic outcome can be variable and the volume and projection of the reconstructed breast can be limited. Furthermore, the effects of radiotherapy to the final aesthetic result are significant where implants have been used. The pros and cons of implant-based reconstruction need to be clearly outlined to the patient prior to surgery.

Procedure

The principal consideration of an implant-based reconstruction is whether there is adequate implant cover beneath the mastectomy skin flaps. The placement of the implant in the subpectora space (posterior to the pectoralis major) is deemed the gold standard. However, this space is limited and therefore tissue expanders are often used to create a larger submuscular space.

The access to the subpectoral space is carried out by a muscle-splitting approach along the fibres of pectoralis major or via its lateral free border with the chest wall (Fig. 6.3). Careful submuscular dissection is performed with special attention to haemostasis Once the implant is positioned in place, muscle fibres are closed over it for complete coverage. Postoperatively, the tissue expander is gradually filled with saline over several weeks, until the desired volume is reached. A number of adjustable implants/expanders (e.g. Becker adjustable implant) allow for a single stage procedure, where the injection port can be removed once the desired volume is reached.

The standard approach is a two-staged procedure where at the second stage, adjustments the implant capsule (capsulotomy) can be made and the tissue expander is a replaced for a definitive fixed volume implant. The critical area of inadequate muscle cover is the inferior border of pectoralis major, where additional implant cover is achieved using a dermal sling as part of a Wise pattern mastectomy or an acellular dermal allograft (e.g. Alloderm). This also allows the use of fixed-volume implants in the immediate reconstruction setting and allows the implant to sit lower on the chest wall thus achieving a better natural shape.

Implants may also be used to augment an autologous reconstruction (specially an LD flap) in cases where the volume of autologous tissue available may not be adequate to achieve symmetry with the contralateral breast.

Additional procedures that may become necessary

- Contralateral symmetrization surgery
- Capsulotomy and replacement of tissue expander implant for a definitive implant (two-stage reconstruction)

Serious/frequently occurring risks

- Wound infection
- Periprosthetic infection
- Bleeding and haematoma formation
- Seroma
- Capsular contracture (may be de novo or as consequence of periprosthetic infection or concurrent postoperative chest wall radiotherapy)
- Postoperative pain
- Implant/tissue expander failure (rare)
- Poor cosmetic outcome
- Need for revision surgery to improve cosmetic outcome (estimated 40% risk of requiring further surgery over a 4-year period)

Blood transfusion necessary

- None

Type of anaesthesia/sedation

- General anaesthesia

Follow-up/need for further procedure

- Wound check to ensure healing of mastectomy scar
- Review of histology and plans for adjuvant therapies
- Serial instillation of saline into the expander implant to achieve the desired volume and projection

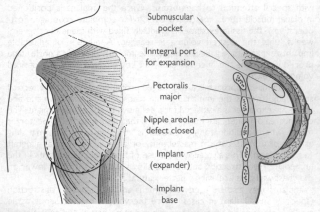

Fig. 6.3 Implant-reconstruction post skin-sparing mastectomy.

Reproduced with permission from Chaudry MA and Winslet MC. *Oxford Specialist Handbook of Surgical Oncology. 2009. Oxford: Oxford University Press, p.140, Figure 2.18.*

Reference

1. Clinical Effectiveness Unit, The Royal College of Surgeons of England, Association of Breast Surgery at the British Association of Surgical Oncology, British Association of Plastic, Reconstructive and Aesthetic Surgeons, Royal College of Nursing, and The NHS Information Centre for health and social care. *Second National Mastectomy and Reconstruction Audit*, NHS National Information Centre, 2009.

Deep inferior epigastric perforator flap (DIEP flap)

Description

Attempts at reducing the donor site morbidity from transverse rectus abdominis myocutaneous (TRAM) flaps led to the development of muscle-sparing techniques and later the deep inferior epigastric perforator (DIEP) free flap. It was first described by Allen and Treece in 1992.[1] Today, DIEP represents the gold standard method for autologous free flap breast reconstruction, using abdominal tissue.

Potentially any woman who has had a mastectomy is candidate for DIEP flap reconstruction. Relative contraindications include a history of heavy smoking, previous long transverse or oblique abdominal incisions or where one or both deep inferior epigastric vessels have been ligated. The need for post-mastectomy radiotherapy has been shown in several series to result in an inferior cosmetic results in all reconstruction, although autologous reconstructions are deemed more resistant. There is as yet no concrete evidence to suggest radiotherapy may lead to delayed flap necrosis and thus it is not considered a contraindication.

Procedure

The DIEP flap is based on the deep inferior epigastric vessels, from which two rows of arteries and veins perforate the rectus abdominis muscle on each side to supply the ipsilateral skin and subcutaneous fat. Preoperative cross-sectional imaging has been shown to help accelerate flap harvesting and to potentially identify a dominant superficial inferior epigastric systems. Preoperative markings delineate the boundaries of the breast/mastectomy cavity and the length of abdominal flap. The latter is similar to the marking of an abdominoplasty.

The abdominal flap is harvested with identification of the lateral and medial rows of the deep inferior epigastric perforators. These are then traced down to their origin, between the fibres of the rectus abdominis muscle and with full preservation of muscle function and innervation. With the vascular pedicle to the free flap isolated, it is transported to the chest and a microvascular anastomosis is fashioned to the internal mammary (and occasionally the thoracodorsal) vessels. For a bilateral reconstruction, tissue from the two halves of the abdomen needs to be harvested on separate perforator pedicles.

The flap is appropriately inset in the mastectomy cavity and the skin envelope resected to fit the mastectomy flaps. The incised anterior rectus sheath is reapproximated using a non-absorbable suture. The umbilicus is sutured in its new position and the abdominal wound closed over two suction drains.

Higher-level postoperative care is essential for regular monitoring of flap viability in the first 24–48h. Low index of suspicion should be kept for a possible haematoma and/or problems with the vascular anastomosis. Early return to theatre for an exploration is an important determinant of salvaging a threatened free flap.

Limited restriction of activity with graded physiotherapy (i.e. raising arms, lifting etc.) for at least 6 weeks postoperatively is associated with a reduction in recipient complication rates.

Additional procedures that may become necessary
- If an adequate calibre perforator vessel is absent—conversion of the procedure to a free TRAM flap

Serious/frequently occurring risks
Complications of a DIEP flap reconstruction are divided into general, donor site, and flap-related problems
- General complications
  - Deep vein thrombosis ± pulmonary embolism (long procedure and prolonged immobility)
  - Basal atelectasis/postoperative pneumonia (poor respirator function and splinting of diaphragm due to donor site pain and tightness of abdominal closure)
- Donor site complications
  - Seroma
  - Haematoma
  - Wound dehiscence and wound infection
  - Umbilical necrosis (1–5%)
  - Pain and discomfort due to tightness of abdominal wound
  - Abdominal hernia (0.6–1.4%)
- Flap related complications
  - Haematoma
  - Thrombosis
  - Early re-exploration for flap related problems (6%)
  - Partial (2.5%) or complete flap failure (1%)
  - Fat necrosis and loss of flap volume (13%)

Blood transfusion necessary
- None (but group and save is needed)

Type of anaesthesia/sedation
- General anaesthesia (often local anaesthetic has to be infiltrated at donor site on completion of the procedure)

Follow-up/need for further procedure
- Meticulous wound care and maintenance of physiology to optimize flap perfusion and reduce donor/recipient site complications in the perioperative and the immediate postoperative period
- Routine postoperative wound check
- Following an immediate reconstruction, review of final histology and plans for an any adjuvant treatment is needed
- Nipple-areolar reconstruction

Reference
1. Allen RJ, Treece P. Deep inferior epigastric perforator flap for breast reconstruction. *Ann Plast Surg* 1994;**32**:32.

Excision biopsy of breast lump/ lumpectomy

Description

The outcome of the triple assessment for a breast lesion dictates the surgical therapy that ensues. In some circumstances, the preoperative assessment may yield inconclusive or indeterminate results thus requiring an excision biopsy to confirm the histological diagnosis. Where a lesion is preoperatively proven to be benign, decision to excise the lesion may be due to patient preference, the size of the lesion (e.g. a large (>2cm) fibroadenoma) or suspicious clinical features. Both approaches involve an excision of the target lesion with minimal disruption of surrounding normal breast tissue.

Current guidelines of the Association of Breast Surgery recommend that a preoperative diagnosis is achieved in over 90% of cases and that excision biopsy is confined to no greater than 25g of tissue.[1] Small impalpable lesions may need to be preoperatively localized using ultrasound marking and/or wire-guided techniques.

Indications for an excision biopsy/lumpectomy

- Excision of a proven benign lesion due to:
  - Patient preference
  - Large lesions resulting in a cosmetic defect
  - Suspicious clinical history
- Lesions with indeterminate or atypical histology (B3) on preoperative assessment (e.g. ADH, ALH, ductal hyperplasia of usual type) or suspicious clinical features
- Presence of a radial scar (associated with presence of atypia or malignancy)[2,3]

Serious/frequently occurring risks

- Infection
- Bleeding
- Poor cosmetic outcome
- Need for further surgery

Blood transfusion necessary

- None

Type of anaesthesia/sedation

- General anaesthesia (generally allows for faster lesion localization and better patient compliance)
- Local anaesthesia feasible for small but easily palpable lesions (infiltration of local anaesthesia may result in the lesion becoming difficult to find)

Follow-up/need for further procedure

- Routine wound check (this can be performed safely by the community team/GP) in benign cases
- Multidisciplinary review of histology, specially where preoperative assessment was suspicious or indeterminate
- Further excision may be required if malignancy is confirmed and microscopic resection margins are deemed inadequate

References

1. Association of Breast Surgery. Surgical guidelines for management of breast cancer. *Eur J Surg Oncol* 2009;**35**(Suppl 1):1–22.
2. Radial scar—also known as a complex sclerosing lesion.
3. Kennedy M, Masterson AV, Kerin M, *et al*. Pathology and clinical relevance of radial scars: a review. *J Clin Pathol* 2003;**56**(10):721–4.

Surgery for nipple discharge (microdochectomy/major duct excision)

Description

Nipple discharge accounts for approximately 5% of breast clinic referrals, of which 5% may be caused by underlying *in situ* or malignant disease. Nipple discharge may be coloured, from a single or multiple ducts. Serosanguinous/bloody discharge from a single duct may be associated with a papilloma, ductal hyperplasia, or carcinoma. More commonly the discharge is found to be physiological and associated with underlying duct ectasia.

The assessment of nipple discharge aims to differentiate between benign physiological discharge and ductal pathology. The principal mode of investigation remains the 'triple assessment'. This is augmented by a number of non-surgical techniques that include ductoscopy, ductography, and ductal lavage, but these are seldom used in routine practice. The surgical management of nipple discharge can be diagnostic as well as therapeutic. The two main approaches include microdochectomy (the approach for a single duct discharge) or major duct excision.

Indications

Microdochectomy
- Persistent blood-stained single duct discharge (in woman of child-bearing age planning to breastfeed)
- Presence of ductal lesion identified or ductography or ductoscopy

Major duct excision
- Persistent multiple duct discharge (may be bloody or non-blood stained)
- Persistent single duct discharge in a woman of non-childbearing age
- Treatment of recurrent periductal mastitis
- Management of physiological nipple inversion

Technique

Due to the abundance of ductal flora, antibiotic prophylaxis is often used. There is no evidence to support the routine use of antibiotic therapy postoperatively.

The approach to the mammary ducts can be achieved either via a radial incision or more commonly using a circumareolar incision (typically three-fifths to half of the areolar circumference). In a microdochectomy, it is important to express the duct discharge in theatre in order to identify the offending duct. The duct is then isolated using a lacrimal probe or via injection of methylene blue into the duct.

Ductoscopy can also be used to illuminate the relevant duct. A 2–3cm length of the duct is isolated and excised. Care should be taken to prevent excision/damage to the neighbouring normal ducts.

In a total duct excision (Hadfield's procedure), all ducts are excised from the underside of the nipple. The specimen includes the surrounding breast tissue to a depth of approximately 2cm behind the NAC (Fig. 6.4).

A purse-string dermal suture behind the nipple can be used to minimize nipple inversion. Incisions are closed in layers using absorbable suture.

Additional procedures that may become necessary
- Failure to identify the single duct in microdochectomy—conversion to a major duct excision
- If malignancy is histologically confirmed—an appropriate oncological resection

Serious/frequently occurring risks[1]
- Change/reduction in sensation of nipple (up to 40%)
- Nipple inversion and poor cosmesis
- Nipple ischaemia (<1%)
- Recurrent discharge
- Difficulty/problems breastfeeding

Blood transfusion necessary
- None

Type of anaesthesia/sedation
- General anaesthesia

Follow-up/need for further procedure
- Routine postoperative wound check
- Review of histology and plans for further treatment
- Assessment of cure from symptoms (i.e. persistent discharge)

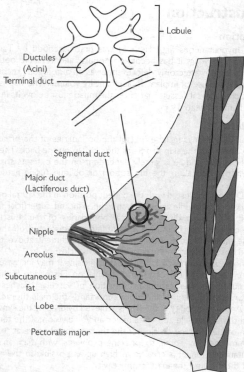

Fig. 6.4 Key breast anatomy.

Reproduced with permission from Gardiner MD and Borley NR. *Training in Surgery*. 2009. Oxford: Oxford University Press, p.43, Figure 3.2.

Reference

1. Dixon JM (ed.) *A Companion to Specialist Surgical Practice—Breast Surgery*. Edinburgh: Elsevier, 2006, p265.

Latissimus dorsi myocutaneous flap reconstruction

Description

The LD myocutaneous flap (Fig. 6.5) was first described by Tansini in 1896. Over the years it has become a popular and versatile option for covering a large mastectomy defect, either as an autologous reconstruction or with the use of implant to augment its volume. The flap is based on the thoracodorsal vessels that enter the muscle just below its insertion into the humoral head.

Procedure

Preoperative markings include that of the boundaries of the breast/mastectomy cavity and the skin paddle of the LD flap on the back. The orientation of the skin paddle is largely dependent on the patients shape and may be horizontal (along the bra straps) or oblique (using natural skin folds).

The LD flap is harvested with the patient position in the lateral position. The marked skin paddle is incised and the skin and superficial fascia is dissected off the proximal and distal boundaries of the muscle. The anterior edge of the LD muscle is identified and dissected off the chest wall. The muscle is detached from its distal attachment above the iliac crest and posteriorly from the paravertebral muscles.

The thoracolumbar fascia is left intact as incising it may increase donor site morbidity and the risk of a lumbar herniation. Dissection of the hilum of the muscle involves careful preservation of vascular braches of the pedicle to serratus anterior and more importantly the main thoracodorsal pedicle. Anterior mobility of the flap is achieved by dividing the synsarcosis between the LD muscle and teres major and/or division of the tendinous insertion of LD. Routine division of the thoracodorsal nerve at this point is recommended by some to prevent problems with flap animation. A subcutaneous tunnel is created as high up as possible in the axilla to transmit the flap into the mastectomy cavity.

The donor site is closed in layers over suction drains. The flap is appropriately inset, the skin paddle trimmed and sutured to the mastectomy flaps. In an implant-augmented reconstruction, the LD muscle provides total muscle coverage of the implant. An extended LD reconstruction is a variation that aims to provide a larger volume of tissue for a complete autologous reconstruction.[1] This approach harvests a greater degree of subfascial fat but also recruits serratus, scapular, and iliac fat pads to gain additional autologous volume.

Postoperative care involves careful observation for flap viability in the first 24–48h, good level of hydration and oxygenation and gradual mobilization of the patient.

Additional procedures that may become necessary

- Nipple–areolar reconstruction
- Contralateral symmetrization procedure

Serious/frequently occurring risks

Complication can be divided into donor site and flap-related problems:
- Flap-related
  - Haematoma
  - Partial or complete flap failure (<1%)
  - Thrombosis
  - Fat necrosis
  - Muscle atrophy and asymmetry due to loss of flap volume
  - Flap animation (as result of tethering of the LD muscle and intact function of thoracodorsal nerve)
- Donor site
  - Skin flap necrosis
  - Wound dehiscence
  - Seroma formation
  - Haematoma formation
  - Arm weakness (related to absence of a functional LD muscle)
  - Chronic donor site pain

Blood transfusion necessary
- None
- Group and save

Type of anaesthesia/sedation
- General anaesthesia (with infiltration of local anaesthetic for postoperative analgesia)

Follow-up/need for further procedure
- Routine postoperative check to ensure satisfactory wound healing and removal of suction drains from the donor site if still *in situ*
- Drainage of donor site seroma (or haematoma)
- If an expander implant is used in a two-stage procedure, tissue expansion is commenced once wounds have healed
- In the immediate reconstruction setting, the final histology and the plans for adjuvant treatment are reviewed and discussed with the patient
- Nipple–areolar reconstruction can be planned for a later date

Huddersfield Health Staff Library
Royal Infirmary (PGMEC)
Lindley
Huddersfield
HD3 3EA

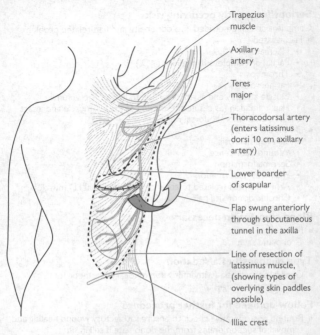

Trapezius muscle

Axillary artery

Teres major

Thoracodorsal artery (enters latissimus dorsi 10 cm axillary artery)

Lower boarder of scapular

Flap swung anteriorly through subcutaneous tunnel in the axilla

Line of resection of latissimus muscle, (showing types of overlying skin paddles possible)

Illiac crest

Fig. 6.5 Latissimus dorsi (LD) flap.

Reproduced with permission from Chaudry MA and Winslet MC. *Oxford Specialist Handbook of Surgical Oncology.* 2009. Oxford: Oxford University Press, p.137, Figure 2.15.

Reference

1. Delay E, Gounot N, Bouillot A, *et al.* Autologous latissimus breast reconstruction: a 3-year clinical experience with 100 patients. *Plast Reconstr Surg* 1998;**102**(5):1461–78.

Mastectomy

Description

Mastectomy is the removal of all breast tissue and some overlying skin including the NAC (Fig. 6.6). Historically, Halstedian theory dictated that breast cancer is a locoregional disease and therefore surgery would include a radical excision of all breast tissue and locoregional axillary nodes, as well as the underlying chest wall musculature (pectoralis major and minor).

More recently Fisherian theory of breast cancer has changed the paradigm of treatment from a locoregional disease to that of systemic control. For this locoregional control would again take the shape of excising breast tissue and relevant regional lymph nodes, while maintaining the integrity of the underlying structures posterior to the mammary gland.

Indications for mastectomy:

- Large tumour where breast-conserving surgery not feasible or likely to result poor cosmetic outcome
- Inflammatory carcinoma
- Multicentricity (tumour deposits in more than one quadrant of the breast)
- Risk-reducing surgery (e.g. BRCA gene mutation carriers)
- Patient preference

Modern-day practice encompasses the following mastectomy techniques:

- *Simple mastectomy:* involves excision of the breast, the overlying skin and NAC only
- *Modified radical mastectomy (Patey's mastectomy):* involves excision of the breast, overlying skin including NAC and axillary node dissection (division of pectoralis minor is seldom required)
- *Skin-sparing mastectomy:* this approach removes all breast tissue (± relevant axillary glands), while maintaining maximum amount of chest wall skin required for a subsequent reconstruction
- *Subcutaneous (nipple-sparing) mastectomy:* this technique removes all subcutaneous breast tissue while preserving the NAC. Controversy remains regarding the oncological safety of preserving the nipple. Intra-operative frozen section analysis of retro-areolar tissue may be used to ensure clear resection margins although the false-negative rate of this technique has been questioned. Therefore this approach is often used selectively, especially in risk-reducing surgery or where the risk of recurrence is estimated to be low. Careful counselling of the patient regarding the risks of local recurrence is the key
- *Wise pattern mastectomy:* this technique amalgamates the standard Wise pattern reduction mammoplasty skin excision and a skin-sparing mastectomy to ultimately reduce the skin envelope of a large breast

Technique

- Following appropriate preoperative planning and skin marking (this would include consideration for reconstruction, degree of skin involvement by tumour etc.), dissection is carried out through the skin and dermis. The 'mastectomy' plane of dissection and the thickness of the mastectomy skin flaps are dependent on the adiposity of the patient

- Careful marking of the breast boundaries is vital in order to prevent over-dissection of the mastectomy cavity, especially if immediate reconstruction is planned. Adherence to the correct plane of dissection ensures adequate oncological resection yet preserving the subdermal vascular plexus that is vital to for skin flap viability. Posterior dissection in the retromammary space should ensure preservation of the fascia over pectoralis major muscle. Dissection of the axillary tail would give access to the contents of the axilla where concurrent axillary surgery can be performed through the same wound
- In skin-sparing mastectomy, the dissection of breast tissue is carried out through a circumareolar incision. In a subcutaneous (nipple-sparing approach), a subareolar incision would allow dissection of the NAC free from the remaining breast tissue. The remainder of the dissection is carried out as previously outlined
- Meticulous haemostasis is mandatory. Use of closed suction drains in the mastectomy cavity is a universally practice. Closure of the wound is carried out in layers using absorbable sutures

Additional procedures that may become necessary

- If there is involvement of the chest wall—(partial) excision of the underlying pectoralis muscle
- Breast reconstruction which may be immediate or delayed—current NICE and British Association of Surgical Oncology guidelines recommend all women being offered reconstructive options if considered for a mastectomy

Serious/frequently occurring risks

- Seroma
- Haematoma
- Mastectomy flap necrosis
- Wound infection (usually consequent to the flap necrosis)
- Poor cosmetic outcome

Blood transfusion necessary

- Group and save is sufficient

Type of anaesthesia/sedation

- General anaesthesia
- Postoperative analgesia—there are several options
  - Local anaesthetic skin infiltration, bathing the mastectomy cavity with local anaesthetic fluid infused via the cavity drains
  - Regional nerve blocks (e.g. paravertebral blocks)

Follow-up/need for further procedure

- Routine postoperative check to ensure satisfactory wound healing ± removal of suction drains
- Review of histology and plans of adjuvant treatment
- Plastic surgical review *if immediate reconstruction* undertaken
- Planning for nipple–areolar reconstruction
- Counselling and planning for a delayed reconstruction

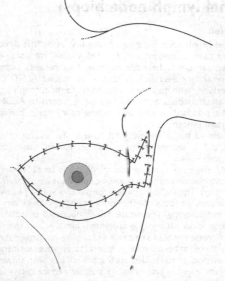

Fig. 6.6 Simple mastectomy with lateral fish tail extension (to remove redundant lateral skin flap).

Reproduced with permission from Chaudry MA and Winslet MC. *Oxford Specialist Handbook of Surgical Oncology*. 2009. Oxford: Oxford University Press p.127 Figure 2.11.

Sentinel lymph node biopsy

Description

The sentinel lymph node is defined as the first node that directly drains the primary tumour. Evidence to date has shown that up to 85% of all stage breast cancers to be node negative, thus patients undergoing an unnecessary axillary clearance. Furthermore, routine ALND carries significant morbidity with no impact on survival. Sentinel lymph node biopsy (SLNB) is an alternative, minimally invasive approach to ALDN that has become the standard of care in prognosticating early, clinically node-negative breast cancer.

The results of the ALMANC trial have so far shown overall lower morbidity and a shorter hospital stay in patient undergoing SLNB compared with ALND.[1]

Currently, the only absolute contraindications to SLNB are clinically node-positive disease and the presence of previous mastectomy (without axillary surgery). The standard of care for patients with a positive sentinel lymph node (tumour focus of >0.2mm) is to undergo an axillary clearance or axillary radiotherapy. The oncological implications of isolated tumour cells (tumour focus <0.2mm) is currently unknown and therefore such patients are treated as SLNB negative and require no further surgery.

Recently, there has been growing interest in techniques for intraoperative analysis of sentinel lymph nodes. Such approach has been shown to avoid repeat surgery, improve patient satisfaction and reduce delays to adjuvant treatment. The techniques used include frozen section analysis and more recently, molecular techniques such as reverse transcriptase polymerase chain reaction (RT-PCR).

Procedure

Current NICE guidelines recommend that SLNB is carried out by a team that is validated in the use of the technique as identified by the NEW START programme.[2,3] This programme has standardized the protocol for sentinel node mapping. It involves dual localization of the sentinel lymph node(s) using technetium-99 labelled nanocolloid and Paten V blue dye.

Access to the axilla can be incorporated into the WLE scar or via a small (commonly <5cm) de novo incision in the axilla. Minimal disruption of the axillary contents is the key. Using a handheld γ-probe, any hot (measured γ-radiation count >x10 background) and/or blue node is excised for histological (or intraoperative) analysis. Meticulous haemostasis is mandatory. The routine use of a suction drain is not indicated. Closure of the wound in layers follows standard practice.

Additional procedures that may become necessary

- Axillary node clearance in sentinel lymph node-positive patients
- Adjuvant chemotherapy or radiotherapy

Serious/frequently occurring risk[1]

- Wound infection
- Haematoma and seroma formation
- Axillary vein thrombosis (in deeper dissections)

- Lymphoedema (overall rate = 5%)[2]
- Sensory loss (intercostobrachial nerve palsy—1% at 12 months)[2]
- Shoulder stiffness (<10%)[2]
- Allergy to Paten V blue dye (0.9%)[4]
- Permanent skin staining with blue dye (<1%)
- Failure to localize the sentinel node (false negative rate <5%)

Blood transfusion necessary

- None necessary

Type of anaesthesia/sedation

- General anaesthesia (with infiltration of local anaesthetic into wound for postoperative analgesia)

Follow-up/need for further procedure

- Routine postoperative wound check
- Assessment of histology and plans for adjuvant treatment
- Aspiration of seroma or haematoma (if symptomatic)

References

1. National Institute for Health and Clinical Excellence *NICE Guidance: Early and Locally Advanced Breast Cancer*. London: NICE 2009.
2. Manse RE, Fallowfield L, Kissin M. et al. Randomized multicenter trial of sentinel node biopsy versus standard axillary treatment in operable breast cancer: the ALMANAC Trial. *J Natl Cancer Inst* 2006;**98**(9):599–609.
3. Raven Department of Education. *NEW START Sentinel Lymph Node Biopsy Training Programme*. Royal College of Surgeons, England (Programme now closed).
4. Barthelmes L, Goyal A, Newcombe RG, et al. and NEW START and ALMANAC study groups. Adverse reactions to patent blue V dye—The NEW START and ALMANAC experience. *Eur J Surg Oncol* 2010;**36**(4):399–403.

Transverse rectus abdominis myocutaneous flap (TRAM flap)

Description

The TRAM flap is an axial pattern pedicle flap popularized following its first description by Hartrampf in 1982.[1] It utilizes a paddle of skin and underlying rectus abdominis muscle, which is mobilized on its pedicle, the deep superior epigastric vessels.

However, it carries two main disadvantages. First, harvesting of significant amounts of rectus sheath and rectus abdominis muscle results in loss of abdominal wall integrity and potential for development of a hernia. The second is the relative unpredictability of the blood supply of any skin harvested beyond the muscle boundary.

Nonetheless, it provides ample tissue for autologous reconstruction of a breast, negating the need for augmentation with an implant. Modifications of this technique include muscle-sparing and the free TRAM flaps, the former resulting in lower risk donor site morbidity related to the abdominal wall. The current practice of using DIEP free flaps has become the gold standard of autologous breast reconstruction using abdominal tissue, and TRAM flaps are seldom used.

Procedure

The TRAM flap (Fig. 6.7) can be used in both the immediate and delayed reconstruction setting. The preoperative skin marking on the abdomen involves a symmetrical abdominal skin ellipse similar to that of an abdominoplasty, within which the skin paddle of the flap is delineated. The myocutaneous flap on the one side of the abdomen provides autologous tissue for the contralateral breast reconstruction.

Careful dissection of skin and dermis preserves the midline-perforating vessels above and below the umbilicus, as well as the subdermal plexus that ensures maximal viability of the skin paddle. Inferiorly, the belly of rectus abdominis is isolated and transected, with ligation of the inferior epigastric vessels. Superiorly the anterior rectus sheath is divided and the muscle and the overlaying fat and skin are elevated. A subcutaneous tunnel from the abdominal wound to the mastectomy cavity transmits the flap, which is then appropriately inset and sutured to the mastectomy skin flaps.

The donor site defect is closed by approximating the anterior rectus sheet superiorly with non-absorbable suture (e.g. no 1. nylon). The defect in the inferior part of the rectus sheath is repaired with a tension free mesh closure. Transposition of the umbilicus on its stalk to its new position concludes closure of the superficial abdominal wound layers. Use of a closed suction drain in the abdominal wound is routine practice.

Serious/frequently occurring risks

These can be *divided into flap related* or donor site related complications:
- Donor site
  - Haematoma
  - Seroma

- Abdominal wound infection and/or dehiscence
- Abdominal wall weakness or frank hernia formation
- Dehiscence/necrosis of umbilicus
- Flap related
  - Partial or total flap failure
  - Poor cosmetic outcome
  - Fat necrosis and loss of flap volume (often related to flap blood supply)
  - Upper abdominal bulging and discomfort related to subcutaneous tunnelling of the flap

Blood transfusion necessary

- Group and save

Type of anaesthesia/sedation

- General anaesthesia (with infiltration of local anaesthetic to donor site wound for postoperative analgesia)

Follow-up/need for further procedure

- Routine postoperative check to ensure adequate wound healing
- Interval check to ensure satisfactory cosmetic outcome/degree of symmetry with contralateral breast and planning for nipple reconstruction

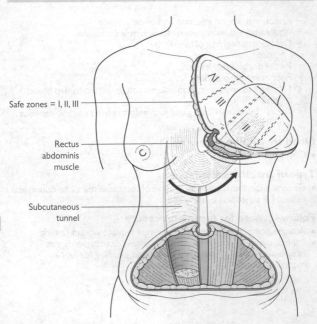

Safe zones = I, II, III

Rectus abdominis muscle

Subcutaneous tunnel

Fig. 6.7 TRAM flap.

Reproduced with permission from Chaudry MA and Winslet MC. *Oxford Specialist Handbook of Surgical Oncology*. 2009. Oxford: Oxford University Press, p.138, Figure 2.16

Reference

1. Hartrampf CR, Scheflan M, Black PW. Breast reconstruction with a transverse abdominal island flap. *Plast Reconstr Surg* 1982;**69**(2):216–25.

Wide local excision of breast tumour

Description

Wide local excision is a term that is synonymous with breast-conserving surgery (BCS), whereby an oncological resection is performed while maintaining as normal a breast shape (Fig 6.8). There are no national guidelines regarding the thickness of resection of margins and locally agreed protocols are followed. Generally, the aim is to achieve macroscopic resection margins of at least 1cm and microscopic resection margins of 1mm and 2mm for invasive and *in situ* carcinoma, respectively. Evidence to date supports the fact that overall local recurrence and survival rates in BCS with postoperative radiotherapy are comparable with that of mastectomy alone.

The principal determinant of a satisfactory cosmetic outcome following a WLE is the proportion of breast tissue that is excised in relation to the total breast size. A resection of greater than 20% of the breast volume significantly impacts the aesthetic outcomes. Therefore recently, a number of plastic surgical techniques have been amalgamated with the oncological breast surgery, with the aim to widen the spectrum of applicability of BCS. These approaches are collectively termed 'oncoplastic breast surgery' and use a myriad of volume displacement, volume replacement and mammoplasty techniques to achieve the optimal aesthetic outcome while avoiding a mastectomy.

Contraindications to a WLE (or BCS) include multicentricity (presence of cancer in more than one quadrant), a high tumour to breast volume ratio (relative contraindication), and inflammatory carcinoma.

Technique

Small, impalpable lesions may require preoperative localization (e.g. ultrasound marking or wire-guided localization). An appropriately placed incision is a key principle in oncoplastic surgery. This minimizes poor cosmetic outcomes and allows for maximum access to the lesion. The full thickness resection aims to achieve macroscopically clear radial margins, and anterior (skin) and posterior (chest wall) margins may be considered less important as postoperative radiotherapy is planned.

Although a number of surgeons would leave the cavity unfilled, this almost always results in poor cosmetic outcomes especially after radiotherapy. Use of oncoplastic techniques with volume displacement techniques helps to obliterate this potential cavity.[1] Where a long subcutaneous tunnel to the lesion is created or where oncoplastic techniques are used to fill the excision cavity, use of titanium clips (e.g. Ligaclips™) help in directing radiotherapy planning.

Careful haemostasis is mandatory. Use of closed suction drains is sometimes required, especially to drain large areas of subcutaneous undermining. The wound is closed in layers using absorbable suture.

Additional procedures that may become necessary

- Concurrent axillary surgery (sentinel node biopsy or axillary clearance as indicated)
- Contralateral symmetrization surgery (performed as an immediate or delayed procedure)
- Reoperative surgery if adequate macroscopic margins not achieved

Serious/frequently occurring risks

- Seroma or haematoma formation
- Wound infection (or development of an infected seroma or haematoma)
- Fat necrosis (specially in volume displacement oncoplastic techniques)
- Poor scaring/cosmetic outcome (this may be exaggerated after radiotherapy)
- Change in sensation of nipple (where periareolar/circumareolar incision used)
- Loss of nipple viability (complication of mammoplasty techniques in oncoplastic surgery)

Blood transfusion necessary

- Not required/group and save

Type of anaesthesia/sedation

- General anaesthesia
- Local anaesthesia (± sedation) may be feasible in selective cases

Follow-up/need for further procedure

- Routine postoperative check to ensure adequate wound healing/ management of haematoma or seroma formation
- Review of histology and planning for adjuvant treatment
- Long-term review of cosmetic outcomes and requirements for contralateral symmetrization surgery

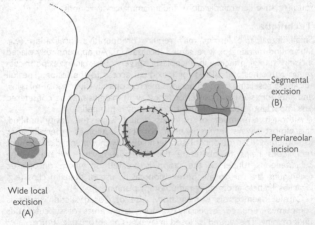

Fig. 6.8 Breast local excision—(a) wide local excision, (b) segmental excision.
Reproduced with permission from Chaudry MA and Winslet MC. Oxford Specialist Handbook of Surgical Oncology. 2009. Oxford: Oxford University Press, p121, Figure 29.

Reference

1. Clough KB, Kaufman GJ, Nos C, et al. Improving breast cancer surgery: a classification and quadrant per quadrant atlas of oncoplastic surgery. *Ann Surg Oncol* 2010;**17**(5):1375–91.

Hepato-pancreatico-biliary surgery

Cholecystectomy

Description

Cholecystectomy refers to surgical removal of the gallbladder for symptomatic cholelithiasis, acalculous cholecystitis, and gallbladder tumours, or polyps. It is also performed along with other surgical procedures such as hepatectomy for primary or secondary liver tumours, as a part of pancreatic resection for tumours of the pancreas or periampullary lesions, for neuroendocrine tumours of the bowel and along with gastric bypass for morbid obesity.

Simple cholecystectomy for symptomatic cholelithiasis is performed laparoscopically in the majority of cases. The procedure is usually performed with four ports, i.e. two 12mm ports (first port is usually inserted the umbilical skin fold and the second is located in the epigastric region) and two 5mm ports (one in the right subcostal region in the mid-clavicular line and the other port is usually located in the right subcostal region in the anterior axillary line) (Fig. 7.1).

This procedure can also be performed with three ports and with a single umbilical port (single incision laparoscopic surgery). The procedure generally takes 30–60min and local anaesthetic infiltration is used to all port sites for postoperative analgesia.

Additional procedures that may become necessary

- Conversion to open procedure
  - In the event of excessive uncontrolled haemorrhage
  - Unclear anatomy in Calot's triangle
  - Inability to demonstrate the critical view of safety
  - For suspected bile duct injury, or injury to small or large bowel during the procedure
- Intraoperative cholangiogram (IOC) is performed routinely in some units, while other units have a more selective policy in that IOC is performed for delineating anatomy or suspected common bile duct (CBD) stones

Benefits

- Treatment of symptomatic cholelithiasis
- Prevention of complications of cholelithiasis (cholecystitis, pancreatitis, obstructive jaundice, cholangitis, recurrent hospital admissions for pain and inflammation)

Alternative procedures/conservative measures

- For patients who are unsuitable/unfit for surgery, ERCP and wide sphincterotomy may prevent further attacks of pancreatitis and/or cholangitis
- Conservative treatment of acute cholecystitis includes antibiotics, analgesia, and low-fat diet
- Percutaneous radiologically guided cholecystostomy may be required for patients with gallbladder empyema who do not respond to conservative measures and who are unfit for surgery

Serious/frequently occurring risks

- Bleeding
- Bile leak/collection
- Stone spillage into the peritoneal cavity intra-operatively
- Conversion to open procedure (~2–15%)
- CBD injury (0.4%–0.6%[1–3])
- Injury to the hepatic artery during dissection of Calot's triangle
- Small/large bowel injury
- Port site hernia
- Wound/port site infection
- Retained stone/jaundice
- Chest infection

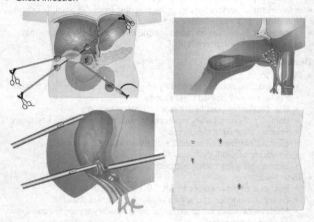

Fig. 7.1 Laparoscopic cholecystectomy showing port placement, anatomy, and technique.

Reproduced with permission from Longmore M, Wilkinson IB, Davidson EH et al. *Oxford Handbook of Clinical Medicine*, 8th edition. 2010. Oxford: Oxford University Press, p.637.

References

1. Gurusamy KS, Davidson BR; Surgical treatment of gallstones. *Gastroenterol Clin North Am* 2010;**39**(2):229–44, viii.
2. Flum DR, Dellinger EP, Cheadle A. et al. Intraoperative cholangiography and risk of common bile duct injury during cholecystectomy. *JAMA* 2003;**289**:1639–44.
3. Ros A, Gustafsson L, Krook H. et al. Laparoscopic cholecystectomy versus mini-laparotomy cholecystectomy: a prospective, randomized, single blind study. *Ann Surg* 2001;**234**(6) 741–9.

Endoscopic retrograde cholangio-pancreatography (ERCP)

Description

ERCP is an endoscopic procedure, usually performed in the endoscopy department. It refers to visualization of the ampulla of Vater (Fig. 7.2) via a side-viewing endoscope and the cannulation of the bile duct/pancreatic duct for visualization of the biliary and pancreatic ductal systems for diagnostic and therapeutic purposes.

Additional procedures that may become necessary

- In the event of perforation/on-going bleeding from the ampulla urgent laparotomy and suture/repair with drainage may be necessary
- In the event of inability to cannulate the bile duct, the sphincter may need to be cut (sphincterotomy)

Benefits

- *Diagnostic:*
  - Obstructive jaundice secondary to gallstones/periampullary tumours
  - Recurrent or retained CBD stones
  - Bile duct injury post laparoscopic cholecystectomy
  - Benign/malignant biliary strictures for biliary brushings and cytology
  - Primary sclerosing cholangitis
  - Chronic pancreatitis to define ductal stricture/obstruction
  - Sphincter of Oddi dysfunction
  - Bile sampling for biliary microlithiasis
- *Therapeutic:*
  - Retrieval of retained/recurrent CBD stones
  - Biliary stenting for cholangitis and/or obstructive jaundice
  - Mesh metal stent for palliation of periampullary tumours/carcinoma of head of pancreas
  - Treatment of bile leak post liver resection/cholecystectomy
  - Sphincterotomy for therapeutic trial of sphincter of Oddi dysfunction
  - Therapeutic trial with pancreatic stent prior to pancreatic duct
  - Drainage surgery in chronic pancreatitis

Alternative procedures/conservative measures

- Magnetic resonance cholangiopancreatography (MRCP) is a alternative imaging modality to visualize the gallbladder and bile ducts for diagnostic purposes, however, it lacks the therapeutic potential of ERCP
- In the event of failure to cannulate the CBD, a percutaneous transhepatic cholangiogram with drainage may be required, especially for patients with obstructive jaundice

Serious/frequently occurring risks[1,2]

- Pancreatitis (7%). Majority managed with conservative management
- Bleeding
- Cholangitis
- Perforation
- Aspiration
- Mortality (0.1%)

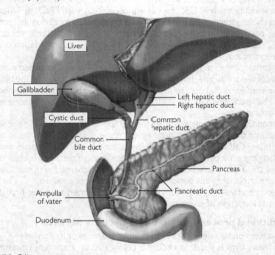

Fig. 7.2 Biliary anatomy.

Reproduced with permission from O'Connor IF and Urdang M. *Oxford Handbook of Surgical Cross-Cover*. 2008. Oxford: Oxford University Press, p.50, Figure 2.3.

References

1. Vandervoort J, Soetikno RM, Tham TCK, *et al*. Risk factors for complications after performance of ERCP. *Gastrointest Endosc*. 2002;**56**(5):656.
2. Chapman RW. Complications of ERCP. In: Green J. Guidelines on complications of gastrointestinal endoscopy. London: British Society of Gastroenterology, 2006:20–5.

Common bile duct exploration

Description

CBD exploration (CBDE) is usually carried out for complicated gallstone disease with CBD calculi. The procedure can either be performed laparoscopically (where expertise is available), or via a subcostal incision in combination with an open cholecystectomy. CBDE is indicated in the event of an inability to clear CBD stones endoscopically with ERCP or when an open cholecystectomy is planned due to previous upper abdominal procedures precluding a laparoscopic approach. It may also become necessary when stones are incidentally discovered on an IOC during a laparoscopic cholecystectomy.[1]

Laparoscopic exploration can be performed via a transcystic route or via a choledochotomy using a operative choledochoscope and specialized stone-retrieving baskets (Fig. 7.3).[2] Laparoscopic choledochotomy should only be performed if the CBD diameter is >8mm on preoperative ultrasound scan.

Open CBDE is usually indicated for multiple CBD calculi or for impacted calculi, or for proximal or intrahepatic stone disease. A T-tube is often left in the CBD at the end of the procedure (Fig. 7.4). A postoperative cholangiogram is performed, usually on day 7, and if the CBD is clear of all calculi the T-tube is removed. Patients can be discharged with the T-tube, and the cholangiogram performed as a outpatient procedure.

Perioperative prophylactic antibiotics are indicated with the first dose given at induction of anaesthesia.

Additional procedures that may become necessary

- Conversion to open procedure if laparoscopic exploration fails
- A biliary bypass if the procedure is performed for recurrent common duct calculi, for ductal stones secondary to ampullary stenosis, diverticulum, or impaired duct motility

Benefits

- CBDE aims to clear the biliary tree of all stone disease and hence prevents further complications, namely biliary obstruction and sepsis

Alternative procedures/conservative measures

- CBD calculi discovered incidentally by intraoperative cholangiography during laparoscopic cholecystectomy can also be treated with ERCP and sphincterotomy postoperatively

Serious/frequently occurring risks[1,3]

- Injury to the CBD
- Biliary stricture
- Bile leak/collection
- Retained stone
- Infection
- Bleeding
- DVT/pulmonary embolism
- Chest infection

Blood transfusion necessary

- Group and save, but transfusion is usually not required

Type of anaesthesia/sedation

- General anaesthesia

Follow-up/need for further procedure

Patients will require follow-up in the surgical clinic at 2–3 months posoperatively with repeat liver function tests ± further imaging as indicated.

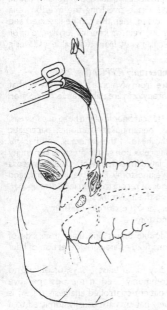

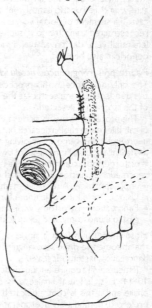

Fig. 7.3 Basket retrieval of CBD calculi.

Reproduced with permission from Dennison AR and Maddern GJ. *Operative Solutions in Hepatobiliary and Pancreatic Surgery.* 2010. Oxford: Oxford University Press, p.230, Figure 4.20.

Fig 7.4 T-tube placement and subhepatic drain postoperatively.

Reproduced with permission from Dennison AR and Maddern GJ. *Operative Solutions in Hepatobiliary and Pancreatic Surgery.* 2010. Oxford: Oxford University Press, p.232, Figure 4.23.

References

1. Ricardi R, Islam S, Canete JJ, et al. Effectiveness and long term results of laparoscopic common bile duct exploration. *Surg. Endosc* 2003;**17**.19–22.
2. Petelin JB. Clinical results of common bile duct exploration. *Endosc Surg Allied Technol* 1993;**1**(3):125–9.
3. Cuschieri A, Lezoche E, Morino M, et al. E.A.E.S. multicentre prospective randomized trial comparing two stage v/s single stage management of patients with gallstone disease and ductal calculi. *Surg Endosc* 1999;**13**(10):952–7.

Pancreatico-duodenectomy

Description

Pancreatico-duodenectomy resections include the following.

Whipple's procedure (Fig. 7.5)

This involves resection of the pancreatic head, entire duodenum, distal stomach including the pylorus and antrum, along with the gallbladder and the distal bile duct and all the lymph nodes around the porta, hepatic artery, and retropancreatic lymphatic tissue overlying the inferior vena cava. If a segment of portal vein is involved, then this can be resected and reconstructed using the long saphenous vein or internal jugular vein, or left renal vein, or, if available, a vascular graft from a suitable cadaveric donor can also be used.

Pylorus-preserving pancreaticoduodenectomy (PPPD) (Fig. 7.6)

The only difference in this procedure from Whipple's procedure is that the duodenum is transected at the prepyloric area and hence no portion of the stomach is resected.

This procedure is usually performed for carcinoma of the head of pancreas, distal bile duct cholangiocarcinomas, periampullary tumours, pancreatic neuroendocrine tumours involving the head of the pancreas, and benign/malignant duodenal tumours. Following resection gastrointestinal continuity is restored, most commonly with an isolated loop Roux-en-Y duct to mucosa pancreaticojejunostomy, choledochojejunostomy, gastrojejunostomy, and jejunojejunostomy. Alternative methods of reconstruction include:

• Using a single loop of jejunum for all the anastomosis
• Pancreatico-gastrostomy with Roux-en-Y hepaticojejunostomy, gastrojejunostomy, and jejunojejunostomy

Most units use at least a single or double drains one from each side of the abdomen to drain serosanguineous fluid to aid early detection of bile/pancreatic anastomotic leaks.

Patients will require an inpatient stay for at least 7 days, usually up to 10–14 days. Epidural analgesia is commonly used in the postoperative phase and if this is contraindicated, patient-controlled analgesia (PCA) is preferred. Immediately postoperatively patients are usually admitted to a high-dependency area for observation for a period of 24–48h. Intravenous proton pump inhibitors are used in most units and octreotide may also be given postoperatively. Drain fluid amylase is measured on day 5 from the pancreatic drain, which aids early detection of pancreatic leaks.

Additional procedures that may become necessary

• Portal vein resection in the case of limited involvement of the portal vein, for attempted curative resection

Benefits

• Resection offers *the only chance* of cure for these cancers
• May resolve pain in patients with chronic pancreatitis when *there is* imaging evidence of obstruction/stricture in the pancreatic head
• Long-term relief from sepsis and biliary obstruction

Alternative procedures/conservative measures

- Palliative bypass procedure including Roux-en-Y choledochojejunostomy, gastrojejunostomy, and jejuno-jejunostomy for inoperable tumours
- In presence of peritoneal disease or extrapancreatic disease resection should not be performed
- For tumours deemed inoperable on preoperative staging scans, biliary and duodenal obstruction can be treated with mesh metal stents introduced endoscopically or percutaneously

Serious/frequently occurring risks[1,2]

- Intraoperative bleeding
- Anastomotic leak
  - Pancreatic anastomosis (pancreatic fistula)—drainage of >10mL of amylase-rich fluid on day 5 or for more than 5 days (7–14%)
  - Choledochojejunostomy—bile leak (1–3%)
  - Jejuno-jejunostomy—bile leak/small bowel contents
  - Gastrojejunostomy (<1%)
- Postoperative bleeding
  - Gastroduodenal artery stump/pseudoaneurysm
  - Portal vein bleed
  - Anastomotic bleed causing haematemesis/melaena/haemobilia
  - Bleeding from mesenteric vessels around resected duodenojejunal flexure
- Delayed gastric emptying (30%, higher incidence with pylorus preserving pancreatico-duodenectomy)
- Wound infection/intra-abdominal collections
- DVT/pulmonary embolism/cardiorespiratory complications
- Chyle leak—incidence depends on extent of lymphadenectomy
- Roux loop obstruction due to anastomotic stricture/kink
- Pancreatic exocrine insufficiency/diabetes
- Irresectability
- Recurrence
- Incisional hernia and chronic wound pain
- Morbidity 30–40%
- Mortality 2–5%

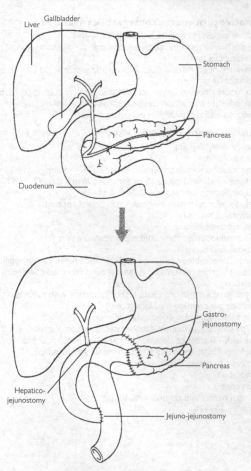

Fig. 7.5 Whipple's procedure showing anastomoses and Roux-en-Y.

Reproduced with permission from Bloom S and Webster G. *Oxford Handbook of Gastroenterology and Hepatology*. 2006. Oxford: Oxford University Press, p.639, Figure 2.31.

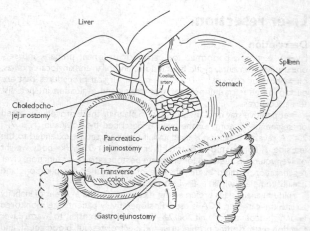

Fig. 7.6 Pylorus-preserving pancreatico-duodenectomy (PPPD).

Reproduced with permission from Chaudry MA and Winslet MC. *Oxford Specialist Handbook of Surgical Oncology.* 2009. Oxford: Oxford University Press, p.390, Figure 7.6.

References

1. Cooperman AM, Kini S, Snacy H, *et al.* Current surgical therapy for carcinoma of the pancreas. *J Clin Gastroenterol* 2000;**31**:107–13.
2. Yeo CJ, Cameron JL, Lillemoe KD, *et al.* Pancreaticoduodenectomy with or without distal gastrectomy and extended retroperitoneal lymphadenectomy for periampullary adenocarcinoma, part 2: randomized controlled trial evaluating survival morbidity and mortality. *Ann Surg* 2002;**236**:355–56; discussion 356–8.

Liver resection

Description

Liver resection is performed for benign or malignant primary and secondary liver tumours, cystic liver lesions, and hilar cholangiocarcinomas, or gallbladder cancers.[1–6] These are major surgical procedures that are performed after careful preoperative staging and evaluation in specialist tertiary centres.

Preoperative staging scans are useful in planning these procedures based on segmental anatomy of the liver as described by Couinaud (Figs. 7.7, 7.8). A reverse L-incision is used and, if required, can be extended to the left side. A minimum of 30% total liver volume or 0.5mL/kg body weight of liver volume is required for adequate postoperative liver function. Liver regeneration is rapid in the absence of sepsis/other complications and usually complete within 6–8 weeks postoperatively.

Epidural analgesia is preferred but if contraindicated/in event of inability to site the catheter, PCA is used. Postoperatively patients are monitored in a high-dependency unit for 24–48h prior to transfer to ward. Liver function tests, clotting profile, urea and electrolytes, full blood count, and lactate are monitored to assess the function of the liver remnant in the postoperative period. Abdominal drains placed at laparotomy may aid early detection of bile leak, particularly after major liver resections. Many patients are managed on an enhanced-recovery after surgery (ERAS) programme, with early mobilization, feeding, and prompt drain removal.[7]

Additional procedures that may become necessary

- Diaphragmatic involvement may require resection along with the liver tumour and is not a contraindication to surgery
- Limited resectable extrahepatic disease is resected along with the liver tumour particularly for colorectal liver secondaries
- Limited involvement of portal vein or inferior vena cava or adrenal gland is resected along with the liver tumours
- Extrahepatic widespread nodal disease or peritoneal disease discovered at laparotomy is a contraindication to further surgery
- Additional lesions detected at laparotomy/intraoperative ultrasound are resected or ablated with RFA, particularly for colorectal liver secondaries or resected later with a staged resection strategy

Benefits

- Liver resection offers the only chance for potential cure at present with reported 5-year survival following surgery of ~40% (colorectal metastases)

Alternative procedures/conservative measures

- RFA offers an alternative strategy for small accessible lesions particularly for unfit patients or recurrent tumours following resection where further surgery is not feasible
- Alcohol ablation is another alternative particularly in patients with primary liver tumours on the background of cirrhosis
- Chemotherapy is useful for colorectal liver secondaries as both adjuvant/neoadjuvant as well as palliative treatment option
- Liver transplantation is considered for patients <65 years with small primary tumours with a background of liver cirrhosis
- Mesh metal stent placed percutaneously/endoscopically is a useful adjunct in palliation of extensive/inoperable hilar cholangiocarcinomas
- Recurrent disease in large bowel detected at laparotomy is resected if resectable

Serious/frequently occurring risks

- Bleeding during surgery and postoperatively from the transected liver surface
- Low CVP anaesthesia, meticulous surgical technique and use of topical haemostatic agents such as Tachosil® and tissue glue/Surgicel® are useful adjuncts to prevent excessive blood loss
- Bile leak, usually from the raw liver surface or from a biliary reconstruction post-resection. Managed conservatively with biliary stent placed endoscopically or percutaneously
- Liver failure (small-for-size syndrome) particularly after extended liver resections. Managed conservatively in conjunction with hepatology colleagues
- Wound/chest infections/pleural effusions: use of perioperative prophylactic antibiotics and aggressive chest physiotherapy with good analgesia are helpful in preventing these complications
- Intra-abdominal collections/ascites: these are managed conservatively with radiologically placed percutaneous drains
- Perioperative venous thromboembolism. Routine use of preventive measures such as thromboembolism stockings, subcutaneous enoxaparin and early mobilization reduces the likelihood of these complications
- Overall morbidity is 7–14%
- Overall mortality in most units <2%

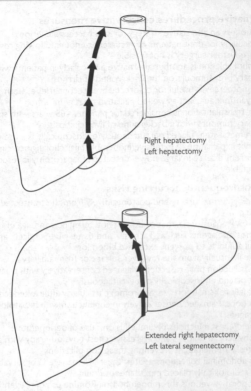

Right hepatectomy
Left hepatectomy

Extended right hepatectomy
Left lateral segmentectomy

Fig. 7.7 Resection planes for right and left hepatectomy (top image) and extended right hepatectomy and left lateral segmentectomy (bottom image).

Reproduced with permission from Sutcliffe RP, Antoniades CG, Deshpande R, et al. *Oxford Specialist Handbook of Liver and Pancreatobiliary Surgery*. 2010. Oxford: Oxford University Press, p.7, Figure 1.4.

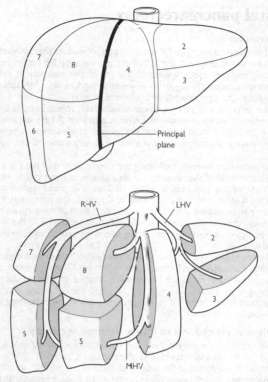

Fig. 7.8 Segments of the liver according to Couinard. LHV = left hepatic vein, MHV = middle hepatic vein, RHV = right hepatic vein.

Reproduced with permission from Sutcliffe RP, Antoniades CG, Deshpande R, et al. *Oxford Specialist Handbook of Liver and Pancreatobiliary Surgery* 2010. Oxford: Oxford University Press, p.3, Figures 1.1 and 1.2.

References

1. Trotter JF, Everson GT. Benign focal lesions of the liver. *Clin Liver Dis* 2001;**5**:17–42.
2. Bruix J, Sherman M, Llovet JM, et al. Clinical management of hepatocellular carcinoma. Conclusions of the Barcelona 2000 EASL conference. *J Hepatol* 2001;**35**:421–30.
3. Makuchi M, Sano K. The surgical approach to HCC: our progress and results in Japan. *Liver Transplant* 2004;**10**:S46–52.
4. Belghiti J, Hiramatsu K, Benoist S, et al. Seven hundred and forty seven hepatectomies in the 1990's: an update to evaluate the actual risk of liver resection. *J Am Coll Surg* 2000;**191**:38–46.
5. House MG, Ito H, Fong Y, et al. Survival after hepatic resection for metastatic colorectal cancer: trends in outcomes for 1,600 patients during two decades at a single institution. *J Am Coll Surg* 2010;**210**(5):744–52, 752–5.
6. Tsoulfas G, Pramateftakis MG, Kanellos I. Surgical treatment of hepatic metastases from colorectal cancer. *World J Gastrointest Oncol* 2011;**3**(1):1–9.
7. Hendry PO, van Dam RM, Bukkems SF, et al. Randomized clinical trial of laxatives and oral nutritional supplements within an enhanced recovery after surgery protocol following liver resection. *Br J Surg* 2010;**97**(8):1998–206.

Distal pancreatectomy

Description

Distal pancreatectomy (Fig. 7.9) is usually performed for potentially resect-able tumours of the body and tail of the pancreas, or for benign lesions including complex cystic lesions of the tail of the pancreas. It can be performed laparoscopically or as an open procedure via a left subcostal extended to the right or a bilateral subcostal incision.

If the lesions are large, or a cancer is suspected, splenectomy is usually performed to ensure adequate lymph node clearance. A splenectomy may also be required if there is injury to the splenic vessels during a attempted spleen-sparing procedure, or if the lesion is very close to the splenic hilum.

The procedure involves mobilizing the splenic flexure of the colon and the greater curve of the stomach including ligation of short gastric vessels. The neck of the pancreas is mobilized from the portal vein and the pancreas is usually divided at the level of the neck. The pancreatic stump is oversewn or stapled, depending on the preference of the surgeon. If the pancreatic duct is visualized, it is suture-ligated separately. If the spleen is to be resected, early ligation of the splenic vessels helps to minimize blood loss.

All patients are prophylactically vaccinated against capsulated organisms including *Haemophilus influenza* B, *Meningococcus* C, and pneumococcus at least 2 weeks prior to the procedure if feasible, or prior to discharge following operation if splenectomy is performed. Lifelong antibiotic prophylaxis is also required to minimize the risk of overwhelming post-splenectomy infections (OPSI).

Additional procedures that may become necessary

- Splenectomy—the patient should be consented for this regardless of whether or not a spleen-preserving procedure is intended
- Tumour involvement of the colonic splenic flexure, adrenal, diaphragm, renal vessels, or left kidney may necessitate an en-bloc resection of the involved organs, particularly if the procedure is performed with curative intent for adenocarcinoma/cystic carcinoma of the body and tail of the pancreas, or for large neuroendocrine tumours involving the body and tail of the pancreas
- A total pancreatectomy for tumours with more extensive involvement, including the neck and the head of the pancreas

Benefits

- For tumours involving the body and tail of pancreas, this procedure offers the only possibility of cure. In the case of benign lesions, distal pancreatectomy may be performed to improve symptoms

Alternative procedures/conservative measures

- For tumours causing duodenal or upper jejunal obstruction, bypass/ duodenal stenting may need to be considered
- There may be a place for further adjuvant chemotherapy postoperatively depending on the histology of the resected specimen

Serious/frequently occurring risks

- Bleeding
  - Intraoperative
  - Postoperative—usually due to slippage of ligatures on the splenic vessel stump or due to pseudoaneurysm involving the splenic vessel stump secondary to a pancreatic stump leak
- Infection
  - Wound infection
  - Chest infections—often collapse consolidation the left lung base due to the laparotomy incision, pain and subsequent basal atelectasis
  - Intra-abdominal collections due to leak from the pancreatic stump
- Fistula
  - Pancreatic fistula incidence is as high as 30%, due to a leak from the pancreatic stump
  - Small bowel or colonic fistula due to damage to the left colon or bowel during surgery
- Endocrine insufficiency and risk of diabetes mellitus or, if the patient is already diabetic at presentation, then worsening of the diabetes postoperatively
- Mortality—<2%
- Morbidity—25–30%

Blood transfusion necessary

- Blood transfusion may become necessary and hence cross-matched blood should be routinely available

Type of anaesthesia/sedation

- General anaesthesia
- Epidural analgesia is usually preferred for postoperative pain relief
- If cannulation of the epidural space fails or is contraindicated, FCA is preferred. A nasogastric tube is routinely inserted and removed within 24h postoperatively

Follow-up/need for further procedure

- Patients are usually followed up in the surgical clinic at 3-monthly intervals with follow-up CT scans if the surgery was for malignancy

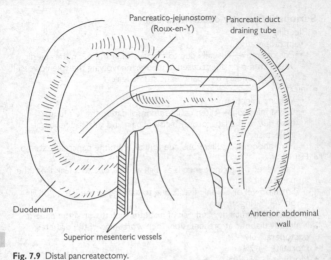

Fig. 7.9 Distal pancreatectomy.
Reproduced with permission from Chaudry MA and Winslet MC. *Oxford Specialist Handbook of Surgical Oncology*. 2009. Oxford: Oxford University Press, p.393, Figure 7.7.

Upper gastrointestinal and bariatric surgery

Bleeding peptic ulcer—oversewing

Description

Approximately 80–85% of upper gastrointestinal haemorrhage stops spontaneously and only conservative therapy is needed. The remaining 15–20% require surgical intervention.[1,2] Upper gastrointestinal endoscopy is the first-line treatment for bleeding peptic ulcer. Various endoscopic methods are available, including injection of adrenaline into the ulcer, and the use of clips, thermoprobe, or laser.

Indications for surgical intervention are:[1–4]

- Requirement of a 6-unit or more transfusion of packed red cells (4 units in the elderly)
- Visible vessel at the base of the ulcer
- Inability to control bleeding endoscopically
- Two or more episodes of re-bleeding

The position of the ulcer should ideally be identified with endoscopy prior to surgical intervention. The gastroduodenal artery runs along the posterior aspect of the first part of duodenum and thus a posterior wall ulcer must be assumed to involve this artery. An upper midline incision is made. In the case of duodenal ulcers a longitudinal pyloroduodenotomy is made. The gastroduodenal artery is under-run proximally and distally. A third suture may be inserted to control the transverse pancreatic branch of the artery. The pyloroduodenotomy is closed transversely (Fig. 8.1).

In the case of gastric ulcers the management depends on the size and position of the ulcer. Smaller ulcers may be sufficiently managed with under-sewing of the bleeding vessel. Very large ulcers may warrant a subtotal gastrectomy.[4] Sufficient biopsies should be taken of gastric ulcers in order to exclude malignancy.

The patient may require intensive care unit (ITU)/high-dependency unit (HDU) care postoperatively depending on their comorbidities. They will also have a nasogastric tube and intra-abdominal drains *in situ*.

Additional procedures that may become necessary

- Subtotal gastrectomy

Benefits

- *Therapeutic*: to control haemorrhage

Alternative procedures/conservative measures

- *Conservative*: management involves supportive therapy only. Although the bleed may stop spontaneously
- *Medical*: all patients should undergo an upper gastrointestinal endoscopy to investigate the cause and site of bleeding, with a potential attempt to endoscopically arrest the bleeding
- *Radiological*: angiographic identification of the bleeding vessel and subsequent embolization is another option in centres where interventional radiology is available

Serious/frequently occurring risks

- *Specific*: uncontrollable haemorrhage resulting in death, re-bleeding—will usually occur within the first 72h and carries a significant mortality, leak from site of pyloromyotomy
- *General*: infection—chest/intra-abdominal/urinary/systemic, DVT/pulmonary embolism/cerebrovascular accident (CVA)
- *Late*: incisional hernia, recurrent ulceration at site of pyloromyotomy or elsewhere, pyloric stenosis

Blood transfusion necessary

- Cross-match 4–6 units (dependent on starting haemoglobin)
- In patients with significant bleeding blood products such as platelets or FFP are likely to be required

Type of anaesthesia/sedation

- General anaesthesia

Follow-up/need for further procedure

- Hospital stay after this procedure will be approximately 1 week
- Patients with peptic ulcer disease will require either medical management or if that fails, a definitive surgical procedure. This will include testing for the presence of *Helicobacter pylori* and subsequent eradication
- Gastric ulcers may prove to be malignant and patients may require further surgery for definitive management of their cancer
- All patients will require further upper gastrointestinal endoscopy

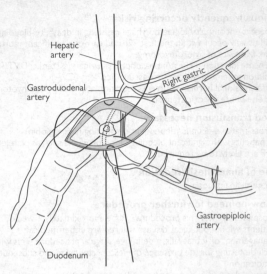

Fig. 8.1 Oversewing of bleeding peptic ulcer.

References

1. Sung JJ, Tsoi KK, Ma TK, et al. Causes of mortality in patients with peptic ulcer bleeding: a prospective cohort study of 10,428 cases. *Am J Gastroenterol* 2010;**105**(1):84–9.
2. Rockall TA, Logan RF, Devlin HB, et al. Variation in outcome after acute upper gastrointestinal haemorrhage. The National Audit of Acute Upper Gastrointestinal Haemorrhage. *Lancet* 1995;**346**(8971):346–50.
3. Rockall TA. Management and outcome of patients undergoing surgery after acute upper gastrointestinal haemorrhage. Steering Group for the National Audit of Acute Upper Gastrointestinal Haemorrhage. *J R Soc Med* 1998;**91**(10):518–23.
4. Cheung FK, Lau JY. Management of massive peptic ulcer bleeding. *Gastroenterol Clin North Am* 2009;**38**(2):231–43.

Heller's cardiomyotomy for achalasia of the cardia

Description

Achalasia is a condition that causes reduced peristalsis of the oesophagus and a high lower oesophageal sphincter (LOS) pressure. The purpose of surgery is to reduce the LOS pressure by dividing the muscle wall, without breaching the inner mucosa. The oesophageal wall consists of overlying adventitia, longitudinal and circular muscles, the muscularis propria layer followed by the submucosa and innermost mucosal layer. A longitudinal incision is made through the adventitia and muscle layers down to submucosa, starting above the LOS and extending down onto the stomach for approximately 3–7cm. This is now most commonly performed laparoscopically, although classically it was an open procedure. An endoscope may be introduced to ensure mucosal integrity on completion of the procedure.

A partial fundoplication may also be performed to prevent excessive acid reflux.

Additional procedures that may become necessary

- Conversion to open procedure
- A thoracoscopic approach—if a more extensive myotomy is required

Benefits

- *Therapeutic*: to improve symptoms of dysphagia

Alternative procedures/conservative measures

- *Conservative*: eating slowly, chewing well, and raising the head of the bed when sleeping
- *Medical*: reduce contractility of the LOS. Treatment includes calcium channel blockers and nitrates. Botulinum toxin (Botox®) can be injected into the LOS to paralyse the muscles and hold it shut
- *Surgical/endoscopic*: pneumatic dilatation of the LOS by oesophagogastroduodenoscopy (OGD) can also be used. This has a risk of perforation and may require repeating

Serious/frequently occurring risks[1–4]

- Early:
  - *General*: DVT/pulmonary embolism, infection (wound/systemic/chest)
  - *Specific*: perforation of oesophagus/stomach, inadequate length of myotomy
- Late:
  - *General*: port site and incisional hernia
  - *Specific*: acid reflux, recurrence of symptoms—due to aperistaltic oesophagus or to scarring following surgery where subsequent dilatation may be required

Blood transfusion necessary

- Group and save

Type of anaesthesia/sedation

- General anaesthesia

Follow-up/need for further procedure

- Even after successful treatment, patient swallowing may deteriorate over time, necessitating further dilatation or a second myotomy
- Some physicians recommend repeated endoscopy to assess for any oesophageal damage secondary to acid reflux

References

1. Costantini M, Zaninotto G, Guirroli E, et al. The laparoscopic Heller-Dor operation remains an effective treatment for esophageal achalasia at a minimum 6-year follow-up. Surg Endosc 2005;**19**(3):345–51.
2. Luckey AE 3rd, DeMeester SR. Complications of achalasia surgery. Thorac Surg Clin 2006;**16**(1):95–8.
3. Mattioli S, Ruffato A, Lugaresi M, et al. Long-term results of the Heller-Dor operation with intraoperative manometry for the treatment of esophageal achalasia. J Thorac Cardiovasc Surg 2010;**140**(5):962–9.
4. Ferulano GP, Dilillo S, D'Ambra M, et al. Short and long term results of the laparoscopic Heller-Dor myotomy. The influence of age and previous conservative therapies. Surg Endosc 2007;**21**(11):2017–23.

Feeding jejunostomy

Description

A feeding jejunostomy may be used as a route to provide enteral feed when it is not possible to administer food via the oesophagus or stomach or where supplemental oral intake is required. Oral feeding may not be possible due to pathology in the oesophagus or stomach, or following recent surgery with an oesophageal anastomosis.[1] Jejunal feeding is also usually employed in patients with neurological deficits.

A small midline incision is made above the umbilicus and a loop of jejunum identified and delivered through the wound. A fine-bore feeding tube is inserted into the lumen of the jejunum. The tube is then fed through the abdominal wall and a fixation device is attached to the skin. This procedure can also be performed laparoscopically.

Additional procedures that may become necessary

- None

Benefits

- *Diagnostic*: to allow enteral feeding while bypassing the oesophagus and stomach

Alternative procedures/conservative measures

- *Conservative*: nasojejunal tube feeding
- *Surgical*: jejunal extension from percutaneous endoscopic gastrostomy (PEG), total parenteral nutrition via a CVC

Serious/frequently occurring risks[2]

- *Early*: tube dislocation/blockage, bowel ischaemia, abdominal wall abscess formation, tube slippage/tearing through of jejunal sutures, intra-abdominal leakage of feed
- *Late*: diarrhoea or constipation, abdominal cramping, nausea and vomiting, tube migration, enterocutaneous fistulas

Blood transfusion necessary

- Group and save

Type of anaesthesia/sedation

- Local anaesthesia/regional anaesthesia (spinal/epidural)/general anaesthesia

Follow-up/need for further procedure

- The tube should not be removed for 10 days to allow time for a tract to develop
- When the jejunostomy is no longer required it can be removed on the ward or in outpatients without any need for local anaesthesia or a further procedure

References

1. Wakefield SE, Mansell NJ, Baigrie RJ, et al. Use of a feeding jejunostomy after oesophagogastric surgery. Br J Surg 1995;82:811–13.
2. Tapia J, Murguia R, Garcia G, et al. Jejunostomy techniques, indications, and complications. World J Surg 1999;23(6):596–602.

Gastrectomy

Description

This procedure is broadly divided into a subtotal or total gastrectomy and can be performed laparoscopically or as an open procedure. An upper midline incision is made for open procedures. In a total gastrectomy the entire stomach is removed and an anastomosis fashioned between the distal oesophagus and a jejunal loop forming a Roux-en-Y reconstruction, leaving a blind duodenal stump. The same reconstruction is performed in a subtotal gastrectomy with the jejunal loop being anastomosed onto the remaining stomach (Fig. 8.2). This is otherwise known as a Bilroth II procedure. In a Bilroth I procedure enough upper duodenum remains to anastomose directly onto the stomach.

Most gastrectomies are performed for gastric cancer. Segmental resection of the stomach can also be performed, for example, in the resections of gastrointestinal stromal tumours. In these procedures the stomach wall is closed primarily and no anastomosis is fashioned.

Patients undergoing gastrectomy need careful preoperative assessment and often require HDU care in the initial postoperative period. Patients may have abdominal drains, a nasogastric tube and/or a urinary catheter *in situ* in the immediate postoperative period. Depending on their comorbidities they may also require invasive monitoring such as CVCs and arterial cannulation.

Additional procedures that may become necessary

- If the surgery is performed laparoscopically it may become necessary to convert to an open procedure
- When there is invasion of other organs by disease—splenectomy, distal pancreatectomy or transverse colectomy
- Splenectomy for bleeding
- Irresectable cancer will lead to closure without excision
- In nutritionally deplete patients, especially those requiring postoperative chemotherapy—insertion of a feeding jejunostomy to provide supplementary enteral feeding

Benefits

- *Diagnostic*: provide histological tissue and stage disease
- *Therapeutic*: to remove cancer and improve prognosis, to relieve obstruction if present, symptom control

Alternative procedures/conservative measures

- This depends on the indication for surgery. The most common indication is stomach cancer. Surgical resection is the only curative treatment for adenocarcinoma of the stomach
- *Conservative*: symptom control and palliation
- *Radiological/oncological*: chemotherapy, radiotherapy, or a combination of both in a palliative setting

Serious/frequently occurring risks[1-3]

- *General*: bleeding, infection including wound, chest, intra-abdominal and systemic, DVT/pulmonary embolism/CVA/myocardial infarction/acute coronary syndrome (ACS)
- *Specific*: anastomotic leak, anastomotic breakdown, duodenal stump leak, dumping syndrome (more prevalent in total gastrectomy), nausea, vomiting, bloating dizziness, sweating, intolerance of large meals, biliary reflux, incomplete excision, recurrence of disease, vitamin B₁₂ deficiency—necessitating lifelong replacement

Blood transfusion necessary

- Group and save/cross-match 2–4 units

Type of anaesthesia/sedation

- General anaesthesia with or without regional epidural anaesthesia for postoperative pain relief

Follow-up/need for further procedure

- Hospital stay is usually between 7 and 10 days
- Further resection—if surgery is undertaken for cancer, positive resection margins for cancer may require re-resection
- Ongoing outpatient monitoring of disease with CT scanning

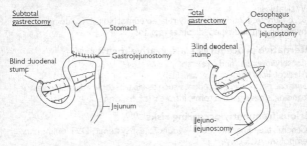

Fig. 8.2 Anatomy post subtotal and total gastrectomy.

References

1. Sasako M, Katai H, Sano T, et al. Management of complications after gastrectomy with extended lymphadenectomy. *Surg Oncol* 2000;9(1):31–4.
2. McCulloch P, Ward J, Tekkis PP, et al. Mortality and morbidity in gastro-oesophageal cancer surgery: initial results of ASCOT multicentre prospective cohort study. *BMJ* 2003;**327**(7425):1192–7.
3. RCSE Clinical Effectiveness Unit/AUGIS/BSG. *National Oesophagogastric Cancer Audit 2009.* Available at: Ɔ www.augis.org/pdf/audits/nhs-ic-og-clinical-audit_2nd_Annual_Report_2009.pdf (accessed 10 May 2011).

Roux-en-Y gastric bypass surgery

Description

Bariatric surgical procedures are divided into malabsorptive procedures and restrictive procedures. Restrictive procedures primarily reduce stomach size, and malabsorptive procedures, while they may also reduce the size of the stomach, primarily act to reduce absorption of ingested food. The commonest bariatric procedure, laparoscopic adjustable gastric banding, is an example of a restrictive procedure. Newer techniques include the sleeve gastrectomy and duodenal switch procedure. Gastric bypass surgery is an example of a mixed restrictive and malabsorptive procedure.

Gastric bypass surgery can be performed either open or laparoscopically. The stomach is divided into a small (~30mL) proximal pouch and a large distal remnant pouch. The gastrointestinal tract is then reconstructed to allow drainage of both segments of stomach via a Roux En-Y reconstruction. This leads to a marked reduction in the functional volume of the stomach and an alteration in the physiological response to food.

Additional procedures that may become necessary

- If performed laparoscopically—conversion to open procedure

Benefits

- Weight loss
- *Secondary*: reduction in obesity related comorbidities including hypertension and type 2 diabetes mellitus

Alternative procedures/conservative measures

- *Conservative*: diet and exercise
- *Medical*: lipid binders (e.g. orlistat)
- *Surgical*: restrictive procedures such as laparoscopic adjustable gastric banding, sleeve gastrectomy, intra-gastric balloon

Serious/frequently occurring risks[1–3]

- *General*: bleeding, infection—wound/chest/systemic, DVT/pulmonary embolism/ACS/CVA
- *Specific*: anastomotic leakage/breakdown, anastomotic ulceration, dumping syndrome—tachycardia, sweating, anxiety, diarrhoea, hyperparathyroidism, inadequate absorption of calcium due to bypass of the duodenum, iron and vitamin B_{12} deficiency, incisional hernias

Blood transfusion necessary

- Group and save/cross-match 2 units

Type of anaesthesia/sedation

- General anaesthesia

Follow-up/need for further procedure

- Routine outpatient review
- Patients require close monitoring by a multidisciplinary team in the initial postoperative period. This includes monitoring and treatment of any psychological sequelae
- After this, follow up of weight loss can be managed in the community by primary care teams

References

1. Lancaster R, Hutter M. Bands and bypasses: 30-day morbidity and mortality of bariatric surgical procedures as assessed by prospective, multi-center, risk-adjusted ACS-NSQIP data. *Surg Endosc* 2008;**22**:2554–63.

2. Pories WJ, Swanson MS, MacDonald KG. *et al*. Who would have thought it? An operation proves to be the most effective therapy for adult-onset diabetes mellitus. *Ann Surg* 1995;**222**:339–52.

3. Talieh J, Kirgan D, Fisher BL. Gastric bypass for morbid obesity: a standard technique by consensus. *Obesity Surg* 1997;**7**:198–202.

Hiatus hernia repair and antireflux surgery

Description

These procedures are used to repair a sliding hiatus hernia or to treat some forms of intractable gastro-oesophageal reflux disease. There are many different types of wrap described. Nissen's is a 360° wrap of fundus around the oesophagus. Other partial wraps (170–270°) have also been described.[1–3] The partial wrap is intended to reduce postoperative dysphagia and bloating.

Prior to undergoing either type of procedure, various investigations need to be undertaken. Preoperative upper gastrointestinal endoscopy is required to assess for oesophagitis or the presence of hiatus hernia. For patients with reflux, oesophageal pH and manometry studies are required to detect the presence and severity of acid reflux, and to detect abnormal contractility of the oesophagus, which may preclude surgical correction.[4] For example, in achalasia, there is abnormal contractility of the LOS and symptoms would not improve and may well deteriorate post-fundoplication.

The procedure is most commonly performed laparoscopically with the patient placed in a modified lithotomy position. The right and left crura are dissected and circumferential dissection of the oesophagus is performed. The hiatus is then closed with sutures. The short gastric vessels may be divided to improve mobilization of the fundus. In Nissen's procedure the mobilized fundus is wrapped 360° around the oesophagus by passing it through the posterior window behind the oesophagus. The wrap is then secured in place on the anterior oesophagus with a varying number of sutures. In a Watson procedure the wrap is wrapped anteriorly through 120° and secured anteriorly (Fig. 8.3).

Additional procedures that may become necessary
- Conversion to open procedure

Benefits
- *Therapeutic*: relieve symptoms and complications of reflux disease

Alternative procedures/conservative measures
- *Conservative*: dietary management
- *Medical*: proton-pump inhibitors, H_2 receptor antagonists
- *Surgical*: endoscopic antireflux procedures

Serious/frequently occurring risks[4,5]
- *Early*: postoperative dysphagia—normal for first 6 weeks, but rarely permanent, pneumothorax, oesophageal perforation, gas bloat syndrome, epigastric pain, splenic or hepatic injury, iatrogenic vagotomy
- *Late*: wrap failure, recurrence of symptoms, hiatal stenosis, ongoing dysphagia

Blood transfusion necessary
- Group and save

Type of anaesthesia/sedation
- General anaesthesia

Follow-up/need for further procedure
- Soft diet for 6 weeks postoperatively
- Follow-up at 4 weeks after the surgery
- Revision surgery is rarely required for recurrence
- Routine outpatient review

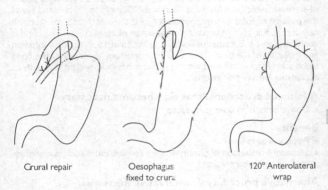

Crural repair   Oesophagus fixed to crura   120° Anterolateral wrap

Fig. 8.3 Fundal wrap in anti-reflux surgery.

References

1. Cai W, Watson DI, Lally CJ, et al. Ten-year clinical outcome of a prospective randomized clinical trial of laparoscopic Nissen versus anterior 180(degrees) partial fundoplication. Br J Surg 2008;**95**(12):1501–5.
2. Watson DI, Jamieson GG, Lally C, et al. Multicenter, prospective, double-blind, randomized trial of laparoscopic nissen vs anterior 90 degrees partial fundoplication. Arch Surg 2004;**139**(11):1160–7.
3. Stewart GD, Watson AJ, Lamb PJ, et al. Comparison of three different procedures for antireflux surgery. Br J Surg 2004;**91**(6):724–9.
4. Peters JH, DeMeester TR. Indications, benefits and outcome of laparoscopic Nissen fundoplication. Dig Dis 1996;**14**(3) 169–79.
5. DeMeester TR, Bonavina L, Albertucci M. Nissen fundoplication for gastroesophageal reflux disease. Evaluation of primary repair in 100 consecutive patients. Ann Surg 1986;**204**(1):9–20.

Laparoscopic adjustable gastric banding

Description

Bariatric surgical procedures are grossly divided into malabsorptive procedures and restrictive procedures. Restrictive procedures primarily reduce stomach size, and malabsorptive procedures, while they may also reduce the size of the stomach, primarily act to reduce absorption of ingested food. Laparoscopic adjustable gastric banding is an example of a restrictive procedure.

In laparoscopic adjustable gastric banding an inflatable silicone band is placed around the fundus of the stomach. This produces a proximal pouch of stomach, which can hold approximately 120g of food. The band slows the passage of food into the remainder of the stomach and the stomach registers as full, giving the patient a sensation of early satiety. The band is connected to a subcutaneous port in the abdominal wall to allow inflation and deflation of the band. This allows the optimum 'tightness' of the band to be achieved, i.e. the level which produces optimum weight loss with an acceptable level of side effects.

Additional procedures that may become necessary

- Conversion to an open procedure

Benefits

- *Primary*: weight loss
- *Secondary*: resolution of obesity-related comorbidities such as diabetes mellitus and hypertension

Alternative procedures/conservative measures

- *Conservative*: diet and exercise
- *Medical*: lipid binders (e.g. orlistat)
- *Surgical*: malabsorptive surgical procedures, sleeve gastrectomy, intragastric balloon

Serious/frequently occurring risks[1–3]

- *General*: bleeding, infection (chest/wound/systemic), DVT/pulmonary embolism/CVA/myocardial infarction
- *Specific*:
  - Early: band slippage, intolerance of band, dysphagia, port site infections, gastro-oesophageal reflux
  - Late: band erosion, port site hernia, diarrhoea

Blood transfusion necessary

- Group and save

Type of anaesthesia/sedation

- General anaesthesia

Follow-up/need for further procedure

- The band is adjusted in outpatients until the optimum tightness of the band is achieved. This can then be adjusted according to the patient's wishes
- Patients may require revision bariatric surgery, commonly a gastric bypass procedure, if weight loss plateaus or the band is not tolerated[2,3]

References

1. Lancaster R, Hutter M. Bands and bypasses: 30-day morbidity and mortality of bariatric surgical procedures as assessed by prospective, multi-center, risk-adjusted ACS-NSQIP data. *Serg Endosc* 2008;**22**:2554–63.
2. Suter M, Calmes JM, Paroz A, *et al.* A 10-year experience with laparoscopic gastric banding for morbid obesity: high long-term complication and failure rates. *Obes Surg* 2006;**16**(7):829–35.
3. O'Brien PE, Dixon JB, Brown W, *et al.* The laparoscopic adjustable gastric band (Lap-Band): a prospective study of medium-term effects on weight, health and quality of life. *Obes Surg* 2002;**12**(5):652–60.

Oesophageal repair

Description

Oesophageal perforation, while rare, is life-threatening, and 90% of cases are secondary to instrumentation of the oesophagus during endoscopy. The remaining 10% are due to Boerhaave's syndrome (oesophageal rupture secondary to vomiting or retching), trauma, or caustic injury secondary to ingestion of substances such as bleach.[1]

Perforations can occur in the neck (cervical), the chest, or in the abdomen. Management depends on the level of the perforation. Diagnosis can be made by direct visualization at endoscopy, water-soluble contrast studies or during contrast CT scanning.[2]

Cervical perforations

This condition is usually dealt with by the ENT department. The perforations are most often treated conservatively but surgical repair may be recommended in the early stages. Later the tissues become friable where only drainage is possible.

Thoracic perforations

Primary repair may be possible in the early stages. In cases of extreme contamination or late intervention, treatment consists of removal of contamination, copious washout, mediastinal drainage, and insertion of a T-tube into the defect. The use of a T-tube creates a controlled fistula.

Abdominal perforations

These are most commonly iatrogenic secondary to surgery. When noted intraoperatively they can be repaired immediately. If they are detected postoperatively, a upper midline laparotomy is required for primary oesophageal repair and peritoneal washout.

Additional procedures that may become necessary

- Feeding jejunostomy
- Drainage gastrostomy
- Insertion of a T-tube for drainage
- Emergency oesophagectomy—if the perforation is extensive or not amenable to repair; carries a high rate of mortality
- Cervical oesophagostomy[3]

Benefits

- *Therapeutic*: to relieve sepsis, This is a life-saving procedure

Alternative procedures/conservative measures

- *Conservative*: antibiotics, antifungal treatment, proton pump inhibitors, total parenteral nutrition, nasogastric tube drainage, palliative care
- *Endoscopic*: covered oesophageal stents

Serious/frequently occurring risks

- *Early*: death (thoracic perforation holds a mortality rate of over 50% for those not explored within 24h and between 10% and 15% for those repaired within 24h[1]), sepsis (intrathoracic/systemic), mediastinitis/

mediastinal collection (may require drainage via mediastinoscopy), acute respiratory distress syndrome, prolonged ITU stay
- *Late*: chronic lung disease, dysphagia, multiple operations

Blood transfusion necessary
- Cross-match 4–6 units

Type of anaesthesia/sedation
- General anaesthesia

Follow-up/need for further procedure
- Prolonged hospital stay
- Repeated imaging and endoscopy to assess the progress of the perforation

References
1. Brinster CJ, Singhal S, Lee L, et al. Evolving options in the management of esophageal perforation. *Ann Thorac Surg* 2004;**77**(4):1475–83.
2. Griffin SM, Lamb PJ, Shenfine J, et al. Spontaneous rupture of the oesophagus. *Br J Surg* 2008;**95**(9):1115–20.
3. Rohatgi A, Papanikitas J, Sutcliffe R, et al. The role of oesophageal diversion and exclusion in the management of oesophageal perforations. *Int J Surg* 2009;**7**(2):142–4.

Oesophageal replacement

Description

The conduit of choice for oesophageal reconstruction is the stomach. However, if the stomach is not available, for example after a total gastrectomy or if pathology involves the stomach and oesophagus, another conduit will be necessary. The commonest indication for this is caustic injury of the oesophagus and stomach. For short defects a free jejunal interposition may be possible, however, larger defects require the colon.

Colonic interposition involves the fashioning of three anastomoses (Fig. 8.4). Ascending or transverse colon is used depending on the length required. The ascending colon is mobilized as an iso-peristaltic loop with a vascular pedicle formed from the middle colic vessels. The caecum is anastomosed to the cervical oesophagus in the neck or the thoracic oesophagus in the chest, forming an oesophagocolic anastomosis. To restore gastrointestinal continuity an ileocolic or colojejunal anastomosis is fashioned.[1]

Jejunal grafts can be used as an iso-peristaltic interposition graft, however, its blood supply limits how high within the thoracic cavity it can be used. If it is required above the level of the aortic arch a vascularized free flap is required. This is technically a much more difficult procedure but may be physiologically preferable and therefore only used where other options are not possible or have failed. An oesophagojejunal anastomosis is fashioned in the chest followed by a jejuno-jejunal anastomosis to restore continuity.[2]

The conduit can be brought up into the neck via the posterior mediastinal, retrosternal, or subcutaneous route. The preferred route is the anatomical route, posterior mediastinal. However if this is not possible alternative routes may become necessary.

Additional procedures that may become necessary

- Although another procedure may not be necessary, the route and choice of interposition conduit may vary intraoperatively

Benefits

- *Therapeutic*: to provide gastrointestinal continuity allowing for enteral feeding

Alternative procedures/conservative measures

- *Conservative*: total parenteral nutrition
- *Endoscopic*: oesophageal stenting
- *Surgical*: long-term feeding jejunostomy

Serious/frequently occurring risks[3]

- *General*: bleeding, infection(wound/chest/systemic), pulmonary embolism/DVT/ACS/CVA
- *Specific*:
  - *Early*: anastomotic leak/breakdown, ischaemic necrosis of conduit
  - *Late*: dumping syndrome, bile reflux, long-term dysphagia (due to poor peristalsis of colon)

Blood transfusion necessary

- Cross-match blood (4–6 units)

Type of anaesthesia/sedation

- General anaesthesia/regional anaesthesia with thoracic epidural insertion is usually performed

Follow-up/need for further procedure

- Follow up is dependent on the indication for surgery
- For cancer patients follow-up is lifelong and may require further oncological treatment dependent on their pathological staging

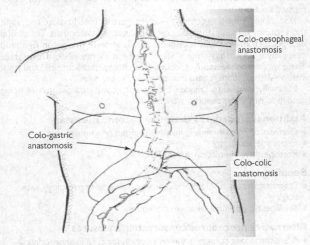

Colo-oesophageal anastomosis

Colo-gastric anastomosis

Colo-colic anastomosis

Fig. 8.4 Right colonic interposition from cervical oesophagus to antrum with colo-colic anastomosis.

Reproduced with permission from McLatchie GR and Leaper DJ. *Oxford Specialist Handbook of Operative Surgery* 2nd edition. 2006. Oxford: Oxford University Press, p.219, Figure 6.6.

References

1. DeMeester TR, Johansson KE, Franze I, et al. Indications, surgical technique, and long-term functional results of colon interposition or bypass. *Ann Surg* 1988;**208**(4):460–74.
2. Sasaki TM, McConnell DB, Moseley HS, et al. Antethoracic jejunal esophagoplasty. An alternate method of repair. *Am J Surg* 1981;**141**(5):534–6.
3. Motoyama S, Kitamura M, Saito R, et al. Surgical outcome of colon interposition by the posterior mediastinal route for thoracic esophageal cancer. *Ann Thorac Surg* 2007;**83**(4):1273–8.

Oesophagectomy (Ivor Lewis/transhiatal/three-stage)

Description

The commonest indication for oesophagectomy is malignant disease, however, occasionally it is needed for benign tumours or strictures. Oesophagectomy may be total or subtotal. The conduit for oesophageal replacement is usually the stomach but colon or vascularized small bowel may be used. Anastomosis may be in the neck or within the thorax. Access to the abdomen is required to mobilize the stomach (or other replacement organs[1]).

Ivor Lewis oesophagectomy involves gastric mobilization and right thoracotomy with intrathoracic oesophagogastric anastomosis. Transhiatal oesophagectomy involves transhiatal mobilization of the oesophagus and oesophagogastric anastomosis via an incision in the neck. Three-stage McKeown oesophagectomy involves laparotomy, thoracotomy, and neck incision with oesophagogastric anastomosis in the neck.

Minimally invasive techniques, thoracoscopy, and laparoscopy are being used in all of the procedures mentioned.

Additional procedures that may become necessary

- Conversion from minimally invasive to open procedure
- Feeding jejunostomy
- Postoperative ventilation in the ITU

Benefits

- *Diagnostic*: histopathological diagnosis of underlying pathology with staging
- *Therapeutic*: potential curative procedure

Alternative procedures/conservative measures

- *Adenocarcinoma*: surgery is the only option for cure in appropriately selected patients
- *Squamous cell carcinoma* (SCC): chemoradiation may be an equivalent treatment
- *Palliative*: oesophageal stents, chemotherapy, and radiotherapy

Serious/frequently occurring risks[2,3]

- *General*: bleeding, infection (wound—including cervical sepsis, chest—increased post-thoracotomy, intra-abdominal, systemic), pulmonary embolism/DVT/CVA/ACS, death
- *Specific*:
  - Early: anastomotic leak/breakdown—leads to a leak of gastric contents into the thoracic cavity. The management depends of the timing and site of the leak. Left pneumothorax, bronchial injury and air leak, recurrent laryngeal nerve injury, chyle leak
  - Late: early satiety, bile reflux, anastomotic stricture

Blood transfusion necessary

- Group and save as a minimum, cross match 4–6 units

Type of anaesthesia/sedation

- General anaesthesia/regional anaesthesia (thoracic epidural usually performed)

Follow-up/need for further procedure

- Patients require a minimum of HDU care postoperatively and many will require a stay in the ITU
- Follow-up is dependent on indication for surgery. For cancer patients follow-up is lifelong, and they may require further oncological treatment dependent on their pathological staging

References

1. Akiyama H. *Surgery for Cancer of the Oesophagus*. Baltimore: Lippincott Williams & Wilkins, 1990.
2. RCSE Clinical Effectiveness Unit/AUGIS/BSG. *National Oesophagogastric Cancer Audit 2009*. Available at: ⅗ www.augis.org/pdf/audits/nhs-ic-og-clinical-audit_2nd_Annual_Report_2009.pdf (accessed 10 May 2011).
3. Griffin SM, Shaw IH, Dresner SM. Early complications after Ivor Lewis subtotal esophagectomy with two-field lymphadenectomy: risk factors and management. *J Am Coll Surg* 2002;**194**(3):285–97.

Oesophagogastroduodenoscopy

Description

OGD is a telescopic examination that is used for direct visualization of the oesophagus, stomach, and the first and second parts of the duodenum (Fig. 8.5). Upper gastrointestinal endoscopy may be diagnostic or therapeutic; emergency or elective. Common indications include gastrointestinal bleeding, dysphagia, vomiting, weight loss, epigastric pain, and reflux symptoms. Various procedures can be performed during an OGD, for example:

- Biopsy
- *Campylobacter*-like organism (CLO) testing
- Management of bleeding ulcers—injection, clips, laser, cryotherapy
- Variceal banding
- Oesophageal stent placement
- Nasogastric/nasojejunal tube placement
- Percutaneous endoscopic gastrostomy
- Balloon dilatation of stricture
- Mucosal resection

Additional procedures that may become necessary

- In an emergency OGD for bleeding—laparotomy for haemostasis
- Biopsy for histology/*H. pylori*

Benefits

- *Diagnostic*: to identify lesion of concern/cause of symptoms or to obtain histology for histopathological analysis
- *Therapeutic*: treatment of strictures, bleeding, malignancy
- Insertion of feeding (nasogastric or nasojejunal) tube

Alternative procedures/conservative measures

- *Radiological*: CT scanning, barium swallow or meal, fluoroscopy, radiological nasogastric or nasojejunal tube placement
- *Conservative*: blind placement of a nasogastric tube, feeding jejunostomy
- *Surgical*: total parenteral nutrition via a central venous line, surgery for treatment of bleeding and strictures

Serious/frequently occurring risks[1,2]

- Bleeding from biopsy site (exceedingly rare), perforation (in diagnostic OGD 1:5000), pain, treatment failure (stent slippage, ongoing bleeding, further structuring), inadequate tissue on biopsy, damage to teeth, aspiration of stomach contents, respiratory depression from sedation

Blood transfusion necessary

- Diagnostic—none
- Therapeutic—group and save/cross-match 4–6 units for acute bleeding. *Additional blood products should be available for the management of* acute gastrointestinal bleeds

Type of anaesthesia/sedation

- Local anaesthesia throat spray or light sedative, very occasionally under general anaesthesia

Follow-up

- This is dependent on the indication and findings of the OGD
- Repeat endoscopy may be required to ensure ulcer healing or to repeat biopsies
- Stents may require replacement or procedures to address tumour overgrowth

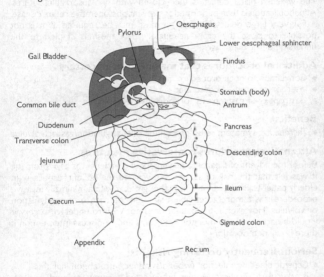

Fig. 8.5 Anatomy of the gastrointestinal tract

References

1. Wolfsen HC, Hemminger LL, Achem SR, et al. Complications of endoscopy of the upper gastrointestinal tract: a single e-center experience. Mayo Clin Proc 2004;79(10):1264–7.
2. Reed WP, Kilkenny JW, Dias CE, et al. A prospective analysis of 3525 esophagogastroduodenoscopies performed by surgeons. Surg Endosc 2004;18(1):11–21.

Paraoesophageal hiatus hernia repair

Description

A paraoesophageal hiatus hernia is uncommon. The gastro-oesophageal junction remains within the abdomen and the stomach herniates beside it into the mediastinum. Repair is usually performed laparoscopically, however, it may be performed via an upper midline incision.[1] The stomach, other herniated contents, and the hernial sac are returned to the abdomen. The hernial sac can then either be circumcised or excised. The widened hiatal defect is then closed with non-absorbable sutures. A fundoplication is then performed to prevent postoperative reflux disease.

For very large defects (>10cm) a mesh may be required as it is not possible to close the crura adequately. The mesh is stapled to the underside of the diaphragm.

Additional procedures that may become necessary

- Conversion to open procedure
- Insertion of mesh—as described
- Gastropexy or gastroplasty for shortened oesophagus

Benefits

- *Therapeutic*: symptom relief, prevention of strangulation/gastric volvulus

Alternative procedures/conservative measures

Before the advent of laparoscopic surgery, if a patient was asymptomatic it was felt that the risk of surgery outweighed the benefit, especially in elderly patients. However, it is now thought that with a minimally invasive procedure it is a more acceptable risk given the chance of strangulation or volvulus. However, if the patient does not wish to undergo surgery it would be acceptable to monitor symptoms and re-discuss intervention if there is any deterioration.

Serious/frequently occurring risks[1–3]

- *General*: bleeding, infection (wound/systemic, intra-abdominal: this is particularly significant if any mesh inserted becomes infected), pulmonary embolism/DVT/CVA
- *Specific*:
  - *Early*: dysphagia, splenic injury, oesophageal perforation
  - *Late*: gas bloat syndrome, epigastric pain, wrap failure, recurrent hernia

Blood transfusion necessary

- Group and save/cross match 2–4 units

Type of anaesthesia/sedation

- General anaesthesia

Follow-up/need for further procedure

- Patients require a soft diet for 6 weeks postoperatively and are seen at 4 weeks postoperatively
- If they are well at this stage the patient can be discharged from follow-up

References

1. Andujar JJ, Papasavas PK, Birdas T, et al. Laparoscopic repair of large paraesophageal hernia is associated with a low incidence of recurrence and reoperation. *Surg Endosc* 2004;**18**(3):444–7.
2. Hashemi M, Sillin LF, Peters JH. Current concepts in the management of paraesophageal hiatal hernia. *J Clin Gastroenterol* 1999;**29**(1):8–13.
3. Fuller CB, Hagen JA, DeMeester TR, et al. The role of fundoplication in the treatment of type II paraesophageal hernia. *J Thorac Cardiovasc Surg* 1996;**111**(3):655–61.

Percutaneous endoscopic gastrostomy

Description

PEG is a method of introducing a feeding tube through the abdominal wall into the stomach for enteral feeding. An endoscope is passed into the stomach and used to transilluminate the abdominal wall. Insufflation distends the stomach and digital pressure is applied to the abdominal wall, which can be visualized indenting on the stomach by the endoscopist.

The PEG tube consists of a silicone tube and a 2cm disc-shaped 'bumper', which abuts the gastric wall. A fine-bore needle is introduced and can be seen entering the stomach on endoscopy; a feeding suture is then passed in through this needle and pulled up through the oesophagus and out through the mouth. The gastrostomy catheter is attached to the feeding suture and pulled down into the stomach. This catheter is passed through the stomach and abdominal wall under direct vision (Fig. 8.6).

Additional procedures that may become necessary

- None

Benefits

- To maintain or supplement nutrition

Alternative procedures/conservative measures

- *Conservative*: nasogastric and nasojejunal feeding. Parenteral nutrition via a CVC is a further method of feeding, however, it should be used only when enteral feeding is not an option
- *Surgical*: jejunostomy. A feeding gastrostomy tube may be inserted at mini-laparotomy if there is obstruction of the oesophagus

Serious/frequently occurring risks[1-3]

- *Early*: bleeding (the gastrostomy tube when inserted can damage to vascular supply surrounding the stomach), pneumoperitoneum and peritonitis, infection at abdominal wall entry site, food/feed leakage into peritoneal cavity, risk associated with sedation
- *Late*: gastric ulcer around site of PEG bumper, tube blockage, migration of tube into gastric wall

Blood transfusion necessary

- None/group and save

Type of anaesthesia/sedation

- Local/general anaesthesia (especially for children/learning difficulties)

Follow-up/need for further procedure

- Regular district nurse/home care and education in use and flushing of tube
- Once the PEG is no longer required it can be removed endoscopically

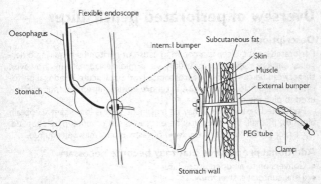

Fig. 8.6 PEG tube placement.

References

1. Zopf Y, Rabe C, Bruckmoser T, et al. Percutaneous endoscopic jejunostomy and jejunal extension tube through percutaneous endoscopic gastrostomy: a retrospective analysis of success, complications and outcome. *Digestion* 2009;**79**(2):92–7.

2. Schrag SP, Sharma R, Jaik NP, et al. Complications related to percutaneous endoscopic gastrostomy (PEG) tubes. A comprehensive clinical review. *J Gastrointestin Liver Dis* 2007;**16**(4):407–18.

3. Figueiredo FA, da Costa MC, Pelosi AD, et al. Predicting outcomes and complications of percutaneous endoscopic gastrostomy. *Endoscopy* 2007;**39**(4):333–8.

Oversew of perforated peptic ulcer

Description

Perforated peptic ulcer is a common cause of peritonitis requiring emergency surgery. Operation is usually via a midline laparotomy, however, surgery can be carried out laparoscopically.[1,2] Small acute duodenal perforations may be closed primarily, but more commonly an omental patch is used to plug the defect.

Perforated gastric ulcers may be malignant so it is important to obtain biopsies. If small, the ulcer may be excised or an omental patch applied. For larger gastric lesions, some form of gastrectomy may be required.

Additional procedures that may become necessary

- Conversion to an open procedure
- Total/subtotal gastrectomy

Benefits

- *Therapeutic*: prevention of further sepsis
- A potentially life-saving procedure

Alternative procedures/conservative measures

- *Conservative*: nasogastric drainage, intravenous antibiotics, and acid suppression with proton pump inhibitors
- Conservative management may be employed in selected patients with minimal symptoms or signs of sepsis. The diagnosis must be confirmed radiologically

Serious/frequently occurring risks[1–3]

- *General*: bleeding, infection (chest, intra-abdominal, systemic), death
- *Specific*:
  - *Early*: leak from site of repair
  - *Late*: recurrent ulceration at site of repair or elsewhere, duodenal stricturing, gastroparesis

Blood transfusion necessary

- Group and save/cross-match 2–6 units depending on starting haemoglobin

Type of anaesthesia/sedation

- General anaesthesia

Follow-up/need for further procedure

- Gastric ulcers may prove to be malignant and patients may require further surgery for definitive management of their cancer
- Further endoscopy will be needed to ensure ulcer healing
- Duodenal ulcers will require proton pump inhibition and *H. pylori* eradication

References

1. Bertleff MJ, Halm JA, Bemelman WA, *et al*. Randomized clinical trial of laparoscopic versus open repair of the perforated peptic ulcer: the LAMA Trial. *World J Surg* 2009;**33**(7):1368–73.
2. Lau WY, Leung KL, Kwong KH, *et al*. A randomized study comparing laparoscopic versus open repair of perforated peptic ulcer using suture or sutureless technique. *Ann Surg* 1996;**224**:131–8.
3. Kocer B, Surmeli S, Solak C, *et al*. Factors affecting mortality and morbidity in patients with peptic ulcer perforation. *J Gastroenterol Hepatol* 2007;**22**(4):565–70.

Sleeve gastrectomy

Description

Bariatric surgical procedures are divided into malabsorptive procedures and restrictive procedures. Restrictive procedures primarily reduce stomach size and malabsorptive procedures, while they may also reduce the size of the stomach, primarily act to reduce absorption of ingested food. Sleeve gastrectomy is an example of a restrictive procedure. It is often used as a bridge procedure in high-risk patients prior to definitive weight loss procedures such as a duodenal switch.

Sleeve gastrectomy is a partial longitudinal gastrectomy. It removes the entire greater curvature of the stomach leaving a gastric volume of approximately 100mL, which drains directly into the duodenum without need for anastomosis. It can be performed laparoscopically or via an upper midline incision.

Additional procedures that may become necessary

- If performed laparoscopically—conversion to open procedure

Benefits

- *Primary*: weight loss
- *Secondary*: resolution of obesity-related comorbidities such as diabetes mellitus and hypertension

Alternative procedures/conservative measures

- *Conservative*: diet and exercise
- *Medical*: lipid binders (e.g. orlistat)
- *Surgical*: malabsorptive surgical procedures, intragastric balloon

Serious/frequently occurring risks[1,2]

- *General*: bleeding, infection (chest/wound/systemic), DVT/pulmonary embolism/CVA/myocardial infarction
- *Specific*:
  - *Early*: staple line leak, splenic injury
  - *Late*: gastric stenosis, gastro-oesophageal reflux, dilatation of the gastric pouch (leading to weight gain), vitamin B_{12} and iron deficiency, port site hernia

Blood transfusion necessary

- Group and save

Type of anaesthesia/sedation

- General anaesthesia

Follow-up/need for further procedure

- Patients require close monitoring by a multidisciplinary team in the initial *postoperative period*
- This includes monitoring and treatment of any psychological sequelae
- Long-term weight loss follow-up may be managed in the community by primary care teams

References

1. Akkary, E., A. Duffy, and R. Bell. Deciphering the sleeve: technique, indications, efficacy, and safety of sleeve gastrectomy. *Obes Surg*, 2008. **18**(10): p. 1323-9.
2. Gumbs, A.A., et al. Sleeve gastrectomy for morbid obesity. *Obes Surg*, 2007. **17**(7): p. 962–9.

Splenectomy

Description

Splenectomy may be required in the treatment of haematological disorders, trauma, or in the case of massive splenomegaly to control symptoms and prevent injury.

Splenectomy is associated with long-term risk of infection so patients require preoperative immunizations where possible and will require lifelong antibiotics prophylaxis.[1] In traumatic splenic injury, splenic conservation should be considered at the time of laparotomy. Splenectomy may be performed laparoscopically or via a left subcostal or upper midline incision.[2]

Additional procedures that may become necessary

- In the case of massive splenomegaly—a long oblique incision, bilateral subcostal incision, or a roof-top incision may be necessary

Benefits

- *Diagnostic*: identify pathological cause of splenic enlargement (lymphoma etc.)
- *Therapeutic*: haematological benefit, control bleeding

Alternative procedures/conservative measures

- This is dependent on the indication for the surgery; medical treatment for haematological conditions is usually exhausted prior to consideration of surgery. In the case of trauma, spleen-preserving procedures are preferred where possible

Serious/frequently occurring risks[3]

- *Early*: bleeding, pancreatic injury (the tail of the pancreas can be damaged during the ligation of the hilar vessels), colonic injury
- *Late*: overwhelming infection (OPSI). This is caused by encapsulated bacteria, including *Streptococcus pneumoniae*. The lifetime risk is approximately 5% with the majority of cases occurring in the first few years post-splenectomy, thromboembolic complications (increased following removal of the spleen due to a rise in the platelet count)

Blood transfusion necessary

- Group and save, cross-matched blood (2–6 units) should be available in cases of massive splenomegaly. In certain haematological conditions, additional blood products (e.g. platelets) should be made available

Type of anaesthesia/sedation

- General anaesthesia

Follow-up/need for further procedure[2]

- In elective splenectomy patients should receive immunizations for *S. pneumoniae*, *Haemophilus influenzae* type B, and *Neisseria meningitidis* 2 weeks prior to surgery
- In the emergency setting, immunizations should be delayed to 2 weeks postoperatively to ensure an adequate immune response

- Patients will require lifelong prophylactic antibiotics (oral phenoxymethylpenicillin or erythromycin)

References

1. Habermalz B, Sauerland S, Decker G, *et al.* Laparoscopic splenectomy: the clinical practice guidelines of the European Association for Endoscopic Surgery (EAES). *Surg Endosc* 2008;**22**(4):821–48.
2. Working Party of the British Committee for Standards in Haematology Clinical Haematology Task Force. Guidelines for the prevention and treatment of infection in patients with an absent or dysfunctional spleen. *BMJ* 1996;**312**(7028):430–4.
3. Cadili A, de Gara C. Complications of splenectomy. *Am J Med* 2008;**121**(5):371–5.

Highly selective vagotomy

Description

Vagotomies are used in the treatment of peptic ulcer disease and their purpose is to abolish vagal stimulation of the parietal cells, thereby decreasing gastric acid secretion.[1] Highly selective vagotomy is rarely performed today as proton pump inhibition can virtually obliterate all gastric acid secretion. Indications for highly selective vagotomy include treatment of complications of increased acid secretion despite proton pump inhibitor treatment and non-compliant patients. This procedure can be performed laparoscopically or via an upper midline incision.

Additional procedures that may become necessary

• None

Benefits

• *Therapeutic*: symptomatic relief, prevention of the complications of peptic ulcer disease, allow for ulcer healing and prevention of further ulceration

Alternative procedures/conservative measures

• *Conservative*: dietary and lifestyle modification (e.g. smoking)
• *Medical*: proton pump inhibitors, H_2 receptor antagonists
• *Surgical*: subtotal gastrectomy—for excision of any concurrent ulcers

Serious/frequently occurring risks[2]

• *Early*: bleeding, infection (wound/chest/systemic), lesser curve necrosis with perforation, gastroparesis
• *Late*: dumping syndrome, delayed gastric emptying, recurrent ulceration, increased susceptibility to gastrointestinal infection

Blood transfusion necessary

• Group and save

Type of anaesthesia/sedation

• General anaesthesia

Follow-up/need for further procedure

• Patients require close follow-up and repeat endoscopy to assess the success of the surgery and monitor for further ulceration or malignancy

References

1. Gilliam AD, Speake WJ, Lobo DN, *et al.* Current practice of emergency vagotomy and Helicobacter pylori eradication for complicated peptic ulcer in the United Kingdom. *Br J Surg* 2003;**90**(1):88–90.
2. Jordan PH, Thornby J. Twenty years after parietal cell vagotomy or selective vagotomy antrectomy for treatment of duodenal ulcer. Final report. *Ann Surg* 1994;**220**(3):283–96.

Transplantation surgery

Introduction

Consenting with a view to procedures involved in transplant surgery is complex and is legislation bound. The HTA 2004[1] and Human Tissue (Scotland) Act (2006)[2] provide a framework for removal, storage, and use of tissues and organs from the deceased and living for specified health-related purposes. The fundamental principle that underpins this Act is the consent in the UK. Consent for removal of organs from the living is covered by the common consent law, but consent for storage and use of organs and tissue is covered by the HTA 2004. For further details, refer to the publications *Codes of Practice on Consent* and *Donation of organs, tissues and cells for transplantation produced by the Human Tissue Authority (HTA)*.[3,4]

References

1. *Human Tissue Act 2004*. Available at: ℘ www.legislation.gov.uk/ukpga/2004/30/contents (accessed 6 May 2011).
2. *Human Tissue (Scotland) Act 2006*. Available at: ℘ www.legislation.gov.uk/asp/2006/4/contents (accessed 6 May 2011).
3. *Human Tissue Authority Code of Practice-Consent*. 2009. Available at: ℘ www.hta.gov.uk/legislationpoliciesandcodesofpractice/codesofpractice/code1consent.cfm (accessed 6 May 2011).
4. *Human Tissue Authority Code of Practice—Donation of Organs, Tissues and Cells for Transplantation* 2009. Available at: ℘ www.hta.gov.uk/legislationpoliciesandcodesofpractice/codesofpractice/code2donationoforgans.cfm (accessed 6 May 2011).

Deceased donor retrieval

Deceased donors have provided the majority of organs transplanted over the last 40 years and include:

- Donation after brain death (DBD; heart-beating donors)
- Donation after cardiac death (DCD; non-heart-beating donors)
- Extended criteria donor (marginal donors)

Description[1,2]

Deceased donors are multiorgan donors in whom laparotomy and thoracotomy is performed to donate the heart, lungs, liver, kidney, pancreas, and small bowel. In DBDs, the patient's cardiorespiratory function is maintained until cold perfusion is set up and adequate dissection done, so that cardiorespiratory arrest coincides with cold perfusion and thus warm ischaemia is avoided. During the procedure, cooling is achieved by two possible techniques: (a) open technique—rapid access laparotomy; and (b) minimal access—intra-aortic balloon catheter technique via a femoral vessel approach, done after cardio-respiratory arrest. Following this, the organs retrieved as discussed in the consent. These patients are exsanguinated and careful suturing, application of dressing, and cleaning are a must to ensure dignity and respect.

Additional procedures that may become necessary

- Frozen section due to suspected occult malignancy

Benefits

- Multiple organs benefiting a possible number of recipients

Serious/frequently occurring risk

- Bleeding
- Damage to viscus, lead to termination of retrieval process
- Damage to organs retrieved

Blood transfusion necessary

- None

Type of anaesthesia/sedation

- *DBDs*: general cessation on commencement of perfusion and exsanguination
- *DCDs*: none

References

1. Forsythe LR. *A Companion to Specialist Surgical Practice Transplantation*, 4th edn. London: WB Saunders/Elsevier, 2009.
2. Danovitch GM. *Handbook of Kidney Transplantation*, 5th edn. Philadelphia: Lippincott Williams & Wilkins, 2010.

Live donor retrieval

Live donor kidney retrieval: laparoscopic donor nephrectomy

Description

The procedure involves keyhole surgery with three to four port sites (two 12mm ports) and a 6–7cm Pfannenstiel incision (organ retrieval/hand-assisted approach), where initially under anaesthesia a laparoscopy is performed followed by dissection of the kidney, then under upmost precautions ligation of the ureter, renal artery and vein with a view to no damage to any of these structures, so as to use the organ for transplantation.

Additional procedures that may become necessary
- Insertion of an arterial line
- Insertion of central venous line, trans-oesophageal Doppler probe for fluid management
- Insertion of urinary catheter

Benefits
- To donate the kidney as a gift for treating renal failure

Alternative procedures/conservative measures
- Open donor nephrectomy

Serious/frequently occurring risk[1]
- Pain, bleeding, scarring, neurovascular injury, visceral injury, vascular injury
- Conversion to open surgery (1/100)
- Adhesion formation (3/100)
- Thromboembolic disease (1/300), myocardial infarction
- Port site hernia, incisional hernia
- Mortality (1/3000)

Blood transfusion necessary
- Very small possibility, cross-match 3 units

Type of anaesthesia/sedation
- General anaesthesia
- Transversus abdominis plane (TAP) blocks or PCA

Follow-up/need for further procedure
- At 1 month, 6 months, and 1 year postoperatively so as to assess renal function (urea and electrolytes (U&E)), blood pressure, full blood count (FBC), and urine for proteinuria and haematuria and annually thereafter

Live donor kidney retrieval: open donor nephrectomy

Description

Traditionally performed through a loin incision (possible of 11th rib excision) or through a mini-incision (subcostal or anterior), complication profile is similar to the previous procedure with an increased incidence of more pain, longer in-hospital stay, and increased risk of pneumothorax.[1]

Live donor liver retrieval

Description

The procedure involves a laparotomy with a reverse L or roof-top incision and midline extension, where in most cases a right hepatectomy (left lobectomy or left lateral segmentectomy (segments II and III), in case of a child recipient), is performed. The liver grows back to 89% of original volume by 6 months.

Additional procedures that may become necessary

- Insertion of an arterial line
- Insertion of central venous line, trans-oesophageal Doppler probe for fluid management
- Insertion of urinary catheter
- Insertion of epidural catheter

Benefits

- To donate a lobe of the liver as a gift for treating end-stage liver disease and hepatic failure

Serious/frequently occurring risk[2]

- Pain, bleeding, scarring, neurovascular injury, visceral injury, vascular injury
- Adhesion formation (3/100)
- Thromboembolic disease (1/300), myocardial infarction
- Incisional hernia
- Bile leak
- Liver failure (small-for-size)
- *Mortality*: right lobe donation—0.23–0.5%,[3] left lobe donation—0.05–0.21%, overall 0.2%

Blood transfusion necessary

- Cross-match 6 units

Type of anaesthetic/sedation

- General anaesthesia
- TAP blocks or PCA or epidural for analgesia

Follow-up/need for further procedure

- At 1 month, 6 months, and 1 year postoperatively in order to assess liver function, blood pressure, FBC, international normalized ratio (INR), and annually thereafter

Live donor pancreas retrieval

A laparoscopic or hand-assisted distal pancreatectomy is performed, where the distal half of pancreas is resected and used for transplantation. These are not performed frequently due to high morbidity and mortality. Complications range from high rates of conversion to open surgery, bleeding, damage to visceral structures, splenectomy (20%), reoperation for intra-abdominal collections, and pseudocyst; 5% develop diabetes mellitus and require insulin postoperatively.[4]

Live donor lung retrieval

Very limited numbers, where donor donates a single lobe of lung for organ transplantation. Morbidity occurs in 20%, with the most common being the need for prolonged thoracostomy for persistent air leaks or drainage.

Live donor small bowel retrieval

An operation in its infancy. Only 32 have been reported in the intestinal transplant registry.[5] The procedure involves a laparotomy and small bowel resection and primary anastomosis. Mortality estimates are difficult due to small numbers, and taking care to avoid small bowel syndrome in the donor is of upmost importance.

References

1. Nanidis T, Antcliffe D, Kokkinos C et al. Laparoscopic versus open live donor nephrectomy in renal transplantation: a meta-analysis. *Ann Surg* 2008;**247**(1):58–70.
2. Chan SC, Fan ST, Lo CM, et al. Toward current standards of donor right hepatectomy for adult-to-adult live donor liver transplantation through the experience of 200 cases. *Ann Surg* 2007;**245**(1):110–17.
3. Iida T, Ogura Y, Oike F et al. Surgery-related morbidity in living donors for liver transplantation. *Transplantation* 2010;**89**(10):1276–82.
4. Reynoso JF, Gruessner CE, Sutherland DE et al. Short- and long-term outcomes for living pancreas donors. *J Hepatobiliary Pancreat Sci* 2010;**17**:92–6.
5. Grant D, Abu-Elmagd K, Reyes J et al. 2003 Report of the Intestine Transplant Registry. *Ann Surg* 2005;**241**(4):607–13.

General complications in transplant surgery

These vary from organ to organ and are related to graft function, side effects of immunosuppression, ischaemia-reperfusion injury, and can be organ specific.

- Delayed graft function: the transplanted organ does not work straightaway and does vary with the type of donor (rarely seen in live donor transplants, never seen with pancreas transplants). It could be related to acute tubular necrosis, intravascular volume contraction, urine leak, ureteric obstruction, rejection or nephrotoxicity. The need for interim dialysis should be discussed
- Acute rejection
- Primary non-function
- Electrolyte and acid–base balance
- Infection: inevitable consequence following immunosuppression and thus patients are at higher risk of cytomegalovirus (CMV), polyoma virus, hepatitis B, hepatitis C as well as bacterial and other opportunistic infections
- Malignancy: 3.5-fold higher than age-matched controls, commonest are skin cancers, Kaposi's sarcoma, and post-transplant lymphoproliferative disease (PTLD)
- Hyperlipidaemia
- Chronic transplant dysfunction (chronic allograft nephropathy), leading cause of graft loss after 1 year
- Recurrent and *de novo* renal disease; focal segmental glomerulosclerosis, membranoproliferative glomerulonephritis types I and II, IgA nephropathy, Henoch–Schönlein purpura, membranous nephropathy, haemolytic uremic syndrome, diabetes
- Complications of immunosuppression

Immunosuppression

Description

There is an ever-increasing range of agents, but most agents are used to prevent rejection act predominantly on T cells via different sites during T-cell activation. Protocols vary in different units but involve a combination of agents. Over the decades the immunosuppressive regimens have become more sophisticated, allowing for long-term graft survival and balancing efficacy versus toxicity, side effects, and tolerable immunosuppressive combination regimens.

Principles of immunosuppression

- Same for all types of organ transplantation
- The aim is to maximize graft protection and minimize side effects
- Most regimens are based on calcineurin blockade and include steroids and antiproliferative agents
- The need for immunosuppression is maximum in the first 3 months but indefinite treatment is needed
- Immunosuppression increases risk of infections and malignancy

Standard recommended regimen

- Anti-CD-25 monoclonal antibodies—target activated T-cells, e.g. basiliximab
- Corticosteroids—via widespread anti-inflammatory action. e.g. prednisolone
- Antiproliferative agents: preventing lymphocyte proliferation, e.g. mycophenolate mofetil and azathioprine
- Calcineurin inhibitors: block IL-2 gene transcription, e.g. tacrolimus and ciclosporin
- Other agents such as mTOR inhibitors (sirolimus and everolimus), monoclonal antibodies (OKT3) and polyclonal antibodies (antilymphocyte globulins) also play a role

Additional procedures that may become necessary

- Peripheral and central venous access for monoclonal antibodies
- Prophylactic antibiotics and antiviral drugs

Benefits

- Prevention and treatment of rejection

Alternative procedures/conservative measures

- Not applicable

Serious/frequently occurring risk

Non-specific

- *Infection*: high risk of opportunistic infections, viral—CMV and polyoma virus are a major problem, Bacterial and fungal infections are common, risk of infection is highest in the first 6 months, chemo-prophylaxis is important in high-risk patients

- *Malignancy*: increased risk of skin cancers (SCC most common), increased risk of PTLD
- New-onset diabetes mellitus (NODM): 20% become hyperglycaemic while 10% require treatment

Specific

- *Corticosteroids*: hypertension, dyslipidaemia, diabetes, osteoporosis, avascular necrosis, cushingoid appearance
- *Azathioprine*: leucopenia, thrombocytopenia, hepatotoxicity, gastrointestinal symptoms
- *Mycophenolate mofetil (MMF)*: leucopenia, thrombocytopenia, gastrointestinal symptoms
- *Ciclosporin*: nephrotoxicity, hypertension, dyslipidaemia, hirsutism, gingival hyperplasia
- *Tacrolimus*: nephrotoxicity, hypertension, dyslipidaemia, alopecia, neurotoxicity, diabetes
- *Anti-CD25 monoclonal antibody*: none described

Follow-up/need for further procedure

Unit protocols usually twice a week for first month, thereafter once a week for next 2 months with gradual spacing out, where by the end of 1 year should be every 3–4 months.

Transplant recipient

Renal transplant

Description

Kidney transplantation is an elective (live donor) or emergency (DCD/ DBD) procedure performed in a patient who has undergone extensive and careful preoperative assessment and preparation. This organ transplant releases the patient from dietary and fluid restriction, need for dialysis and physical constraints imposed by the need for dialysis, in addition a better quality of life, improved survival, and being more cost-effective.

The procedure is performed under general anaesthesia and involves central line insertion, urinary catheter insertion followed by a Rutherford–Morrison incision (oblique incisions from the symphysis in the midline curving laterally and superiorly in the direction of the iliac crest), an extraperitoneal dissection using meticulous aseptic technique, and perfect haemostasis. The iliac vessels are then exposed and the renal vein anastomosis performed end to side to the external iliac vein, while the renal artery either to the external iliac artery (end to side) or the internal iliac artery (end to end) and ureter to urinary bladder over a double JJ stent. Drains may or may not be used; closed systems are preferred. This is followed by closure of deep layers with non-absorbable suture and of skin with subcutaneous dissolvable suture. An Opsite™ dressing is preferred as it allows postoperative ultrasound scanning without disturbing the dressing.

Additional procedures that may become necessary

In the case of re-transplantation, patients need to be consented for transplant nephrectomy, bilateral dissections or extensive retroperitoneal dissection for access to the inferior vena cava (IVC) and possible groin dissection for saphenous vein harvesting in case vessel reconstruction is required.

Benefits
- To treat renal failure and remove the need for dialysis

Alternative procedures/conservative measures
- Continue with dialysis

Serious/frequently occurring risk[1]
- *Surgical complications*: wound infections (2%), vascular complications (renal artery thrombosis 1%, renal vein thrombosis 5%, renal artery stenosis 10%), urological complications 5% (urinary leaks, ureteric obstruction), lymphoceles causing pain, ureteric obstruction, oedema of ipsilateral leg, bleeding, visceral injury, neurovascular injury, pain and mortality (1%)
- Immunosuppression complications (◻ see 'Immunosuppression', p.276)
- *Delayed graft function*: DBD (30%), DCD (50%) and live donors (5%), and associated need for dialysis post-transplantation
- *Primary non-function*: graft survival at 1 year 90% and 75% at 5 years, while patient survival 90% at 1 year and 80% at 5 years
- Acute rejection 10–12%
- Recurrent disease
- Urinary tract infection

- Infections and malignancy
- Fluid retention, polyuria
- Chronic transplant dysfunction (chronic rejection, chronic allograft nephropathy), which is the leading cause of graft loss after 1 year

Blood transfusion necessary
- Cross-matched antibody, CMV-negative blood: 3 units

Type of anaesthetic/sedation
- General anaesthesia
- TAP blocks and PCA for postoperative analgesia
- Patients at higher risk: American Society of Anaesthesiologists (ASA) grade III onwards and general risk of myocardial infarction; DVT should be discussed

Follow-up/need for further procedure
- Intense transplant unit protocols, discharged usually after day 7, thereafter usually twice a week for first month, thereafter once a week for next 2 months with gradual spacing out, where by the end of 1 year should be every 3–4months checking for FBC, renal profile and drug levels
- Flexible cystoscopy under local anaesthesia for JJ stent removal at 4 weeks

Pancreas transplant
Description
Pancreas transplantations are performed in three distinct clinical scenarios:
- Simultaneous pancreas-kidney (SPK) (Fig. 9.1)
- Pancreas after kidney transplant
- Pancreas transplant alone

The procedure involves a midline laparotomy and most centres perform the whole organ transplant with a segment of duodenum. The pancreas graft is placed intraperitoneally usually on the right side. The donor vessels of the pancreas are anastomosed to the recipient's iliac vessels and exocrine secretions are most commonly dealt with by anastomoses of the graft duodenum to the small bowel (enteric drainage) often via a Roux-en-Y. Occasionally it may be anastomosed to the urinary bladder (urinary drainage). The pancreas graft functions immediately after revascularization. In an SPK, the kidney is then transplanted either intraperitoneally on the left side, or extraperitoneally as in a standard kidney-alone transplantation. The patients are initially managed postoperatively on ITU.

Additional procedures that may become necessary
- Insertion of central line, arterial line, and urinary catheter
- Between a fifth to a quarter of patients require a re-laparotomy to deal with complications

Benefits
- To treat diabetes and renal failure (SPK)

Alternative procedures/conservative measures
- Renal transplant in an SPK may be placed extraperitoneally as described previously

Serious/frequently occurring risk[2]
- *Infective*: systemic infections (opportunistic associated with immunosuppression), local infections (wound infection 10%, peritonitis, localised/intra-abdominal collections, enteric and pancreatic fistula)
- *Vascular*: haemorrhage (early-allograft vessels, late rupture of pseudo-aneurysm), thrombosis (allograft arterial or venous thrombosis 5%)
- *Allograft pancreatitis*: reperfusion injury or reflex pancreatitis (0.3–0.6%) (especially after bladder drainage)
- *Complications specific to bladder drainage*: chronic dehydration, acidosis, recurrent UTI, haematuria, chemical cystitis, urethral strictures, urethral disruption
- *Anastomotic leak*: 1.1–1.3%
- *Acute rejection*: 10–20%
- *Mortality*: 5%, after SPK, 1-year patient survival is 95% and 1-year graft survival of pancreas is 85%, while kidney is 95%. 5-year patient survival after SPK is 86% and graft survival is 71%

Blood transfusion necessary
- Cross-matched antibody, CMV negative blood: 6 units

Type of anaesthetic/sedation
- General anaesthesia with TAP blocks and PCA for post op analgesia. (patients are of higher risk, ASA grade III onwards and general risk of MI, DVT should be discussed)

Follow-up/need for further procedure
- Intense unit protocols, discharged usually after 7–10 days, thereafter usually twice a week for first month, thereafter once a week for next 2 months with gradual spacing out, where by the end of 1 year should be every 3–4 months, checking for FBC, renal profile, drug levels and blood sugar monitoring
- Flexible cystoscopy under local anaesthesia for JJ stent removal at 4 weeks (SPK patients)

Liver transplant

Description

A liver transplantation is the most effective way of treating end-stage liver failure and is performed via a transverse upper abdominal incision with a midline extension. There are generally four types of liver grafts:
- Whole organ
- Reduced size
- Split
- Live donor liver transplant

In the case of the IVC replacement technique, the recipient initially undergoes a hepatectomy, where the CBD and hepatic artery are divided followed by IVC clamping and division above and below the liver (Fig. 9.2a). Sometimes the creation of a veno-venous bypass is necessary (IVC and portal vein to axillary or internal jugular vein). The portal vein is then clamped and divided, allowing the recipient liver to be removed. The donor liver is placed *in-situ* allowing supra- and infra-caval anastomosis, then portal vein and hepatic artery anastomosis thereafter permitting graft reperfusion. Finally, biliary drainage is re-established via a duct-to-duct anastomosis.

Alternatively, the piggyback technique (Fig. 9.2b) may be preferred in which diseased native liver is dissected off leaving the vena cava intact and the suprahepatic vena cava of the donor is anastomosed end to side to the anterior wall of the recipient vena cava. The patients are managed postoperatively on ITU.

Additional procedures that may become necessary
- Insertion of central line, arterial line, and urinary catheter
- Repeated assessment of coagulation
- Increased risk of re-explorations to deal with complications

Benefits
- To treat end-stage liver disease and liver failure

Serious/frequently occurring risk[2]
- Haemorrhage
- Infection and malignancy
- Primary non-function: 5–10%
- *Vascular complications*: hepatic artery thrombosis—4–10% in adults and 9–42% in paediatric patients, which is associated with 80% mortality, hepatic artery stenosis—11–13%, pseudoaneurysm—2%, portal vein complications—1–13% (thrombosis and stenosis), IVC and associated hepatic vein complications—1–4% (thrombosis and stenosis)
- *Biliary complications*: 20% involve more commonly biliary stenosis and less frequently bile leaks
- *Acute rejection*: 15–20% in first 3 months
- *Complications from immunosuppression*: hypertension, nephrotoxicity
- Pleural effusions, lung collapse on the right side
- *Mortality*: 30 day mortality rate 10–15%, 1-year survival for elective liver transplants in adults is 90% and 70% at 5 years

Blood transfusion necessary
- Cross-matched antibody, CMV-negative blood 20 units
- Coagulopathy correction is appropriately carried out with FFP, cryo-precipitate, and platelets as necessary; and adequate units kept ready in the blood bank

Type of anaesthetic/sedation
- General anaesthesia with epidural/patient-controlled anagesia (PCA) for postoperative analgesia (patients at higher risk—ASA grade III onwards and general risk of myocardial infarction, DVT should be discussed)

Follow-up/need for further procedure
- Intense transplant unit protocols, usually twice a week for first month, thereafter once a week for next 2 months with gradual spacing out, where by the end of 1 year should be every 3–4 months checking for FBC, liver profile, INR, renal profile, and drug levels

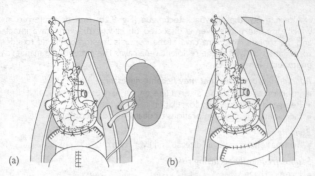

Fig. 9.1 (a) Simultaneous kidney/pancreas transplant with bladder drainage and (b) to small bowel Roux-en-Y loop.

Reproduced with permission from Torpey N, Moghal NE, Watson E, *et al. Oxford Specialist Handbook of Renal Transplantation*. 2010. Oxford: Oxford University Press, p.414, Figure 20.1a and b.

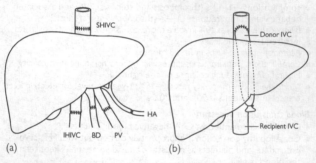

Fig. 9.2 Orthotopic liver transplant showing (a) standard IVC replacement technique and (b) piggyback technique. SH/IHVC, supra-/infrahepatic IVC; BD, bile duct; HA, hepatic artery; PV, portal vein.

Reproduced with permission from Sutcliffe RP, Antoniades CG, Deshpande R, *et al. Oxford Specialist Handbook of Liver and Pancreatobiliary Surgery*. 2010. Oxford: Oxford University Press, p.113, Figure 5.3a and b.

References

1. Danovitch GM. *Handbook of Kidney Transplantation*, 5th edn. Philadelphia: Lippincott Williams & Wilkins, 2010:181–217.
2. Forsythe JLR. *A Companion to Specialist Surgical Practice Transplantation*, 4th edn. WB: Saunders/Elsevier, 2009:141–97.

Vascular access

Description

Vascular access involves creation of an arteriovenous fistula (Fig. 9.3), where the named vein is anastomosed to the named artery end to side with a view to creating a high-flow system so as to needle for haemodialysis (first described by Bresica et al. (1966)) Preferably the non-dominant hand and distal site are used first.

They are classified as:

- *Primary access*: radio-cephalic (RC AVF) (cephalic vein to radial artery), brachio-cephalic (BC AVF) (cephalic vein to brachial artery)
- *Secondary access*: brachio-basilic (BB AVF) (basilic vein to brachial artery as first stage (anastomosis), second stage (superficialization of the vein) or combined procedure)
- *Tertiary access*: brachio-axillary PTFE graft (BA graft), axillo-axillary PTFE loop graft (AA Graft), thigh loop PTFE graft (femoro-femoral)

Additional procedures that may become necessary

- Preoperative ultrasound duplex or venogram—to assess veins peripherally or centrally, especially for secondary and tertiary access

Benefits

- To provide access for haemodialysis

Alternative procedures/conservative measures

- Permacath™ insertion as an interim temporary measure until the fistula matures and can be used for dialysis

Serious/frequently occurring risk

- Infection, bleeding, neurovascular injury, scarring
- Immediate thrombosis—5%
- Failure to mature
- Lymphatic leak, lymphoceles formation, arm swelling, poor wound healing
- Steal syndrome—5%
- Failure at 1 year: RC AVF 10–20%, BC AVF 20–30%, BB AVF 30%, Grafts 40%

Blood transfusion necessary

- None for primary and secondary access
- Group and save for tertiary access

Type of anaesthetic/sedation

- RC AVF, BC AVF, first-stage BB AVF under LA infiltration
- Second-stage BB AVF, Combined BB under GA or LA with a brachial plexus block
- Tertiary access under GA

Follow-up/need for further procedure

- Six week and 3 months so as to assess AVF is maturing, though further may be required

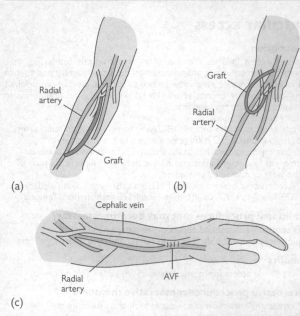

Fig. 9.3 Permanent vascular access for haemodialysis: (a) forearm straight PTFE graft, (b) forearm loop PTFE graft, (c) radial arterio-venous fistula.

Reproduced with permission from Levy J, Brown E, Daley C, et al. Oxford Handbook of Dialysis 3rd edition. 2009. Oxford: Oxford University Press, p.107, Figure 2.5.

Reference

1. *Vascular Access Society Guidelines.* 2007. Available at: ℘ www.vascularaccesssociety.com (accessed 11 May 2011).

Peritoneal dialysis access

Description

The procedure involves placing a peritoneal dialysis catheter, so it lies in the sump of the pelvis and can be used to place peritoneal dialysis fluid in the abdominal cavity where the peritoneum lining acts as a partially permeable membrane and can thus be used for dialysis. The catheter is tunnelled out through the abdominal wall usually on the side opposite to the dominant hand. The procedure can be done either with a peritoneoscopic technique or laparoscopic technique or open surgery.[1]

Additional procedures that may become necessary

- Adhesionolysis

Benefits

- To provide access for peritoneal dialysis

Alternative procedures/conservative measures

- Haemodialysis

Serious/frequently occurring risk

- Infection, bleeding, visceral injury, scarring, adhesions
- Failure, including catheter dysfunction
- Tract infections and peritonitis (peritoneal dialysis peritonitis)
- Fluid leak (wound (more common with open procedure), chest and scrotum)
- Hernia (groin and wound)
- Laparoscopic conversion to open 1%

Blood transfusion necessary

- None

Type of anaesthetic/sedation

- General/local anaesthesia and sedation

Follow-up/need for further procedure

- Continuous ambulatory peritoneal dialysis (CAPD) training clinic (Fig. 9.4)

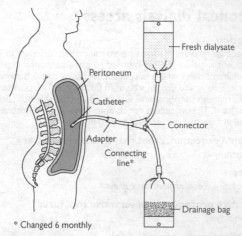

* Changed 6 monthly

Fig. 9.4 CAPD technique and system.

Reproduced with permission from Levy J, Brown E, Daley C, et al. *Oxford Handbook of Dialysis* 3rd edition. 2009. Oxford: Oxford University Press, p.239, Figure 4.6.

Reference

1. Renal Association. *Peritoneal Access Guidelines*. Renal Association, 2009. Available at
   ℅ www.renal.org/Clinical/GuidelinesSection/PeritonealAccess.aspx (accessed 11/May 2011).

Laparoscopic surgery

Introduction to laparoscopic surgery

Laparoscopic surgery is a minimal-access surgical technique that involves insufflation of the abdominal cavity with carbon dioxide to allow diagnosis and treatment of intra-abdominal pathologies. The first published laparoscopic procedure in humans dates back to 1910 and is credited to Hans Christian Jacobaeus (Stockholm, Sweden). Since that initial procedure, laparoscopic surgery encountered many controversies before being accepted as a safe alternative to traditional open techniques. The introduction of gas insufflation, improvement of optics, and development of laparoscopic instruments have been key to the modernization of the technique.

There are specific issues regarding laparoscopic surgery that should be considered at disclosure. The specific complications relating to each procedure are discussed in the relevant section. The aim of this chapter is to provide an overview of the issues relating to laparoscopy in general.

Explaining laparoscopic surgery to patients

Laparoscopic surgery can be described to patients as 'keyhole surgery', as this is a term that most patients are familiar with. It is also important to break down the steps of an operation. For general surgical laparoscopy this would include:

- This procedure is performed under general anaesthesia
- Once asleep, a small cut is usually made in the region of the belly button (umbilicus)
- A small plastic sheath is inserted into the abdomen and gas is pumped into the abdominal cavity. (The gas used is carbon dioxide because it is highly soluble and rapidly excreted by the body)
- The gas pumped into the abdomen elevates the front of your abdominal wall away from internal organs. This creates the necessary space for us to obtain good views and perform the operation
- Further small incisions of 5–10mm are made through in which we place further plastic sheaths. Through these plastic sheaths, we insert our instruments
- Most often two further incisions are made, however, this number can vary depending on the pathology identified and the intended operation. The location of these incisions depends on the indications for the procedure and also the pathology identified

Conversion to an open procedure is often wrongly included as a risk when patients are being consented for a laparoscopic operation. This is not a risk and should be included as part of the standard operation (i.e. laparoscopic procedure ± conversion to open). The percentage rate of conversion depends on the procedure being undertaken and the experience of the surgeon performing the operation. The important point to emphasize to the patient is that if the operation cannot be safely completed laparoscopically, it will be necessary to convert to open. When consenting, one should also demonstrate the potential incision sites for the open version of the same operation to the patient. This ensures that the patient is fully informed prior to the procedure and aware of the possible outcomes.

Advantages of laparoscopic surgery

Laparoscopic surgery is considered the gold standard technique for chole-cystectomy and fundoplication.[1,2] Laparoscopic appendicectomy is considered the gold standard technique for resection of the appendix in women of childbearing age.[3] It is advocated, but not currently considered the gold standard for male patients, obese patients, and elderly patients. There have been mixed results reported with laparoscopic appendicectomy in pregnant women and the technique should be used with caution in this cohort of patients. Laparoscopic colorectal surgery is an evolving technique and the oncological safety profile cannot be proven as conclusive long-term data do not yet exist.[4]

Major advantages of laparoscopic surgery over open surgery

- Excellent visualization of the abdomen and pelvis
- Smaller scars/cosmetic benefit
- Reduced rates of wound infection
- Reduced postoperative pain[5]
- Reduced postoperative drug requirements
- Shorter hospital stay
- Earlier return to activities of daily living[6]
- Decreased postoperative ileus[5]

References

1. Bittner R. The standard of laparoscopic cholecystectomy. *Langenbecks Arch Surg* 2004;**389**:157–63.
2. Salminen PT, Hiekkanen HI, Rantala AP, et al. Comparison of long-term outcome of laparoscopic and conventional nissen fundoplication: a prospective randomized study with an 11-year follow-up. *Ann Surg* 2007;**246**:201–6.
3. Vettoretto N, Agresta F. A brief review of laparoscopic appendectomy: the issues and the evidence. *Tech Coloproctol* 2011;**15**:1–6.
4. Künzli BM, Friess H, Shrikhande SV. Is laparoscopic colorectal cancer surgery equal to open surgery? An evidence based perspective. *World J Gastrointest Surg* 2010;**2**(4):101–8.
5. Le Blanc-Louvry I, Coquerel A, Koning E, et al. Operative stress response is reduced after laparoscopic compared to open cholecystectomy: the relationship with postoperative pain and ileus. *Dig Dis Sci* 2000;**45**:1703–13.
6. Raymond TM, Kumar S, Dastur JK, et al. Case controlled study of the hospital stay and return to full activity following laparoscopic and open colorectal surgery before and after the introduction of an enhanced recovery programme. *Colorectal Dis* 2010;**12**(10):1001–6.

Complications of laparoscopic surgery

General complications

Complications of laparoscopic surgery are primarily related to the surgery or due to the secondary effects of the pneumoperitoneum. Potential risks/complications include:

- Infection
- Bleeding/haematoma
- Thromboembolism
- Adhesion formation
- Port site hernia formation
- Basal atelectasis/pneumonia
- Damage to surrounding structures/Iatrogenic injury
  - Solid organ damage
  - Small bowel/colon
  - Major vascular injury
  - Bile duct injuries
  - Bladder

The injuries can occur during trocar insertion (increased risk with Veress needle), due to electrocautery conductivity or as a result of technical failure. Such injuries can go unrecognized at the time of laparoscopy, and therefore a high index of clinical suspicion is necessary in postoperatively unwell patients.

(Complications related to specific procedures are listed under the relevant chapters.)

Complications due to pneumoperitoneum

When absorbed, the systemic effects of carbon dioxide, the gas used for insufflation of the abdomen, include:

- Increase in $PaCO_2$
- Increase in respiratory rate
- Myocardial instability/cardiac dysrhythmia
- Decrease in pH

Abdominal compartment syndrome is a rare, serious complication as a result of intra-abdominal hypertension. It is most commonly due to prolonged carbon dioxide insufflation, and if it is unrecognized, it can lead to severe organ dysfunction.

Cardiac complications

- Increased venous return
- Decreased cardiac output (CO)
- Increased systemic vascular resistance
- Increased risk of bradycardia (vagal stimulation)
- Gas embolism

Respiratory complications

- Ventilation/perfusion mismatching
- Displacement of the diaphragm
- Pneumothorax
- Pneumomediastinum
- Respiratory failure

New techniques in laparoscopic surgery

Description

Laparoscopic surgery techniques continue to evolve and operating through a single trans-umbilical incision is gaining prominence. The single port technique is most commonly known as single incision laparoscopic surgery (SILS™) or laparoendoscopic single site (LESS) surgery. To date, operations performed via the single port technique include:

- Appendicectomy
- Cholecystectomy
- Nephrectomy
- Colonic resection
- Antireflux surgery
- Bariatric—gastric band placement and gastric bypass
- Inguinal hernia repair

Single port surgery is technically more demanding than traditional laparoscopic surgery and is currently practised by experts in certain centres on select patients. The single port technology has also led to innovation with regards to instruments (e.g. curved/reticulating versions) and camera systems (e.g. flexible). The main demonstrable advantage of single port surgery is that the end cosmetic result is (virtually) scarless. However, given the technique is relatively new, there is no level I evidence proving its efficacy/superiority to traditional laparoscopic surgery. However, it is important to monitor further developments and it remains to be seen whether SILS™ and LESS are adopted in mainstream surgical practice.

Urological surgery

Antegrade image-guided nephrostomy/ insertion of ureteric stent

Description

Antegrade nephrostomy insertion is a radiologically guided procedure, commonly performed under fluoroscopic and/or ultrasound guidance. A percutaneous tube is placed within the renal pelvis or calyceal system and acts as a conduit for urinary drainage in the presence of ureteric obstruction, antegrade instillation of contrast medium, or placement of an antegrade ureteric stent. The commonest emergency indication for placement of a nephrostomy is in the obstructed, infected kidney where the retrograde approach carries a theoretical risk of both increased pyelovenous pressures with bacterial translocation into the systemic circulation[1] and placing a potentially septic and hypotensive patient under general anaesthesia. To facilitate this procedure safely, the INR clotting result required should be <1.5.

The procedure is either performed with the patient supine, lateral position or prone and local anaesthetic is administered through the tract site. The kidney is punctured under ultrasound or fluoroscopic guidance and contrast medium injected to fill the pelvicalyceal system. A guide-wire is introduced, over which a nephrostomy tube or antegrade stent may be placed.

Additional procedures that may become necessary

- Pyelography
- Antegrade ureteric stent placement at the time of nephrostomy insertion or as a separate procedure
- Repeat procedure to remove the nephrostomy under fluoroscopic guidance
- Percutaneous nephrolithotomy (PCNL)[2]

Benefits

- *Diagnostic*: a descending pyelogram can identify the level of ureteric obstruction, filling defects and anomalies, allowing for a 'road-map' of the upper urinary tract for further treatment
- *Therapeutic*: to provide a tract prior to PCNL, to dissolve renal calculi, to obtain direct access to the upper urinary tract for various endourological procedures including placement of a ureteric stent, deliver chemotherapeutic agents to the renal collecting system, provide prophylaxis after resection for local chemotherapy in patients with tumours of the renal pelvis, to act as a conduit for urinary drainage

Alternative procedures/conservative measures

- *Medical*: systemic antibiotics until resolution of sepsis and then consider a retrograde approach, in rare circumstances haemofiltration may be *required to stabilize patient prior to intervention*
- *Surgical*: for staghorn renal calculi, consider flexible ureteroscopy and stone fragmentation, for obstructed renal tract consider retrograde stent insertion, for palliative setting of ureteric obstruction, consider long-term retrograde ureteric stents/metal ureteric stents/ureteric diversion procedures ± re-implantation[3,4]

Serious/frequently occurring risks

- Bleeding (including haematuria), infection (often a profound septic response can occur resulting in further intravenous antibiotic administration), post-procedure pain, urinoma, renal parenchymal injury, peri-renal haematoma formation, deterioration in renal function
- Need for further procedure to resolve cause of obstruction
- Dislodgement/blockage of nephrostomy
- Need for further procedure to change nephrostomy or to internalize ureteric stent)

Blood transfusion necessary

- None/group and save

Type of anaesthesia/sedation

- Local anaesthesia
- Regional/general anaesthesia (if nephrostomy tract is created prior to PCNL)

Follow-up/need for further procedure

- Monitor patient until sepsis has resolved prior to internalization of ureteric stent
- Consider definitive treatment for underlying cause of obstruction
- May require exchange/removal of ureteric stent

References

1. Mariappan P, Smith G, Bariol SV, et al. Stone and pelvic urine culture and sensitivity are better than bladder urine as predictors of urosepsis following percutaneous nephrolithotomy: a prospective clinical study. *J Urol* 2005;**173**(5):1610–4.
2. Motola JA, Smith AD. Therapeutic options for the management of upper tract calculi. *Urol Clin North Am* 1990;**17**(1):191–206.
3. Clayman RV, Kavoussi LR. Endosurgical techniques for noncalculous disease. In: Walsh PC, Retik AB, Vaughan ED, et al. (eds) *Campbell's Urology*, 7th edn. Philadelphia, PA: WB Saunders, 1992:2235–45.
4. Tanaka T, Yanase M, Takatsuka K. Clinical course in patients with percutaneous nephrostomy for hydronephrosis associated with advanced cancer. *Hinyokika Kiyo* 2004;**50**(7):457–62.

Circumcision (foreskin of the penis)

Description

Circumcision of the male foreskin involves surgical removal of the fold of skin covering the glans penis. The procedure can be performed at any age, however, it is most commonly performed in infancy, childhood, and in middle age.

Many cultures have historically used circumcision as a rite of passage, a mark of cultural identity[1] or for hygienic reasons. Medical indications for circumcision are limited to phimosis, paraphimosis, balanitis xerotica obliterans (BXO), recurrent balanitis, harvesting of tissue for hypo/epispadias repair or for tissue biopsy of adherent penile malignancy.

There are numerous techniques for performing a circumcision (e.g. cuff technique (Fig. 11.1), bipolar scissor circumcision) and the choice often depends on the surgeon. There are numerous devices that aid in this process (e.g. Plastibell circumcision device), and the foreskin is removed and often sent for histological examination. The wound may be closed with absorbable or non-absorbable sutures depending on the technique employed. The penis itself may become swollen postoperatively for up to 3 weeks and the wound may take 4–6 weeks to heal.[2]

Additional procedures that may become necessary

- Frenuloplasty
- Preputial adhesiolysis
- Preputioplasty (if an underlying hypospadias is identified and the foreskin is to be preserved)[3]
- Meatal dilatation meatotomy

Benefits

- *Diagnostic*: BXO, biopsy of underlying penile malignancy
- *Therapeutic*: phimosis, paraphimosis, BXO, posthitis
- *Reconstructive*: tissue grafting in the repair of hypo/epispadias
- Religious/cultural/hygiene[4]

Alternative procedures/conservative measures

- *Conservative*: poor anaesthetic risk or in patients with long-term suprapubic catheter in place where urethral passage of urine is no longer an issue. General foreskin and penile hygiene. Gentle retraction of foreskin in cases of phimosis. *Disadvantage*: underlying pathology not addressed and recurrence common
- *Medical*: antibiotics for recurrent balanitis. *Disadvantage*: underlying pathology not addressed and recurrence common
- *Surgical*: frenuloplasty (for painful or bleeding frenulum during intercourse or retraction of foreskin), preputial adhesiolysis (for preputial adhesions limiting retraction of foreskin), dorsal slit (for acute non-retractile paraphimosis)

Serious/frequently occurring risks

- *Common*: bleeding (which may necessitate reoperative intervention and ligation of frenular artery), pain, scar, prolonged wound healing/dressings, infection (local/systemic), persistence of absorbable sutures

- *Occasional*: cosmetic dissatisfaction (requiring further procedure to remove excess skin at a later date), tender scar
- *Rare*: identification of underlying malignancy requiring further intervention, urethral injury (resulting in urethrocutaneous fistula) on performing dorsal slit or ligating frenular artery, tattooing from dyed sutures, Fournier's gangrene[4]

Blood transfusion necessary

- None

Type of anaesthesia/sedation

- General anaesthesia
- Very occasionally under spinal/epidural local anaesthesia (without adrenaline/ephedrine) for those unfit for general anaesthesia
- Local anaesthetic infiltration as a penile block (at base of penis) or circumferential ring block (around foreskin)

Follow-up/need for further procedure

- None or review in outpatient clinic for review of wound and histology
- If associated with underlying malignancy (penile/foreskin), further surgical intervention/systemic treatment may need initiating, necessitating referral to specialist urological services

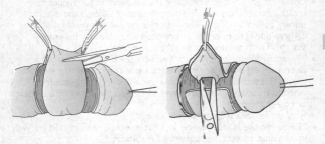

Fig. 11.1 Cuff technique for circumcision of foreskin of the penis.

Reproduced with permission from Reynard J, Mark S, Turner K, *et al. Oxford Specialist Handbook of Urological Surgery*. 2008. Oxford: Oxford University Press, p.614, Figures 9.1 and 9.2.

References

1. Robinson R, Makin E, Wheeler R. Consent for non-therapeutic male circumcision on religious grounds. *Ann R Coll Surg Engl* 2009;**91**(2):152–4.
2. Elder JS. Circumcision. *BJU Int* 2007;**99**(6):1553–64.
3. Munro NP, Khan H, Shaikh NA, *et al.* Y-V preputioplasty for adult phimosis: a review of 89 cases. *Urology* 2008;**72**(4):913–20.
4. Warner E, Strashin E. Benefits and risks of circumcision. *Can Med Assoc J* 1981;**125**(9):967–76, 992.

Cystectomy (radical)

Description

Although most bladder malignancies are non-muscle invasive at diagnosis (75%), tumours which are muscle invasive, associated with diffuse carcinoma *in situ* (CIS), or do not respond to conventional transurethral resection or intravesical chemotherapy require special attention.

Radical cystectomy does provide a potentially curative option for these patients. The procedure is performed in a supine patient where a midline lower abdominal transperitoneal approach is used. The bladder is taken off is lateral pedicles and midline urachus, and in men, the prostate gland in its entirety is also removed. In women, the anterior pelvic compartment is also removed (anterior vaginal wall/uterus) and effectively an anterior pelvic exenteration performed. During the procedure, bilateral pelvic lymphadenectomy is also performed.

The ureters are divided close to the bladder and these are brought forward to anastomose to the chosen form of urinary diversion (Fig. 11.2). Urinary diversion techniques include:[1]

- Ileal conduit urinary diversion: this is the most popular form of urinary diversion where a segment of ileum is isolated and the distal end brought out as a stoma. The ureters are anastomosed to the proximal end of the ileal segment
- Continent urinary diversion: there are a number of techniques to create a neo-bladder avoiding the presence of a stoma and external urinary collection device. The principles involve manipulation of small or large bowel to re-create an orthotopic neo-bladder for urinary storage. This is anastomosed to the native urethra
- Ureterosigmoidostomy urinary diversion: the oldest form of urinary diversion methods where the ureters are anatomized to the sigmoid colon. This technique is particularly useful in developing countries where the social stigma and community support in stoma care is poor or non-existent

Indications for radical cystectomy include:

- Muscle-invasive bladder cancer without evidence of metastasis (or with low-volume, resectable locoregional metastases)
- Superficial bladder tumours refractory to cystoscopic resection, intravesical chemotherapy or immunotherapy, bladder tumour not amenable to transurethral resection of bladder tumour (TURBT), or invasive tumour involving the prostatic urethra
- G3pT1 tumour unresponsive to intravesical bacille Calmette Guérin (BCG) vaccine therapy
- CIS refractory to intravesical immunotherapy or chemotherapy
- Palliation for pain, bleeding, or urinary frequency
- Primary adenocarcinoma, squamous cell carcinoma, or sarcoma
- Rarely, radical cystoprostatectomy is indicated for salvage treatment *for recurrent prostate cancer or intractable haematuria* following primary therapy with radiation

The decision behind radical cystectomy is ideally made within a multidisciplinary setting, and the patient may be offered other treatment options to secure oncological control. This can include external beam radiotherapy,

TURBT, or intravesical/systemic chemotherapy. Patients are counselled pre- and postoperatively with close liaison with cancer nurse specialists' and stoma care nurses (if necessary) throughout their journey.

Additional procedures that may become necessary

- Postoperative pelvic and abdominal drains
- Urethrectomy (for anterior urethral disease)
- Pelvic lymphadenopathy
- Neo-adjuvant chemotherapy
- Adjuvant chemo-radiotherapy
- Alternative urinary diversion technique

Benefits

- *Diagnostic*: allows histopathological grading and staging of disease where in certain circumstances upstaging of disease is seen
- *Therapeutic*: the procedure is performed for curative intent and oncological control
- *Functional*: continent diversion procedures in younger patients aim to restore functional 'storage' capacity

Alternative procedures/conservative measures

- *Conservative/palliative*: in patients with poor anaesthetic risk or in patients with poor quality of life, palliative care may be the appropriate management plan
- *Chemotherapy*: this may be in the form of systemic or intra-vesical chemotherapy either in the neoadjuvant or adjuvant setting
- *Radiotherapy*: in patients with poor anaesthetic risk or who have poor survival outcomes on preoperative risk stratification may be appropriate for radiotherapy
- *Surgery*: regular debulking TURBT in patients who are not suitable for cystectomy. Alternatively the approach used for cystectomy can vary to include laparoscopic and robot assisted radical cystectomy
- *Urinary diversion techniques*: neo-bladder formation, ileal conduit, ureterosigmoidostomy, cutaneous ureterostomy

Serious/frequently occurring risks

Complications from radical cystectomy are high and serious complications can affect up to 25% of patients postoperatively.[2–5]

- *General*: need for reoperation (10%), bleeding requiring reoperation or blood transfusion, thromboembolic event, wound infection and sepsis requiring intravenous or oral antibiotics, wound dehiscence (10%), prolonged intestinal ileus or obstruction (10%), rectal injury (4%), cardio-respiratory event, long-term erectile dysfunction, death (perioperative period: 1%)
- *Specific*: need for ureteric stent insertion, erectile dysfunction, dry orgasm where no semen is produced or ejaculation, need for self-catheterization if neo-bladder/conduit fails to empty effectively, need for urethrectomy, incontinence of urine, local cancer recurrence or distant metastases, incisional hernia, deteriorating renal function, rectal injury requiring colostomy, difficulty in females with intercourse due to painful shortened or narrowed vagina

- *Ileal conduit*: prolonged ileus, urinary leak requiring percutaneous drain or defunctioning nephrostomy, uretero-ileal or enteral anastomotic leak, uretero-ileal anastomotic stricture, pyelonephritis and ascending urinary tract infections, skin excoriation, stomal prolapse or stenosis, metabolic dysfunction (hyperchloraemic acidosis, B_{12} deficiency), adenocarcinoma (5%—long-term risk in bowel mucosa)
- *Continent urinary diversion*: urinary leak requiring percutaneous drainage or defunctioning nephrostomy, pelvic abscess formation, orthotopic neo-bladder and urinary tract calculus formation, catheterizing problems and stomal stenosis, urinary incontinence, nocturnal enuresis, pouch-ureteric reflux, ascending urinary tract infections, uretero-pouch anastomotic strictures, neo-bladder rupture (early/late), metabolic dysfunction (hyperchloraemic acidosis, B_{12} deficiency), adenocarcinoma (5%—long-term risk in bowel mucosa)
- *Ureterosigmoidostomy*: frequent ascending urinary tract infections, long-term risk of deteriorating renal function, frequent diarrhoea and watery stools, malignant transformation of urothelium (adenocarcinomas)[1]

Blood transfusion necessary
- Cross-match 2–6 units

Type of anaesthesia/sedation
- General anaesthesia
- Epidural anaesthesia often administered preoperatively as a method of postoperative pain control

Follow-up/need for further procedure
- Patients will often spend the initial postoperative period on the ITU/HDU
- Drains will need removal when output decreases
- Stoma nurse follow-up/continence nurse follow-up/urology cancer nurse support
- Outpatient follow-up with regular surveillance imaging and serum electrolyte review (serum creatinine, potassium, bicarbonate and vitamin B_{12})
- Multidisciplinary team review of histopathological results from resected specimen to determine postoperative surveillance or treatment plan
- Need for adjuvant chemo/radiotherapy in select cases

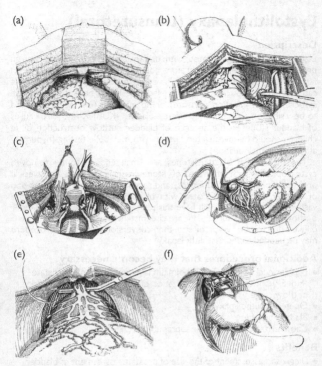

Fig. 11.2 (a) Perivesical space developed to mobilize bladder anteriorly. (b) Incision of endopelvic fascia and division of pubourethral and puboprostatic ligaments. (c) In females, division of the posterior fornix of the vagina. (d) Dissection around the dorsal venous complex of the prostate. (e) Ligation of the dorsal venous complex of the prostate. (f) Oversewing of dorsal venous complex and division of urethra.

Reproduced with permission from McLatchie GR and Leaper DJ. *Oxford Specialist Handbook of Operative Surgery* 2nd edition. 2006. Oxford: Oxford University Press, p.505, Figure 13.7.

References

1. Reynard J, Brewster S, Biers S, eds. *Oxford Handbook of Urology*. Oxford: Oxford University Press, 2006, pp258–65

2. British Association of Urological Surgery. *Procedure Specific Consent Forms for Urological Surgery—Radical Cystectomy and Ileal Conduit (Male)*. Available at: ℘ www.baus.org.uk (accessed 17 May 2011).

3. British Association of Urological Surgery. *Procedure Specific Consent Forms for Urological Surgery—Radical Cystectomy and Formation of New Bladder with Bowel (Female)*. Available at ℘ www.baus.org.uk (accessed 17 May 2011).

4. British Association of Urological Surgery. *Procedure Specific Consent Forms for Urological Surgery—Radical Cystectomy and Ileal Conduit (Female)*. Available at: ℘ www.baus.org.uk (accessed 17 May 2011).

5. British Association of Urological Surgery. *Procedure Specific Consent Forms for Urological Surgery—Radical Cystectomy and Formation of New Bladder with Bowel (Male)*. Available at: ℘ www.baus.org.uk (accessed 17 May 2011).

Cystolitholapaxy (transurethral)

Description

Bladder calculi are associated with urinary stasis secondary to benign prostatic enlargement and therefore commoner in men over the age of 50. In a subgroup of patients who have long-term urethral or suprapubic catheters *in situ*, up to 25% develop bladder calculi. These stones may be associated with infection (struvite) or no infection (uric acid) and tend to be visible on a plain kidney–ureter–bladder (KUB) X-ray. Rare causes of bladder stones in the absence of bladder outflow obstruction or in children should be investigated further with metabolic testing (hyperparathyroidism, malnutrition).[1]

The majority of bladder stones are small enough to be removed cystoscopically with the use of stone-crushing forceps, intravesical pneumatic or ultrasonic lithotripsy and recently lasers.[2] As the formation of bladder calculi is associated with bladder outflow obstruction, the vast majority of patients will have this procedure combined with bladder outflow obstruction surgery. In rare circumstances when stone retrieval is difficult due to poor vision or size, then conversion to an open procedure may be needed (open cystolitholapaxy).

Additional procedures that may become necessary

- Bladder neck incision/TURP/holmium laser enucleation of prostate (HoLEP)/photo-selective vaporization of the prostate (PVP) (bladder outflow surgery)
- Open cystolitholapaxy
- Bladder biopsies
- Catheterization (urethral or suprapubic)

Benefits

- *Diagnostic*: assessment of the size of prostate, assessment of bladder neck for outflow obstruction
- *Therapeutic*: remove bladder calculi in isolation or combined with bladder outflow surgery, reduce risk of urinary tract infections, symptomatic improvement

Alternative procedures/conservative measures

- *Conservative*: encourage fluid intake, and bladder emptying exercises (largely ineffective), monitor calculus if asymptomatic and patient high risk for surgery
- *Medical*: α-blocker and 5-α-reductase inhibitors as medical treatment for bladder outflow obstruction may improve symptoms, but will not treat bladder calculus. Prophylactic antibiotics to prevent secondary infection. Stone dissolution therapy does not work particularly well with bladder calculi
- *Surgical*: open cystolitholapaxy involves open surgery and the *propensity to have further* complications associated with intra-abdominal surgery, percutaneous (with the aid of a 30F sheath) and even laparoscopic cystolitholapaxy has been described with good outcomes

Serious/frequently occurring risks

- *Common*: bleeding (haematuria), dysuria, painful passage of stone fragments, catheter-associated discomfort
- *Occasional*: urinary tract infections requiring oral or intravenous antibiotics, recurrence, residual fragments necessitating further procedure, trauma to urethra and bladder causing haematuria
- *Rare*: haematuria and clot retention necessitating further cystoscopy and washout, injury to urethra necessitating catheterization (up to 2 weeks), urethral stricture formation, perforation of the bladder and/or urethra necessitating catheterization or open surgical repair[3]

Blood transfusion necessary

- None/group and save

Type of anaesthesia/sedation

- Regional/general anaesthesia

Follow-up/need for further procedure

- Routine outpatient follow-up with X-ray KUB, flow-rate (urine) on arrival (FROA) and residual volume (RV)
- May need to return for bladder outflow surgery at later date

References

1. Westenberg A, Harper M, Zafirakis H, et al. Bladder and renal stones: management and treatment. *Hosp Med* 2002.**63**(1):34–41.
2. Isen K, Em S, Kilic V, et al. Management of bladder stones with pneumatic lithotripsy using a ureteroscope in children. *J Endourol* 2008;**22**(5):1037–40.
3. British Association of Urological Surgery. *Procedure Specific Consent Forms for Urological Surgery—Cystolithopaxy or 'Rigid' Cystoscopy and Bladder Stone Removal*. Available at: ℘ www.baus.org.uk (accessed 17 May 2011).

Cystoscopy (flexible)

Description

This is a telescopic examination of the bladder with the use of a thin fibreoptic flexible telescope (Fig. 11.3). The procedure allows direct visualization of the urethra and bladder for diagnostic or follow-up purposes in an outpatient setting using local anaesthetic lubricating jelly. The flexible cystoscope is introduced into the urethra under sterile conditions, and although the procedure is principally diagnostic, biopsies, diathermy and laser can be undertaken due to the presence of a working channel. The flexible cystoscope has the ability to deflect 270°, and therefore the user is able to retrovert the scope and view the bladder neck.

It is important that the urine of the patient is tested to ensure there is no evidence of active urinary tract infection, which precludes this examination (unless in certain circumstances where it is performed under antibiotic cover).

Indications for flexible cystoscopy include:
- Visible haematuria
- Persistent non visible haematuria
- Irritative lower urinary tract symptoms (LUTS)
- Recurrent urinary tract infections
- Establish diagnosis of stricture
- Assess transurethral size of prostate gland
- Follow-up surveillance of patients with previously diagnosed and treated bladder cancer
- Cystoscopic removal of ureteric stents
- Cystoscopic insertion of urethral catheter/suprapubic catheter

Additional procedures that may become necessary
- Biopsy of bladder mucosal lesion
- Removal of ureteric stent
- Urethral dilatation
- Diathermy/laser ablation of bladder lesion
- Photography of bladder or urethral lesion
- Active bladder filling to measure FROA and post-void residual (PVR) volume
- Insertion of urethral/suprapubic catheter

Benefits
- *Diagnostic*: diagnostic and follow-up direct examination of bladder
- *Therapeutic*: biopsy, removal of ureteric stent, diathermy/laser ablation of bladder lesion

Alternative procedures/conservative measures
- *Radiological*: for patients who are unable to tolerate flexible cystoscopy due to poor mobility, contractures or the extremely frail and elderly patient, consider ultrasound KUB/CT urogram/contrast CT abdomen and pelvis (▶▶the diagnostic yield of these investigations is poor for small lesions within the bladder)

- *Surgical*: for patients unable to tolerate flexible cystoscopy (paediatric patients/pain) consider general anaesthesia/regional anaesthesia and rigid cystoscopy ± bladder biopsies

Serious/frequently occurring risks

- *Common*: bleeding (haematuria), dysuria
- *Occasional*: urinary tract infections requiring oral or intravenous antibiotics,[1,2] trauma to urethra, prostate or bladder resulting in haematuria
- *Rare*: haematuria and clot retention necessitating further cystoscopy and washout, need for catheterization (temporary), urethral stricture formation[3]

Blood transfusion necessary

- None

Type of anaesthesia/sedation

- Local anaesthetic lubricating gel

Follow-up/need for further procedure

- Dependent on the indication and findings of cystoscopy
- If a bladder tumour or a suspicious area is identified within the bladder, urgent follow-up with transurethral resection of bladder tumour or rigid cystoscopy and bladder biopsies may be required

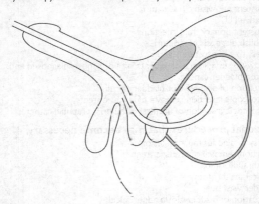

Fig. 11.3 Flexible cystoscope.

Reproduced with permission from Reynard J, Mark S, Turner K. et al. *Oxford Specialist Handbook of Urological Surgery*. 2008. Oxford: Oxford University Press, p.21, Figure 2.3.

References

1. Almallah YZ, Rennie CD, Stone J, et al. Urinary tract infection and patient satisfaction after flexible cystoscopy and urodynamic evaluation. *Urology* 2000;**56**(1):37–9.
2. Clark KR, Higgs MJ. Urinary infection following out-patient flexible cystoscopy. *Br J Urol* 1990;**66**(5):503–5.
3. British Association of Urological Surgery. *Procedure Specific Consent Forms for Urological Surgery—(Flexible) Cystoscopy +/- Biopsy or Stent Removal.* Available at: ꙮ www.baus.org.uk (accessed 17 May 2011).

Cystoscopy (rigid)—diagnostic

Description

This is a telescopic examination of the bladder with the use of a rigid telescope. The procedure allows direct visualization of the urethra and bladder for diagnostic or therapeutic purposes. It is carried out under regional or general anaesthesia and will therefore require the patient to be admitted in a day-case/inpatient setting.

The rigid cystoscope is a rigid metal instrument introduced into the urethra under sterile conditions, and although the procedure is principally diagnostic, it is used as an adjunct or precursor to a therapeutic procedure (e.g. cystolithalopaxy/TURP/ureteric stent insertion). Biopsies, cystodiathermy and ureteric (JJ) stent insertion can be undertaken due to the presence of a working channel (and in certain cystoscopes, a deflecting bridge).

The rigid cystoscope has the ability to be fitted with telescopes of varying deflection angle (0/30/70/120°), and therefore the user is able to view the bladder neck, bladder trigone, or urethra accordingly. It is important that the urine is tested to ensure there is no evidence of active urinary tract infection, which precludes this examination (unless in certain circumstances where it is performed under antibiotic cover).

Indications for rigid cystoscopy[1] include:
- Visible haematuria
- Persistent non-visible haematuria
- Irritative LUTS
- Recurrent urinary tract infections
- Establish diagnosis of stricture
- Assess size of prostate gland
- Follow-up surveillance of patients with previously diagnosed and treated bladder cancer
- Evacuation of bladder clot/bladder calculi
- Cystoscopic insertion/removal of ureteric stents
- Cystoscopic insertion of urethral catheter/suprapubic catheter

Additional procedures that may become necessary
- Biopsy of bladder mucosal lesion
- Insertion/removal of ureteric stent
- Urethral dilatation
- Optical urethrotomy
- Bladder washout
- Evacuation of bladder clot/bladder calculi
- Diathermy/laser ablation of bladder lesion
- Insertion of urethral/suprapubic catheter

Benefits
- *Diagnostic*: diagnostic and follow-up examination of bladder
- *Therapeutic*: for indications as listed

Alternative procedures/conservative measures

- *Radiological*: for patients who are unable to tolerate a general or flexible cystoscopy due to poor mobility, contractures, and the extremely frail and elderly patient who s not fit for a general/regional anaesthesia, consider ultrasound KUB/CT urogram/contrast CT abdomen and pelvis (▶▶the sensitivities of these investigations are poor for small lesions within the bladder)
- *Surgical*: for patients unable to tolerate rigid cystoscopy consider flexible cystoscopy

Serious/frequently occurring risks

- *Common*: bleeding (haematuria) dysuria, temporary insertion of urethral catheter
- *Occasional*: urinary tract infections requiring oral or intravenous antibiotics, trauma to urethra, prostate or bladder resulting in haematuria, diagnosis of bladder mucosal lesion/stone requiring treatment
- *Rare*: haematuria and clot retention necessitating further cystoscopy and washout, need for catheterization (temporary), urethral stricture formation, perforation of urethra/bladder necessitating temporary catheter insertion or open procedure to repair defect in bladder
- Complications associated with subsequent specific procedure performed[1,2]

Blood transfusion necessary

- None/group and save (depending on subsequent therapeutic procedure)

Type of anaesthesia/sedation

- Regional/general anaesthesia (rarely, rigid cystoscopy can be performed under local anaesthetic lubrication in women)

Follow-up/need for further procedure

- Dependent on the indication and findings of cystoscopy or therapeutic procedure

References

1. Lee CS, Yoon CY, Witjes JA. The past present and future of cystoscopy: the fusion of cystoscopy and novel imaging technology. *BJ J Int* 2008;**102** 9 Pt B):1228–33.
2. British Association of Urological Surgery. *Procedure Specific Consent Forms for Urological Surgery—(Rigid) Cystoscopy Including Biopsy if Required*. Available at: ℜ www.baus.org.uk (accessed 17 May 2011).
3. Stav K, Leibovici D, Goren E. et al. Adverse effects of cystoscopy and its impact on patients' quality of life and sexual performance. *Isr Med Assoc J* 2004 6(8):474–8.

Epididymal cyst excision

Description

An epididymal cyst is also known as a spermatocoele (when there are spermatozoa contained within the cystic fluid).[1] These slow-growing cystic swellings are derived from the collecting tubules of the epididymis and are often asymptomatic. They lie within the scrotum, vary in size and are felt separately from (above and behind) the testis. They are often multiple cysts, bilateral and multiloculated. Transillumination is possible and characteristic of larger cysts. Some can cause testicular pain, become large and cause a dragging sensation, become infected, or there may be cyst haemorrhage resulting in pain. These cysts are commonly diagnosed on clinical findings, however prior to surgical intervention, it is prudent to confirm this diagnosis with ultrasound.

A midline or transverse scrotal incision is performed. The dartos and tunica vaginalis are opened and the testis is delivered into the wound. The testis is inspected, a hydrocoele is excluded or repaired, and the epididymis is isolated with the cyst. The cyst is ideally enucleated or separated off the epididymis taking care not to damage it. The testis is returned to the scrotum after haemostasis is secured and the wound closed in layers with absorbable sutures.

Additional procedures that may become necessary

- Hydrocoele repair (Lord's/Jaboulay procedure)
- Multiple epididymal cyst excision
- Epididymectomy (in circumstances where multiple epididymal cysts obscure normal epididymal tissue)
- Epididymal/testicular biopsy

Benefits

- *Diagnostic*: histopathological confirmation of benign epididymal cyst can be performed after removal, removal of equivocal cystic swellings on examination or ultrasound scan for diagnosis
- *Therapeutic*: alleviate pain (although this may persist despite removal), remove unsightly swelling, decrease dragging sensation, or prevent recurrent infections of cyst

Alternative procedures/conservative measures

- *Conservative*: analgesia, scrotal support, monitor asymptomatic cyst if causing no symptoms
- *Surgical*: aspiration of cyst (high recurrence rates, and risk of introducing sepsis into cyst), sclerotherapy of cysts,[2] epididymectomy for recurrent cysts refractory to multiple surgical exploration and excision, however, there is a risk of sub-fertility (unilateral) and infertility (bilateral)

Serious/frequently occurring risks

- *Occasional*: bleeding (scrotal haematoma resulting in either slow resorption or further procedure to evacuate clot), chronic scrotal or testicular pain (up to 5% cases), infection (wound/epididymo-orchitis necessitating antibiotic therapy), non-resolution of symptoms, recurrence of epididymal cysts
- *Rare*: epididymal scarring/damage resulting in sub-fertility[3]

Blood transfusion necessary

- None

Type of anaesthesia/sedation

- Local/regional/general anaesthesia

Follow-up/need for further procedure

- Scrotal support for up to one week
- Warm sit down bath after 48h to soak and remove dressing
- No follow-up required unless indicated

References

1. Walsh TJ, Seeger KT, Turek PJ. Spermatocele in adults: when does size matter? *Arch Androl* 2007;**53**(6):345–8.
2. Beiko DT, Morales A. Percutaneous aspiration and sclerotherapy for treatment of spermatoceles. *J Urol* 2001;**166**(1):137–9.
3. British Association of Urological Surgery. *Procedure Specific Consent Forms for Urological Surgery—Removal of Epididymal Cyst.* Available at: ℛ www.baus.org.uk (accessed 17 May 2011).

Huddersfield Health Staff Libra
Royal Infirmary (PGMEC)
Lindley
Huddersfield
HD3 3EA

Extracorporeal shockwave lithotripsy

Description

Extracorporeal shockwave lithotripsy (ESWL) is a non-invasive technique whereby externally focused shockwaves are targeted at renal calculi within the urinary tract allowing for stone fragmentation. The three principal methods of shockwave generation are electrohydraulic, electromagnetic, and piezoelectric energy. The effectiveness of ESWL is dependent on the size of the stone, location of stone (lower pole calculi and calculi within a calyceal diverticulum have worse outcomes), obesity, renal anatomy, and stone composition (cystine and calcium oxalate monohydrate are difficult stones to fragment).

ESWL is used for renal stones <2cm size (stone-free rate: 80% for stones <1cm, 60% for stones 1–2cm and 50% for stones >2cm) and ureteric stones <1cm in size.

The patient is given analgesia or sedation pre-procedure and occasionally oral antibiotics, they are positioned supine, prone or in the lateral position to focus the stone under fluoroscopic/ultrasound guidance. Treatment is commenced at low energy and increased throughout the treatment session.

Contraindications to treatment include:
- Pregnancy
- Uncorrected coagulopathy
- Use of anticoagulation
- Active urinary tract infection
- Abdominal aortic aneurysm

It is key to remind the patient that more than one ESWL session may be required to achieve stone fragmentation.

Additional procedures that may become necessary

- Pre-ESWL ureteric stent placement for larger calculi >1cm (to facilitate passage of stone fragments) and prevent a *steinstrasse* ('stone street' line of obstructing stone fragments in ureter)

Benefits

- *Therapeutic*: achieve stone fragmentation (non-invasive method)

Alternative procedures/conservative measures

- *Conservative*: stones can be managed conservatively if asymptomatic, not causing pain, are non-obstructing and not acting as a focus for recurrent urinary tract infections. Occasionally a ureteric stent is inserted in an emergency setting, which may allow passage of calculi up to 1cm in size (European Association of Urology (EAU) guidelines[1]) without the need for treatment
- *Medical*: α-blocker (tamsulosin) to aid the passage of lower third ureteric calculi, medical stone dissolution therapy (primary treatment in combination with ESWL) in patients with uric acid stones unfit for surgery or in whom ESWL is contraindicated

- *Surgical*: rigid cystoscopy and ureteric stent insertion (to facilitate stone passage), rigid ureteroscopy and stone basketing/fragmentation (ureteric calculi), flexible ureteroscopy and stone fragmentation

Serious/frequently occurring risks

- *Common*: haematuria (visible/non-visible), renal angle tenderness, renal colic (as stone fragments pass), urinary tract infection necessitating oral/intravenous antibiotics (infectious stones that cause a transient bacteriuria/bacteraemia)
- *Occasional*: failure to fragment calculi, need for repeat ESWL sessions,[2,3] recurrence, peripheral oedema, perirenal haematoma formation (0.5%), need for surgical intervention (ureteroscopy and stone fragmentation or cystoscopy and ureteric stone insertion)
- *Rare*: acute renal impairment (those with a history of ischaemic heart disease, type 2 diabetes mellitus, pre-existing chronic kidney disease, solitary kidney), *steinstrasse* ('stone street' line of obstructing stone fragments in ureter), severe renal tract sepsis/pyonephrosis necessitating nephrostomy insertion[4]

Blood transfusion necessary

- None

Type of anaesthesia/sedation

- Oral/intramuscular analgesia/sedation/(general anaesthesia in children)

Follow-up/need for further procedure

- Follow-up KUB X-ray to confirm position and size of stone
- CT KUB to assess stone fragmentation
- Outpatient clinic appointment as required
- Metabolic stone risk factor analysis (serum uric acid/calcium/24h urinary collection) in recurrent stone formers

References

1. Türk C, Knoll T, Petrik A, *et al.* EAU Clinical Guidelines—Guidelines on Urolithiasis. Arnhem, The Netherlands: European Association of Urology 2011.
2. Perry KT, Smith ND, Weiser AC, *et al.* The efficacy and safety of synchronous bilateral extracorporeal shock wave lithotripsy. *J Urol* 2000;**164**(3 Pt 1):644–7.
3. Abdel-Khalek M, Sheir KZ, Mokhtar AA, *et al.* Prediction of success rate after extracorporeal shock-wave lithotripsy of renal stones—a multivariate analysis model. *Scand J Urol Nephrol* 2004;**38**(2):161–7.
4. British Association of Urological Surgery *Procedure Specific Consent Forms for Urological Surgery—Extra-Corporeal Shock Wave Lithotripsy (ESWL)*. Available at: ℜ www.baus.org.uk (accessed 17 May 2011).

Frenuloplasty

Description
An abnormally short 'bow-stringing' frenulum on the ventral aspect of the glans penis restricts normal retraction of the foreskin. The condition known as frenulum breve can result in difficult painful foreskin retraction, a bleeding frenulum, chronic frenular scarring, and painful intercourse. It can co-exist with phimosis in which case circumcision is the treatment of choice, however, in isolation, frenuloplasty may be sufficient to relieve symptoms.[1]

The frenulum is divided either with a scalpel or diathermy and occasionally a haemostatic suture or a running suture is placed when sufficient frenular release/laxity is achieved. Often a V-Y-plasty or Z-plasty is required to allow sufficient length. The wound is closed with absorbable sutures.

Additional procedures that may become necessary
- Circumcision of foreskin of penis
- Preputioplasty

Benefits
- *Therapeutic*: to regain sufficient length to the frenulum to allow painless retraction of the foreskin

Alternative procedures/conservative measures
- *Conservative*: observation and moisturizer use to aid retraction of foreskin during sexual intercourse. Gentle retraction of foreskin to limit of frenular stretch (poor results)
- *Surgical*: circumcision is often the treatment of choice in patients who have associated phimosis or who have frenular contracture or scarring post-frenuloplasty

Serious/frequently occurring risks
- *Occasional*: bleeding (classically from frenular artery and may require ligation), pain; scarring; infection necessitating antibiotic treatment, need for circumcision if suboptimal improvement in symptoms, persistent suture present (delayed reabsorption of suture requiring removal)
- *Rare*: altered penile sensation, scar tissue tenderness which may persist, cosmetic dissatisfaction[2]

Blood transfusion necessary
- None

Type of anaesthesia/sedation
- Local anaesthesia

Follow-up/need for further procedure
- Warm bath to loosen dressing over penis after 48h
- Follow-up not required unless specifically indicated

References
1. Rajan P, McNeill SA, Turner KJ. Is frenuloplasty worthwhile? A 12-year experience. *Ann R Coll Surg Engl* 2006;**88**(6):583–4.
2. British Association of Urological Surgery. *Procedure Specific Consent Forms for Urological Surgery—Frenuloplasty*. Available at: ✋ www.baus.org.uk (accessed 17 May 2011).

Hydrocoele repair

Description

A hydrocoele is an abnormal collection of fluid between the parietal and visceral layer of the tunica vaginalis. They vary in size and are usually painless unless associated with underlying painful testicular pathology. Clinical examination reveals a uni- or bilateral scrotal lump, which is smooth to touch with a palpable superior margin. The underlying testis is often difficult to palpate and it will transilluminate on shining a light from the side of the lesion.

Causes of hydrocoele formation are:

- Primary: these idiopathic masses develop over a long period of time with no underlying testicular pathology
- Secondary: infection (epididymo-orchitis/filariasis/tuberculosis/syphilis), trauma, tumour (underlying testicular malignancy)

Surgical treatment of a hydrocoele usually follows ultrasound confirmation of the diagnosis and sonographic examination of the underlying testis to exclude testicular malignancy. A midline raphe incision or a transverse scrotal incision is used and deepened dividing the dartos muscle and the tunica vaginalis. Fluid is then aspirated and the hydrocoele is usually repaired via one of the following techniques:[1]

- *Lord's plication technique* is usually performed for smaller or medium hydrocoeles whereby the tunica vaginalis is plicated. Advantages include decreased bleeding, a smaller incision and decreased trauma to surrounding scrotal tissue.
- *Jaboulay eversion procedure* is usually performed for larger hydrocoeles, and involves excision and eversion of the hydrocoele sac (Fig. 11.4).

Additional procedures that may become necessary

- Scrotal drain insertion
- Scrotoplasty (plastic surgical technique to reduce the amount of redundant scrotal skin associated with large hydrocoeles)
- *Rare*: need for testicular surgery/biopsy/orchidectomy if underlying tumour identified (if no preoperative ultrasound performed)

Benefits

- *Diagnostic*: hydrocoele fluid or tunica can be examined histologically for evidence of tumour, filariasis infection, microscopy, and culture of fluid in cases of infection or for cytology
- *Therapeutic*: remove hydrocoele, allow symptomatic relief, aid passage of urine (buried penis)

Alternative procedures/conservative measures

- *Conservative*: analgesia, scrotal support, monitor asymptomatic hydrocoele if not causing symptoms
- *Surgical*: aspiration of cyst (high recurrence rates, and risk of introducing sepsis into hydrocoele

Serious/frequently occurring risks

- *Occasional*: bleeding (scrotal haematoma resulting in either slow resorption, lump in scrotum or need for further procedure to evacuate clot), chronic scrotal or testicular pain (up to 5% cases),

infection (wound/epididymo-orchitis necessitating antibiotic therapy), non-resolution of symptoms, recurrence of hydrocoele
• *Rare*: need for further therapy for abnormal testicle (in cases where malignancy is suspected or diagnosed intraoperatively)[2]

Blood transfusion necessary
• None

Type of anaesthesia/sedation
• Local anaesthesia (with cord block for small hydrocoeles)/regional anaesthesia/general anaesthesia

Follow-up/need for further procedure
• Scrotal support for up to one week
• Warm sit down bath after 48h to soak and remove dressing
• No follow-up required unless indicated

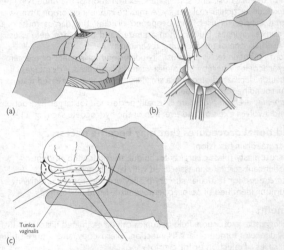

Tunica
vaginalis

Fig. 11.4 Lord's procedure for hydrocoele repair: (a) A skin incision is made and the hydrocoele delivered into the wound; (b) the tunica vaginalis is opened and the hydrocoele fluid drained. The testis is then delivered and the tunica inverted; (c) the inverted tunica vaginalis is plicated along its length allowing it to concertina behind the testis. The testis is then replaced into the scrotum and the dartos muscle and skin closed.

Reproduced with permission from Reynard J, Mark S, Turner K, et al. Oxford Specialist Handbook of Urological Surgery. 2008. Oxford: Oxford University Press, pp. 619 and 621, Figures 9.4, 9.6, and 9.7.

References
1. Lau ST, Lee YH, Caty MG. Current management of hernias and hydroceles. *Semin Pediatr Surg* 2007;**16**(1):50–7.
2. British Association of Urological Surgery. *Procedure Specific Consent Forms for Urological Surgery—Hydrocoele Repair*. Available at: ℘ www.baus.org.uk (accessed 17 May 2011).

Intravesical injection of botulinum toxin-A

Description

Overactive bladder (OAB) is a symptom complex that includes urgency with or without urge incontinence, nocturia, and frequency of urination. Classically OAB is associated with detrusor overactivity. The diagnosis is made from history, exclusion of other causes of bladder/prostate/urethral pathology (urinary tract infection/bladder outflow obstruction) and/or urodynamics investigation.[1]

Treatment classically involves behavioural modification and medical treatment of which anti-cholinergic drugs are the mainstay of treatment.

Intravesical botulinum toxin-A represents a new therapeutic modality in patients with urodynamics-proven detrusor overactivity in whom conventional therapy has failed.[2,3] Its use has also been shown to be effective in patients with similar symptoms from a neuropathic bladder secondary to an underlying neuromuscular disorder. Its action is to inhibit acetylcholine release at the neuromuscular junction reducing muscle contractility. This not only potentially increases bladder capacity, but reduces urgency.

Botulinum toxin-A is injected directly into the bladder submucosa or detrusor muscle under rigid or flexible cystoscopic guidance.[1] The bladder trigone is avoided[3] and up to 20 aliquots of 1mL injections are administered. Effects of botulinum toxin-A last between 6 and 12 months, and repeat procedures may be necessary when the effects diminish (dosage can increase depending on response). In up to 5% cases, detrusor paralysis can result in significant bladder residual volumes, necessitating intermittent self-catheterization (ISC). This should be taught to all patients preoperatively.

Additional procedures that may become necessary

- Hydro-distension of bladder
- Bladder biopsies
- Need to teach ISC

Benefits

- Decrease symptoms of overactive bladder (particularly urge incontinence) resistant to medical therapy and behavioural modification advice

Alternative procedures/conservative measures

- *Conservative*: dietary and fluid intake advice (modify fluid intake, avoiding stimulants, bladder training), pelvic floor exercises, biofeedback training, high-frequency electrical stimulation (stimulation and strengthening of pelvic floor musculature)
- *Medical*: (up to 50% response rate) anticholinergic drugs (oxybutyrin, solifenacin, terfenadine, tolterodine, trospium chloride), tricyclic antidepressants, desmopressin, baclofen
- *Surgical*: neuromodulation, auto-augmentation (detrusor myomectomy—excision of detrusor muscle over dome of bladder), augmentation enterocystoplasty (clam ileocystoplasty—bi-valving of bladder with anastomosis of detubularized segment of ileum), conduit diversion (incontinent ileal conduit, sacral nerve stimulation (SNS)

Serious/frequently occurring risks

- Cystoscopy
  - *Common*: bleeding (haematuria), dysuria, temporary insertion of urethral catheter
  - *Occasional*: urinary tract infections requiring oral or intravenous antibiotics, trauma to urethra, prostate or bladder resulting in haematuria, diagnosis of bladder mucosal lesion/stone requiring treatment
  - *Rare*: haematuria and clot retention necessitating further cystoscopy and washout, need for catheterization (temporary), urethral stricture formation, perforation of urethra/bladder necessitating temporary catheter insertion or open procedure to repair defect in bladder
- Botulinum toxin-A
  - Need for repeat treatment, failure to improve symptoms, acute retention of urine, need for ISC, febrile illness, proximal myopathy, flu-like symptoms, (rare: swallowing/breathing difficulties/headache/diarrhoea)
  - *Rare*: recurrence as noted[1-5]

Blood transfusion necessary

- None

Type of anaesthesia/sedation

- Local/general anaesthesia

Follow-up/need for further procedure

- Follow-up in 6–12 weeks to assess response
- Teach patients ISC as necessary pre- or postoperatively
- Follow up patients in 6 months to assess response or need for re-injection/repeat procedure

References

1. Dowson C, Khan MS, Dasgupta P, *et al.* Repeat botulinum toxin-A injections for treatment of adult detrusor overactivity. *Nat Rev Urol* 2010;**7**(12):661–7.
2. Smaldone MC, Ristau BT, Leng WW. Botulinum toxin therapy for neurogenic detrusor overactivity. *Urol Clin North Am* 2010;**37**(4):567–80.
3. Abdel-Meguid TA. Botulinum toxin-A injections into neurogenic overactive bladder--to include or exclude the trigone? A prospective, randomized, controlled trial. *J Urol* 2010;**184**(6):2423–8.
4. Drake JM. Intravesical botulinum toxin for lower urinary tract dysfunction. *F1000 Med Rep* 2010;**2**.pii:6.
5. Kuo HC, Liao CH, Chung SD. Adverse events of intravesical botulinum toxin A injections for idiopathic detrusor overactivity: risk factors and influence on treatment outcome. *Eur Urol* 2010;**58**(6):919–26.

Nephrectomy (simple/partial/radical/ nephro-ureterectomy)

Description

This is the surgical removal of the kidney (simple), kidney and its surrounding Gerota's fascia (radical), part of the kidney (partial), or the kidney and ureter (nephroureterectomy). The latter three procedures are performed for renal cancer. The procedure can be performed both as an open or laparoscopic procedure and the kidney can be approached retroperitoneally with the patient in the lateral position, or transperitoneally with the patient supine with a slight tilt towards the operating surgeon.

Indications for nephrectomy include renal cell carcinoma (radical nephrectomy, partial nephrectomy), transitional cell carcinoma (TCC) of the renal collecting system or ureter (nephroureterectomy), a symptomatic non-functioning kidney with or without a staghorn calculus or persistent haemorrhage following renal trauma.

Radical nephrectomy may involve exploration of the renal vein or IVC to achieve tumour clearance from the associated vein. If significant tumour thrombus exists (particularly in the vena cava), it may be that cardiothoracic support is necessary with extracorporeal cardiopulmonary bypass.

Partial nephrectomy is a treatment option to preserve nephron function and is suitable in certain smaller peripheral tumours which may be exophytic in nature. If there is any concern where oncological control may be compromised, then a radical nephrectomy or other forms of nephron-sparing surgery (e.g. RFA, cryotherapy) should be performed as appropriate.

All patients prior to surgery should have their case discussed in a multidisciplinary team meeting with a surgeon, radiologist, oncologist, and histopathologist present.

Postoperatively a drain may be placed in situ, a chest X-ray performed and a catheter may be left in situ for 10–14 days (post-nephro-ureterectomy). Routine chest physiotherapy is essential with early mobilization to reduce respiratory and thromboembolic complications following surgery and must be emphasized to the patient preoperatively.

Additional procedures that may become necessary

- Urethral catheterization
- Abdominal drain insertion
- Conversion to open procedure (if laparoscopic)
- Conversion to radical nephrectomy (if partial nephrectomy)
- Need for future therapy/surveillance (flexible cystoscopy for TCC surveillance/surveillance CT scans)

Benefits

- *Diagnostic*: remove offending pathology and provide histopathological diagnosis for staging and further treatment planning
- *Therapeutic*: to improve symptoms, prevent further haemorrhage (traumatic/debulking tumour load), curative procedure in cancer surgery, cytoreductive nephrectomy in larger tumours

Alternative procedures/conservative measures

- *Conservative*: patients with smaller tumours, <3cm in size, with regular surveillance CT/ultrasound scans to ensure no increase in size. The older patient with multiple comorbities may not be suitable for surgical intervention and potentially can be managed conservatively
- *Radiological*: segmental renal artery embolization
- *Nephron sparing surgery*: radiofrequency ablation (CT guided), cryotherapy (laparoscopic), partial nephrectomy
- *Surgical*: partial nephrectomy, radical nephrectomy
- *Oncological*: molecular-targeted therapies (e.g. tyrosine kinase inhibitors), immunotherapy, radiotherapy

Serious/frequently occurring risks

- *Common*: temporary insertion of urinary catheter, insertion of wound drain
- *Occasional*: bleeding which may require further surgery or blood transfusion, infection of wound necessitating antibiotic therapy, inadvertent injury to diaphragm or opening of pleura necessitating insertion of intercostals drain, need for adjuvant therapy for cancer control, chronic pain at incision site, numbness and paraesthesia along incision, incisional hernia which may require further surgery, ileus (particularly if transperitoneal approach)
- *Rare*: injury to adjacent visceral structures including blood vessels, spleen, liver, pancreas, lung or bowel, which requires further treatment or surgery, alternative diagnosis on histopathological diagnosis other than cancer, cerebrovascular event, cardiopulmonary event, thromboembolic event, ITU/HDU admission, death
- *Partial nephrectomy*: need for radical nephrectomy, local recurrence, inadequate oncological clearance with need for further therapy
- *Nephroureterectomy*: recurrence of disease elsewhere within the urinary tract, need for surveillance cystoscopy and upper tract imaging
- *Laparoscopic*: conversion to open procedure, shoulder tip pain, abdominal bloating, port site hernia[1-5]

Blood transfusion necessary

- Group and save/cross-match 2–6 units depending on patient

Type of anaesthesia/sedation

- General anaesthesia (with regional anaesthesia for postoperative pain relief)

Follow-up/need for further procedure

- Removal of drain when volumes decrease
- Remove of urinary catheter 10–14 days postoperatively from nephroureterectomy (to allow bladder wall healing)
- Outpatient review with histology
- *Oncological follow-up*
- Surveillance CT/ultrasound/chest radiograph or cystoscopy for TCC

References

1. British Association of Urological Surgery. *Procedure Specific Consent Forms for Urological Surgery—Radical Nephrectomy.* Available at: ℔ www.baus.org.uk (accessed 17 May 2011).
2. British Association of Urological Surgery. *Procedure Specific Consent Forms for Urological Surgery—Partial Nephrectomy.* Available at: ℔ www.baus.org.uk (accessed 17 May 2011).
3. British Association of Urological Surgery. *Procedure Specific Consent Forms for Urological Surgery—Nephroureterectomy.* Available at: ℔ www.baus.org.uk (accessed 17 May 2011).
4. British Association of Urological Surgery. *Procedure Specific Consent Forms for Urological Surgery—Laparoscopic Radical Nephrectomy.* Available at: ℔ www.baus.org.uk (accessed 17 May 2011).
5. British Association of Urological Surgery. *Procedure Specific Consent Forms for Urological Surgery—Cystoscopy Laparoscopic Simple Nephrectomy.* Available at: ℔ www.baus.org.uk (accessed 17 May 2011).

Optical internal urethrotomy

Description

Stricturing disease of the urethra is a pathological process that involves fibrotic scar tissue formation within the tissues surrounding the urethra resulting in a narrowing of the lumen. Patients can present with decreased flow, incomplete bladder emptying, dysuria, haematuria, recurrent urinary tract infections and obstructive uropathy. Diagnosis is made with history, clinical examination (external urethral meatus), flow-rate studies, retrograde/antegrade urethrography, or urethroscopy.

Disease processes that cause urethral stricture formation include:
• Infection (gonococcal urethritis)
• Inflammation (BXO resulting in meatal or submeatal stenosis)
• Trauma (pelvic fractures, urethral instrumentation including post-transurethral resection of the prostrate (TURP), cystoscopy, catheterization, post radical prostatectomy)

Optical urethrotomy is an endoscopic procedure whereby the urethral stricture is visualized and incised with a knife or laser. It is best suitable for short (<1.5cm) strictures with minimal peri-urethral fibrosis, or for first time stricture presentation in the younger patient. The urethra re-epithelializes following incision of the stricture. Often, a catheter is placed between 3 and 5 days following the procedure and a trial of voiding is performed as an outpatient. In certain circumstances (particularly patients with recurrent strictures, the younger patient,[1] or a patient with a long segment stricture) ISC or referral for excision and re-anastomosis/urethroplasty (free-tissue transfer technique) is advised.

Additional procedures that may become necessary
• Urethral catheterization
• Suprapubic catheterization
• Urethral dilatation (in certain circumstances dilatation with a urethral sound will sufficiently open a stricture—beware of false passage creation, and avoid causing urethral trauma that may convert a short stricture into a longer stricture in the long term)
• Bladder biopsies
• Need for future therapy (ISC/referral for urethroplasty)
• Meatotomy/meatal dilatation (for distal meatal strictures where the urethra cannot be cannulated with the optical urethrotome)

Benefits
• *Diagnostic*: diagnose underlying stricture, length of stricture and proximity to external urethral sphincter
• *Therapeutic*: to improve symptoms associated with urethral stricture and prevent complications from bladder outflow obstruction

Alternative procedures/conservative measures
• *Conservative*: manage patient conservatively with regular urine flow-rate examination, residual volume measurements, and monitor serum creatinine and evidence of upper tract dilatation on ultrasonography in the patient who wishes no further treatment and is asymptomatic.

In patients who are able to perform ISC, this is an option to prevent further re-stricturing. It requires good hand–eye coordination and dexterity and may be difficult in the older patient

- *Medical*: in patients with BXO and meatal stenosis may require topical steroid treatment to limit the progression of disease. If this fails, formal circumcision of the foreskin may be necessary
- *Surgical*:
  - Urethral dilatation (beware of false passage creation/stricture progression/conversion of short stricture into longer segment stricture—restructure rates are higher if associated with bleeding)
  - Suprapubic catheter insertion (to avoid trauma to stricture or urethra, and to provide a conduit for antegrade and retrograde urethrography to plan future treatment
  - In males—Excision and primary reanastomosis of urethra
  - Tissue transfer procedure (urethroplasty with buccal or pedicled skin flap). The latter two techniques should be performed following adequate imaging of urethra in younger patients or in patients with recurrent stricture formation who do not wish to have repeat dilatation/urethrotomy procedures. These are often carried out in specialist centres that deliver a urethral reconstruction service. In these circumstances, a urethrogram is a useful adjunct in delineating stricture anatomy[2]

Serious/frequently occurring risks
- *Common*: bleeding (haematuria), dysuria, temporary insertion of urethral catheter
- *Occasional*: urinary tract infections requiring oral or intravenous antibiotics, trauma to urethra, prostate or bladder resulting in haematuria, recurrence of stricture, need to biopsy lesion in bladder, need for further therapy (including ISC, referral for specialist stricture treatment—urethroplasty/excision and anastomosis, need to insert suprapubic catheter
- *Rare*: haematuria and clot retention necessitating further cystoscopy and washout, failure of procedure due to complete urethral occlusion, false passage creation or perforation of urethra/bladder necessitating prolonged period of catheterization or conversion to open procedure to repair defect in bladder, erectile dysfunction, decreased continence (if stricture involves or lies adjacent to external urethral sphincter)[1]

Blood transfusion necessary
- None/group and save

Type of anaesthesia/sedation
- Regional or general anaesthesia

Follow-up/need for further procedure

- Dependent on findings of stricture
- If catheter inserted, trial without catheter can be scheduled between 24h and 5 days post optical urethrotomy
- Review in outpatient clinic with flow rate assessment, RV, and symptomatic review
- Referral to learn ISC
- Referral for definitive surgical procedure for stricture

References

1. British Association of Urological Surgery. *Procedure Specific Consent Forms for Urological Surgery—Cystoscopy and Optical Internal Urethrotomy.* Available at: ℘ www.baus.org.uk (accessed 17 May 2011).
2. Wong SS, Narahari R, O'Riordan A, *et al.* Simple urethral dilatation, endoscopic urethrotomy, and urethroplasty for urethral stricture disease in adult men. *Cochrane Database Syst Rev* 2010;**4**:CD006934.
3. Zehri AA, Ather MH, Afshan Q. Predictors of recurrence of urethral stricture disease following optical urethrotomy. *Int J Surg* 2009;**7**(4):361–4.

Orchidectomy (simple/sub-capsular/radical) ± insertion of silicone implant

Description

Orchidectomy is performed for both testicular and non-testicular pathology. The approach used varies depending on the underlying disease process that requires attention. Unilateral or bilateral orchidectomy can be performed. Three approaches are commonly used to remove the testicle or testicular tissue:

- *Radical inguinal orchidectomy:* this is the approach used for (suspected) testicular malignancy. An inguinal incision is used, the external oblique aponeurosis opened and the spermatic cord isolated and ligated. The testis is then mobilized from the scrotum via the superficial inguinal ring and removed. This technique allows ligation of the testicular lymphatics high up the spermatic cord. Cross-clamping of the cord early in the procedure avoids spread during testicular manipulation and avoids scrotal skin metastasis if a scrotal approach was used. Occasionally the opposite testis is biopsied if clinically small, abnormal on ultrasound or clinical examination or there is a history of maldescent. Patients should have a chest X-ray and serum tumour markers (β-human chorionic gonadotrophin (hCG), α-fetoprotein (AFP) and lactate dehydrogenase (LDH)) measured prior to radical orchidectomy. Their diagnosis should be correlated with findings on ultrasound[1]

- *Simple orchidectomy:* this is performed via vertical or horizontal scrotal incision. The testis is delivered and a transfixion suture used to secure the cord on its removal. This approach is used for removing the testicle when cancer is not suspected (i.e. severe epididymo-orchitis with abscess formation, infarcted testis secondary to torsion, tuberculous orchitis, chronic testicular pain)

- *Subcapsular orchidectomy:* this technique is used to achieve castrate levels of testosterone by removal of the functioning testicular tissue in an attempt to achieve hormonal control for advanced prostate cancer. It is performed via a midline scrotal approach and both testicles are treated. The tunica albuginea is opened, and the seminiferous tubules removed. The capsule is then closed with preservation of the epididymis and testicular appendages. Rapid drop in serum testosterone levels are expected to <0.2nmol/L within 8h of subcapsular orchidectomy

In cases where the patient requests a testicular implant, a silicone implant may be inserted and secured to the scrotum. This is contraindicated in the presence of active sepsis and great care must be taken in handling the implant to avoid contamination. Where bilateral orchidectomy is performed, or in the younger patient who is likely to require chemotherapy, hormone therapy and/or sperm banking with pre- and postoperative counselling may be required.

Additional procedures that may become necessary

- Scrotal drain insertion
- Need for further treatment (chemotherapy/radiotherapy)

- Need for further investigations (staging CT scan)
- Insertion of testicular prosthesis (generally avoid in the infected setting of infection or if chemotherapy/radiotherapy may be given)
- *Rare*: need for further testicular surgery/biopsy/orchidectomy if underlying tumour identified during scrotal exploration

Benefits

- *Diagnostic*: histopathological evaluation of testicular specimen and spermatic cord and allow future treatment planning
- *Therapeutic*: remove diseased or symptomatic testicle

Alternative procedures/conservative measures

- *Conservative*: benign conditions: analgesia, antibiotics, scrotal support, monitor asymptomatic or minimally symptomatic patients, serial radiological intervention to characterize lesions of the testis in unconvincing cases, no testicular prosthesis insertion
- *Medical*: for treatment of advanced/metastatic prostate cancer—luteinizing hormone-releasing hormone agonists, oestrogens, antiandrogens, 5-α-reductase inhibitors
- *Surgical*: testicular biopsy prior to formal orchidectomy

Serious/frequently occurring risks

- *Occasional*: bleeding (scrotal haematoma resulting in either slow resorption, lump in scrotum, or need for further procedure to evacuate clot), chronic scrotal pain (up to 5% cases), infection (wound necessitating antibiotic therapy), non-resolution of symptoms, infertility/sub-fertility, if performed for malignancy the need for further therapy (chemo-radiation), the need to biopsy other testicle if small, abnormal, or history of maldescent of testis
- *Rare*: unsuspected diagnosis on histopathological diagnosis of malignancy, need for further therapy for abnormal testicle (in cases where malignancy is suspected or diagnosed intraoperatively)
- *Insertion of testicular prosthesis*: abnormal position or lie of implant (in particular may be high riding in warm weather), palpable suture (may be painful), imperfect cosmetic result, prosthesis infection and pyo-scrotum requiring drainage or/and removal of testicular implant, bleeding requiring implant removal, leakage of silicone-based fluid from implant within scrotum, unknown long-term effects of silicone-based implants[2–4]

Blood transfusion necessary

- None/group and save

Type of anaesthesia/sedation

- Local anaesthesia with cord block (regional anaesthesia/general anaesthesia

Follow-up/need for further procedure

- Dependent on underlying indication for orchidectomy
- No follow-up in benign cases unless patient requests testicular implant insertion
- Prostate-specific antigen (PSA)/serial tumour markers/staging CT/chest radiograph in patients with malignancy

References

1. Aparicio J, Díaz R. Management options for stage I seminoma. *Expert Rev Anticancer Ther* 2010;**10**(7):1077–85.
2. British Association of Urological Surgery. *Procedure Specific Consent Forms for Urological Surgery—Simple Orchidectomy*. Available at: ℜ www.baus.org.uk (accessed 17 May 2011).
3. British Association of Urological Surgery. *Procedure Specific Consent Forms for Urological Surgery—Insertion of Testicular Prosthesis*. Available at: ℜ www.baus.org.uk (accessed 17 May 2011).
4. British Association of Urological Surgery. *Procedure Specific Consent Forms for Urological Surgery—Radical Orchidectomy +/– Silicone Implant*. Available at: ℜ www.baus.org.uk (accessed 17 May 2011).

Percutaneous nephrolithotomy

Description

Percutaneous nephrolithotomy (PCNL) is a percutaneous endoscopic technique that facilitates direct access into the kidney via a tract between the skin and the renal collecting system. It has been developed to remove upper urinary tract calculi that are not amenable to other treatment modalities (ESWL/flexible ureteroscopy and stone fragmentation).

Indications for PCNL include:
- Stone size >2cm (symptomatic or associated with urinary tract sepsis)
- Stones that have failed ESWL or retrograde flexible ureteroscopy and stone fragmentation
- Stag-horn calculi
- Symptomatic calculi located within a calyceal diverticulum

Initially the collecting system is filled via cystoscopic cannulation of the ureter and fluid instilled into the renal collecting system. The patient is then repositioned (traditionally in the prone position, however, recently increasing data are available for supine procedures) for PCNL and under ultrasound or fluoroscopic guidance, a renal calyx is punctured and a guide-wire threaded into the collecting system. Serial dilators are passed over the guide-wire to create a tract through which a nephroscope is advanced, and fragmentation of the renal calculus is performed with laser or ultrasonic lithotripsy. A nephrostomy tube is placed post-procedure and occasionally a ureteric stent is placed. More recently, 'tubeless' PCNL has been practised.

Outcomes are good for small stones (90–95% stone clearance), staghorn calculus clearance combined with postoperative ESWL for fragments is in the order of 80–85%.

Additional procedures that may become necessary

- Cystoscopy and bladder biopsy
- Retrograde ureteric stent insertion
- Antegrade ureteric stent insertion
- Nephrostomy insertion
- Flexible renoscopy and stone fragmentation via PCNL tract

Benefits

- *Diagnostic*: obtain samples of stone which can be sent for biochemical analysis
- *Therapeutic*: remove symptomatic renal calculi, remove source of infection, prevent further stone burden development

Alternative procedures/conservative measures

- *Conservative*: dietary advice, fluid intake advice
- *Medical*: medical stone dissolution and expulsive therapy, treatment of *underlying cause of stone formation*
- *Surgical*: ESWL, retrograde ureterorenoscopy and stone fragmentation, Retrograde ureteric stent insertion with ESWL, open/laparoscopic pyelolithotomy[1]

Serious/frequently occurring risks

- *Common*: insertion of ureteric stent and urethral catheter that will need removal as separate procedure, bleeding (haematuria), passage of stone fragments, post-procedure discomfort
- *Occasional*: the need for more than one puncture site to gain access to kidney and adequate stone clearance, incomplete stone removal, the need for further procedure for complete stone clearance, recurrence of new calculi, pleural effusions compromising respiratory function or necessitating the placement of an intercostal drain
- *Rare*: severe bleeding requiring transfusion of blood or blood products, embolization of kidney, or as a final resort require nephrectomy,[2] damage to adjacent organs (lung/bowel/spleen/liver) necessitating further emergency treatment, cardiovascular compromise (due to fluid absorption from irrigation solution[3,4])

Blood transfusion necessary

- Group and save/(rarely cross-match)

Type of anaesthesia/sedation

- Local anaesthesia (very rarely performed in supine unfit patient)/regional anaesthesia/general anaesthesia

Follow-up/need for further procedure

- Will require analgesia on ward postoperatively with subsequent removal of nephrostomy and catheter
- KUB X-ray to identify residual stone fragments[5]
- May require removal of ureteric stent
- May require further treatment (further PCNL/ESWL/retrograde ureterorenoscopy) for residual stone fragments
- Outpatient review with imaging as required on discharge

References

1. Srisubat A, Potisat S, Lojanapiwat B, et al. Extracorporeal shock wave lithotripsy (ESWL) versus percutaneous nephrolithotomy (PCNL) or retrograde intrarenal surgery (RIRS) for kidney stones. *Cochrane Database Syst Rev* 2009;4:CD007044.
2. Rastinehad AR, Andonian S, Smith AD, et al. Management of hemorrhagic complications associated with percutaneous nephrolithotomy. *Endourol* 2009;23(10):1763–7.
3. British Association of Urological Surgery. *Procedure Specific Consent Forms for Urological Surgery—Percutaneous Nephrolithotomy (PCNL)*. Available at: ℜ www.baus.org.uk (accessed 17 May 2011).
4. Srinivasan AK, Herati A, Okeke Z, et al. Renal drainage after percutaneous nephrolithotomy. *J Endourol* 2009;23(10):1743–9.
5. Skolarikos A, Papatsoris AG. Diagnosis and management of postpercutaneous nephrolithotomy residual stone fragments. *J Endourol* 2009;23(10): 751–5.

Preputial adhesiolysis

Description

The prepuce, mucosal surface of the foreskin, and the glans penis have a common epithelium. The process of gradual separation and subsequent keratinization between the two layers takes place at any time between late gestation and adolescence. The term preputial adhesion is frequently used and there is often coexistent smegma (a white congealed discharge from the coronal glands and breakdown products of the preputial adhesions) which may act as a source of infection in cases of recurrent balanitis. Parents often worry about significant ballooning of the penis during urination.

Up to 60% of children between the ages of 6 and 9 years are unable to completely retract their foreskin; however, this disappears by the age of 17 years.

Patients or parents who do not wish for circumcision may choose release of preputial adhesions as a therapeutic option. This involves drawing back the foreskin and, using either blunt or sharp dissection, the foreskin is peeled away from the glans penis to the level of the coronal sulcus. If adhesions are fibrotic, dense or bleed excessively, then conversion to a formal circumcision may be advocated. Often petroleum jelly is placed on the exposed glans and the parents or patient is taught to pull the foreskin back regularly to prevent further adhesion formation, although no evidence exists to suggest this as a primary therapy for phimosis or preputial adhesions.

Additional procedures that may become necessary

- Preputioplasty
- Circumcision of foreskin
- Frenuloplasty

Benefits

- *Diagnostic*: in adults to identify any underlying pathology on foreskin or glans (i.e. malignancy) causing adhesion
- *Therapeutic*: prevent recurrent episodes of balanoposthitis, ballooning of penis on urination

Alternative procedures/conservative measures

- *Conservative*: no treatment, most cases of childhood adhesions are physiological and separation takes place over time, there is no evidence to suggest gentle foreskin retraction prevents phimosis
- *Medical*: antibiotics and analgesia or topical anti-inflammatory agents for recurrent balanoposthitis
- *Surgical*: circumcision of foreskin

Serious/frequently occurring risks

- *Common*: temporary bleeding or oozing of serosanguineous (straw-coloured) fluid from raw surface of penis, temporary tenderness over penis

- *Occasional*: infection of glans penis requiring antibiotic therapy, need for future circumcision, recurrence of adhesions requiring repeat procedure
- *Rare*: cosmetic dissatisfaction, hyperaesthesia and sensitive glans penis post-procedure[1]

Blood transfusion necessary
- None

Type of anaesthesia/sedation
- Local anaesthesia/regional anaesthesia/general anaesthesia

Follow-up/need for further procedure
- Outpatient review if required on discharge
- Analgesia
- Encourage moisturizer use over glans penis

Reference
1. British Association of Urological Surgery. *Procedure Specific Consent Forms for Urological Surgery—Freeing of Preputial Adhesions.* Available at: ℜ www.baus.org.uk (accessed 17 May 2011).

Prostatectomy (radical)

Description

Radical prostatectomy is the surgical removal of the entire prostate gland including its capsule. It is performed with curative intent for patients with localized prostate cancer with an appropriate life expectancy (>10 years) and who have a good performance status. Excision of the prostatic urethra and seminal vesicles is included in the specimen and commonly, the procedure includes simultaneous pelvic lymph node dissection either as a diagnostic (staging) marker or for therapeutic intent. Care is taken to reduce the risk of injury to the neurovascular bundle that runs inferolateral to the prostate, the external urethral sphincter that lies distal to the verumontanum and the rectum posteriorly. If the presence of palpable disease extends laterally, the neurovascular bundle may be sacrificed to avoid compromise in cancer control.

The procedure itself can be performed open, laparoscopic, or robotic. The open technique can be performed retropubic (Fig. 11.5) or transperineal. The transperineal technique does not allow for lymph node dissection.[1]

After removal of the specimen, reconstruction of the bladder neck is performed with an anastomosis to the urethra. This is performed over a catheter which is traditionally left *in situ* for approximately 2 weeks. A drain is commonly placed following the procedure and removed 1–2 days following the operation (when drain volumes are minimal). Patients are sent home with their catheter *in situ*, which is commonly removed between 7 and 21 days; a cystogram is required only if there is a documented urine leak or if there are catheter-related problems. Some institutions routinely perform cystograms prior to catheter removal.

Characteristically the decision behind radical prostatectomy is made in a multidisciplinary setting and the patient may be offered other treatment options to secure oncological control. This can include external beam radiotherapy, active surveillance, and brachytherapy. Patients are counselled pre- and postoperatively with close liaison with the cancer nurse specialists throughout their journey.

Additional procedures that may become necessary

- Pelvic lymph node dissection
- Abdominal drain insertion
- Urethral catheter placement
- Postoperative radiotherapy/hormone therapy/chemotherapy (based on local policy)
- Postoperative cystogram prior to catheter removal

Benefits

- *Diagnostic*: allows histopathological grading and staging of disease where in certain circumstances upstaging of disease is seen
- *Therapeutic*: the procedure is performed for curative intent and cancer control

Alternative procedures/conservative measures

- *Conservative*: some patients may be suitable for an active surveillance protocol where PSA is monitored and interval re-biopsy is performed to identify change or upstaging of disease

- *Medical*: hormonal therapy in either tablet or injection form may be used in a neo-adjuvant setting prior to further treatment or as a disease control measure in certain subgroup of patients
- *Radiotherapy*: external beam radiotherapy to the prostate with curative intent may offer oncological control, Brachytherapy is whereby permanent implantable radioactive 'brachytherapy' seeds are placed within the prostate and is used to achieve oncological control
- *Surgical*: the surgical approach can vary between open retropubic, open transperineal, laparoscopic, and robotic prostatectomy[1]

Serious/frequently occurring risks

- *General*: postoperative pain, chronic wound or pelvic pain, wound infection requiring a period of antibiotics (oral/intravenous), incisional hernia, chest infection, cardiovascular event including myocardial infarction, deep vein thrombosis, pulmonary embolism, HDU/ITU admission, death (1:500 cases)
- *Common*: temporary insertion of urethral catheter and abdominal drain, impotence due to unavoidable peri prostatic neurovascular bundle injury (70–90%), failure to produce semen during orgasm, sub-fertility
- *Occasional*: bleeding and blood loss requiring transfusion or further surgery to control bleeding, urinary incontinence requiring the use of incontinence pads or further surgery (5% patients beyond 6 months require >1 pad/day), residual cancer outside the prostate requiring a period of observation or treatment recurrent disease, the need for radiotherapy/hormone therapy, postoperative catheter displacement requiring further procedure to reinsert catheter, postoperative urine or lymphatic collection requiring percutaneous or open drainage, bladder neck stenosis (5–8% of patients 2–6 months postoperatively)
- *Rare*: injury to rectum necessitating temporary colostomy, transperineal approach—rectovesical fistula requiring further treatment, ureteric injury requiring reimplantation/primary anastomosis/JJ stenting[2,3]

Blood transfusion necessary

- Group and save/cross-match 2–4 units (depending on starting haemoglobin)

Type of anaesthesia/sedation

- General anaesthesia (often combined with regional anaesthesia for pain relief postoperatively)

Follow-up/need for further procedure

- Removal of abdominal/perineal drain 1–2 days post-procedure (or when volume from drain decreases)
- Removal of urethral catheter between 7 and 21 days (either with or without cystogram prior to trial of voiding)
- Outpatient review at 4–6 weeks with repeat PSA
- Multidisciplinary team review with histology
- Possible need for adjuvant radiotherapy or hormone therapy in the future
- Erectile dysfunction clinic for support with erectile dysfunction

- Continence nurse regarding postoperative urinary incontinence
- Postoperative support and counselling with cancer nurse specialist/oncology/urology

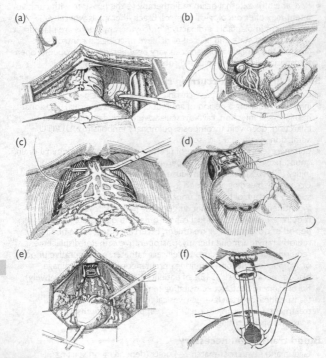

Fig. 11.5 Stages of a radical retropubic prostatectomy. (a) incision of endopelvic fascia and lateral dissection of prostate; (b) dissection of dorsal venous complex between pubic arch and urethra; (c) suture ligation of dorsal venous complex; (d) sharp division of urethra to create urethral stump; (e) retrograde dissection of prostate off Denonvilliers fascia; (f) anastomosis of bladder neck to urethral stump.

Reproduced with permission from McLatchie GR and Leaper DJ. *Oxford Specialist Handbook of Operative Surgery* 2nd edition. 2006. Oxford: Oxford University Press, p.509, Figure 13.8.

References

1. Reynard J, Brewster S, Biers, eds. *Oxford Handbook of Urology*. Oxford: Oxford University Press, 2006, p222.
2. *British Association of Urological Surgery. Procedure Specific Consent Forms for Urological Surgery—Radical Retropubic Prostatectomy and Pelvic Lymph Node Dissection.* Available at: ℘ www.baus.org.uk (accessed 17 May 2011).
3. British Association of Urological Surgery. *Procedure Specific Consent Forms for Urological Surgery—Radical Perineal Prostatectomy.* Available at: ℘ www.baus.org.uk (accessed 17 May 2011).

Retrograde pyelogram ± retrograde insertion of ureteric stent

Description

The ureters are tubular structures that run between the renal pelvis and the posterior-inferior wall of the bladder. They have the potential to obstruct due to intraluminal pathology (calculi clots), mucosal or intramural pathology (TCC, fibroepithelial polyps), or extramural pathology (retroperitoneal fibrosis/retroperitoneal lymphadenopathy). The result is that renal drainage is compromised and this can lead to obstructive uropathy, deteriorating renal function and occasionally sepsis secondary to pyonephrosis.

Retrograde pyelography is the process by which contrast medium is instilled into the ureter and the pattern of filling is observed on fluoroscopy to identify pathology. Cystoscopy is performed and a ureteric catheter is placed down the cystoscope and gently inserted into the ureter by 1–2cm. Contrast medium is then pushed into the ureter and the pattern of ureteric filling is noted (noting irregularities, filling defects, etc.). The ureteric catheter is advanced further to the upper ureter and the renal pelvis is filled (looking for evidence of hydronephrosis and pelviureteric junction obstruction). The ureteric catheter is then withdrawn and subsequent drainage is visualized live on fluoroscopy.

Retrograde ureteric stent insertion may be necessary as a measure to relieve obstruction. Here a guide-wire is placed via cystoscopy into the kidney and a hollow tube is railroaded into the kidney. Most stents utilized are JJ stents (Figs. 11.6, 11.7), which have a pigtail coil proximally in the kidney and another in the bladder to avoid stent migration.

Indications for ureteric stent insertion include:
• Relief of obstruction (calculi, strictures—benign/malignant)
• Prevention of obstruction (post-ureteroscopy)
• Passive dilation of ureter (pre-ureteroscopy)
• Long-term management of obstruction (patients receiving chemotherapy/radiotherapy)
• Post-ureteric surgery/injury (ensure antegrade flow of urine and healing of ureter around stent
• Prior to pelvic surgery to aid identification of ureter intraoperatively
• Following endopyelotomy (for pelviureteric junction obstruction)

Stents can be made from a multitude of materials, which include biodegradable to short-term or long-term metallic stents. In certain circumstances short segment ureteric Memokath® stents are inserted for up to 5 years in the treatment of short-segment ureteric strictures.

Additional procedures that may become necessary
• Retrograde pyelography (if stent only)
• Retrograde stent insertion (if pyelography only)
• Diagnostic/therapeutic ureteroscopy (stone fragmentation/endopyelotomy)
• Biopsies of bladder/ureter
• Antegrade percutaneous nephrostomy ± antegrade stent insertion

Benefits
- *Diagnostic*: in adults to identify any underlying pathology of bladder/ureter/renal pelvis/kidney
- *Therapeutic*: to improve the drainage of the kidney and prevent deteriorating renal function or obstructive uropathy

Alternative procedures/conservative measures
- *Conservative*: in a non-functioning/poorly functioning kidney in the presence of obstruction, if the patient is asymptomatic then observation may be all that is necessary with renal function measurement and serial radiological imaging
- *Radiology*: alternatives to retrograde pyelography include CT urogram, IVU, MAG3 renogram, CT KUB, ultrasound KUB
- *Medical*: antibiotics for recurrent obstruction associated with sepsis
- *Surgical*: nephrostomy and antegrade stent insertion, primary ureteroscopy and stone fragmentation or biopsies, endopyelotomy, pyeloplasty, ureterolysis, ureteric bypass surgery (all dependent on underlying pathology in question)

Serious/frequently occurring risks
- *Common*: bleeding (haematuria), dysuria, temporary insertion of urethral catheter, temporary discomfort from stent causing pain, frequency, urgency, and haematuria, further procedure to remove stent (usually flexible cystoscopy, however, occasionally under general anaesthesia), use of X-ray imaging and associated radiation
- *Occasional*: urinary tract infections requiring oral or intravenous antibiotics, trauma to urethra, prostate or bladder resulting in haematuria, diagnosis of bladder mucosal lesion/stone requiring treatment, difficulty in passing stent necessitating either nephrostomy and antegrade stenting or open surgery, need to perform ureterorenoscopy
- *Rare*: stent encrustation, haematuria and clot retention necessitating further cystoscopy and washout, need for catheterization (temporary), urethral stricture formation, perforation of urethra/bladder necessitating temporary catheter insertion or open procedure to repair defect in bladder, contrast-associated allergic reaction/sensitivity
- Complications associated with subsequent specific procedure performed[1,2]

Blood transfusion necessary
- None

Type of anaesthesia/sedation
- Local anaesthesia (rarely performed via flexible cystoscopy)/regional anaesthesia/general anaesthesia

Follow-up/need for further procedure
- *Outpatient review or inpatient follow-up*, depending on the underlying pathology
- Stent change or removal date must be documented and discussed with patient
- Some patients may require anti-cholinergic medication for severe stent symptoms

- Stent advice sheet (coping with a ureteric stent)
- Analgesia

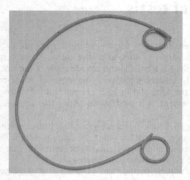

Fig. 11.6 JJ stent.
Reproduced with permission from Reynard J, Brewster S, and Biers S. *Oxford Handbook of Urology* 2nd edition. 2009. Oxford: Oxford University Press, p.690, Figure 17.10.

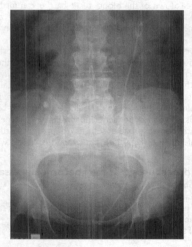

Fig. 11.7 KUB radiograph demonstrating a JJ stent *in situ*.
Reproduced with permission from Reynard J, Brewster S, and Biers S. *Oxford Handbook of Urology* 2nd edition. 2009. Oxford: Oxford University Press p.443, Figure 9.13.

References

1. British Association of Urological Surgery. *Procedure Specific Consent Forms for Urological Surgery—(Rigid) Cystoscopy and Stent Procedure*. Available at: ℜ www.baus.org.uk (accessed 17 May 2011).
2. British Association of Urological Surgery. *Procedure Specific Consent Forms for Urological Surgery—(Rigid) Cystoscopy and Retrograde Pyelogram*. Available at: ℜ www.baus.org.uk (accessed 17 May 2011).

Scrotal exploration for suspected torsion of testis

Description

The commonest indication for an emergency scrotal exploration is to exclude the diagnosis of torsion of the testis. Acute testicular torsion results when there is a twist in the blood supply of the testicle and epididymis, and must be suspected in any patient with acute-onset testicular pain between the ages of 10 and 30, in particular if there is a history of testicular maldescent. It is worthwhile noting that any age group can be affected.

Clinical examination may reveal a swollen testis, which is exquisitely tender and in an abnormal lie within the hemi-scrotum. There may be a reactive hydrocoele and the patient may present with referred abdominal pain or autonomic symptoms (i.e. vomiting).

Surgical exploration of the hemi-scrotum is an emergency. Delay in de-torting the testicle can result in permanent ischaemic damage resulting in atrophy, loss of testosterone production, and infertility or subfertility. There is a theory that antibodies directed at the contralateral testicle during the breakdown of the blood–testis barrier can further compound fertility. Both testes must be fixed in the presence of torsion, as the bell-clapper deformity that predisposes to this condition is likely to be bilateral.[1]

A midline vertical scrotal incision is used access each testicle. The testis in question is delivered into the wound. If it is torted, then the torsion should be corrected and the testis placed in a warm, saline-soaked swab for 10min. If the testis still appears black, then trans-scrotal orchidectomy should be performed with a transfixion suture securing the cord. If however, it pinks up, then fixation should be performed bilaterally. How this is done is surgeon dependent. Most will use a three-point fixation technique with non-absorbable sutures to prevent further torsion in two planes of rotation (Fig. 11.8). The wound is closed with absorbable sutures.

Additional procedures that may become necessary

- Orchidectomy
- Bilateral fixation of testicles
- Excision of hydatid of Morgagni or appendix epididymis (appendages which are able to tort and cause testicular pain)
- Insertion of scrotal drain

Benefits

- *Diagnostic*: to identify the cause of acute scrotal pain. To exclude the diagnosis of acute testicular torsion
- *Therapeutic*: prevent further testicular ischaemia, salvage the testicle and prevent further torsion bilaterally

Alternative procedures/conservative measures

- *Conservative*: observation in cases of testicular torsion risks the loss of testicle

- *Medical*: in cases where the history is longstanding or if symptoms, signs, urine dipstick testing suggest epididymo-orchitis, antibiotic therapy may be indicated with sonographic examination of testicles
- *Surgical*: Exploration is the only true method of reliably excluding testicular torsion. Ultrasound scanning may add time, delay the diagnosis and prolong testicular ischaemia. Only use this when the history and clinical findings are not suggestive or equivocal[2]

Serious/frequently occurring risks

- *Common*: discomfort
- *Occasional*: wound infection, haematoma, uncomfortable palpable sutures, granuloma formation
- *Rare*: further torsion despite fixation

Blood transfusion necessary

- None

Type of anaesthesia/sedation

- Regional anaesthesia/general anaesthesia

Follow-up/need for further procedure

- Outpatient review if required on discharge
- Analgesia
- If the diagnosis is epididymo-orchitis, treatment with antibiotics may be indicated and follow-up ultrasound necessary

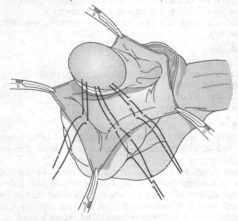

Fig. 11.8 Three-point testicular suture fixation of testis.

Reproduced with permission from Reynard J, Mark S, Turner K, et al. *Oxford Specialist Handbook of Urological Surgery*. 2008. Oxford: Oxford University Press, p.10, Figure 8.58.

References

1. Frank JD. Fixation of the testis. *Br J Urol Int* 2002;**89**:331–33.
2. British Association of Urological Surgery. *Procedure Specific Consent Forms for Urological Surgery—Exploration of Scrotum for Suspected Torsion of Testis*. Available at: ℘ www.baus.org.uk (accessed 17 May 2011).

Suprapubic catheter insertion (cystoscopic/blind/ultrasound guided)

Description

Suprapubic catheterization is a technique used to allow for bladder emptying in circumstances where urethral catheterization is not possible, tolerated or at the patient's choice to manage their lower urinary tract symptoms.

The catheter is situated approximately 2–3cm above the symphysis pubis and recent British Association of Urological Surgeons (BAUS) guidelines[1] have standardized care associated with its insertion, use, and follow-up care.

Indications

- For acute or chronic urinary retention where urethral catheterization is difficult or potentially dangerous
- Neurological disease (i.e. multiple sclerosis/spinal cord injury)
- Long term urethral catheter use resulting in ventral penile split/patulous urethra
- Intractable urinary incontinence
- Following operative intervention (i.e. stress urinary incontinence procedures/colorectal surgery/post-TURP in patients with large bladder residuals)
- In cases of urethral trauma
- Palliative use (in elderly patient care and comfort)
- Urodynamic investigation (in cases where urethral catheterization is not possible)

Contraindications

- Known bladder malignancy
- Unexplained haematuria (exclude bladder malignancy)
- Pelvic fractures (relative)
- Coagulopathy (relative)
- Lower abdominal surgery (relative)

Technique

- *Closed technique (blind)*: in cases of acute or chronic urinary retention where the bladder is palpable, and there is no evidence of lower abdominal surgery
- *Ultrasound guided*: in cases where there is evidence of lower abdominal surgery, or a bladder that is not palpable, or difficult body habitus
- *Cystoscopic bladder filling*: in cases where there is evidence of lower abdominal surgery, difficult body habitus, a bladder that is not palpable or identifiable easily on ultrasound scan. The patient is given general anaesthesia and active bladder filling with cystoscopic views of suprapubic catheterization is performed
- *Open*: this is used again for difficult cases where an open cystotomy is performed and the catheter placed and secured within the bladder under direct vision. Often the catheter can be tunnelled subcutaneously to one side for comfort

Suprapubic catheter sets and equipment vary but the principle of aspiration of urine with a needle prior to introduction of trocar or guide-wire is essential to ensure adequate placement.

Additional procedures that may become necessary

- Insertion of urethral catheter
- Washout of bladder/clots
- Cystoscopy guided
- Biopsy of bladder mucosal lesion

Benefits

- *Diagnostic*: identify cause of obstruction (cystoscopic), when used as part of urodynamics, to identify underlying bladder behaviour as a cause of symptoms
- *Therapeutic*: to aid bladder drainage for indications as listed

Alternative procedures/conservative measures

- Management conservative without catheter
- Urethral catheterization
- Suprapubic aspiration (in acute setting)
- Flexible cystoscopy-guided catheter insertion
- *Surgical*: open cystotomy and tunnelled suprapubic catheterization, permanent urinary diversion procedure

Serious/frequently occurring risks

- *Common*: bleeding (haematuria), dysuria, temporary insertion of urethral catheter in addition to suprapubic catheter, need for regular change of suprapubic catheter (3–4 monthly)
- *Occasional*: urinary tract infections requiring oral or intravenous antibiotics, trauma to urethra, prostate or bladder resulting in haematuria, diagnosis of bladder mucosa lesion/stone requiring treatment, blocking of catheter requiring flushing regularly, bladder discomfort, urgency, pain, or bladder stone formation requiring treatment
- *Rare*: haematuria and clot retention necessitating further cystoscopy and washout, need for catheterization (temporary), urethral stricture formation, perforation of urethra/bladder necessitating temporary catheter insertion or open procedure to repair defect in bladder, injury to surrounding organs and viscera that results in requiring additional surgery (bowel perforation)[2]

Blood transfusion necessary

- None/group and save (depending on context of insertion)

Type of anaesthesia/sedation

- Local anaesthesia/regional anaesthesia/general anaesthesia

Follow-up/need for further procedure

- Dependent on indication for suprapubic catheterization
- First catheter change usually performed in hospital at 8–12 weeks (as per local policy)
- Subsequent catheter changes can take place in the community (usually every 3 months)
- Re-referral if complications with suprapubic catheter (i.e. blockage, recurrent infections, bypassing)

References

1. Harrison SC, Lawrence WT, Morley R, et al. British Association of Urological Surgeons' suprapubic catheter practice guidelines. *BJU Int* 2010;**107**:77–85.
2. British Association of Urological Surgery. *Procedure Specific Consent Forms for Urological Surgery—Suprapubic Catheter Insertion (Cystostomy)*. Available at: ℅ www.baus.org.uk (accessed 17 May 2011).

Transrectal ultrasound ± guided biopsies of the prostate gland

Description

The commonest indication for transrectal ultrasound is to evaluate the prostate gland and via guided biopsies, it is the commonest method of diagnosing prostate cancer. Images of the prostate are obtained, following which accurate derived prostate volume can be calculated, and cysts, abscesses, and calcifications within the prostate including peripheral zone lesions suggestive of malignancy or inflammation can be identified.

The indications for transrectal ultrasound include:

- Accurate prostate volume measurements
- Seminal vesicle and ejaculatory duct assessment in male infertility
- Suspected prostatic abscess
- Investigation in chronic pelvic pain for prostatic cysts or calculi
- Abnormal digital rectal examination (DRE) may mandate biopsies
- Elevated PSA (exception is very high PSA with abnormal DRE suggestive of metastatic prostate cancer) mandates biopsy
- Previously normal biopsies with rising PSA
- As part of active surveillance plan to re-biopsy patient
- Brachytherapy planning for prostate cancer

Commonly a patient is counselled for a TRUS ± biopsies prior to the procedure. If biopsies are anticipated, then a prophylactic course of oral antibiotics is started 1 day prior to the procedure and continued for 3–5 days.

The procedure is carried out with a patient in left lateral position or in lithotomy position. An ultrasound probe is introduced into the rectum (Fig. 11.9) and the prostate is visualized in two planes for measurement of volume. Needle-guided biopsies are taken and a minimum of six cores obtained, three from each lobe. The increased number of biopsies improves the sensitivity of the test, however, it also increases the complication profile. Targeted biopsies of prostatic lesions are also taken as required, and seminal vesicle biopsies can add information regarding the stage of disease if prostate cancer is implicated.

Additional procedures that may become necessary

- Biopsies of prostate gland
- Aspiration of cyst of prostate gland
- Aspiration of abscess of prostate gland
- Volume measurements

Benefits

- *Diagnostic*: identify cause of symptoms, measure volume of prostate to plan treatment, identify cause of raised PSA, histopathological identification of prostate cancer, inflammation or benign adenomatous change, grading of prostate cancer, and upstaging of disease in patients on active surveillance protocol
- *Therapeutic*: aspiration of symptomatic prostate cyst or abscess

Alternative procedures/conservative measures

- *Conservative*: PSA follow-up and serial DRE, clinical and biochemical diagnosis of prostate cancer
- Medical: antibiotics and anti-inflammatory agents in patients with prostatitis
- *Radiology*: increasing evidence has been published suggesting the incorporation of MRI prior to TRUS biopsies to diagnose and map prostate cancer (particularly in younger patients with a palpable nodule—T2 disease)
- *Surgery*: Patients who undergo TURP may have their prostate chips reviewed histopathologically for underlying prostate cancer

Serious/frequently occurring risks

- *Common*: bleeding for up to 3 weeks post-procedure (haematuria, per rectal bleeding (significant rectal bleeding 0.5%), haematospermia), dysuria, vasovagal event immediately post-procedure
- *Occasional*: acute retention of urine necessitating temporary insertion of urethral catheter, infection, and life-threatening septicaemia, requiring intravenous antibiotics and hospital admission (septicaemia 0.5%)
- *Rare*: haematuria and clot retention necessitating further cystoscopy and washout, acute prostatitis/chronic prostatitis and chronic pain[1,2]

Blood transfusion necessary

- None

Type of anaesthesia/sedation

- Local anaesthesia/regional anaesthesia/general anaesthesia

Follow-up/need for further procedure

- Dependent on indication for TRUS and biopsy
- Review in outpatient clinic with outcome of histopathology
- Discussion at local/regional multidisciplinary team meeting with histopathology

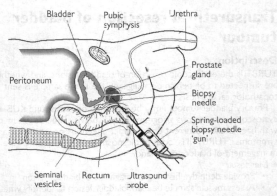

Fig. 11.9 Transrectal ultrasound-guided biopsy of prostate gland: an ultrasound probe is inserted into the rectum to guide the biopsy needle into the correct position where several core biopsies are taken from the prostate.

Reproduced with permission from Reynard J, Brewster S and Biers S. *Oxford Handbook of Urology* 2nd edition. 2009. Oxford: Oxford University Press, p.303, Figure 7.7.

References

1. Rodriguez LV, Terris MK. Risks and complications of transrectal ultrasound guided prostate needle biopsy: a prospective study and review of the literature. *J Urol* 1998;**160**(6 Pt 1):2115–20.

2. Ecke TH, Gunia S, Bartel P, et al. Complications and risk factors of transrectal ultrasound guided needle biopsies of the prostate evaluated by questionnaire. *Urol Oncol* 2008;**26**(5):474–8.

Transurethral resection of bladder tumour

Description

TURBT is the endoscopic resection of bladder lesions, and whether they are suspected to be benign or malignant, the tissue sample is sent for histopathological diagnosis.

Primary bladder tumours may be identified on ultrasound KUB, flexible cystoscopy, intravenous urogram, or CT pelvis. Patients often present with haematuria, recurrent urinary tract infections or lower urinary tract symptoms. TURBT has both a diagnostic and therapeutic role in the management of bladder malignancy.

- *Diagnostic:*
  - Provide definitive histological diagnosis of bladder lesion
  - Assess muscle sample beneath bladder lesion to identify whether muscle invasive
  - Biopsy separate areas of bladder to assess the presence of CIS
  - Biopsy the prostatic urethra if radical surgery is considered
  - Allows re-staging of tumour in cases of recurrence
- *Therapeutic:*
  - To achieve visual tumour resection and surrounding margin clearance in Ta/T1 disease (associated with adequate treatment in 70% new cases)
  - Decrease chance of tumour recurrence
  - Decrease chance of tumour progression of primary tumour
- *Palliative:* palliative debulking TURBT followed by radiotherapy in the elderly unfit patient with muscle invasive bladder cancer[1]

All TURBT procedures must be preceded by an examination under anaesthesia to identify whether the bladder has a mass present, and whether it is fixed or mobile. TURBT is the mainstay of treatment in patients with superficial bladder tumours (TCC) with recurrences not amenable to ablative treatment via flexible cystoscopy.

Additional procedures that may become necessary

- Random bladder biopsies
- Prostatic urethral loop biopsies
- Postoperative adjuvant intravesical chemotherapy (mitomycin C)
- Urethral catheterization with irrigation

Benefits

- *Diagnostic:* histopathological diagnosis, grading and staging of tumour, allows planning of further treatment, allows re-staging in recurrences
- *Therapeutic:* for first presentation superficial tumours may be therapeutic if macroscopic clearance is achieved
- Improvement in lower urinary tract symptoms associated with bladder tumour (i.e. strangury, haematuria, dysuria, recurrent urinary tract infections, urgency, etc.)

Alternative procedures/conservative measures

- *Conservative/palliative:* if tumour burden is small and the patient is not suitable for anaesthesia, then symptomatic control may be appropriate

- Flexible cystoscopy and diathermy destruction of tumour/laser tumour destruction in patients who are high risk for general/regional anaesthesia or have very small superficial recurrences on check cystoscopy
- Radiotherapy
- Chemotherapy
- Combination chemo-radiotherapy (therapeutic or palliative)
- Radical cystectomy (see ☐ p.290)
- Urinary diversion procedure
- Palliative care

Serious/frequently occurring risks

- *Common*: bleeding (haematuria), dysuria, temporary insertion of urethral catheter with bladder irrigation, need for the administration of intravesical chemotherapy to prevent recurrence, need for regular check cystoscopy
- *Occasional*: urinary tract infections requiring oral or intravenous antibiotics, no guarantee that this one procedure can prevent recurrence or cure, incomplete tumour resection in larger tumours, trauma to urethra, prostate or bladder resulting in haematuria, need for further definitive therapy
- *Rare*: haematuria and clot retention necessitating further cystoscopy and washout, urethral stricture formation, perforation of urethra/bladder necessitating temporary catheter insertion or open procedure to repair defect in bladder[2,3]
- *Mitomycin C (intravesical postoperative)*: transient irritative LUTS (15%), rash over genitalia or palms of hands, (rare: systemic toxicity)

Blood transfusion necessary

- Group and save/cross-match (depending on preoperative haemoglobin and tumour mass)

Type of anaesthesia/sedation

- Regional anaesthesia/general anaesthesia

Follow-up/need for further procedure

- Dependent on indication for TURBT
- Review in outpatient clinic with outcome of histopathology
- Discussion at local/regional multidisciplinary team meeting with histopathology
- Check flexible cystoscopy follow-up/general anaesthesia check cystoscopy (first check) depending on local policy
- May require interval tumour re-resection depending on histology or tumour burden

References

1. Hollenbeck BK, Miller DC, Taub D, et al. Risk factors for adverse outcomes after transurethral resection of bladder tumors. *Cancer* 2006;**106**(7):1527–35.
2. British Association of Urological Surgery. *Procedure Specific Consent Forms for Urological Surgery—Transurethral Resection of Bladder Tumour*. Available at: ℘ www.baus.org.uk (accessed 17 May 2011).
3. Nieder AM, Meinbach DS, Kim SS, et al. Transurethral bladder tumor resection: intraoperative and postoperative complications in a residency setting. *J Urol* 2005;**174**(6):2307–9.

Transurethral resection of prostate gland/open prostatectomy (transperineal/Millen's)

Description

Surgery for benign occlusive prostate disease categorized into two groups, endoscopic surgery and open surgery. Endoscopic treatment includes bladder neck incision, bladder neck resection, TURP, laser vaporization of prostate (i.e. PVP), and laser enucleation of prostate (i.e. HoLEP). Open surgery includes transvesical prostatectomy and simple retropubic (Millen's) prostatectomy. Although laser enucleation is gaining popularity as a treatment modality, particularly for larger prostates that would usually be subjected to open surgery, the vast majority of urologists perform TURP as the gold standard surgical treatment.

TURP is an endoscopic procedure that utilizes a cutting loop via a resectocope to shave away prostate chips. The prostate tissue is resected to the capsule and the chips are washed out of the bladder to undergo histopathological analysis.

Indications for TURP

- Lower urinary tract symptoms refractory to medical management and lifestyle advice
- Obstructive uropathy secondary to occlusive prostate disease (high pressure-chronic retention)
- Recurrent acute retention of urine
- Bladder stones secondary to occlusive prostate disease
- Haematuria secondary to benign prostatic enlargement

Open suprapubic/transvesical (Freyer) prostatectomy is ideally suited approach for median lobe enlargement. The bladder is opened and the adenoma within the median lobe is enucleated (Figs. 11.10, 11.11).

Simple (Millen's) prostatectomy: the prostate is exposed via a Pfannenstiel or lower midline incision, the dorsal vein complex is suture ligated and the capsule opened. The adenoma is then developed by finger dissection and the adenoma enucleated.

In both procedures a catheter is left for 5 days and a drain is left *in situ* for 24–48h.[5]

Indications for open prostatectomy

- Large prostate (>100mL)
- Patient habitus or limited hip abduction which does not facilitate positioning for TURP
- Failed TURP secondary to bleeding
- Large bladder calculi necessitating open cystolithotomy combined with prostatectomy

Open simple prostate surgery is not advised in patients with prostate cancer, or in patients who have had a previous prostatectomy.

Additional procedures that may become necessary

- Bladder biopsies
- Prostatic urethral biopsies
- Bladder neck incision
- Transrectal ultrasound and biopsies under general anaesthesia (abnormal prostate on rectal examination)
- Urethral catheterization with irrigation
- Suprapubic catheter for patients with high preoperative residual volumes

Benefits

- *Diagnostic*: histopathological diagnosis of prostate tissue, assess response of symptoms to bladder outflow surgery
- *Therapeutic*: to treat occlusive prostate for indications as listed

Alternative procedures/conservative measures

- *Conservative*: lifestyle changes, dietary and fluid intake advice
- *Medical*: α-antagonists, 5-α-reductase inhibitors, hormone treatment in patients with prostate cancer can reduce prostate volume and either improve symptoms or render the patient catheter free
- *Surgical*: bladder neck incision, bladder neck resection, transurethral resection of prostate gland, laser vaporization of prostate (i.e. PVF), and laser enucleation of prostate (i.e. HoLEP), radical prostatectomy in prostate cancer patients suitable for this mode of treatment

Serious/frequently occurring risks

- *Common*: bleeding (haematuria), dysuria, frequency, temporary insertion of urethral catheter with irrigation, no semen production (retrograde ejaculation ~20% if transurethral incision of bladder neck, 75–80% if TURP), non-resolution of symptoms
- *Occasional*: urinary tract infections requiring oral or intravenous antibiotics, trauma to urethra, prostate or bladder resulting in haematuria, diagnosis of bladder mucosal lesion/stone requiring bleeding requiring return to theatre/further cystoscopy and washout/blood transfusion, impotence (20%), incontinence of urine (temporary/permanent), need for repeat procedure (10%), failure to void necessitating further catheterization
- *Rare*: urethral stricture formation, perforation of urethra/bladder necessitating temporary catheter insertion or open procedure to repair defect in bladder, transurethral resection syndrome (absorption of irrigation fluid causing confusion, congestive cardiac failure, dilutional hyponatraemia), finding of unsuspected cancer in removed prostate tissue necessitating further treatment[2-4]
- *Open prostatectomy*: need for temporary urethral catheterization, need for temporary wound drain, retrograde ejaculation and associated sub-fertility, frequency, urgency of urination, bleeding requiring further surgery or transfusion of blood, impotence (10%), wound infection requiring antibiotics, incisional hernia, incontinence of urine (temporary/permanent), need for intensive care admission (cardiovascular/respiratory/neurological compromise/death)[5]

Blood transfusion necessary

- Group and save/cross-match (depending on preoperative haemoglobin)

Type of anaesthesia/sedation

- Regional anaesthesia/general anaesthesia

Follow-up/need for further procedure

- Dependent on indication for prostate surgery
- Review in outpatient clinic with outcome of histopathology with repeat flow rate and residual volume assessment
- Discussion at local/regional multidisciplinary team meeting with histopathology if necessary

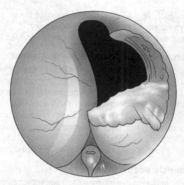

Fig. 11.10 Transurethral resection of prostate gland: beginning of lateral lobe resection.

Reproduced with permission from Blandy, Notley and Reynard, *Transurethral resection*, 5th edition. 2005, Taylor & Francis, London.

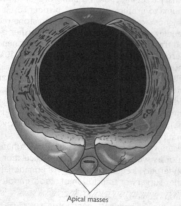

Apical masses

Fig. 11.11 Transurethral resection of prostate gland: completed prostate resection cavity.

Reproduced with permission from Blandy, Notley and Reynard, *Transurethral resection*, 5th edition. 2005, Taylor & Francis, London.

References

1. Smith RD, Patel A. Transurethral resection of the prostate revisited and updated. *Curr Opin Urol* 2011;**21**(1):36–41.

2. British Association of Urological Surgery. *Procedure Specific Consent Forms for Urological Surgery—Simple (Millen's) Retropubic Prostatectomy*. Available at: ℘ www.baus.org.uk (accessed 17 May 2011).

3. British Association of Urological Surgery. *Procedure Specific Consent Forms for Urological Surgery—Transurethral Incision or Resection of the Prostate (Cancer)*. Available at: ℘ www.baus.org.uk (accessed 17 May 2011).

4. British Association of Urological Surgery. *Procedure Specific Consent Forms for Urological Surgery—Transurethral Incision or Resection of the Prostate*. Available at: ℘ www.baus.org.uk (accessed 17 May 2011).

5. Rassweiler J, Teber D, Kuntz R, et al. Complications of transurethral resection of the prostate (TURP)—incidence, management, and prevention. *Eur Urol* 2006;**50**(5):969–79; discussion 980.

Ureterorenoscopy (diagnostic/therapeutic)

Description

Ureterorenoscopy can be performed in an antegrade or retrograde fashion. Classically retrograde ureterorenography is performed with a rigid ureteroscope or flexible ureteroscope. A rigid ureteroscope is a straight instrument is able to negotiate the length of the ureter. They vary in size and number of working channels. They are ideal to exclude ureteric pathology and to treat intraluminal pathology. A flexible ureteroscope has the advantage of a flexible tip which allows for controlled deflection of the end of the scope. It is ideal to diagnose or treat renal pelvis or calyceal lesions or calculi.

The patient is supine with the legs elevated (lithotomy position). Cystoscopic cannulation of the ureter is performed with a guide-wire (or sometimes two) placed into the kidney. This safety guide-wire acts as a route for the rigid or flexible ureteroscope. Fluoroscopy is used as an adjunct to 'screen' the ureteroscope and check its position (Fig. 11.12). Once the procedure is complete, a ureteric stent may be placed postoperatively.

Additional procedures that may become necessary

- Endoscopic lithotripsy
- Retrograde endopyelotomy (laser)
- Endoscopic incision of ureteric strictures
- Dilatation of ureteric strictures
- Placement of ureteric stent (Memokath®)
- Treatment of calyceal diverticular lesions
- Treatment of malignant urothelial tumours
- Treatment of benign tumours or bleeding lesions

Benefits

- *Diagnostic:*
  - Investigation of abnormal radiological findings, i.e. filling defects
  - Determine the aetiology of ureteric obstruction
  - Identifying cause of positive urinary cytology results, culture results, or other test results (if normal cystoscopic findings)
  - Evaluation of ureteric injury
- *Therapeutic:*
  - Endoscopic lithotripsy
  - Retrograde endopyelotomy (laser)
  - Endoscopic incision of ureteric strictures
  - Dilatation of ureteric strictures
  - Placement of ureteric stent (Memokath®)
  - Treatment of calyceal diverticular lesions
  - Treatment of malignant urothelial tumours
  - Treatment of benign tumours or bleeding lesions

Alternative procedures/conservative measures

- *Conservative*: in a non-functioning/poorly functioning kidney in the presence of obstruction, if the patient is asymptomatic then observation may be all that is necessary with renal function measurement and serial radiological imaging, spontaneous stone passage
- *Medical*: medical expulsive therapy for stone passage
- *Radiology*: alternatives to retrograde pyelography include CT urogram, IVU, MAG3 renogram, CT KUB, ultrasound KUB
- *Surgical*: nephrostomy and antegrade ureterorenoscopy (all dependent on underlying pathology in question, ESWL/PCNL

Serious/frequently occurring risks

- *Common*: bleeding (haematuria), dysuria, temporary insertion of urethral catheter, insertion of ureteric stent with need to remove/exchange this, no guarantee of cure
- *Occasional*: urinary tract infections requiring oral or intravenous antibiotics, trauma to urethra, prostate, bladder or ureter resulting in haematuria, recurrence of stricture in ureter, need to biopsy lesion in bladder or ureter, need for further therapy, failure to pass the ureteroscope due to narrow ureter necessitating further procedure, stone recurrence, incomplete stone clearance
- *Rare*: haematuria and clot retention necessitating further cystoscopy and washout, false passage creation or perforation of urethra/bladder/ureter necessitating prolonged period of catheter insertion/stent/conversion to open procedure to repair defect (ileal loop interposition), need for nephrostomy[1–4]

Blood transfusion necessary

- None

Type of anaesthesia/sedation

- Regional/general anaesthesia

Follow-up/need for further procedure

- Follow-up is dependent on underlying pathology
- Radiological follow-up scans
- Removal of stent as outpatient
- Failed procedure may necessitate nephrostomy or antegrade stent insertion

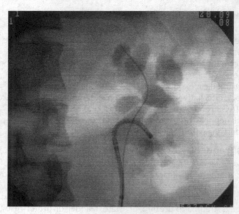

Fig. 11.12 Fluoroscopic view of flexible ureterorenoscopic fragmentation of intrarenal calculi.

Reproduced with permission from Reynard J, Brewster S, and Biers S. *Oxford Handbook of Urology* 2nd edition. 2009. Oxford: Oxford University Press, p.425, Figure 9.6.

References

1. British Association of Urological Surgery. *Procedure Specific Consent Forms for Urological Surgery—Ureteroscopy +/– Biopsy.* Available at: ℜ www.baus.org.uk (accessed 17 May 2011).
2. British Association of Urological Surgery. *Procedure Specific Consent Forms for Urological Surgery—Ureteroscopic Stone Removal.* Available at: ℜ www.baus.org.uk (accessed 17 May 2011).
3. Fuganti PE, Pires S, Branco R, et al. Predictive factors for intraoperative complications in semirigid ureteroscopy: analysis of 1235 ballistic ureterolithotripsies. *Urology* 2008;**72**(4):770–4.
4. Geavlete P, Georgescu D, Niță G, et al. Complications of 2735 retrograde semirigid ureteroscopy procedures: a single-center experience. *J Endourol* 2006;**20**(3):179–85.

Urethral dilation (cystoscopy—male/female)

Description
Stricturing disease of the urethra is a pathological process that involves fibrotic scar tissue formation within the tissues surrounding the urethra resulting in a narrowing of the lumen. Patients can present with decreased flow, incomplete bladder emptying, dysuria, haematuria, recurrent urinary tract infections and obstructive uropathy. Diagnosis is made with history, clinical examination (external urethra meatus), flow-rate studies, retrograde/antegrade urethrography, or urethroscopy.

Disease processes that cause urethral stricture formation include:
- Infection (gonococcal urethritis)
- Inflammation (BXO resulting in meatal or submeatal stenosis)
- Trauma (pelvic fractures, urethral instrumentation including post-TURP, cystoscopy, catheterization, post-radical prostatectomy)

Urethral dilation is a process whereby sounds of increasing diameter are passed along the urethra with lubrication in an attempt to open a stricture or narrowing of the urethra. It is designed to stretch the urethra with minimal scarring.[1]

Additional procedures that may become necessary
- Urethral catheterization
- Suprapubic catheterization
- Optical urethrotomy
- Bladder biopsies
- Future therapy (ISC/referral for urethroplasty)
- Meatotomy/meatal dilatation (for distal meatal strictures where the urethra cannot be cannulated with the optical urethrotome)

Benefits
- *Diagnostic*: diagnose underlying stricture, length of stricture, and proximity to external urethral sphincter
- *Therapeutic*: to improve symptoms associated with urethral stricture and prevent complications from bladder outflow obstruction

Alternative procedures/conservative measures
- *Conservative*: manage patient conservatively with regular urine flow-rate examination, residual volume measurements and monitor serum creatinine and evidence of upper tract dilatation on ultrasonography in the patient who wishes no further treatment and is asymptomatic. In patients who are able to perform ISC, this is an option to prevent further re-stricturing. It requires good hand–eye coordination and dexterity and may be difficult in the older patient
- *Medical*: patients with BXO with meatal stenosis may require topical steroid treatment to limit the progression of disease
- *Surgical*:
  - Optical urethrotomy
  - Suprapubic catheter insertion (to avoid trauma to stricture or urethra, and to provide a conduit for antegrade and retrograde urethrography to plan future treatment

- In males, excision and primary reanastomosis of urethra
- Tissue transfer procedure (urethroplasty with buccal or pedicled skin flap). The latter two techniques should be performed following adequate imaging of urethra, in younger patients or in patients with recurrent stricture formation who do not wish to have repeat dilatation/urethrotomy procedures. These are often carried out in specialist centres that deliver a urethral reconstruction service

Serious/frequently occurring risks

- *Common*: bleeding (haematuria), dysuria, temporary insertion of urethral catheter
- *Occasional*: urinary tract infections requiring oral or intravenous antibiotics, trauma to urethra, prostate or bladder resulting in haematuria, recurrence of stricture (this is particularly so if bleeding is associated with urethral dilation as it implies that there has been further trauma to the urethra), need to biopsy lesion in bladder, need for further therapy (including ISC, optical urethrotomy, referral for specialist stricture treatment—urethroplasty/excision and anastomosis, need to insert suprapubic catheter
- *Rare*: haematuria and clot retention necessitating further cystoscopy and washout, failure of procedure due to complete urethral occlusion, false passage creation or perforation of urethra/bladder necessitating prolonged period of catheter insertion or conversion to open procedure to repair defect in bladder, erectile dysfunction, decreased continence (if stricture involves or lies adjacent to external urethral sphincter)[2–4]

Blood transfusion necessary

- None

Type of anaesthesia/sedation

- Local/regional or general anaesthesia

Follow-up/need for further procedure

- Dependent on findings of stricture
- If catheter inserted, trial without catheter can be scheduled between 24h and 5 days post-procedure
- Review in outpatient clinic with flow rate assessment, RV, and symptomatic review
- Referral to learn ISC
- Referral for definitive surgical procedure for stricture

References

1. Wong SS, Narahari R, O'Riordan A, et al. Simple urethral dilatation, endoscopic urethrotomy, and urethroplasty for urethral stricture disease in adult men. *Cochrane Database Syst Rev* 2010;4:CD006934.
2. British Association of Urological Surgery. *Procedure Specific Consent Forms for Urological Surgery—(Rigid) Cystoscopy and Urethral Dilation in Women + Biopsy if Required*. Available at: ℜ www.baus.org.uk (accessed 17 May 2011).
3. British Association of Urological Surgery. *Procedure Specific Consent Forms for Urological Surgery—(Rigid) Cystoscopy and Urethral Dilation in Men + Biopsy if Required*. Available at: ℜ www.baus.org.uk (accessed 17 May 2011).
4. British Association of Urological Surgery. *Procedure Specific Consent Forms for Urological Surgery—Cystoscopy and Optical Internal Urethrotomy*. Available at: ℜ www.baus.org.uk (accessed 17 May 2011).

Vasectomy

Description

Vasectomy is the surgical procedure by which a section of the vas deferens is removed from each side to achieve permanent sterility. Although it is deemed that every man of legal age and able to give consent can decide in favour of vas ligation for the purpose of sterilization, there are certain preconditions that many surgeons or physicians look for. This is primarily to provide weight towards their decision prior to offering the operation. These include:

- A certain number of children are required in the family of the patient
- A stable relationship is required
- Ideally the partner should accompany the man during the consultation or ideally back the decision for vasectomy

The procedure can be carried out under local or general anaesthesia depending on patient preference. The vas is palpated and the cord is infiltrated with local anaesthetic. Once the vas deferens is isolated through the skin, it is clamped and the scrotal skin incised over a distance of 0.5–1.0cm. The vas is then separated from its overlying sheath and divided between two clips. A segment might be sent for histopathology to confirm it is truly vas deference that has been ligated. Both ends can be ligated or coagulated by diathermy to occlude the lumen. The wound is closed with a single absorbable suture.[1]

Fo low-up of patients must be accurate and patients must be told to continue using barrier contraception or for partner to use oral contraception until two negative semen samples are achieved on two different tests spaced 2 weeks apart (usually 12 and 14 weeks, as per local policy).

Additional procedures that may become necessary

- Nil

Benefits

- *Diagnostic*: histopathological confirmation of benign vas deferens tissue is important in documenting accurate ligation of the structure
- *Therapeutic*: as a permanent method of contraception

Alternative procedures/conservative measures

- Other forms of contraception (male or female) including barrier contraceptive, oral contraceptive agents and implantable contraceptive agents
- *Surgical*: female laparoscopic tubal ligation

Serious/frequently occurring risks

- *Common*: irreversible procedure, scrotal bruising and pain, two semen samples required demonstrating the absence of live sperm before unprotected intercourse
- *Occasional*: bleeding (scrotal haematoma resulting in either slow re-absorption or further procedure to evacuate clot)

- *Rare*: infection, (wound/epididymo-orchitis necessitating antibiotic therapy), spontaneous rejoining of the two ends of the vas deferens resulting in fertility and pregnancy (1:2000), chronic scrotal or testicular pain (up to 5% cases), sperm granuloma formation, persistence of non-motile sperm[2,3]

Blood transfusion necessary

- None

Type of anaesthesia/sedation

- Local/regional/general anaesthesia

Follow-up/need for further procedure

- Scrotal support for up to one week
- Warm sit down bath after 48h to soak and remove dressing
- Follow-up with semen analysis at 12 and 14 weeks (to ensure azoospermia) as per local policy. Patient to continue using other forms of contraceptive until this is achieved

References

1. Cook LA, Pun A, van Vliet H, et al. Scalpel versus no-scalpel incision for vasectomy. *Cochrane Database Syst Rev* 2007;**2**:CD004112.
2. Adams CE, Wald M. Risks and complications of vasectomy. *Urol Clin North Am* 2009;**36**(3):331–6.
3. British Association of Urological Surgery. *Procedure Specific Consent Forms for Urological Surgery—Vasectomy*. Available at: ℘ www.baus.org.uk (accessed 17 May 2011).

Orthopaedic surgery

Achilles tendon repair

Description

Most Achilles tendon problems arise due to overuse injuries and are multifactorial. However, in a trauma setting a true rupture is the most common presentation.

There is still debate regarding open repair and the associated risk of wound complications (reported as up to 4%) and conservative splinting and the risk of re-rupture reported as 3.5% in operative patients versus 12% in non-operative patients.[1,2]

Open repair is typically performed under general anaesthesia, with the patient prone. If the tendon ends can be approximated a primary repair is achieved and the skin closed with either absorbable subcuticular or non-absorbable sutures. Postoperative rehabilitation programmes vary with some groups preferring cast or brace immobilization for 6–8 weeks; however, the period of immobilization necessary has not been clearly defined.

Additional procedures that may become necessary
- Tendon grafting

Benefits
- *Therapeutic*: mechanical improvement

Alternative procedures/conservative measures
- *Conservative*: cast immobilization, functional bracing
- *Surgical*: percutaneous repair

Serious/frequently occurring risks
- *Common*: re-rupture, wound break down, pain, bleeding, stiffness
- *Occasional*: DVT, nerve injury
- *Rare*: tendon lengthening

Blood transfusion necessary
- None/group and save

Type of anaesthesia/sedation
- Generally under general anaesthesia
- Spinal/regional anaesthesia if unfit for general anaesthesia

Follow-up/need for further procedure
- Follow up at two weeks for wound review and change of cast

References
1. Khan RJ, Fick D, Keogh A, *et al*. Treatment of acute achilles tendon ruptures. A meta-analysis of randomized, controlled trials. *J Bone Joint Surg Am* 2005;**87**(10):2202–10.
2. American Academy of Orthopaedic Surgeons. *The Diagnosis and Treatment of Acute Achilles Tendon Rupture. Guideline and Evidence Report*. Rosemont, IL: American Academy of Orthopaedic Surgeons, 2009.

Ankle fractures

Description

Ankle fractures are a common injury among the young and elderly, often resulting from a combination of rotation and abduction or adduction forces. Stable fractures, i.e. those with isolated lateral malleolus fractures that are in a good position with an intact syndesmosis, may be managed conservatively. If there is failure to achieve or maintain reduction, or there is an unstable fracture pattern, operative intervention is indicated.

Open reduction and internal fixation should be planned once the soft tissues allow, i.e. swelling will allow soft tissue closure postoperatively and fracture blisters are intact or not near the planned incision. Fixation is often carried out with a locking compression plate or one-third tubular plate ± lag screw insertion. The medial malleolus can often be fixed with cannulated screws or partially threaded cancellous screws. The syndesmosis is checked and one or two screws inserted as needed if unstable. The case is usually performed under general anaesthesia with tourniquet control. Closure is with absorbable subcuticular sutures.

Additional procedures that may become necessary

- Syndesmosis screw insertion

Benefits

- *Therapeutic*: mechanical improvement

Alternative procedures/conservative measures

- Conservative: casting
- Surgical: external fixation

Serious/frequently occurring risks[1,2]

- *Common*: infection (1.5%)
- *Occasional*: malunion, non-union (1% at 5 years)
- *Rare*: failure of metal work, pulmonary embolism (0.5%)

Blood transfusion necessary

- Group and save

Type of anaesthesia/sedation

- Generally under general anaesthesia
- Spinal/regional anaesthesia if unfit for general anaesthesia

Follow-up/need for further procedure

- Follow up at two weeks for wound review and change of cast
- Removal of syndesmosis screw typically at 9 weeks

References

1. ScoHoo NF, Krenek L, Eagan MJ, et al. Complication rates following open reduction and internal fixation of ankle fractures. *J Bone Joint Surg Am* 2009;**91**:1042–9.
2. Marx RC, Mizel MS. What's new in foot and ankle surgery. *J Bone Joint Surg Am* 2010;**92**(2): 512–23.

Anterior cruciate ligament repair

Description

The anterior cruciate ligament (ACL) is integral in stabilizing the knee. The ACL-deficient knee has been linked to an increased rate of degenerative osteoarthritic changes and meniscal injuries. These injuries are most often a result of contact injuries with a rotational component and low-velocity, non-contact, deceleration forces.

Primary suture repair of the ACL used to be performed but due to failure rates of up to 100% it has now been abandoned for reconstructive techniques.

ACL reconstruction can be performed with the use of either autograft (bone-patellar tendon-bone or hamstring tendon autograft) or allograft tissue.[1] It is currently unclear if the outcomes of these two methods differ significantly. These techniques are usually performed using an arthroscopic approach under general anaesthesia.

Additional procedures that may become necessary

- Open reconstruction, meniscal tear repair/resection

Benefits

- *Therapeutic*: mechanical improvement

Alternative procedures/conservative measures

- *Conservative*: functional bracing
- *Surgical*: open repair

Serious/frequently occurring risks[1–3]

- *Common*: re-rupture (8%), anterior knee pain (6%)
- *Occasional*: anterior knee numbness (1.5%)
- *Rare*: DVT

Blood transfusion necessary

- Group and save

Type of anaesthesia/sedation

- Generally under general anaesthesia
- Spinal/regional anaesthesia if unfit for general anaesthesia

Follow-up/need for further procedure

- Removal of sutures by general practitioner or practice nurse
- Structured physiotherapy protocol, working especially on quadriceps and hamstring strengthening and stabilization
- Routine follow-up in orthopaedic outpatients at 6 weeks to assess progress

References

1. Carey JL, Dunn WR, Dahm DL, et al. A systematic review of anterior cruciate ligament reconstruction with autograft compared with allograft. *J Bone Joint Surg Am* 2009;**91**(9):2242–50.
2. Poolman RW, Abouali JA, Conter HJ, et al. Overlapping systematic reviews of anterior cruciate ligament reconstruction comparing hamstring autograft with bone-patellar tendon-bone autograft: why are they different? *J Bone Joint Surg Am* 2007;**89**(7):1542–52.
3. Geib TM, Shelton WR, Phelps RA, et al. Anterior cruciate ligament reconstruction using quadriceps tendon autograft: intermediate-term outcome. *Arthroscopy* 2009;**25**(12):1408–14.

Carpal tunnel decompression

Description

Carpal tunnel syndrome results from compression of the median nerve as it enters the palmar surface of the hand under the flexor retinaculum. It typically presents with pain, paraesthesia, and hypoaesthesia over the radial three and a half fingers, often at night. Electrophysiological tests (nerve conduction studies) are often performed to support the clinical diagnosis.

Surgery usually involves local or regional anaesthesia as a day case. An incision is made over the flexor retinaculum with or without tourniquet control, with complete division of the retinaculum to ensure release. Closure is typically with interrupted non-absorbable sutures, and dressing with a bulky bandage and early mobilization.

Additional procedures that may become necessary

- Internal neurolysis
- Epineurotomy
- Tenosynovectomy

Benefits

- *Therapeutic*: pain relief, restoration of median nerve function

Alternative procedures/conservative measures[1,2]

- *Conservative*: avoidance of precipitating activities, splinting
- *Medical*: analgesia and corticosteroid injection may be beneficial
- *Surgical*: endoscopic carpal tunnel release

Serious/frequently occurring risks[1]

- *Common*: recurrence of pain, scar, pilar pain (pain in the heel of the scar on pressure)
- *Occasional*: damage to median nerve and its branches, infection

Blood transfusion necessary

- None/group and save

Type of anaesthesia/sedation

- Generally under local/regional anaesthesia
- General anaesthesia for secondary revision or other complex cases

Follow-up/need for further procedure

- Removal of sutures by general practitioner or practice nurse
- Routine follow-up in orthopaedic outpatients at 3 months to assess progress

References

1. Scholten RJ, Mink van der Molen A, Uitdehaag BM, *et al*. Surgical treatment options for carpal tunnel syndrome. *Cochrane Database Syst Rev* 2007;**4**:CD003905.
2. American Academy of Orthopaedic Surgeons. *Clinical Practice Guidelines on the Treatment of Carpal Tunnel*. Rosemont, IL: American Academy of Orthopaedic Surgeons, 2008.

Clavicle fractures

Description

Clavicle fractures are common fractures accounting for up to 12% of all fractures. They can be divided into lateral, middle, and medial third fractures, with approximately 80% being middle third fractures. Of middle third clavicle fractures, there is approximately 15% prevalence of non-union of fractures treated without surgery and a 2% rate of non-union of fractures treated with plate fixation.[1]

Indications for operative treatment of acute midshaft clavicular fractures include open fractures, fractures with compromised skin due to severe fracture displacement ('tented skin'), and fractures associated with vascular or neurological injury. Other acute fracture indications that are proposed are initial clavicular shortening of 2cm, and comminuted fractures with a displaced transverse fragment.

Lateral third fractures that do go on to form a painful/symptomatic non-union may require fixation with either a synthetic sling or a hook plate. The latter can limit shoulder abduction and will usually need to be removed at around 8 weeks.

The procedure is carried out under general anaesthesia, with plate or intramedullary fixation, with subcuticular absorbable sutures to close. A period of support from a sling postoperatively is usual with rehabilitation as per local protocol.

Additional procedures that may become necessary

- Removal of metal work at a later date

Benefits

- *Therapeutic*: mechanical improvement

Alternative procedures/conservative measures

- *Conservative*: broad arm sling[1]
- *Surgical*: intramedullary fixation

Serious/frequently occurring risks[2,3]

- *Common*: malunion, non-union (2.2%)
- *Occasional*: hardware prominence requiring removal, plate failure, infection
- *Rare*: supraclavicular neuroma, subclavian vein injury

Blood transfusion necessary

- Group and save

Type of anaesthesia/sedation

- General anaesthesia

Follow-up/need for further procedure

- Removal of sutures/wound review by general practitioner or practice nurse
- Routine follow-up in fracture clinic at 4 weeks to assess progress

References

1. Canadian Orthopaedic Trauma Society. Nonoperative treatment compared with plate fixation of displaced midshaft clavicular fractures. A multicenter, randomized clinical trial. *J Bone Joint Surg Am* 2007;**89**:1–10.
2. Bahk MS, Kuhn JE, Galatz LM, *et al.* Acromioclavicular and sternoclavicular injuries and clavicular glenoid, and scapular fractures. *J Bone Joint Surg Am* 2009;**91**:2492–510.
3. Zlowodzki M, Zelle BA, Cole PA, *et al.* Treatment of acute midshaft clavicle fractures: systematic review of 2144 fractures: on behalf of the Evidence-Based Orthopaedic Trauma Working Group. *J Orthop Trauma* 2005;**19**:504–7.

Distal radius fractures

Description

Distal radius fractures are a common injury, particularly in the elderly. Several options exist for treatment. Non-operative management consists of closed treatment with casting. Operative treatment options include Kirschner (K) wire insertion, external fixation, arthroscopic-assisted external fixation, and various methods of open reduction and internal fixation. Indications that have been suggested for operative intervention are radial shortening, >2mm articular step, volar tilt of >10°, and dorsal tilt >10°.

The operation is usually carried out under general anaesthesia with tourniquet control. The method of fixation is defined by the fracture pattern, and currently despite multiple prospective meta-analyses including a Cochrane review, no specific type of fixation has been proven to be advantageous.[1,2] The volar approach is favoured over a dorsal incision due to the soft tissue interposition between the plate and the tendons, minimizing adhesions. Skin closure is usually with absorbable subcuticular sutures.

Additional procedures that may become necessary

- Bone grafting
- Nerve decompression

Benefits

- *Therapeutic*: mechanical improvement

Alternative procedures/conservative measures

- Conservative: casting
- Surgical: K-wiring, external fixation (bridging and non-bridging)

Serious/frequently occurring risks[1-3]

- *Common*: malunion, non-union
- *Occasional*: damage to tendons, infection (1–2%)
- *Rare*: failure of metal work

Blood transfusion necessary

- None/group and save

Type of anaesthesia/sedation

- Generally under general anaesthesia
- Spinal/regional anaesthesia if unfit for general anaesthesia

Follow-up/need for further procedure

- Follow up at two weeks for wound review and change of cast
- Removal of K-wires in fracture clinic, typically at 6 weeks
- Routine follow-up in fracture clinic at 3 months to assess progress

References

1. Liporace FA, Adams MR, Capo JT, *et al.* Distal radius fractures. *J Orthop Trauma* 2009;**23**(10):739–48.
2. American Academy of Orthopaedic Surgeons. *The Treatment of Distal Radius Fractures: Guideline and Evidence Report.* Rosemont, IL: American Academy of Orthopaedic Surgeons, 2009.
3. MacKenney PJ, McQueen MM, Elton R. Prediction of instability in distal radial fractures. *J Bone Joint Surg Am* 2006;**88**:1944–51.

Extracapsular neck of femur fractures

Description

Neck-of-femur fractures are relatively common. Approximately 50% are extracapsular. Fixation was traditionally with dynamic hip screw, with good long-term results. More recently the cephalomedullary devices have gained popularity, particularly with intertrochanteric and reverse oblique fractures; however, there is currently no consensus on which fixation method is better with a recent prospective blinded study showing no significant benefit of one treatment modality over the other.[1,2]

The procedure is usually carried out on a traction table under general anaesthesia or spinal/epidural. The prosthesis is inserted and skin closure is with clips or subcuticular sutures.

The emphasis postoperatively is mobilization to help prevent further complications such as pressure sore and infections, which will severely increase morbidity. At this time bone-protecting agents, if not contraindicated, should be commenced.

Benefits

- *Therapeutic*: mechanical improvement

Alternative procedures/conservative measures

- *Surgical*: intramedullary fixation

Serious/frequently occurring risks

- *Common*: need for revision (approx 4–6%), DVT (4%)
- *Occasional*: periprosthetic fracture approx 2–4%)
- *Rare*: infection (superficial 2%, deep 1%)

Blood transfusion necessary

- Group and save

Type of anaesthesia/sedation

- Generally under general anaesthesia
- Spinal/regional anaesthesia if unfit for general anaesthesia

Follow-up/need for further procedure

- Removal of sutures by general practitioner or practice nurse
- Routine follow-up in fracture clinic at 6–8 weeks to assess progress

References

1. Adams CI, Robinson CM, Court-Brown CM, et al. Prospective randomized controlled trial of an intramedullary nail versus dynamic screw and plate for intertrochanteric fractures of the femur. *J Orthop Trauma* 2001;**15**:394–400.
2. Nikolaou VS, Papathanasopoulos A, Giannoudi PV. What's new in the management of proximal femoral fractures? *Injury* 2008;**39**(12): 309–18.

Ganglion excision

Description

Ganglions are commonly found on the dorsum of the hand over the scapholunate ligament (approx 70% of all ganglions) and are a mucinous filled cyst typically adjacent to joint capsule or the tendon sheath. They may present just as a soft swelling or can cause mild aching.

Options for treatment include aspiration and injection of hyaluronidase; however, the recurrence rate is approximately 50%.[1,2] Surgery for a dorsal ganglion usually involves local or regional anaesthesia as a day case. An incision is made directly over the ganglion, with the cyst being mobilized down to the joint capsule, with its capsular extensions then being excised. Closure is typically with interrupted non-absorbable sutures, and dressing with a bulky bandage and early mobilization.

Additional procedures that may become necessary
- Nil

Benefits
- *Therapeutic*: pain relief

Alternative procedures/conservative measures
- *Conservative*: observation
- *Medical*: needle aspiration followed by 3 weeks immobilization
- *Surgical*: arthroscopic excision

Serious/frequently occurring risks[1,2]
- *Common*: recurrence (up to 50%)
- *Rare*: damage to digital nerves (<1%), Infection (<1%)

Blood transfusion necessary
- None/group and save

Type of anaesthesia/sedation
- Generally under local/regional anaesthesia
- General anaesthesia for secondary revision or other complex cases

Follow-up/need for further procedure
- Removal of sutures by general practitioner or practice nurse
- Routine follow-up in orthopaedic outpatients at 3 months to assess progress

References
1. Kang L, Akelman E, Weiss AP. Arthroscopic versus open dorsal ganglion excision: a prospective, randomized comparison of rates of recurrence and of residual pain. *J Hand Surg Am* 2008;**33**(4):471–5.
2. Thornburg LE. Ganglions of the hand and wrist. *J Am Acad Orthop Surg* 1999;**7**(4):231–8.

Hallux valgus correction

Description

Hallux valgus occurs with lateral deviation of the great toe and medial deviation of the first metatarsal. Commonly the deformity is characterized by progressive subluxation of the first metatarsophalangeal joint. Patients typically present with pain centred over the medial eminence caused by irritation of the dorsal cutaneous nerve of the great toe or an inflamed or thickened bursa overlying the area.

There are multiple operations available for the correction of hallux valgus, the details of which are outside the scope of this book;[1-3] however, the majority require an osteotomy. Closure is typically with interrupted non-absorbable sutures, dressing with a bulky bandage and walking is encouraged with a heel-bearing shoe. At approximately 6 weeks, metatarsophalangeal and interphalangeal joint movement is initiated.

Additional procedures that may become necessary
- K-wire insertion

Benefits
- *Therapeutic*: pain relief

Alternative procedures/conservative measures
- *Conservative*: use of a wider toe box, padding of the affected area
- *Medical*: analgesia if required
- *Surgical*: osteotomy of the cuneiform, arthrodesis of the metatarsophalangeal joint, excisional arthroplasty

Serious/frequently occurring risks[2,3]
- *Common*: recurrence (10%)
- *Occasional*: avascular necrosis of the metatarsal head, non-union
- *Rare*: damage to digital nerves (<1%), infection (<1%)

Blood transfusion necessary
- None

Type of anaesthesia/sedation
- General/regional anaesthesia

Follow-up/need for further procedure
- Follow up at two weeks for wound review and change of cast
- Removal of K-wires at 6 weeks

References
1. The American Academy of Orthopaedic Surgeons. Instructional course lectures—hallux valgus. *J Bone Joint Surg Am* 1995;**78**;932–66.
2. Easley ME, Trnka HJ. Current concepts review: hallux valgus part II: operative treatment. *Foot Ankle Int* 2007;**28**(6):748–58.
3. Robinson AH, Limbers JP. Modern concepts in the treatment of hallux valgus. *J Bone Joint Surg Br* 2005;**87**(8):1038–45.

Hip arthroscopy

Description

Hip arthroscopy allows thorough visualization of the acetabular labrum, femoral head, and acetabular chondral surfaces, as well as of the fovea, ligamentum teres, and adjacent synovium. This procedure was initially only performed at specialist centres; however, like most advances in surgery, it is becoming more widespread although it remains technically complex.

Access to the hip joint is difficult because of the resistance to distraction resulting from the large muscular envelope, the strength of the iliofemoral ligament, and the negative intra-articular pressure. The procedure involves general anaesthesia, with the use of a traction table to distract the hip. A guide-wire and sequential dilation under image intensifier control allow suitable port placement. A number of therapeutic procedures can be carried out including removal of loose bodies, debridement of acetabular and femoral head chondral flap lesions, and repair of labral tears. At the end of the procedure, the arthroscopic fluid is drained out of the joint and the incisions are closed with sutures, skin glue or Steri-strips.

Postoperatively, patients can mobilize fully weightbearing as their pain allows, initially with crutches and without them after a few days.

Additional procedures that may become necessary

- Labral debridement
- Synovial biopsy
- Removal of loose bodies
- Correction of femoro-acetabular impingement

Benefits

- *Diagnostic*: biopsy if suspicion of chronically infected or inflamed joint
- *Therapeutic*: pain relief, mechanical improvement

Alternative procedures/conservative measures

- *Conservative*: include physiotherapy/prescribed exercise and other lifestyle changes
- *Medical*: analgesia and anti-inflammatories are the mainstay of first-line treatment. Corticosteroids or hyaluronic acid may be injected into the knee joint
- *Surgical*: total hip replacement (THR), hip resurfacing

Serious/frequently occurring risks[1-3]

- *Common*: recurrence of pain, scar, damage to nerves
- *Occasional*: guide-wire failure, haemarthrosis, infection
- *Rare*: DVT

Blood transfusion necessary

- None/group and save

Type of anaesthesia/sedation

- Generally under general anaesthesia
- Very occasionally under spinal/epidural/local anaesthesia in those unfit for general anaesthesia

Follow-up/need for further procedure
- Removal of sutures by general practitioner or practice nurse
- Routine follow-up in orthopaedic outpatients at 6 weeks to assess progress

References

1. McCarthy JC, Lee J. Hip arthroscopy: indications, outcomes, and complications. *J Bone Joint Surg Am* 2005;**87**:1137–45.
2. Clarke MT, Arora A, Villar RN. Hip arthroscopy: complications in 1054 cases. *Clin Orthop* 2003;**406**:84–8.
3. Griffin DR, Villar RN. Complications of arthroscopy of the hip. *J Bone Joint Surg Br* 1999;**81**:604–6.

Hip resurfacing

Description

Hip resurfacing arthroplasty involves removal of the diseased or damaged surfaces of the head of the femur and the acetabulum. The hip is then fitted with a non-cemented monoblock acetabular component combined with a metal-on-metal bearing made from cobalt-chromium alloy to form a pair of metal bearings. This is generally performed under general anaesthesia, with closure of the skin by subcuticular sutures or surgical clips.

The procedure was popularized by the reported ease of revision to total hip arthroplasty, the reduced risk of dislocation due to larger bearing size (0.05% in the first year), and decreased risk of loosening due to the use of metal-on-metal bearing surfaces, avoiding the wear debris associated with polyethylene. However, this is now being challenged with revision rates of 14% being reported. [1,2]

Another concern with these devices is the possibility of metal degradation products being absorbed into the body and their local and systemic effects. The implications of this are presently unknown.

Additional procedures that may become necessary
- Conversion to total hip arthroplasty

Benefits
- *Therapeutic*: pain relief, mechanical improvement

Alternative procedures/conservative measures
- *Conservative*: physiotherapy/prescribed exercise and other lifestyle changes
- *Medical*: analgesia and anti-inflammatories are the mainstay of first-line treatment. Corticosteroids or hyaluronic acid may be injected into the hip joint
- *Surgical*: hip arthroscopy (although not currently indicated for moderate to severe osteoarthritis, may be beneficial in other aetiologies), THR

Serious/frequently occurring risks[3,4]
- *Common*: pain, scar, revision of prosthesis (loosening, periprosthetic fracture), exposure to metal ions, pseudo-tumour formation
- *Occasional*: bleeding, infection, dislocation (0.05% in the first year)
- *Rare*: DVT, pulmonary embolism

Blood transfusion necessary
- Group and save

Type of anaesthesia/sedation
- Generally under general anaesthesia
- Very occasionally under spinal/epidural with sedation in those unfit for general anaesthesia

Follow-up/need for further procedure

- Removal of surgical clips by general practitioner or practice nurse
- Routine follow-up in orthopaedic outpatients at 6 weeks to assess progress

References

1. American Academy of Orthopaedic Surgeons. *Modern Metal-on Metal Hip Resurfacing: A Technology Overview*. Rosemont, IL: American Academy of Orthopaedic Surgeons, 2009.
2. National Institute for Clinical Excellence. *Guidance on the Use of Metal on Metal Hip Resurfacing Arthroplasty*. London: NICE, 2002.
3. Hing CB, Back DL, Bailey M, et al. The results of primary Birmingham hip resurfacings at a mean of five years. An independent prospective review of the first 230 hips. *J Bone Joint Surg Br* 2007;**89**(11):1431–8.
4. Amstutz HC, Le Duff MJ. Eleven years of experience with metal-on-metal hybrid hip resurfacing: a review of 1000 conserve plus. *J Arthroplasty* 2008;**23**(6 Suppl 1):36–43.

Humeral supracondylar fracture (paediatric)

Description

Supracondylar fractures of the humerus are a common paediatric injury. Classically Gartland II and III type fractures (displaced) are managed operatively, usually with closed reduction and percutaneous pinning. Gartland I type fractures (undisplaced) are managed conservatively with an above-elbow cast.

There is still debate regarding the wiring technique, with opinion split between lateral entry and medial/lateral entry. Lateral entry advocates state that there is a reduced risk of inadvertently damaging the ulnar nerve, while advocates of medial/lateral entry point to a possible benefit with increased mechanical strength. [1–3]

The procedure involves general anaesthesia and K-wire insertion under image intensifier guidance. The wires are dressed and the elbow is immobilized in an above-elbow cast.

Additional procedures that may become necessary

- Opening of fracture site to reduce fragments

Benefits

- *Therapeutic*: pain relief, mechanical improvement

Alternative procedures/conservative measures

- *Conservative*: manipulation and above elbow cast

Serious/frequently occurring risks[2,3]

- *Common*: loss of reduction (3%)
- *Occasional*: damage to nerves (2%), conversion to open reduction
- *Rare*: infection (<1%)

Blood transfusion necessary

- None

Type of anaesthesia/sedation

- General anaesthesia

Follow-up/need for further procedure

- Follow-up and review of fracture position and pin sites at 1 week in fracture clinic
- Removal of K-wires at 4 weeks

References

1. Zenios M, Ramachandran M, Milne B, *et al*. Intraoperative stability testing of lateral-entry pin fixation of pediatric supracondylar humeral fractures. *J Pediatr Orthop* 2007;**27**(6):695–702.
2. Omid R, Choi PD, Skaggs DL. Supracondylar humeral fractures in children. *J Bone Joint Surg Am* 2008;**90**(5):1121–32.
3. Brauer CA, Lee BM, Bae DS, *et al*. A systematic review of medial and lateral entry pinning versus lateral entry pinning for supracondylar fractures of the humerus. *J Pediatr Orthop* 2007;**27**(2):181–6.

Knee arthroscopy

Description

Knee arthroscopy is usually performed under general anaesthesia as a day case procedure. A small incision is made in the knee and saline is pumped into the joint space to facilitate visualization. An arthroscope, attached to a video camera is inserted through a second small incision. Some loose debris may be flushed out through the cannula along with the irrigation fluid, but consent must include the possibility for the need to carry out other procedures such as meniscal tear excision.

Debridement is often performed at the same time as washout; this involves the use of instruments to remove damaged cartilage or bone. At the end of the procedure, the saline is drained out of the joint, local anaesthetic is often added at this point and the incisions are closed with sutures, skin glue, or Steri-strips.

Additional procedures that may become necessary

- Meniscal tear excision/repair
- Synovial biopsy
- Removal of loose bodies

Benefits

- *Diagnostic*: biopsy if suspicion of chronically infected or inflamed joint
- *Therapeutic*: pain relief, mechanical improvement

Alternative procedures/conservative measures[1,2]

- *Conservative*: physiotherapy/prescribed exercise and other lifestyle changes
- *Medical*: analgesia and anti-inflammatories are the mainstay of first-line treatment. Corticosteroids or hyaluronic acid may be injected into the knee joint
- *Surgical*: if there is a knee-joint effusion, fluid around the knee may be aspirated with a needle to reduce pain and swelling. After arthroscopy, if these therapies do not work, a knee replacement may be necessary for severe osteoarthritis (approximately 10%)

Serious/frequently occurring risks

- *Common*: recurrence of pain, scar
- *Occasional*: haemarthrosis, infection <1%[3]
- *Rare*: DVT (0.5%)

Blood transfusion necessary

- None/group and save

Type of anaesthesia/sedation

- Generally under general anaesthesia
- Very occasionally under spinal/epidural/local anaesthesia in those unfit for a general anaesthesia

Follow-up/need for further procedure

- Removal of sutures by general practitioner or practice nurse
- Routine follow-up in orthopaedic outpatients at 6 weeks to assess progress

References

1. Moseley JB, O'Malley K, Petersen NJ, *et al*. A controlled trial of arthroscopic surgery for osteoarthritis of the knee. *New Engl J Med* 2002;**347**:81–8.
2. National Institute for Health and Clinical Excellence. *Arthroscopic Knee Washout, With or Without Debridement, for the Treatment of Osteoarthritis: Guidance*. London: NICE, 2007.
3. Montgomery S, Campbell J. Septic arthritis following arthroscopy and intra-articular steroids. *J Bone Joint Surg Br* 1989;**71**:540.

Total hip arthroplasty

Description

Elective THR is carried out to relieve discomfort and disability caused by arthropathies (including osteoarthritis and rheumatoid arthritis) of the hip. THR is considered to be one of the most effective orthopaedic procedures performed at the present time.

There are a number of surgical approaches to the hip, with the posterior approach remaining the most common for elective primary THR. There is good evidence to support the combined use of antibiotic impregnated cement and systemic antibiotics to reduce infection.[1-3] This is generally performed under general anaesthesia, with closure of the skin by subcuticular sutures or surgical clips.

There are a large number of prosthesis designs, bearing materials and fixation modalities. Many of these have specific complications, e.g. ceramic-on-ceramic bearing surfaces have an increased risk of squeaking and cracking. Metal-on-metal has the possible risk of metal ion exposure. The rate of revision as reported by the Swedish Joint Registry is approximately 6% at 7 years.

Additional procedures that may become necessary

- Fixation of intraoperative femoral fracture

Benefits

- *Therapeutic*: pain relief, mechanical improvement

Alternative procedures/conservative measures

- *Conservative*: physiotherapy/prescribed exercise and other lifestyle changes
- *Medical*: analgesia and anti-inflammatories are the mainstay of first-line treatment. Corticosteroids or hyaluronic acid may be injected into the hip joint
- *Surgical*: hip arthroscopy (although not currently indicated for moderate to severe osteoarthritis, may be beneficial in other aetiologies), hip resurfacing, osteotomy, and arthrodesis

Serious/frequently occurring risks

- *Common*: pain, scar, revision of prosthesis
- *Occasional*: bleeding, infection (superficial 2% and deep 0.2%[1,3]), intraoperative femoral fracture, dislocation (5%), damage to sciatic nerve, leg length discrepancy
- *Rare*: DVT, pulmonary embolism (0.4% even in the untreated patient[4])

Blood transfusion necessary

- Group and save

Type of anaesthesia/sedation

- Generally under general anaesthesia
- Very occasionally under spinal/epidural with sedation in those unfit for general anaesthesia

Follow-up/need for further procedure

- Removal of surgical clips by general practitioner or practice nurse
- Routine follow-up in orthopaedic outpatients at 6 weeks

References

1. Hanssen AD, Osmon DR, Nelson CL. Prevention of deep periprosthetic joint infection. *J Bone Joint Surg Am* 1996;**78**(3):458-71.
2. British Orthopaedic Association. *Primary Total Hip Replacement: A Guide To Good Practice*. London: British Orthopaedic Association, 2006.
3. AlBuhairan B, Hind D, Hutchinson A. Antibiotic prophylaxis for wound infections in total joint arthroplasty: a systematic review. *J Bone Joint Surg Br* 2008;**90**(7):915–19.
4. Lie SA, Engesaeter LB. Early post-operative mortality after 67 548 total hip replacements. *Acta Orthop Scand* 2002;**73**(4):392–9.

Total knee arthroplasty

Description

Severe pain and disability with accompanying radiological changes in the knee are almost always the indications for total knee arthroplasty, in patients where conservative treatment has failed or is futile. Occasionally there may be an indication to replace a knee because of progressive deformity and/or instability, and pain may not necessarily be the most significant factor.

This is generally performed under general anaesthesia. A midline incision is made with intraoperative tourniquet to aid the surgical field. There are multiple implants available, varying in fixation, whether cruciate sparing or sacrificing, constraint, and composition. Even though for a true total knee replacement all three compartments—medial, lateral and patellofemoral—are resurfaced, commonly, depending on surgeon preference or patella condition, the patellofemoral compartment may not be resurfaced.

There is good evidence to support the combined use of antibiotic impregnated cement and systemic antibiotics to reduce infection.[1,2] The routine use of drains is still a matter of debate. Closure of the skin is by subcuticular sutures or surgical clips.

Postoperatively the patient is either mobilized with physiotherapy or continuous passive movement machines immediately or on day 1 postoperatively.

Additional procedures that may become necessary

- Fixation of intraoperative femoral or tibial fracture

Benefits

- *Therapeutic*: pain relief, mechanical improvement

Alternative procedures/conservative measures

- *Conservative*: physiotherapy/prescribed exercise and other lifestyle changes
- *Medical*: analgesia and anti-inflammatories are the mainstay of first-line treatment. Corticosteroids or hyaluronic acid may be injected into the hip joint
- *Surgical*: knee arthroscopy, unicompartmental arthroplasty, osteotomy, and arthrodesis

Serious/frequently occurring risks[1-3]

- *Common*: pain, scar, revision of prosthesis (approximately 1.4% at 8 years)
- *Occasional*: vascular injury (0.1%), infection (1% at 1 year), intraoperative femoral or tibial fracture, dislocation, damage to common peroneal nerve (0.58%[4])
- *Rare*: DVT, pulmonary embolism

Blood transfusion necessary

- Group and save

Type of anaesthesia/sedation

- Generally under general anaesthesia
- Spinal/epidural with sedation in those unfit for general anaesthesia

Follow-up/need for further procedure

- Removal of surgical clips by general practitioner or practice nurse
- Routine follow-up in orthopaedic outpatients at 6 weeks

References

1. American Academy of Orthopaedic Surgeons. Instructional course lectures—common complications of total knee arthroplasty. *J Bone Joint Surg Am* 1997;**79**:278–311.
2. British Orthopaedic Association. *Knee Replacement: A Guide To Good Practice*. London: British Orthopaedic Association, 1999.
3. Deirmengian CA, Lonner JH. What's new in adult reconstructive knee surgery. *J Bone Joint Surg Am* 2009;**91**(12):3008–18.
4. Mont MA, Dellon AL, Chen F, *et al*. The operative treatment of peroneal nerve palsy. *J Bone Joint Surg Am* 1996;**78**:863–9.

Intracapsular neck of femur fractures—hemiarthroplasty

Description

For intracapsular fractures, the Garden classification is the most commonly used: I, incomplete; II, complete but non-displaced; III, complete, partially displaced; and IV, complete and fully displaced.[1]

Classically displaced intracapsular neck of femur fractures are managed with hemiarthroplasty, either cemented or uncemented.[2] There is still debate about the use of cemented prosthesis and their potential for better functional results balanced with the risk of intraoperative hypotension.[3] Total hip arthroplasty may be considered in those patients with good preoperative function and existing osteoarthritis; however, there are concerns over an increased risk of postoperative dislocation.

The bipolar prosthesis has a theoretical advantage in that it is designed to move on its inner bearing, in addition to articulating at the prosthesis–acetabulum interface. The purpose of this design is to achieve less acetabular wear, less pain, lower dislocation rates, and increased range of motion. However, bipolar prostheses are more expensive and it is still unclear whether or not the inner bearing loses mobility with time and becomes stiff, thereby minimizing the advantage of this design.

Benefits

- *Therapeutic*: mechanical improvement

Alternative procedures/conservative measures

- *Surgical*: bipolar hemiarthroplasty, total hip arthroplasty

Serious/frequently occurring risks

- *Common*: dislocation (5%), pain (5% at 24 months)
- *Occasional*: DVT, pulmonary embolism (1–5%), need for revision
- *Rare*: infection (1%)

Blood transfusion necessary

- Group and save

Type of anaesthesia/sedation

- Generally under general anaesthesia
- Spinal/regional anaesthesia if unfit for general anaesthesia

Follow-up/need for further procedure

- Removal of clips by general practitioner or practice nurse
- Routine follow-up in orthopaedic outpatients at 6–8 weeks to assess progress

References

1. Garden RS. Reduction and fixation of subcapital fractures of the femur. *Orthop Clin North Am* 1974;**5**:633.
2. Frihagen F, Nordsletten L. Madsen JE. Hemiarthroplasty or internal fixation for intracapsular displaced femoral neck fractures: randomized controlled trial. *BMJ* 2007;**335**:1251–4.
3. Khan RJ, MacDowell A, Crossman P, *et al.* Cemented or uncemented hemiarthroplasty for displaced intracapsular fractures of the hip—a systematic review. *Injury* 2002;**33**(1):13–17.

Intracapsular neck of femur fractures— cannulated screws

Description

For intracapsular fractures, the Garden classification is the most commonly used: I, incomplete; II, complete but non-displaced; III, complete, partially displaced; and IV, complete and fully displaced.

Typically cannulated screws are used for undisplaced or minimally displaced intracapsular fractures, as the blood supply is likely to be sufficient, in patients with good-quality bone to prevent avascular necrosis, although this is still one of the major postoperative risks. The procedure involves the patient positioned on a traction table, then, with image intensifier guidance, insertion of three cannulated screws, usually positioned in an inverted triangle with the lowest screw being inserted above the lesser trochanter.

The wound is closed in layers with subcuticular sutures or surgical clips to the skin. Weightbearing status is usually partial to full.

Additional procedures that may become necessary

- Hemiarthroplasty

Benefits

- *Therapeutic*: mechanical improvement

Alternative procedures/conservative measures

- *Conservative*: skin traction
- *Surgical*: dynamic hip screw with derotation screw

Serious/frequently occurring risks[1-3]

- *Common*: revision at 10 years (33%), avascular necrosis (10%)
- *Occasional*: malunion and non-union (5–10%)
- *Rare*: infection 1%

Blood transfusion necessary

- Group and save

Type of anaesthesia/sedation

- Generally under general anaesthesia
- Spinal/regional anaesthesia if unfit for general anaesthesia

Follow-up/need for further procedure

- Removal of staples by general practitioner or practice nurse
- Routine follow-up in orthopaedic outpatients at 6 weeks to assess progress

References

1. Nikolaou VS, Papathanasopoulos A, Giannoudis PV. What's new in the management of proximal femoral fractures? *Injury* 2008;**39**(12):1309–18.
2. Parker MJ. The management of intracapsular fractures of the proximal femur. *J Bone Joint Surg Br* 2000;**82**(7):937–41.
3. Parker MJ, Tagg CE. Internal fixation of intracapsular fractures. *J R Coll Surg Edinb* 2002;**47**(3):541–7.

Intramedullary nail fixation of femoral fractures

Description

Intramedullary nail fixation of a femoral fracture has become gold standard when compared with plate fixation or conservative treatment in the majority of cases. The benefits over plate fixation include reduction of extensive soft tissue dissection with the increased risk of infection and quadriceps scarring.

Intramedullary nailing can be performed as either retrograde or antegrade and can be reamed or unreamed. The debate surrounding reamed versus unreamed is ongoing.[1] The negative effects proposed for reaming are elevated intramedullary pressures, elevated pulmonary artery pressures, and increased fat embolism. However, reaming allows the use of larger nails and the overall outcome of bone growth and blood supply does not differ, with the latter being re-established at approximately 11 weeks.

Additional procedures that may become necessary

- Utilization of skeletal traction pin intraoperatively

Benefits

- *Therapeutic*: mechanical improvement

Alternative procedures/conservative measures

- *Conservative*: skin traction
- *Surgical*: external fixation, plate fixation

Serious/frequently occurring risks[2]

- *Common*: malunion and non-union (2%)
- *Occasional*: infection
- *Rare*: compartment syndrome, fat embolism, DVT, pulmonary embolism

Blood transfusion necessary

- Group and save

Type of anaesthesia/sedation

- Generally under general anaesthesia
- Spinal/regional anaesthesia if unfit for general anaesthesia

Follow-up/need for further procedure

- Removal of staples by general practitioner or practice nurse
- Routine follow-up in fracture clinic at 6 weeks to assess progress

References

1. Rudloff MI, Smith WR. Intramedullary nailing of the femur: current concepts concerning reaming. *J Orthop Trauma* 2009;**23**(5 Suppl):S12–17.
2. Giannoudis PV, Pape HC, Cohen AP, et al. Review: systemic effects of femoral nailing: from Küntscher to the immune reactivity era. *Clin Orthop Relat Res* 2002;**404**:378–86.

Intramedullary nail fixation of tibial fractures

Description
Intramedullary nail fixation of a tibial shaft fracture has become gold standard when compared to plate fixation or conservative treatment in the majority of cases. Fractures close to the mortise, the knee and multi-segmental fractures will likely benefit from plating or the use of external fixation devices.

Tibial intramedullary nails are often used in open fractures, using less soft tissue stripping, which allows concomitant soft tissue coverage. Conservative management of tibial fractures still has an important role to play in those who have significant comorbidities; however, nailing allows early mobilization, avoiding the stiffness of the ankle and the knee associated with full leg casting.[1]

The debate surrounding reamed versus unreamed is ongoing. The negative effects proposed for reaming are elevated intramedullary pressures, elevated pulmonary artery pressures, and increased fat embolism. However, reaming allows the use of larger nails and the overall outcome of bone growth and blood supply does not differ with the latter being re-established at approximately 11 weeks.

Additional procedures that may become necessary
- Poller screw insertion in more proximal fractures

Benefits
- *Therapeutic*: mechanical improvement

Alternative procedures/conservative measures
- *Conservative*: cast immobilization
- *Surgical*: external fixation, plate fixation

Serious/frequently occurring risks
- *Common*: anterior knee pain (50%), malunion and non-union (4%[2,3])
- *Occasional*: infection (2%)
- *Rare*: compartment syndrome, fat embolism, DVT, pulmonary embolism

Blood transfusion necessary
- Group and save

Type of anaesthesia/sedation
- Generally under general anaesthesia
- Spinal/regional anaesthesia if unfit for general anaesthesia

Follow-up/need for further procedure
- Removal of staples by general practitioner or practice nurse
- Routine follow-up in fracture clinic at 6 weeks to assess progress

References

1. Eone LB, Sucato D, Stegemann PM, et al. Displaced isolated fractures of the tibial shaft treated with either a cast or intramedullary nailing. An outcome analysis of matched pairs of patients. *J Bone Joint Surg Am* 1997;**79**(9):1336–41.
2. Väistö O, Toivanen J, Kannus P. et al. Anterior knee pain and thigh muscle strength after intramedullary nailing of tibial shaft fractures: a report of 40 consecutive cases. *J Orthop Trauma* 2004;**18**(1):18–23.
3. Toivanen JA, Väistö O, Kannus P, et al. Anterior knee pain after intramedullary nailing of fractures of the tibial shaft. A prospective, randomized study comparing two different nail-insertion techniques. *J Bone Joint Surg Am* 2002;**84**(4):580–5

Trigger finger release

Description

Trigger finger results from localized tenosynovitis of the superficial and deep flexor tendons adjacent to the A1 pulley at the metacarpal head. This inflammation causes nodular enlargement of the tendon (commonly in the ring and middle fingers), causing a painful clicking as the nodule moves through the pulley.

Surgery usually involves local or regional anaesthesia as a day case. An incision is made over the A1 pulley with tourniquet control, care is taken to visualize the digital nerves and release the A1 pulley and then to assess if there is any further triggering. Closure is typically with interrupted non-absorbable sutures, and dressing with a bulky bandage and early mobilization.

Additional procedures that may become necessary

- Excision of small piece of tendon sheath if passage of tendon is still restricted after release of A1 pulley

Benefits

- *Therapeutic*: pain relief, mechanical improvement

Alternative procedures/conservative measures

- *Conservative*: physiotherapy, typically by splinting the distal interphalangeal joint of the affected finger
- *Medical*: analgesia and corticosteroid injection may be beneficial
- *Surgical*: percutaneous release of the A1 pulley

Serious/frequently occurring risks[1,2]

- *Common*: recurrence (3%)
- *Occasional*: bowstringing of tendons
- *Rare*: damage to digital nerves, infection

Blood transfusion necessary

- None/group and save

Type of anaesthesia/sedation

- Generally under local/regional anaesthesia
- General anaesthesia for secondary revision or other complex cases

Follow-up/need for further procedure

- Removal of sutures by general practitioner or practice nurse
- Routine follow-up in orthopaedic outpatients at 6 weeks to assess progress

References

1. Turowski general anaesthesia, Zdankiewicz PD, Thomson JG. The results of surgical treatment of trigger finger. *J Hand Surg Am* 1997;**22**(1):145–9.
2. Ryzewicz M, Wolf JM. Trigger digits: principles, management, and complications. *J Hand Surg Am* 2006;**31**(1):135–46.

Plastic surgery

Carpal tunnel decompression

Description

Carpal tunnel syndrome is caused by compression of the median nerve at the wrist. Treatment options include splinting, corticosteroid injection, ultrasound therapy, and surgery.

Surgery is considered the definitive treatment, with ~70–97% success rates reported.[1,2] The procedure, which can be open or endoscopic, may be performed under tourniquet control typically with a local/regional block. Endoscopic techniques may have higher chance of nerve injury.

For open release, the skin is incised between the hypothenar and thenar eminences. The carpal tunnel is decompressed through incising the transverse carpal ligament and the tunnel examined for any abnormalities or mass lesions. Synovectomy of flexor tendons may also be performed. The skin is then closed and a dressing applied. A splint may then be applied for 1–2 weeks. Prophylactic antibiotics may be given.

Additional procedures that may become necessary

• Splinting

Benefits

• *Therapeutic*: relieve pain and paraesthesia; improve grip strength
• *Diagnostic*: carpal tunnel is examined for any abnormalities/lesions

Alternative procedures/conservative measures[1–3]

• *Conservative*: splinting may be of benefit in milder cases or during pregnancy. Recovery may also be spontaneous. *Disadvantages*: short-term efficacy only
• *Medical*: ultrasound therapy. *Disadvantages*: limited evidence of efficacy
• *Surgical*: steroid injections. *Disadvantages*: short-term efficacy only; risk of median nerve injury

Serious/frequently occurring risks[1,2]

• *Common*: bleeding; scarring; pain (particularly scar and pillar pain—may persist for ~6/12); stiffness; grip/pinch/pincer weakness
• *Occasional*: infection; ongoing symptoms/recurrence of symptoms
• *Rare*: chronic regional pain syndrome; median/ulnar nerve injury; ulnar artery injury; flexor tendon laceration; bow stringing of flexor tendons

Blood transfusion necessary

• None/group and save

Type of anaesthesia/sedation

• Local
• Regional or general anaesthesia (if pathology, e.g. synovitis/tumours, suspected in carpal tunnel)

Follow-up/need for further procedure

• Removal of sutures in 10–14 days
• Routine outpatient review
• Physiotherapy as required

References

1. Huisstede B, Randsdorp M, Ccert J, et al. Carpal tunnel syndrome: Part II: effectiveness of surgical treatments—a systematic review. *Arch Phys Med Rehabil* 2010;**91**(7):1005–24.
2. Ono S, Clapham P, Chung K. Optimal management of carpal tunnel syndrome. *Int J Gen Med* 2010;**3**:255–61.
3. Huisstede B, Hoogvliet P, Randsdorp M, et al. Carpal tunnel syndrome: Part I: effectiveness of non-surgical treatments—a systematic review. *Arch Phys Med Rehabil* 2010;**91**(7):981–1004.

De Quervain's tenosynovitis decompression

Description

De Quervain's tenosynovitis is caused by entrapment and inflammation of the tendons within the first dorsal compartment of the wrist due to thickening of the sheath. Treatment options include splinting, corticosteroid injections and surgical release of the compartment.

Steroid injections are commonly the first-line treatment for de Quervain's tenosynovitis (cure rate of 62–93% reported[1]) with surgery reserved for those unresponsive to conservative management.

Surgical release is generally performed under tourniquet control under local/regional anaesthesia, typically through a transverse incision within the skin crease overlying the first dorsal compartment. The compartment is exposed and incised dorsally. The tendons (of extensor pollicis brevis and abductor pollicis longus) are then examined with any septum present divided and full release of the tendons ensured. The sheath may then be left open or partially excised. The skin is closed and a dressing applied with or without the addition of a splint (typically for 10–14 days). Sutures are removed at 10–14 days. Prophylactic antibiotics may be given.

Additional procedures that may become necessary

- Splinting

Benefits

- *Therapeutic*: reduce symptoms (pain and swelling)
- *Diagnostic*: aid confirmation of diagnosis of de Quervain's tenosynovitis

Alternative procedures/conservative measures[1]

- *Conservative*: splinting. *Disadvantages*: highly variable efficacy reported (good results reported in patients with minimal symptoms)
- *Medical*: non-steroidal anti-inflammatory drugs (in conjunction with other treatment) *Disadvantages*: no significant difference in outcome noted
- *Surgical*: intra-sheath corticosteroid injections. *Disadvantages*: temporary worsening of symptoms (~3–10 days postinjection); skin depigmentation; fat atrophy

Serious/frequently occurring risks

- *Common*: bleeding; infection; scarring (particularly hypertrophic scars); pain (particularly of scar); superficial radial nerve injury; neuritis; paraesthesia
- *Occasional*: tendon subluxation;[2] ongoing symptoms/recurrence; neuroma; prolonged/delayed wound healing

Blood transfusion necessary

- None/group and save

Type of anaesthesia/sedation

- Local/regional/general anaesthesia

Follow-up/need for further procedure
- Removal of sutures in 10–14 days
- Routine outpatient review
- Physiotherapy as required

References
1. Ilyas A. Nonsurgical treatment for de Quervain's tenosynovitis. *J Hand Surg Am* 2009;**34**(5):928–9.
2. Littler J, Freedman D, Malerich M. Compartment reconstruction for de Quervain's disease. *J Hand Surg Br* 2002;**27**(2):242–4.

Digital replantation

Description

Digital amputation may result from various causes including crush injuries, lacerations, and avulsions. Replantation is not indicated in all amputations and type of injury, length of extraction, cold/warm ischaemia, level of amputation, contamination of wound and digit, patient factors (age, co-morbidities, social history) and patient choice must be considered.

Typically such operations are performed under general anaesthesia, although, often axillary/infraclavicular blocks may be used as an adjunct to limit arterial spasm via sympathetic blockade. The wound and amputated digit(s) are thoroughly debrided and injured structures identified and assessed before being repaired in a systematic approach as outlined here.

The bone of the amputated stump is shorted (typically between 5 and 10mm) to reduce tension of subsequent neurovascular anastomoses and improve survival of the replant. The bone ends are then fixed either with K-wires, intramedullary screws, or plates. The extensor tendons, followed by flexor tendons, are then repaired. Arteries are subsequently explored with segments with intimal damage resected, due to the tendency for thrombosis.

A tension-free repair is crucial to minimize thrombosis risk. If too much length has been lost to achieve a tension-free arterial anastomosis, a vein graft (positioned in reverse) should be employed. Once repaired, the digital nerves are examined, damaged ends excised and healthy ends then realigned and repaired, again under no tension. Where this is not possible, a nerve graft may be used, with the donor nerve either being from an amputated digit unsuitable for replantation, or from the sural or lateral antebrachial cutaneous nerve. Alternatively, nerve grafting may be delayed until the replant has healed. The veins are then repaired, requiring ideally two veins per artery repaired.

Where primary repair is not possible, vein grafting may be performed with a minimum of one vein per artery repaired. The skin wounds are loosely closed following achievement of haemostasis. Where skin loss has occurred, skin grafting may be required.

The digit(s) are then dressed with sterile, non-compressive, bulky dressings together with a plaster splint to position the wrist in slight extension. Fingertips are left visible for postoperative assessment and the hand elevated on a soft pillow.

The patient must be kept warm, and should avoid caffeine, chocolate, and smoking, as these can cause vasoconstriction and thus compromise the replant. Patients are kept nil by mouth for 24–48h postoperatively due to this being the period of greatest risk of thrombosis. Doppler pulse, oxygen saturation, digital colour, capillary refill time, and temperature are often monitored hourly for the first 24h and then performed every 2h for the subsequent 48h. Prophylactic intravenous antibiotics are also given in addition to tetanus prophylaxis (where appropriate). As pain and anxiety increase sympathetic tone, thus resulting in vasoconstriction, adequate analgesia ± anxiolytics is required. For the same reason, adequate hydration must be maintained.

In order to reduce thrombosis risk, perioperative anticoagulation is sometimes given, the choice of which depends on surgeon, surgical unit and injury type. Dressings are assessed daily, typically changed on postoperative day 2/3 and the digit cleaned of any coagulated blood, which could potentially cause a tourniquet effect.

Rehabilitation typically involves 2 weeks of immobilization followed by active and passive movement of the uninvolved digits, elbow and shoulder. All digits are actively mobilized at weeks 3–4. Strict adherence to physiotherapy is essential, as directed by specialist hand therapists. Specialized splints may also be given.

Additional procedures that may become necessary

- *Grafts*: vein/nerve/skin
- Use of leeches postoperatively (if venous congestion is thought to be present, leeches may be used to remove blood from the digit, while also promoting bleeding through an anticoagulant present in their saliva)

Benefits

- *Diagnostic*: assess extent of injury and whether replantation is appropriate
- *Therapeutic*: aim to restore function of the amputated digit(s) and thus overall hand function, although recovery is prolonged and digits with poor sensation and stiffness function poorly

Alternative procedures/conservative measures[1,2]

- *Surgical*: where replantation is inappropriate/not possible, simple debridement, shortening and closure of the stump or conversion to a ray amputation may be performed *Disadvantages*: depending on the digit(s) affected hand function may be significantly reduced—in particular, thumb amputations due to loss of opposition; aesthetic alteration; phantom pain; stiffness

Serious/frequently occurring risks[3,4]

- *Common*: bleeding; pain; scarring; prolonged wound healing/dressings; infection (local/systemic); stiffness and restricted range of mobility; reduced function (motor and sensory) of digit(s)/hand; cold intolerance
- *Occasional*: tendon ruptures; tendon adhesions; bony malunion/non-union; capsular contraction; complete or partial loss of replant
- *Rare*: chronic regional pain syndrome

Blood transfusion necessary

- Group and save

Type of anaesthesia/sedation

- Generally under general anaesthesia with adjunctive blocks

Follow-up/need for further procedure

- Removal of sutures in 10–14 days
- Close review in outpatient clinic, dressing clinics and hand therapy is required
- Secondary reconstructive operations; secondary tendon/nerve repairs; tenolysis; capsulotomies; osteotomies may be required

References

1. Soucacos P. Indications and selection for digital amputation and replantation. *J Hand Surg Br* 2001;**26**(6):572–81.
2. Thomas F, Kaplan D, Raskin K. Indications and surgical techniques for digit replantation. *Bull Hosp Jt Dis* 2001–2002;**60**(3–4):179–88.
3. Dec W. A meta-analysis of success rates for digit replantation. *Tech Hand Up Extrem Surg* 2006;**10**(3):124–9.
4. Waikakul S, Sakkarnkosol D, Vanadurongwan V, *et al.* Results of 1018 digital replantations in 552 patients. *Injury* 2000;**31**(1):33–40.

Dupuytren's contracture release—regional fasciectomy

Description

Dupuytren's contracture is caused by fibrosis (resulting in thickening and shortening) of the palmar fascia; most commonly affecting the ring and little fingers. Various treatment options exist, however, most require surgical intervention, most commonly regional fasciectomy.

Surgery is indicated when metacarpophalangeal contracture is >30° or with any involvement of an interphalangeal joint. When the interphalangeal joint is involved, a contracture may persist postoperatively. Recurrence is universal and is associated with age of onset and degree of skin involvement.

The procedure is performed under tourniquet control, typically under a regional block or general anaesthesia. In a regional fasciectomy, the skin is incised and affected fascia dissected and excised. The wound is closed with Z-plasty and dressed, with the hand immobilized for a few days. Prophylactic antibiotics are typically given.

Additional procedures that may become necessary

- Splinting for joint contracture
- Full-thickness skin grafting where dermofasciectomy is performed

Benefits

- *Diagnostic*: assess extent of fibrosis
- *Therapeutic*: remove fibrotic fascia and treat joint contracture

Alternative procedures/conservative measures

- *Conservative*: left untreated a Dupuytren's contracture will usually progress. Splinting is also relatively ineffective. *Disadvantages*: disease progression leading to further reduction of joint mobility and hand function
- *Medical*: these treatments have been shown to be largely ineffective
- *Surgical*:
  - Injection with collagenase (*Clostridium histolyticum*) has shown promising results. *Disadvantages*: high recurrence rate of 67% at metacarpophalangeal joint and 100% at proximal interphalangeal joint contractures; swelling; bruising; pain; lymphadenopathy; skin tears[1]
  - Percutaneous needle aponeurotomy may be performed for patients with predominant metacarpophalangeal contractures or those in whom surgery is inappropriate, unfavourable, or unwanted. Results are reasonable with 79% postoperative pain noted at the metacarpophalangeal joint by Foucher et al.[2] *Disadvantages*: high recurrence of 58% with reoperation rates of 24% reported; digital nerve injury
  - Injection with steroids may have a role for small painful nodules in limiting progression temporarily. *Disadvantages*: temporary effects; dermal atrophy; skin depigmentation; tendon rupture

- Fasciotomy and local fasciectomy. *Disadvantages*: high recurrence rate
- Radical fasciectomy. *Disadvantages*: comparable recurrence rates to that of regional fasciectomy with higher complication rates and need for large skin flaps
- Open palm technique (leaving the wound open to heal via secondary intention). *Disadvantages*: prolonged healing time; need for ongoing dressings and splinting
- Dermofasciectomy has reported lower recurrence rates. *Disadvantages*: full-thickness skin grafting/dermal substitute required

Serious/frequently occurring risks[3,4]

- *Common*: bleeding; pain; scarring; recurrence (as previously noted); infection; skin necrosis; numbness; stiffness
- *Occasional*: vascular injury; chronic regional pain syndrome
- *Rare*: pseudoaneurysm; inclusion cyst

Blood transfusion necessary

- None/group and save

Type of anaesthesia/sedation

- Regional/general anaesthesia

Follow-up/need for further procedure

- Removal of sutures in 10–14 days
- Routine outpatient follow-up
- Physiotherapy as required for contracture/stiffness

References

1. Watt A, Curtin C, Hentz V. Collagenase injection as nonsurgical treatment of Dupuytren's disease: 8-year follow-up. *J Hand Surg Am* 2010;**35**(4):534–9e1.
2. Foucher G, Medina J, Navarro R. Percutaneous needle aponeurotomy. Complications and results. *Chir Main* 2001;**20**(3):206–11.
3. Shaw R, Chong A, Zhang A, *et al.* Dupuytren's disease: history, diagnosis and treatment. *Plast Reconstr Surg* 2007;**120**(3):44e–54e.
4. Coert J, Nerin J, Meek M. Results of partial fasciectomy for Dupuytren disease in 261 consecutive patients. *Ann Plast Surg* 2006;**57**(1):13–17.

Extensor tendon repair

Description

Extensor tendon injuries commonly occur with sharp lacerations, crush and punch/bite injuries. Lacerated and ruptured are repaired; either primarily or with the use of a tendon graft/transfer. Tendon grafts may be used for delayed injuries or those with significant tendon loss.

Repairs are performed under a local/regional/general anaesthesia with tourniquet control. Typically antibiotics are given in open wounds and tetanus vaccination (where required).

The wound is closed, dressed and splinted as appropriate. Most tendon injuries require a period of postoperative splinting and physiotherapy for up to 10 weeks.

Additional procedures that may become necessary

- Extension of wound ± debridement
- Tendon grafts—typically using palmaris longus, plantaris, or a long toe extensor
- Local flaps for skin loss
- Fracture fixation

Benefits

- *Therapeutic*: aim to restore function and close open wounds
- *Diagnostic*: exploration of wound to assess injury

Alternative procedures/conservative measures

- *Conservative*: splinting. *Disadvantages*: stiffness; adhesion formation; higher risk of rupture

Serious/frequently occurring risks[1-3]

- *Common*: bleeding; infection; scarring; paraesthesia; contracture; pain (including donor site); joint stiffness; adhesions. weakness
- *Occasional*: rupture; stiffness of adjacent digits (quadriga phenomenon)
- *Rare*: chronic regional pain syndrome

Blood transfusion necessary

- None/group and save

Type of anaesthesia/sedation

- Local/regional/general anaesthesia

Follow-up/need for further procedure

- Removal of sutures in 10–14 days
- Routine outpatient review
- Physiotherapy as required

References

1. Carl H, Forst R, Schaller P. Results of primary extensor tendon repair in relation to the zone of injury and pre-operative outcome estimation. *Arca Orthop Trauma Surg* 2007;**127**(2):115–19.
2. Harz K, Saint-Cyr M, Semmler M, *et al*. Extensor tendon injuries: acute management and secondary reconstruction. *Plast Reconstr Surg* 2008;**121**(3):109e–20e.
3. Rockwell W, Butler P, Byrne B. Extensor tendon: anatomy, injury and reconstruction. *Plast Reconstr Surg* 2000;**106**(7):1592–603.

Flexor tendon repair

Description

Open flexor tendon injuries and those with closed avulsions and functional deficit require surgical repair. Ideally washout is performed immediately with primary repair within 24–72h of injury. Where insufficient distal tendon remains, primary repair may be performed with either an anchor suture in the distal phalanx or with a pullout suture tied over the nail plate.[1,2]

In cases where tendon length is insufficient for primary repair, commonly with delayed or crush injuries repair, using grafts may be required (secondary repair[3]). Where extensive scarring, infection, or secondary rupture has occurred, two-stage grafting techniques using rods and tendon grafts may be performed. In a two-stage procedure, a silicone rod is implanted with any scarred tendon removed and pulley reconstruction performed as required. A 'pseudotendon sheath' subsequently forms over the rod. The second stage is performed 3–5 months later once maximal passive range of motion (ROM) has been achieved. This involves replacement of the rod with a tendon graft. Use of a tendon rod is contraindicated in contaminated wounds.

Repairs are performed under local/regional/general anaesthesia with tourniquet control. Typically antibiotics are given in open wounds and tetanus vaccination (where required). The wound is closed, dressed and splinted as appropriate. Most tendon injuries require a period of post-operative splinting and physiotherapy for up to 10 weeks.

Additional procedures that may become necessary[1,4]

- Extension of wound ± debridement
- Tendon grafting—typically using: palmaris longus or long toe extensor tendons
- Pulley reconstruction using local tissue/tendon grafts
- Neurovascular repair

Benefits

- *Therapeutic*: aim to restore function and close open wounds
- *Diagnostic*: explore wound to assess injury

Alternative procedures/conservative measures

- *Conservative*: splinting. *Disadvantages*: stiffness; adhesion formation; unsuitable for complex cases, open or contaminated wounds
- *Surgical*: arthrodesis of the distal interphalangeal joint may be performed in isolated flexor digitorum profundus rupture. *Disadvantages*: immobile joint

Serious/frequently occurring risks

- *Common*: bleeding; infection; scarring; paraesthesia; tendon rupture; joint contracture; pain; adhesions; stiffness; weakness
- *Occasional*: rupture; bowstringing; stiffness of adjacent digits (quadriga phenomenon); nail deformity (where pullout sutures are used)
- *Rare*: chronic regional pain syndrome

Blood transfusion necessary
- None/group and save

Type of anaesthesia/sedation
- Local/regional/general anaesthesia

Follow-up/need for further procedure
- Removal of sutures in 10–14 days
- Routine outpatient review
- Physiotherapy as required

References

1. Moore T, Anderson B, Seiler J. Flexor tendon reconstruction. *J Hand Surg Am* 2010;**35**(6): 1025–30.
2. Moiemen N, Elliot D. Primary flexor tendon repair in zone 1. *J Hand Surg Br* 2000;**25**(1):78–84.
3. Freilich A, Chhabra A. Secondary flexor tendon reconstruction, a review. *J Hand Surg Am* 2007;**32**(9):1436–42.
4. Lilly S, Messer T. Complications after treatment of flexor tendon injuries. *J Am Acad Orthop Surg* 2006;**14**(7):387–96.

Ganglion cyst—surgical excision

Description

Ganglion cysts are common benign lesions which may be present adjacent to any joint or tendon sheath; ~50–70% found on the dorsal aspect of the wrist. Over 50% of untreated cysts resolve spontaneously.[1] Ganglion cysts may be symptomatic—causing pain, triggering, nerve compression, or limitation of movement due to size/position.

Treatment options include aspiration and surgical excision. Surgical excision has much lower recurrence rates (1–5% for dorsal and 7% for volar wrist ganglia reported[2,3]).

The procedure, which may be open or arthroscopic, is performed under local/regional/general anaesthesia. The base of the ganglion is dissected to its origins and excised. Recent studies have shown comparable recurrence rates and complications of arthroscopic ganglionectomy as compared to open resection.[4]

The defect is closed and dressed and specimen sent for histopathological examination. Immobilization may be required (typically 1–2 weeks).

Prophylactic antibiotics may be given.

Additional procedures that may become necessary

- Splinting

Benefits

- *Diagnostic*: confirm nature of lesion
- *Therapeutic*: improve aesthetics; reduce symptoms (pain/triggering/nerve compression/limitation of movement)

Alternative procedures/conservative measures

- *Conservative*: as noted >50% will spontaneously resolve. If asymptomatic, no excision may be warranted. *Disadvantages*: ongoing/deterioration of symptoms (if present); enlarging ganglion
- *Surgical*: aspiration. *Disadvantages*: high recurrence rates

Serious/frequently occurring risks[1-3]

- *Common*: bleeding; pain; scarring (including hypertrophic scarring); stiffness; infection; recurrence
- *Occasional*: neuroma (particular of radial nerve); weakness; limited range of movement
- *Rare*: damage to palmar cutaneous branch of median nerve and radial artery (with volar ganglia excisions)

Blood transfusion necessary

- None/group and save

Type of anaesthesia/sedation

- Local/regional/general anaesthesia

Follow-up/need for further procedure
- Removal of sutures in 10–14 days
- Routine outpatient review with histopathology results
- Physiotherapy may be required for stiffness

References
1. Gude W, Morelli V. Ganglion cysts of the wrist: pathophysiology, clinical picture and management. *Curr Rev Musculoskelet Med* 2008;**1**:205–11.
2. Edwards S, Johansen J. Prospective outcomes and associations of wrist ganglion cysts resected arthroscopically. *J Hand Surg Am* 2009;**34**(3):395–400.
3. Jebson P, Spencer E. Flexor tendon sheath ganglions: results of surgical excision. *Hand* 2007;**2**:94–100.
4. Rocchi L, Canal A, Fanfani F. *et al*. Articular ganglia of the volar aspect of the wrist: arthroscopic resection compared with open excision. A prospective randomized study. *Scand J Plast Reconstr Surg Hand Surg* 2008;**42**(5):253–9.

Hand fracture reduction: open reduction internal fixation and K-wiring

Description

Metacarpal and phalangeal fractures are common injuries. Closed, undisplaced, stable fractures and those which are stable after reduction under anaesthesia may be managed conservatively with splints.

Where fixation is required, K-wires, tension band wiring or open reduction and internal fixation with the use of plates and screws may be used.

K-wires cause less soft tissue trauma but fracture stability is often less than with open reduction and internal fixation. More accurate alignment of fracture is possible with direct open visualization. In cases where bone loss or significant comminution is present, bone grafting may be required. This may be autogenous, allograft, or synthetic.

Fracture reduction is typically performed under tourniquet control under local/regional /general anaesthesia.

K-wires in the hand are generally removed after ~4 weeks. Plates and screws are left *in situ* permanently unless causing problems or in a child (as leaving the plates in a growing skeleton would lead to growth deformity).

Prophylactic antibiotics are typically given to all patients requiring fixation.

Additional procedures that may become necessary

- Cast/splint
- Bone grafting—if autogenous: common donor sites: ilium, distal radius

Benefits

- *Therapeutic*: reduce fracture to restore anatomy and improve functional outcome
- *Diagnostic*: extent of fracture/involvement of surrounding structures (with open reduction internal fixation)

Alternative procedures/conservative measures[1]

- *Conservative*: closed, undisplaced fractures may be placed in splint/cast applied; displaced fractures may undergo manipulation under anaesthesia with subsequent splinting.
  Disadvantages: if any displacement/rotation, functional outcome may be limited. If manipulation under anaesthesia fails, further procedure as outlined may be required

Serious/frequently occurring risks[2,3]

- *Common*: bleeding; pain; scarring; stiffness; prolonged wound healing/dressings; infection; weakness; adhesions (capsular/tendon)
- *Occasional*: malunion; non-union; surrounding soft tissue injury (including muscle/tendon injury); nerve/vascular injury; loosening of wires (pin site infection)
- *Rare*: amputation; chronic regional pain syndrome

Blood transfusion necessary

- None/group and save

Type of anaesthesia/sedation

- Local/regional/general anaesthesia

Follow-up/need for further procedure

- Removal of sutures in 10–14 days
- Routine outpatient review with removal of K-wires if inserted at ~4 weeks
- Physiotherapy may be required for stiffness

References

1. Bernstein M, Chung K. Hand fractures and their management: an international view. *Injury* 2006;**37**:1043–8.
2. Bushnell B, Draeger R, Crosby C, *et al.* Management of intra-articular metacarpal base fractures of the second through fifth metacarpals. *J Hand Surg Am* 2008;**33**(4):573–83.
3. Freeland A, Orbay J. Extraarticular hand fractures in adults: a review of new developments. *Clin Orthop Relat Res* 2006;**445**:133–45.

Local flaps—advancement, rotational, transpositional

Description

When planning closure of a surgical defect, location, size, tissue characteristics, and aesthetics must be carefully considered. Closure may be achieved through healing by secondary intention, simple side-to-side closure or use of a skin flap or skin graft. Secondary intention healing may be the best option for concave areas such as the medial canthus, preauricular region, or alar groove, with excellent cosmetic results. When direct closure causes excessive skin tension or anatomical distortion, a local flap may be the most appropriate method for closure. Where insufficient movement or tissue is available for a flap closure, skin grafting may be required.

• Advancement flaps: an advancement flap (Fig. 13.1) is a flap created in order to 'slide' the tissue directly over the defect, transferring the tension of the closure to a more suitable site. They include single pedicle, bipedicle, and V-Y flaps. Advancement flaps on the face normally have a random blood supply, whereas on other parts of the body these may be based on perforators
  • Single pedicle flaps—parallel incisions are made, extending from the defect, ideally along relaxed skin tension lines, in order to minimize scarring. With advancement, the skin excess at the base of the flap may then be removed either by excising Burrow's triangles (skin and subcutaneous fat) or by performing bilateral Z-plasties
  • Bipedicle flaps—a bilateral advancement flap follows the same principle as a single pedicle flap
  • V-Y flap[1]—used to convert a V-shaped flap into a Y-shaped suture line by advancing the broad base of the V into the defect and then closing the base primarily
• Rotational flaps: a rotational flap (Fig. 13.2) is created by rotating adjacent tissue in a semicircular arc from a fulcrum point, in order to close a defect. These can also be random flaps or rely on perforators for improved vascular supply. In order to improve lymphatic drainage, the flap is ideally inferiorly based and in general, created to a 4:1 flap:defect ratio to allow sufficient mobility and tension distribution. A standing cone often results at the distal end of the flap, which may be managed with a simple back cut or alternatively by excising a Burrow's triangle. Considerable undermining is required for such flaps
• Transposition flaps: a transposition flap (Fig. 13.3) is one in which the donor tissue is remote from the defect. A Z-plasty (Fig. 13.4) is created using two transposition flaps in order to lengthen a contracted scar or alter the orientation

The flap is sutured in place and dressings applied.

Benefits

• *Therapeutic*: aid healing of wound with minimal scarring/deformity

Alternative procedures/conservative measures

- *Conservative*: allow secondary intention healing. *Disadvantages*: poor cosmetic result; prolonged healing time
- *Surgical*:
  - Skin grafts. *Disadvantages*: poorer cosmetic result, particularly on the face; minimal protection of underlying structures; complications of skin grafts (□ see 'Skin grafts', p.411). Free flaps. *Disadvantages*: complex flaps involving microvascular surgery with greater risk of failure/necrosis; longer operation; need for hospitalization

Serious/frequently occurring risks

- *Common*: bleeding; infection; scarring; pain; paraesthesia
- *Occasional*: partial flap necrosis; poor cosmetic result; distortion of anatomical landmarks
- *Rare*: complete flap necrosis

Blood transfusion necessary

- None/group and save

Type of anaesthesia/sedation

- Depending on the site and size of the flap reconstruction, local or general anaesthesia may be used

Follow-up/need for further procedure

- Suture removal in 5–10 days with follow-up in outpatient clinic to assess healing and outcome

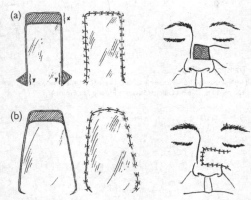

Fig. 13.1 Advancement flap.

Reproduced with permission from McLatchie GR and Leaper DJ. *Oxford Handbook of Operative Surgery*, 2nd edition. 2006. Oxford: Oxford University Press, p.781, Figure 17.7.

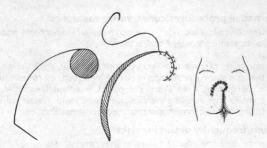

Fig. 13.2 Rotation flap.
Reproduced with permission from McLatchie GR and Leaper DJ. *Oxford Handbook of Operative Surgery*, 2nd edition. 2006. Oxford: Oxford University Press, p.785, Figure 17.8.

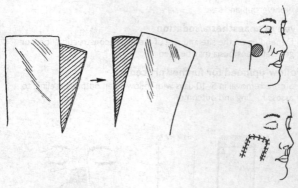

Fig. 13.3 Transposition flap.
Reproduced with permission from McLatchie GR and Leaper DJ. *Oxford Handbook of Operative Surgery*, 2nd edition. 2006. Oxford: Oxford University Press, p.785, Figure 17.9.

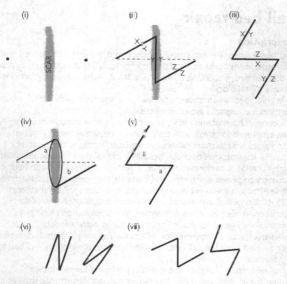

Fig. 13.4 Z-plasty.

Reproduced with permission from Giele H and Cassell O. *Oxford Specialist Handbook of Plastic and Reconstructive Surgery.* 2008. Oxford: Oxford University Press, p.774, Figure 22.14.

Reference

1. Zook E, Van Beek A, Russell R, *et al.* V-Y advancement flap for facial defects. *Plast Reconstr Surg* 1930;**65**(6):786–97.

Nail bed repair

Description

Nail bed injuries are extremely common and are often associated with a subungual haematoma or distal phalanx fracture. Treatment requires repair of the nail bed + splinting of the nail plate if avulsed, typically performed under a digital block.

As nail bed injuries are commonly associated with distal phalanx fractures, radiographs are often necessary.

- *Subungual haematoma management:* conservative management may be employed for small, painless haematomas, when the nail margin and plate are intact and where no displaced fracture is present. For painful haematomas or those typically >25% of the nail, evacuation via trephination is performed by using a heated needle/pin or ophthalmic cautery to penetrate the nail and evacuate the underlying haematoma. ▶▶Although it was previously thought that subungual haematomas 25–50% required avulsion of the nail plate and examination of the nail bed, studies have recently shown that trephination alone gives equivalently good results.[1,2] For haematomas with associated distal phalanx fractures, however, or where the nail margin/plate is disrupted or avulsed from the nail bed, examination and repair of the nail bed is indicated
- *Nail bed repair:*[3,4] repairs are typically performed under local anaesthesia, with the digital tourniquet applied. Absorbable sutures are used with as little debridement performed as possible to minimize nail deformity. Where nail bed avulsion has occurred, a split thickness nail bed graft may be required.[3,4] For defects <50%, the graft may be taken from the same digit. For those >50%, the great toe is typically used. Harvesting of the nail bed is taken, ideally using a microscope (again under digital/regional blockade and tourniquet control) and sutured into place

Once the nail bed is repaired, the tourniquet is released and the digit dressed, typically with an non-adherent dressing. The wound will need to be reviewed in 7–10 days. Antibiotic cover may be given for patients at increased risk of infection or those with an underlying phalanx fracture.

Patients should be informed that approximately three nail cycles (~1 year) are required before reliable assessment of the final nail appearance may be made.

Additional procedures that may become necessary

- Splinting
- Nail bed/skin grafting

Benefits

- *Diagnostic:* assess extent of injury
- *Therapeutic:* repair nail bed, aim to improve cosmesis of subsequent nail growth

Alternative procedures/conservative measures

- *Conservative*: small subungual haematomas/nail bed injuries may be managed conservatively, and often patients with such injuries do not seek medical help. Severe crush injuries with large areas of nail bed loss may be left to heal via secondary intention. *Disadvantages*: ongoing pain; growth distortion of the nail or loss of the nail may occur
- *Surgical*:
  - Trephination of small subungual haematomas as described may be sufficient. *Disadvantages*: if large, an underlying nail bed injury may be missed leading to abnormal nail growth or loss of the nail
  - Grafting—where the nail bed has been avulsed, full-thickness nail bed grafting or split thickness skin graft (STSG) may be performed. *Disadvantages*: donor digit/toe will have subsequent nail deformity (however, inconsequential if used from an amputated digit/toe); non-adherence of growing nail to the skin graft, respectively

Serious/frequently occurring risks[2-4]

- *Common*: bleeding; pain; prolonged wound healing/dressings; abnormal/deformed nail growth
- *Occasional*: infection (local—nail bed/wound); loss of nail with failure of subsequent nail growth
- *Rare*: infection (underlying bone/tendon sheath/hand/systemic)

Blood transfusion necessary

- None/group and save

Type of anaesthesia/sedation

- Generally under digital nerve block
- Occasionally under local/regional/general anaesthesia

Follow-up/need for further procedure

- Dressings are changed after 5–10 days. A protective splint may be required for ~2 weeks postoperatively
- Wound and nail appearance will need outpatient follow-up either with the surgical team or specialist nurse clinic

References

1. Batrick N, Hashemi K, Freij R. Treatment of uncomplicated subungual haematoma. *Emerg Med J* 2003;**20**(1):65.
2. Roser SE. Gellman H. Comparison of nail bed repair versus nail trephination for subungual hematomas in children. *J Hand Surg Am* 1999;**24**(6):1166–70.
3. Brown R, Zook E, Russell R. Fingertip reconstruction with flaps and nail bed grafts. *J Hand Surg Am* 1999;**24**(2):345–51.
4. Hsieh SC. Chen SL, Chen TM, *et al*. Thin split-thickness toenail bed grafts for avulsed nail bed defects. *Ann Plast Surg* 2004;**52**:375–9.

Peripheral nerve repair

Description

Peripheral nerve injuries are common and the degree of injury may vary widely.

- Neurapraxia caused by simple contusion and axonotmesis injuries (those in which endoneurial tubes and neural architecture remain intact) will recover spontaneously, often taking 3–4 months for recovery of a neurapraxic injury and longer for axonotmesis injuries; with regeneration occurring at 1–2mm/day
- Nerve injuries in which the axons, endoneurial tubes, and overall architecture have been disrupted require surgical repair. It is often, however, not possible to distinguish the degree of injury by examination of the patient and thus whether exploration ± repair is warranted. If there is any uncertainty then exploration or nerve conduction studies are performed

Nerve repairs[1,2] may be delayed a few months postinjury, however, for clean, transected nerves, primary, tension-free, reapproximation of nerve ends within 2–3days of injury is preferable. Where a gap is present, due to nerve loss or retraction, a nerve graft (acellular allograft or autograft) or conduit (biological or synthetic tube) may be required to ensure a tension-free repair. Nerve grafts are typically used for larger gaps, with the commonest donor being the sural nerve. Other donor sites include: medial and lateral antebrachial cutaneous nerves. In severe proximal nerve injuries, a nerve transfer may be used.

The procedure is typically performed with tourniquet control under regional/general anaesthesia depending on extent of injury and potential need for nerve grafting. Once repaired, the wound is closed, and the limb is dressed and immobilized using a back-slab/splint. Prophylactic antibiotics are generally given.

Strict adherence to subsequent physiotherapy and sensory re-education is required and the patient must be aware of the prolonged recovery period.

Additional procedures that may become necessary

- Nerve grafting/transfer

Benefits

- *Diagnostic*: assess extent of injury
- *Therapeutic*: aim to regain maximal sensory and/or motor function possible

Alternative procedures/conservative measures

- *Conservative*: spontaneous recovery will occur with neurapraxic and axonotmesis injuries. *Disadvantages*: if the injury involves disruption of the endoneurons/neural architecture and is managed conservatively, recovery of the nerves will not occur thus leading to loss of nerve function (sensory/motor); neuromas may develop; pain

Serious/frequently occurring risks[2]
- *Common*: bleeding; pain; scarring; infection; suboptimal nerve recovery (permanent sensory/motor deficit); neuroma

Blood transfusion necessary
- None/group and save

Type of anaesthesia/sedation
- Regional/general anaesthesia

Follow-up/need for further procedure
- Removal of skin sutures in 10–14 days
- Regular follow-up is required to monitor progress
- Physiotherapy as required

References
1. Isaacs J. Treatment of acute peripheral nerve injuries: current concepts. *J Hand Surg Am* 2010;**35**(3):491–7.
2. Tung T, Mackinnon S. Nerve transfers: indications, techniques and outcomes. *J Hand Surg Am* 2010;**35**(2):332–41.

Skin biopsies

Description

Skin biopsies are performed when diagnosis/removal of a skin lesion is required. The tissue sample is sent to histopathology for analysis, with results usually available between 4 and 10 days. Although many specialties may carry out this procedure, depending on the size of the lesion, wound closure/reconstruction maybe required and hence is commonly performed by plastic surgeons.

There are three main types of skin biopsy: shave/curettage, incisional/punch, and excisional biopsies.

- A *shave/curettage biopsy* involves the removal of a small fragment of the lesion. A shave biopsy uses a scalpel, whereas a curettage biopsy uses a curette
- *Incisional biopsies* involve taking a full thickness skin sample together with underlying subcutaneous fat. They are commonly used to obtain diagnosis of pigmented, inflammatory, and neoplastic lesions. These biopsies maybe elliptical (where a scalpel is used) or cylindrical, termed a 'punch' biopsy (where a circular blade is employed)[1]
- *Excisional biopsies* involve removal of the entire lesion using a 1–3mm margin

Although biopsies are associated with a risk of misdiagnosis, the incidence of inaccurate microstaging and misdiagnosis is higher with shave and curretage biopsies due to the disruption of tissue morphology.[2] Excisional biopsies are therefore the recommended method of choice for most suspicious skin lesions.[3]

Depending on the size of the defect, direct closure or reconstruction using a local flap or skin graft. Once diagnosis is confirmed, further excision may be required.

Additional procedures that may become necessary

Local flap or split thickness skin grafting.
- Further excision/wide local excision if malignancy is detected
- Further investigations/procedures/treatment depending on staging if malignancy is detected

Benefits

- *Therapeutic*: remove lesion, reduce risk of disease progression, possible cure
- *Diagnostic*: identify lesion, aid staging of disease if malignant

Alternative procedures/conservative measures

- *Conservative*: regular monitoring of lesion. *Disadvantages*: if malignant, progression of disease may occur

Serious/frequently occurring risks

- *Common*: bleeding; swelling; pain; scar; prolonged wound healing, infection (local)
- *Occasional*: incomplete resection requiring further excision; misdiagnosis;[2] inaccurate microstaging; recurrence
- *Rare*: infection (systemic)

Blood transfusion necessary
• None

Type of anaesthesia/sedation
• Local anaesthesia
• If an STSG or local flap is required for closure, general anaesthesia or regional block may be used

Follow-up/need for further procedure
• Removal of sutures in 5–10 days depending on site (general practitioner/practice nurse)
• Review in outpatient clinic/referring practitioner with histology results within 2 weeks

References

1. Zuber T. Punch biopsy of the skin. *Am Fam Physician* 2002;**65**(6):1155–8, 1161–2, 1164.
2. Ng J, Swain S, Dowling J, et al. The impact of partial biopsy on histopathologic diagnosis of cutaneous melanoma: Experience of an Australian tertiary referral service. *Arch Dermatol* 2010;**146**(3):234–9.
3. National Comprehensive Cancer Network. NCCN Practice Guidelines in Oncology— V.2.2010. Melanoma. USA: National Comprehensive Cancer Network.

Huddersfield Health Staff Library
Royal Infirmary (PGMEC)
Lindley
Huddersfield
HD3 3EA

Skin cancer—standard surgical excision and Mohs' micrographic surgery

Description

Basal cell carcinomas are the most common type of skin cancer. Although they very rarely metastasize they cause local destruction of tissues, which may lead to serious disfigurement. There are more than a dozen subtypes (Fig. 13.5) with multiple treatment options available. Surgical excision and cryotherapy are the most common treatments.

For high-risk infiltrating or recurrent BCC, cases are often managed by a multidisciplinary team with a plastic surgeon, dermatologist, radiotherapist, and pathologists deciding the most appropriate treatment.

The standard techniques available are as follows:

- Surgical excision using a standard margin
- Mohs' micrographic surgery
- Techniques that do not obtain histological information:
  - Cryosurgery
  - Curettage and electrodessication
  - Radiotherapy
  - Chemotherapy
  - Photodynamic therapy
  - Carbon dioxide laser ablation

Standard surgical excision typically involves a 3–5mm margin, with the specimen sent for histopathological examination. Tumour clearance has been reported as 95% for well-defined lesions <2cm with a 4–5mm margin 5% requiring further resection. Recurrence rates have been reported as <2% at 5years.

Mohs' micrographic surgery (Fig. 13.6) is a staged resection with histological examination and mapping of the surgical margins. This guides the surgeon to resect and re-examine any incomplete margins. Chances of complete excision are increased and review of the literature has reported 5-year cure rates of up to 99% for primary BCCs and between 90% and 96% for recurrent disease.[1,2] It is thus the preferred treatment for high-risk infiltrating BCCs, recurrent BCCs, and BCC near lid margins.

The procedure may be performed as a day-case procedure over several hours or over a number of days.

Disadvantages of Mohs': labour intensive; time consuming; expensive. The defect is then closed primarily, using a local skin flap, skin graft or left to heal by wound contraction and epithelialization.

SCCs (Fig. 13.7) are the second most common form of skin cancer. They cause local destruction and may metastasize.

The standard treatment is surgical excision up to 1cm margin or Mohs' surgery and reconstruction of the defect. Adjuvant radiotherapy is occasionally required with aggressive subtypes in high-risk locations.

Management of lymph node metastasis is with surgical lymphadenectomy and or radiotherapy. Cases are normally managed in the multidisciplinary team setting. Chemotherapy is rarely used.

Melanomas (Fig. 13.8) are rarer skin cancers but have higher local recurrence rates. Tumours >1mm thickness more frequently metastasize.

Treatment is by surgical excision with 1–2cm margin and sentinel node biopsy or regular monitoring of the draining lymph nodes. Management of lymph node metastasis is with surgical lymphadenectomy and/or radiotherapy.

Cases are managed in the multidisciplinary team setting. Chemotherapy may be used in cases with metastases to organs.

Additional procedures that may become necessary

- Reconstruction of defect with skin graft, flap or regular dressings until healed
- Adjuvant radiotherapy
- Rarely chemotherapy

Benefits

- Excision of the tumour and histological examination

Alternative procedures/conservative measures

- *Conservative*: regular observation. *Disadvantages*: disease progression with progressive disfigurement and local destruction
- *Medical*:
  - Radiotherapy may be used as a primary treatment of some BCCs and SCCs in medically unfit patients or cases where resection is impossible or would be difficult to reconstruct. Cure rates have been shown to vary between ~84% and 96% (long-term >4-year results) for primary and recurrent BCCs. *Disadvantages*: expensive and thus typically limited areas with radiotherapy facilities. Higher recurrence rates compared with surgery (7.5% compared with 0.7% at 4 years, respectively); longer healing times; scarring/contractures; pain; dysaesthesia; pruritus; altered pigmentation and telangiectasia (in >65%); radiodystrophy (41% of patients), radionecrosis (5%); fistulae; inferior to surgery/Mohs'[2]
  - Topical chemotherapy such as imiquimod and 5-fluorouracil have reported up to 100% histological clearance in some subtypes of BCCs (such as small, primary, superficial BCCs, although results vary widely throughout the literature).[4] Chemotherapy may be used as an adjuvant therapy to surgery. *Disadvantages*: limited to certain subtypes only; prolonged administration; site reactions common: erythema, oedema, induration, erosion, scaling, crusting, hypopigmentation, pruritus, sensation of burning, paraesthesia, pain; distant reactions: erythema, fatigue, myalgia, arthralgia, lymphadenopathy; high recurrence rates (up to 20% at 2 years)
  - Photodynamic therapy[5]—topical methyl aminolevulinate (MAL) photodynamic therapy is a good treatment option for primary superficial BCCs, and has a reasonable role for primary, low-risk nodular BCCs, with good cosmetic results (89% having 'good or excellent' results) shown. In superficial BCCs, cure rates of 97% at 3 months with 22% recurrence at 48 months has been reported. It may be used in conjunction with other treatments such as curettage or when other modalities are inappropriate. *Disadvantages*: limited data on use; success varies greatly depending on subtype of BCC; repeated treatments; pain; crusting, erythema; inferior to surgery/Mohs'

- *Surgical*:
  - Curettage and electrodessication. Main role being for low-risk primary BCCs with overall cure rates of ~92.3% at 5 years. *Disadvantages*: unsuitable for high-risk and recurrent BCCs (cure rates for recurrent BCCs ~60% at 5 years)
  - Cryosurgery can be used for superficial lesions. High cure rates of ~99% at 5 years have been reported for low-risk BCCs. *Disadvantages*: no histological diagnosis; unsuitable for certain sites on face due to scarring
  - Carbon dioxide laser ablation is at present an uncommon treatment option for treatment of BCCs but may have a role in addition with curettage for large or multiple low-risk BCCs. Results have shown good cosmesis and fast healing times. *Disadvantages*: limited data[6]

Serious/frequently occurring risks

- *Common*: bleeding; pain; scarring; prolonged wound healing/dressings; wound infection
- *Occasional*: incomplete excision (with standard surgical excision); need for skin graft or local/random flap
- *Rare*: recurrence as noted

Blood transfusion necessary

- None/group and save

Type of anaesthesia/sedation

- Local/general anaesthesia

Follow-up/need for further procedure

- Removal of sutures in 10–14 days
- Within 2 weeks for histology results and wound check. This may be sooner if a flap is used

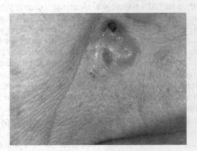

Fig. 13.5 Nodulocystic BCC.

Reproduced with permission from Burge S and Wallis O. *Oxford Handbook of Medical Dermatology*. 2011. Oxford: Oxford University Press, p.328, Figure 17.5.

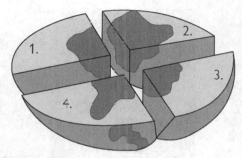

Fig. 13.6 Mohs' micrographic surgery.

Reproduced with permission from Kerawala C and Newlands C. *Oxford Specialist Handbook of Oral and Maxillofacial Surgery*. 2010. Oxford: Oxford University Press, p.154, Figure 3.3.

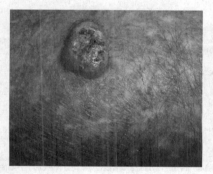

Fig. 13.7 Squamous cell carcinoma.

Reproduced with permission from Burge S and Wallis D. *Oxford Handbook of Medical Dermatology*. 2011. Oxford: Oxford University Press p.329, Figure 17.6.

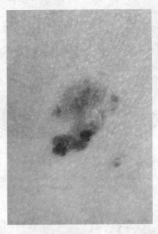

Fig. 13.8 Superficial spreading melanoma.

Reproduced with permission from Burge S and Wallis D. *Oxford Handbook of Medical Dermatology*. 2011. Oxford: Oxford University Press, p.331, Figure 17.7.

References

1. Smeets N, Kuijpers D, Nelemans P, *et al*. Mohs' micrographic surgery for treatment of basal cell carcinoma of the face-results of a retrospective study and review of the literature. *Br J Dermatol* 2004;**151**(1):141–7.
2. Telfer N, Colver G, Morton C. Guidelines for the management of basal cell carcinoma. *Br Assoc Dermatol* 2008;**159**(1):35.
3. Petit J, Avril M, Margulis A, *et al*. Evaluation of cosmetic results of a randomized trial comparing surgery and radiotherapy in the treatment of basal cell carcinoma of the face. *Plast Reconstr Surg* 2000;**105**:2544–51.
4. Beutner K, Geisse J, Helman D, *et al*. Therapeutic response of basal cell carcinoma to the immune response modifier imiquimod 5% cream. *J Am Acad Dermatol* 1999;**41**(6):1002–7.
5. Braathen L, Szeimies RM, Bassett-Seguin N, *et al*. Guidelines on the use of photodynamic therapy for nonmelanoma skin cancer: an international consensus. *J Am Acad Dermatol* 2007;**56**:125–43.
6. Campolmi P, Brazzini B, Urso C, *et al*. CO_2 laser treatment of basal cell carcinoma with intraoperative histopathologic and cytologic examination. *Dermatol Surg* 2002;**28**(10):909–11.

Skin grafts

Description

Skin grafting is the use of skin or skin substitutes to cover a defect where primary closure, secondary intension healing, or local flaps are unavailable or unsuitable. The two main types are: STSG and full thickness skin grafts (FTSGs) as determined by the presence of either partial or full thickness dermis, respectively (Fig. 13.9). Recent advances in manufacture of skin substitutes such as acellular dermal allografts are also available and may also be used, or used in conjunction with STSGs.[1]

- *STSGs*: broad range of potential uses; may be meshed to enable coverage of larger surface areas; potential for use in cavities and for mucosal deficits, resurfacing of muscle flaps and for postsurgical defects at high risk for tumour recurrence (where recurrent tumour may be visible beneath the STSG). As STSGs have less tissue requring revascularization than FTSGs, they may be used on almost any recipient, including those with limited vascularity. Their disadvantages, however, are their poor cosmetic result, owing to abnormal pigmentation (hypo/hyperpigmentation), lack of hair and bulk, abnormally smooth texture and shiny appearance; dryness (xerosis); fragility; limited durability with radiotherapy; greater graft contracture compared with FTSGs and inability to grow with the patient. In addition, the donor site, which heals by epithelialization, is often painful, dry, and cosmetically poor
- FTSGs: most commonly used for facial defects with better cosmetic results possible due to the greater potential for colour, texture and thickness matching. Such desired skin qualities must be carefully considered when choosing the donor site to allow for optimal matching, remembering that skin appendages are retained (hair/arrector pilli/sebaceous glands/sweat glands). FTSGs undergo less contraction during healing and are more likely to grow with the patient. Their main disadvantages are the requirement for well-vascularized, uncontaminated recipient beds and size limitation. Donor sites are typically closed primarily, although, rarely, they may be resurfaced with an STSG from another site

Procedure

The recipient bed is anaesthetized, cleaned and debrided where necessary and meticulous haemostasis achieved. Donor site for either STSG or FTSG harvest must be chosen and agreed on by both surgeon and patient.

STSGs may be taken from various sites, although most commonly the anteromedial thigh is used due to convenience of wound care and lack of interruption to ambulation. The skin is anaesthetized, cleaned and lubricated before being harvested using a hand or electrical dermatome (Fig. 13.10). The graft may be meshed before being applied to the recipient bed and fixed to the surrounding skin. This is then dressed for ~5 days. The donor site is dressed and normally left undisturbed for 10–14 days.

▶▶Meshing increases expansion ratios from 1:1 to up to 6:1 and allows for drainage of serosanguinous fluid thus improving graft survival, particularly useful in contaminated septic wounds. However, cosmesis is poorer with a 'pitted' appearance resulting.[2]

For FTSGs, the donor area is infiltrated with local anaesthesia and excised using a scalpel, closed directly and dressed. The graft is sutured into place and subdermal fat removed to allow better revascularization, normally with a tie over pressure dressing.

Patients must be counselled regarding fragility of the grafts and advised to avoid any excessive activity for 1–2 further weeks. Antibiotics may be given to patients at increased risk of infection, such as immunosuppressed or diabetic patients.

Additional procedures that may become necessary

- Application of VAC dressing—used to minimize shearing forces and fluid collection beneath the graft. If used, a non-adherent material must be placed in between the graft and VAC sponge

Benefits

- *Therapeutic*: cover defect; improve wound healing and cosmesis

Alternative procedures/conservative measures

- *Conservative*: wound healing via secondary-intention. *Disadvantages*: delayed/failure of wound healing; prolonged need for dressings; exposed muscle/soft tissue; infection (local/systemic); water and protein losses (in cases such as burns and ulcers); contracture (particularly problematic if over a joint)
- *Surgical*: flap reconstruction or use of skin substitutes. *Disadvantages*: limited by size

Serious/frequently occurring risks[3]

- *Common*: bleeding; seroma; poor cosmesis; pain; xerosis; graft contracture (greater with STSG than FTSG); poor mechanical durability; sensory disturbance/loss (temporary)
- *Occasional*: infection; incomplete graft take; breakdown of graft; hypertrophic scarring; contractures near free margins may cause cosmetic and/or functional problems (e.g. ectropion when grafts are near the eyelid)[4]
- *Rare*: complete failure of graft survival

Blood transfusion necessary

- None

Type of anaesthesia/sedation

- Local or general anaesthesia may be used, depending on the size and number of wounds

Follow-up/need for further procedure

- Outpatient wound (recipient and donor) review 5–7 and 10–14 days postoperatively
- Removal of sutures in 10–14 days
- If cosmesis is poor, topical treatments (e.g. using steroids), dermabrasion, laser resurfacing or progressive surgical excision may be performed[5]
- Surgical revision for correction of functional contractures may be required[5]

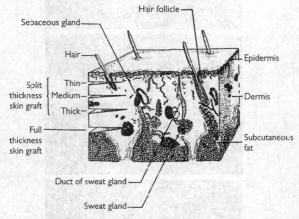

Fig. 13.9 Skin thickness for split-thickness skin grafts (STSG) and full-thickness skin grafts (FTSG).

Reproduced with permission from McLatchie GR and Leaper DJ. *Oxford Handbook of Operative Surgery* 2nd edition. 2006. Oxford: Oxford University Press, p.775, Figure 17.3.

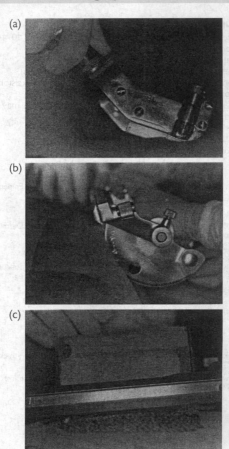

Fig. 13.10 Use of dermatomes for STSGs.

Reproduced with permission from McLatchie GR and Leaper DJ. *Oxford Handbook of Operative Surgery* 2nd edition. 2006. Oxford: Oxford University Press, p.777, Figure 17.4.

References

1. Andreassi A, Bilenchi R, Biagioli M, *et al.* Classification and pathophysiology of skin grafts. *Clin Dermatol* 2005;**23**(4):332–7.
2. Vandeput J, Nelissen M, Tanner J, *et al.* A review of skin meshers. *Burns* 1995;**21**(5):364–70.
3. Ratner D. Skin grafting. *Semin Cutan Med Surg* 2003;**22**(4):295–305.
4. Lutz M, Otley C, Roenigk R, *et al.* Reinnervation of flaps and grafts of the face. *Arch Dermatol* 1998;**134**(10):1271–4.
5. Brenner M, Perro C. Recontouring, resurfacing, and scar revision in skin cancer reconstruction. *Facial Plast Surg Clin North Am* 2009;**17**(3):469–87.e3.

Trigger finger release

Description

Trigger finger is caused by thickening of the flexor tendon impairing gliding within the pulley system. The tendon nodule impinges proximal or distal to the A-1 pulley, causing problems with extending or flexing the finger. Corticosteroid injections are usually the first-line treatment with 73–94% cure rates reported.[1] Splinting has also been shown to be effective with 70–73% success rates reported. Congenital nodules or those unresponsive to non-operative treatment, however, may require surgical release (60–97% cure rates reported).[2,3] Surgery involves either percutaneous or open release of the A-1 pulley, under local/regional/general anaesthesia. In percutaneous release, a small incision is made either using a needle/scalpel with no skin suturing required. Open procedures require a larger skin incision and skin closure but are generally accepted as safer. A dressing is applied. Antibiotics may be given.

Additional procedures that may become necessary
- Splinting

Benefits
- *Therapeutic*: improve mobility; reduce pain; increase grip strength
- *Diagnostic*: synovial tissue may be sent for histopathological examination; tendon gliding may be assessed

Alternative procedures/conservative measures
- *Conservative*: splinting. *Disadvantage*: no significant improvement in grip strength reported; heavily reliant on patient compliance
- *Surgical*: corticosteroid injections.[1] *Disadvantages* (although rare): infection; bleeding; steroid flare; hot flushes; fat atrophy; skin depigmentation; tendon rupture; nerve/vessel damage

Serious/frequently occurring risks[2–4]
- *Common*: bleeding; pain; scarring
- *Occasional*: infection; bowstringing; digital nerve injury; stiffness (~16% for both percutaneous and open release); paraesthesia
- *Rare*: continued/recurrence of triggering (~1% and 2% for percutaneous and open release, respectively); synovial fistula

Blood transfusion necessary
- None/group and save

Type of anaesthesia/sedation
- Local/regional/general anaesthesia

Follow-up/need for further procedure
- Removal of sutures in 10–14 days
- Routine outpatient review

References

1. Peters-Veluthamaningal C, Winters J, Groenier K, *et al.* Corticosteroid injections effective for trigger finger in adults in general practice: a double-blind randomized placebo controlled trial. *Ann Rheum Dis* 2008;**67**(9):1262–6.

2. Dierks U, Hoffmann R, Meek M. Open versus percutaneous release of the A1-pulley for stenosing tenovaginitis: a prospective randomized trial. *Tech Hand Up Extrem Surg* 2008;**12**(3):183–7.

3. Gilberts E, Wereldsma J. Long-term results of percutaneous and open surgery for trigger fingers and thumbs. *Int Surg* 2002;**87**(1):48–52.

4. Will R, Lubahn J. Complications of open trigger finger release. *J Hand Surg Am* 2010;**35**(4):594–6.

Wound exploration, debridement, repair ± closure

Description

Traumatic wounds can occur with burns, crush injuries and sharp lacerations, and may be clean or contaminated. They often require exploration and debridement, repair or reconstruction of underlying structures and closure of the wound. Wound closure may be either immediate or once infection has been eradicated. Estimation of the extent of damage to vital tissues should be made by preoperative examination. The type of repair and reconstruction should be predicted and the patient informed of the possibility of multiple debridements depending on degree of tissue damage or contamination.

Procedure

Wound extension may be necessary and allows for exploration and repair of damaged structures. In some cases tissue that is contaminated, necrotic, or infected may need to be removed and sent for microscopy, culture, and sensitivity analysis. Following debridement, the appropriate structures are repaired or reconstructed. 🕮 See 'Additional procedures that may become necessary', p.417.

The wound is then either closed appropriately or packed with saline gauze or a vacuum-assisted dressing ± applied. A drain may be inserted. Final closure is planned which may be performed in stages following further debridements or dressing changes.

The patient may be given broad-spectrum antibiotics, particularly for contaminated wounds or where infection may have devastating consequences, e.g. where potential extens on to central nervous system, orbit, hand, etc. exists. If necrotizing infection is suspected, immediate involvement of ITU, anaesthetic team, and microbiology is required.

Additional procedures that may become necessary

- Repair of damaged structures
  - Nerves—🕮 see 'Peripheral nerve repair', p.402
  - Tendons—🕮 see 'Flexor tendon repair', p.390/'Extensor tendon repair', p.389
  - Vascular injures—primary repair or vascular grafts
  - Prophylactic compartment release (particularly for reperfusion injuries)

Benefits

- *Diagnostic*: explore wound to assess injury
- *Therapeutic*: reduce risk of infection, assist functional recovery and close wounds (not always immediately)

Alternative procedures/conservative measures

- *Conservative*: healing by secondary intension (repeat dressings and debridement) with or without antibiotics. *Disadvantages*: continuing damage to local structures; infection (local/systemic); chronic pain; poor functional recovery; delayed/failed wound healing; poor cosmesis

Serious/frequently occurring risks

- *Common*: minor bleeding (unless arterial repair); hypertrophic scars; itching and tenderness; infection (local/systemic); delayed wound healing or wound breakdown, requiring repeat dressing changes and/or debridement
- *Occasional*: further surgery (depending largely on wound type, initial injuries and any repairs performed); damage to surrounding soft tissues/structures; ischaemia if vascular injury present
- *Rare*: amputation; overwhelming infection; fatality (in the case of necrotizing infection and some streptococcal infections)

Blood transfusion necessary

- None/group and save/cross-match (dependent on wound type/ severity—e.g. with necrotizing fasciitis; significant trauma/burns). Depends on expected blood loss with debridement

Type of anaesthesia/sedation

- Local, regional, or general anaesthesia may be used depending on size, severity, location, and type of wound(s)

Follow-up/need for further procedure

- Removal of sutures in 10–14 days
- Dependent on wound type/findings/any repairs or other procedures performed
- Simple wound explorations and debridement may only require removal of sutures/change of dressings by practice/district nurse
- Patients with large or complicated wounds or those in whom repairs of any underlying structures or additional procedures were performed may remain in hospital until wounds are closed or require outpatient review and rehabilitation
- Scar, nerve, tendon, or vascular injuries may require secondary surgery

Ear, nose, and throat surgery

Adenoidectomy

Description

The adenoids are a mucosa-associated lymphoid tissue (MALT) located in the roof of the nasopharynx. They are problematic primarily in childhood when repeated upper respiratory tract infections cause hypertrophy, resulting in difficulty with nose breathing. This is less of an issue in adults where the respiratory tract is relatively larger. Indications for adenoidectomy include nasal obstruction causing mouth breathing or snoring, obstructive sleep apnoea (OSA), and glue ear (exacerbated by blockage of the eustachian tube orifices by the adenoids).

During the procedure the patient is supine with shoulder bolsters and a head ring, allowing examination of the nasopharynx under direct vision using a laryngeal mirror and digital palpation of the adenoidal pad and palate to check for submucous cleft palate. The adenoids are removed either with a blade or suction diathermy until a clear view of the posterior choanae is achieved and taking care to avoid damaging the eustachian tube cushions. Haemostasis is achieved with a combination of pressure applied with swabs and diathermy.

Mode of anaesthesia/sedation
• General anaesthesia

Intended benefits
• Improving nose breathing and reducing snoring
• Treatment of OSA
• Treatment of glue ear

Additional procedures that may become necessary
• Often undertaken simultaneously with tonsillectomy and/or grommet insertion if indicated

Alternative procedures/conservative measures
• Conservative management: watch and wait—especially in children whose symptoms may improve with age
  • *Pros*: avoids surgery
  • *Cons*: unlikely to be successful, delays treatment, and prolongs duration of symptoms

Serious/frequently occurring complications
• *Occasional*: primary haemorrhage (within 24h, <1% incidence—this may be even lower with diathermy techniques), infection of the adenoid bed and subsequent offensive breath (usually at 7–10 days postoperatively), pain, damage to teeth
• *Rare*: secondary haemorrhage (after 24h). Velopharyngeal insufficiency (occurs 1 in 3000 cases): fluid or air escapes into the nasopharynx resulting in difficulties with speech (rhinolalia aperta, i.e. nasal voice) and swallowing. Risk is increased for patients with craniofacial deformity such as cleft palate. Adenoidectomy is therefore traditionally not performed in individuals with cleft palate although there is evidence[1]

that partial adenoidectomy may yield symptomatic relief while avoiding adverse effects on the voice. These patients should be referred to specialist centres
- *Very rare*: nasopharyngeal stenosis due to scarring in the adenoid bed

Blood transfusion necessary
- Not usually required
- Consider group and save in children

Follow-up/need for further procedure
- Usually no follow-up unless procedure performed for glue ear or OSA, then review at 2–3 months

Reference
1. Tweedie DJ, Skilbeck CJ, Wyatt ME, et al. Partial adenoidectomy by suction diathermy in children with cleft palate to avoid velopharyngeal insufficiency. *Int J Pediatr Otorhinolaryngol* 2009;**73**(11):1594–7.

Huddersfield Health Staff Library
Royal Infirmary (PGMEC)
Lindley
Huddersfield
HD3 3EA

Cervical lymph node biopsy

Description

Cervical lymph nodes should be managed in the setting of an established neck lump clinic, which will have dedicated clinical, radiological, and histopathological resources. Fine needle aspiration (often ultrasound-guided) must be performed first to exclude SCC, which has a high risk of seeding to the skin during excision biopsy, and, therefore, requires a different pathway of care.

Once this has been done, cervical lymph node biopsy ± panendoscopy can be arranged. Primarily a diagnostic procedure, cervical lymph node biopsy may involve either partial or complete excision of a superficial node. While complete excision should always be attempted and is preferable, this may be precluded by local infiltration of surrounding tissue.

Patients will usually present with a lump in the neck that may or may not be associated with other head and neck symptoms, e.g. hoarse voice. The node is excised through as small an incision as practicable to leave minimal scarring.

Mode of anaesthesia/sedation

- Local anaesthesia for small, superficial nodes
- General anaesthesia for large or deep nodes or those suspected of local infiltration

Intended benefits

- This is a diagnostic procedure necessary to plan further treatment

Additional procedures that may become necessary

- None

Alternative procedures/conservative measures

- An appropriate work-up is mandatory as described, such that a combination of the relevant imaging ± panendoscopy may preclude the need for lymph node biopsy whilst providing sufficient diagnostic information for definitive treatment to be planned. This will depend on the patient's symptoms/presentation

Serious/frequently occurring risks/complications

- *Common*: scarring (including higher risk of wound hypertrophy/keloid in patients with dark skin)
- *Rare*: neurovascular damage. The location of the lymph node, its depth and whether it is infiltrating adjacent tissue will determine the structures at risk:
  - Anterior triangle: carotid sheath and branches of external carotid, internal and external jugular veins, anterior jugular vein, retromandibular vein, vagus nerve, hypoglossal nerve, ansa cervicalis *nerve, nerve to mylohyoid, thyroid and parathyroid glands,* submandibular gland, larynx, trachea, oesophagus

- Posterior triangle: occipital artery, suprascapular artery, superficial cervical artery, external jugular vein, suprascapular vein, transverse cervical vein, spinal root of the accessory nerve, branches of cervical plexus

Blood transfusion necessary

- Not usually required
- Group and save may be required based on local policy

Follow-up/need for further procedure

- Follow up in 10–14 days to discuss histopathology

Combined approach tympanoplasty

Description

Cholesteatoma is an overgrowth of epithelium into a cavity/retraction pocket in the tympanic membrane. This gradually expands into the middle ear and mastoid cavity, eroding the ossicular chain, mastoid air cells, and, in severe cases, into the inner ear.

The middle ear is accessed via a postauricular or endaural (anterior) incision and through the external auditory canal (EAC) by reflection of the tympanic membrane. The cholesteatoma is meticulously removed, taking care to avoid damage to the surrounding structures. The mastoid air cells are eradicated using a drill with progressively smaller burrs to leave a single large mastoid cavity, while preserving the posterior wall of the EAC. The incision is closed and the tympanic membrane replaced and the EAC packed with bismuth iodoform paraffin paste (BIPP)-soaked gauze. This is left in place until follow-up.

Mode of anaesthesia/sedation

- General anaesthesia

Intended benefits

- Clearance of the cholesteatoma and prevention of further disease progression which may result in:
  - Hearing loss
  - Vertigo
  - Tinnitus
  - Chronic ear discharge
  - Facial nerve palsy
- Combined approach tympanoplasty (CAT) may also rarely be performed for placement of a middle ear hearing aid or cochlear implant and severe otitis media

Additional procedures that may become necessary

- Second-look combined approach tympanoplasty to ensure no recurrence of cholesteatoma. The development of high-resolution CT and diffusion-weighted MRI (dwMRI), which can detect minute amounts of cholesteatoma (as little as 2mm diameter in the case of dwMRI) may avoid the need for second-look CAT in the future

Alternative procedures/conservative measures

- Alternatives: atticotomy, attico-antrostomy, small cavity mastoidectomy, modified radical mastoidectomy, radical mastoidectomy, extended modified radical mastoidectomy
- Once the presence of cholesteatoma is established, surgical intervention becomes necessary to prevent extensive damage to the ossicular chain and, eventually, the inner ear if left unchecked. Rarely, patients with high general anaesthetic risk may be managed with suction clearance of as much cholesteatoma as possible and topical antibiotics; however, the disease will inevitably progress

Serious/frequently occurring risks/complications

- Common: recurrence, blood stained auricular discharge (this is not necessarily infective in origin)
- Occasional: wound infection
- Rare: iatrogenic damage of the ossicular chain and hearing loss, vertigo, tinnitus, facial nerve palsy, loss of taste in the tongue, meningitis, cerebral abscess

Blood transfusion necessary

- Not required

Follow-up/need for further procedure

- Follow-up after 2 weeks for removal of the BIPP packs and examination
- Audiometry at 6 weeks
- The patient should not drive for 48h (longer if dizziness persists)
- They should keep the ear dry for 3 months and not fly until advised to do so at review (the exact length of time will vary based on local policy)

Examination of ears and aural toilet

Description
Aural toilet is undertaken for impacted wax that is causing pain and/or hearing loss. It may also be performed in cases of moderate to severe otitis externa where infected debris and discharge is occluding the EAC and impeding the access of topical treatment.

Access to the EAC is gained using an aural speculum and the wax/debris removed using a combination of microsuction, wax hooks, and crocodile forceps. The entire EAC is cleared and examined, taking care to look into the attic for any hidden debris.

Mode of anaesthesia/sedation
- The majority of adults and older children will be able to tolerate this procedure without any anaesthesia/sedation. As such it is usually carried out in the outpatients department
- Most young children and some adults/older children will require general anaesthesia

Intended benefits
- Removal of ear wax
- Reduction of pain
- Improved hearing
- Treatment of otitis externa
- Excision of EAC lesions, e.g. aural polyps

Additional procedures that may become necessary
- Removal of ear wax
- Treatment of otitis externa
- Excision of EAC lesions, e.g. aural polyps

Alternative procedures/conservative measures
- For wax impaction, softening with olive oil/sodium bicarbonate ear drops is an option but has usually been tried before aural toilet is considered

Serious/frequently occurring risks/complications
- *Common*: recurrence of otitis externa, recurrence of wax impaction, trauma to the EAC, which may require a course of ear drops to prevent superimposed infection
- *Rare*: iatrogenic rupture of the tympanic membrane

Blood transfusion necessary
- Not required

Follow-up/need for further procedure
- Usually no follow-up is required unless the case of otitis externa is extremely severe, in which case the patient may already be an inpatient
- Some patients will require aural toilet at 6-monthly intervals if impaction of wax is recurrent

Functional endoscopic sinus surgery

Description

The paranasal sinuses drain via the osteomeatal complex (OMC) (Fig. 14.1). Blockage of the OMC by chronic rhinosinusitis or sinu-nasal polyposis results in symptoms of nasal blockage (difficulty breathing, poor sense of smell and facial pressure). Functional endoscopic sinus surgery (FESS) aims to remove the blockage of the OMC and restore the function of this key area in draining the sinuses. Preoperative CT sinuses (which includes essential coronal views) is mandatory before FESS is performed. Patients with chronic/recurrent sinusitis should also have allergen investigation with skin prick or radioallergosorbent test (RAST) testing.

Mode of anaesthesia/sedation

- General anaesthesia

Intended benefits

- Restore the function of the OMC. Benefits may include:
  - Reduction of nasal obstruction
  - Improved sense of smell
  - Excision of sinu-nasal polyps

Additional procedures that may become necessary

- Septoplasty may also be necessary in cases where nasal septal deviation contributes to nasal obstruction

Alternative procedures/conservative measures

- FESS becomes an option usually when non-surgical intervention has failed. Most individuals requiring FESS will already have undergone medical treatment with topical steroids, systemic antihistamines, antibiotics, and saline douching

Serious/frequently occurring risks/complications

- *Common*: bleeding, infection, recurrence of sinu-nasal polyposis
- *Rare*: cerebrospinal fluid leak (0.2%). Intrusion into the orbit and damage to its contents via the lamina papyracea. Orbital haematoma. Optic nerve damage. Anosmia

Blood transfusion necessary

- Not usually required
- Group and save

Follow-up/need for further procedure

- The patient should undergo a regimen of nasal douching three to four times a day for 2 weeks (there are many commercial brands available, e.g. SinuRinse™, Sterimar™)
- Postoperative antibiotics may be necessary, particularly when infected sinus contents are evacuated
- Patients should be followed up at 6–8 weeks for review of symptoms (and sooner if they have heavy intranasal crusting postoperatively)

- Patients should be aware that ongoing treatment with topical steroids or systemic antihistamines may still be necessary postoperatively (especially in cases of allergic rhinitis)

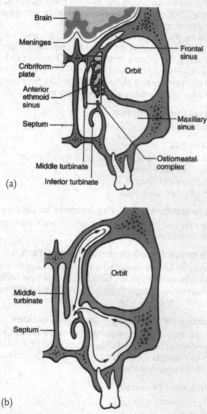

Fig. 14.1 The OMC (a) before and (b) after FESS.

Reproduced with permission from Corbridge R and Steventon N. *Oxford Handbook of ENT and Head and Neck Surgery* 2nd edition. 2010. Oxford: Oxford University Press, p.163, Figure 6.4.

Grommet insertion

Description

Certain middle ear disease warrants grommet (ventilation tube) insertion (Fig. 14.2). This is mainly glue ear/persistent middle ear effusion. Children who will benefit are those with bilateral glue ear documented for 3 months or more and with a hearing loss in the better ear of 25–30dB or worse (averaged over 0.5, 1, 2, and 4kHz).[1] A radial incision is made with a myringotome in the anteroinferior segment of the eardrum and a grommet (or tympanostomy tube) inserted. Any excess middle ear effusion is aspirated. If bleeding occurs, non-ototoxic ear drops are inserted to prevent blockage. The grommet allows for pressure equilibration in the middle ear, and in cases of glue ear compensates for the poorly functioning eustachian tube. The procedure is usually performed in children (80% of whom will experience glue ear). Preoperative tympanometry and audiometry should be performed at least within 3 months of surgery to confirm the need and to establish baseline hearing.

Mode of anaesthesia/sedation

- Can be performed under general or local anaesthesia. Local anaesthesia is usually reserved for adult patients or those in whom general anaesthetic poses a risk (local anaesthetic cream is applied under the microscope, left for 1h then removed using microsuction)

Intended benefits

- Resolve symptoms of persistent middle ear effusion (primarily hearing loss) and prevent progression of disease

Additional procedures that may become necessary

- Adenoidectomy and/or tonsillectomy—performed concomitantly—if there is evidence of adenoidal or tonsillar hypertrophy causing obstruction of the eustachian tube within the nasopharynx

Alternative procedures/conservative measures

- *Conservative*: all patients should undergo a period of at least 3 months watchful waiting. 50% of cases will resolve spontaneously within 3 months. Any evidence of progression of disease as listed however, warrants that surgery be expedited

Serious/frequently occurring risks/complications

- This is generally an uncomplicated procedure. Evidence of an infected effusion intraoperatively may warrant a course of antibiotic and steroid ear drops. The risks of chronic (particularly infected) and persistent middle ear effusion far outweigh those of grommet insertion
- *Rare*: a persistent eardrum perforation after the grommet is extruded. This would require surgical repair

Blood transfusion necessary

- Not required

Follow-up/need for further procedure
- Check of grommets and audiometry at 6–8 weeks
- No swimming for 6 weeks postoperatively but thereafter swimming is permitted, provided there is no underwater diving
- Prevent dirty or soapy water entering the ear with Vaseline-coated cotton balls ± a shower cap
- It is fine to fly with grommets
- Grommets do not need to be removed and most will be extruded after 6–9 months

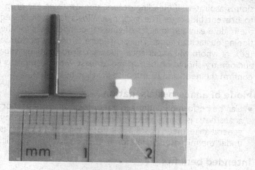

Fig. 14.2 Ventilation tubes: Richards T-tube (left), Shah grommet (centre), Shah mini-grommet (right).

Reference
1. ENT UK. *OME (Glue ear)/Adenoid and Grommet: Position Paper*. ENT UK 2009. Available at: ☞ www.entuk.org (accessed 4 May 2011).

Laryngectomy

Description

Laryngectomy is performed in general for large T3/4 laryngeal tumours (25–60% 5-year survival rate). Smaller T1/2 tumours (80% 5-year survival rate) are usually treated with external beam radiotherapy or with endoscopic laser surgery.

In a total laryngectomy the larynx is excised and the trachea brought out as a stoma to the skin (Fig. 14.3). The pharynx is repaired to conserve the swallowing mechanism. Many varied forms of partial laryngectomy have also been described but the procedure of consent and the risks and benefits associated are similar so only total laryngectomy will be addressed here. Total laryngectomy may also be performed for a dysfunctional larynx (e.g. post-radiotherapy) where airway protection is compromised and the risks of aspiration, subsequent infection, and death are great.

Mode of anaesthesia/sedation
- General anaesthesia

Intended benefits
- Treat laryngeal cancer
- Prevent aspiration

Additional procedures that may become necessary
- Neck dissection in patients with nodal metastases
- Postoperative radiotherapy

Alternative procedures/conservative measures
- Radiotherapy is an alternative option for some T3 tumours. In these cases surgery is held in reserve should radiotherapy fail
- Chemotherapy may also be an option but only as an adjunct to either radiotherapy or surgery

Serious/frequently occurring risks/complications
- *Common complications*: bleeding, pharyngo-cutaneous fistula
- *Major risks*: cardiovascular complications, DVT/pulmonary embolism, chest infection, myocardial infarction, flap failure, inability to vocalize, death

Blood transfusion necessary
- Cross-match 4 units

Follow-up/need for further procedure
- The patient should expect to be in hospital for up to 10–14 days should all go to plan. However, potential complications are numerous and many patients will have a longer inpatient stay. The following needs to be addressed during this time:
  - Immediately postoperatively most patients should be cared for in an HDU or ITU
  - Thromboembolic prophylaxis
  - Early mobilization and chest physiotherapy

- Postoperative assessment by the speech and language therapy team
- Ensure adequate nutrition and electrolyte levels. The dietetics team should be involved immediately postoperatively as the patient will initially require enteral feeding
- Broad-spectrum antibiotics (usually for first 72h postoperatively only)
- Early removal of central and peripheral lines once patient tolerating oral intake
- Removal of urinary catheter once patient is mobilizing
- Flap observation and monitor for pressure sores. Should the flap fail a further free muscle flap may be necessary (e.g. pectoralis major)

- A unique postoperative consideration for laryngectomy is that the patient will be unable to vocalize. They should be provided with pen/pencil and paper immediately postoperatively to account for this. Voice restoration post-laryngectomy can be achieved in a number of ways, all of which involve inducing vibration of the pharyngo-oesophageal segment:
  - Tracheo-oesophageal puncture (TOP): primary puncture is usually done (i.e. at the time of laryngectomy), but secondary puncture is an alternative. A one-way TOP valve is inserted. The patient occludes the tracheostoma, air enters the pharynx via the valve, thereby causing the necessary vibration
  - Oesophageal speech: air is swallowed into the stomach then expelled to cause vibration of the pharyngo-oesophageal segment. Not all patients are able to do this
  - Artificial larynx (e.g. Servox™): in this situation, the source of vibration is external and applied to the neck to cause vibration of the pharynx. The quality of voice is less natural but can still result in effective communication

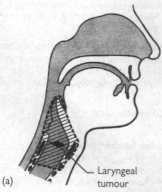

(a)   Laryngeal tumour

Fig. 14.3 *Difference between anatomy in* laryngectomy and tracheostomy: (a) normal anatomy (shaded area is excised in laryngectomy), (b) post-laryngectomy anatomy, (c) post-tracheostomy anatomy.

Reproduced with permission from Corbridge R and Steventon N. *Oxford Handbook of ENT and Head and Neck Surgery* 2nd edition. 2010. Oxford: Oxford University Press, p.227, Figure 12.5 and p.241, Figure 12.14.

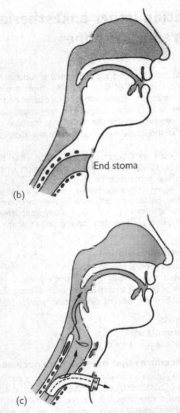

Fig. 14.3 *(Contd.)* Difference between anatomy in laryngectomy and tracheostomy: (a) normal anatomy (shaded area is excised in laryngectomy), (b) post-laryngectomy anatomy, (c) post-tracheostomy anatomy.

Reproduced with permission from Corbridge R and Steventon N. *Oxford Handbook of ENT and Head and Neck Surgery* 2nd edition. 2010. Oxford: Oxford University Press, p.227, Figure 12.5 and p.241, Figure 12.14.

Manipulation under anaesthesia of fractured nasal bones

Description

The left and right nasal bones are prominently embossed on the face. As a result, approximately half of facial bone fractures are nasal fractures. Injury results in distraction, fragmentation, depression, or any combination of these of either or both nasal bones. This may cause nasal obstruction and/or aesthetic compromise for the patient. At the time of injury a nasal septal haematoma should be excluded before the patient is sent home with analgesia.

The patient should then be assessed 5–7 days after the injury once swelling is reduced to decide whether manipulation under anaesthesia is necessary and the procedure performed within 2 weeks (maximum 3 weeks) of the injury before the bones set in their fractured positions. The bones are manipulated digitally and/or using instruments to restore them to their prior alignment (a pre-injury photograph may prove useful). The use of nasal splints is dependent on the unit in which you work and is not universal.

Mode of anaesthesia/sedation

- 0–14 years: always general anaesthesia
- Older than 14 years: depending on your unit's practice, reduction under local and/or general anaesthesia may be offered. Both have been shown as efficacious in providing a good outcome for patients[1]

Intended benefits

- Reduce nasal obstruction
- Improve aesthetic appearance of the nose

Additional procedures that may become necessary

- Nasal septum deviation is common with nasal injury and is a more common cause of nasal obstruction. Patients should be advised prior to manipulation under anaesthesia, therefore, that their nasal obstruction may persist and septoplasty/septo-rhinoplasty may be necessary in the future. They should wait up to 3 months to assess whether the obstruction is problematic enough to warrant surgery, and in young children it should be advised to delay septoplasty till the age of 17. This is because the nose continues to grow and early surgery may cause further aesthetic and functional problems
- Nasal packing for excessive bleeding

Alternative procedures/conservative measures

- No treatment—if the aesthetic appearance of the broken nose and/or any nasal obstruction is not problematic for the patient

Serious/frequently occurring risks/complications

Some pain and minor bleeding is to be expected. Patients should be warned preoperatively that an inadequate postoperative result (either aesthetic or functional) may result

Blood transfusion necessary

- Not usually required

Follow-up/need for further procedure

- No routine follow up. The patient should avoid contact sport for 3–4 weeks
- As mentioned, repeat manipulation under anaesthesia or, more likely septo-rhinoplasty, may be necessary

Reference

1. Atighechi S, Baradaranfar MH, Akbari SA. Reduction of nasal bone fractures: a comparative study of general, local, and topical anesthesia techniques. *J Craniofac Surg* 2009;**20**(2):382–4.

Modified radical mastoidectomy

Description

This is an alternative treatment for cholesteatoma to CAT. The attic cholesteatoma is cleared as in CAT, however, in this instance the head of the malleus and incus are also removed. The mastoid antrum and its air cells are obliterated and a mastoid cavity formed by removing the posterior wall of the ear canal, thus connecting the giant mastoid air cell to the outer world. The common cavity is packed with BIPP soaked gauze.

Mode of anaesthesia/sedation
- General anaesthesia

Intended benefits
- Clearance of the cholesteatoma and prevention of further disease progression which may result in:
  - Hearing loss
  - Vertigo
  - Tinnitus
  - Chronic ear discharge
  - Facial nerve palsy

Additional procedures that may become necessary
- None

Alternative procedures/conservative measures
- Combined approach tympanoplasty, atticotomy, attico-antrostomy, small cavity mastoidectomy, radical mastoidectomy, extended modified radical mastoidectomy

Serious/frequently occurring risks/complications
- *Common*: wound infection
- *Rare*: hearing loss, vertigo, tinnitus, chronic ear discharge, vertigo, loss of taste in the tongue, meningitis, brain abscess

Blood transfusion necessary
- Not required

Follow-up/need for further procedure
- Follow up at 2 weeks for removal of BIPP packing and examination
- Audiometry at 6 weeks
- The patient should not drive for 48h (longer if dizziness persists)
- The patient should keep the ear dry and not fly until advised by their specialist at review
- Mastoid cavities often require long-term toileting as they can accumulate debris or chronically discharge

Myringoplasty

Description

This procedure is performed to repair persistent perforations in the eardrum. Most perforations are small and heal spontaneously after 4–6 weeks, those that do not may require myringoplasty. If there is additional damage to the contents of the middle ear (e.g. ossicular chain) then the procedure to repair these is called tympanoplasty. Only myringoplasty is addressed here. The eardrum is approached via either a postauricular or endaural incision. A piece of graft tissue (usually temporalis fascia) is harvested, the eardrum elevated, and the graft placed underneath the eardrum. The eardrum is replaced and the ear canal packed with BIPP soaked gauze to hold it in place.

Mode of anaesthesia/sedation

- General anaesthesia

Intended benefits

- Prevent repeated middle ear infections
- Improve any hearing loss

Additional procedures that may become necessary

- It may become evident intraoperatively that tympanoplasty is required

Alternative procedures/conservative measures

- Watchful waiting should have been tried for at least 4 weeks before surgery is considered

Serious/frequently occurring risks/complications

- *Common*: Blood-stained, pink aural discharge is common and expected. If this becomes profuse, yellow/green in colour, offensive in smell and if pain increases this is evidence of wound infection and antibiotics are required. Failure of the graft may also occur (20% risk in the UK)
- *Rare*: Facial nerve palsy (temporary or permanent), worsening of any hearing loss

Blood transfusion necessary

- Not required

Follow-up/need for further procedure

- Follow-up at 2 weeks for removal of ear packing and examination
- Audiometry at 6 weeks

Oesophagoscopy and foreign body removal

Description

A foreign body (usually a food bolus) may become lodged in the oesophagus. The patient presents in distress, with pain, the sensation of an obstruction and unable to swallow their own saliva. Obstruction occurs most commonly at sites of normal anatomical narrowing of the oesophagus. These are at the level of cricopharyngeus at the thoracic inlet, at the level of the carina, and at the gastro-oesophageal junction. The first of these is the most common and that with which ENT surgeons are concerned. During the procedure a rigid oesophagoscope is inserted, the foreign body removed with endoscopic instruments, and the whole oesophagus examined for evidence of perforation or further foreign bodies.

Mode of anaesthesia/sedation

- Always performed under general anaesthesia

Intended benefits

- Removal of foreign body
- Prevent aspiration of saliva in a patient unable to swallow

Additional procedures that may become necessary

- None

Alternative procedures/conservative measures

- *Surgical:* removal within 24h is mandatory if the suspected foreign body is sharp e.g. chicken/fish bone
- *Conservative:* should always be attempted first if it is a soft food bolus and the patient is stable. This involves:
  - Keeping the patient calm and ensuring their airway is secure
  - Telling them to spit out any saliva and not to attempt to swallow it
  - Trying to shift the foreign body by encouraging the patient to drink a carbonated drink under observation, e.g. a cola
  - Giving an intravenous smooth muscle relaxant (e.g. hyoscine (Buscopan®) 20mg)—this can be repeated once if there is no improvement after 20–30min
  - Giving an intravenous anxiolytic (e.g. diazepam 5mg)—this should be in an environment with resuscitation equipment at hand such as A&E majors

Serious/frequently occurring risks/complications

- *Common:* minor bleeding, short-lived pain, damage to teeth, temporo-mandibular joint dislocation
- *Rare:* oesophageal perforation and possible mediastinal infection

Blood transfusion necessary
- Not usually required

Follow-up/need for further procedure
- Usually no formal follow-up
- Patients who have had several episodes of oesophageal foreign body should be investigated with barium swallow

Ossiculoplasty

Description

The ossicular chain consists of the malleus, incus, and stapes. It is the mechanism by which sound is conducted and amplified from the eardrum to the inner ear via the footplate of the stapes, which sits in the oval window. Any surgery to alter the configuration of the ossicular chain is known as ossiculoplasty. This may be done in conjunction with surgery to the eardrum (myringoplasty), in which case the procedure is known as a tympanoplasty.

Ossiculoplasty may take several forms but is primarily used in three types of pathology.

Cholesteatoma

It is commonly performed as part of a CAT or modified radical mastoidectomy (MRM), when parts of the ossicular chain have been damaged by the disease and have to be removed along with the cholesteatoma.

Otosclerosis

Stapedectomy is another form of ossiculoplasty and is a surgical treatment for otosclerosis (an osseous dyscrasia of the temporal bone that causes spongiotic then sclerotic changes, which affect the annular ligament and footplate of the stapes, causing gradual fixation and therefore progressive hearing loss). In stapedectomy the stapes is removed and replaced with a prosthesis that restores the conductive function of the ossicular chain.

Ossicular disruption as a result of trauma

Trauma to the head or ear may cause disruption of the ossicular chain and result in conductive hearing loss. In these situations ossicular reconstruction may become necessary after haemotympanum and middle ear effusion/blood are excluded. High-resolution CT of the temporal bone in suspected otosclerosis or ossicular chain disruption will reveal the pathology.

Mode of anaesthesia/sedation

- Usually under general anaesthesia. However, stapedectomy is often performed under local anaesthesia with sedation—the benefit being that the effect of the procedure on hearing can be assessed intraoperatively

Intended benefits

- Improve conductive hearing loss

Additional procedures that may become necessary

- None

Alternative procedures/conservative measures

- Cholesteatoma: combined approach tympanoplasty aims to preserve the ossicular chain. However, certain cholesteatomas will warrant MRM, e.g. attic cholesteatoma, as the ossicular chain has already become involved with the disease and should be removed to minimize risk of recurrence
- Otosclerosis: some patients may choose to have no treatment, a hearing aid is also a conservative option and surgery should only be tried after a hearing aid has been trialled for at least 3 months
- Trauma: immediately following the injury there will be haemotympanum and associated hearing loss. This should be allowed to settle over 6 weeks and the patient reviewed with tympanogram to assess for middle ear effusion/blood. If these are excluded then high-resolution CT of the temporal bones should first be performed to assess the exact nature of the disruption. Surgery should not be rushed into

Serious/frequently occurring risks/complications

- No improvement in hearing, facial nerve palsy, worsening of hearing, vertigo or dizziness, tinnitus, extrusion of prosthesis, a dead ear, scarring (postauricular or endaural), taste disturbance

Blood transfusion necessary

- Not required

Follow-up/need for further procedure

- Follow-up at 2 weeks for removal of aural BIPP dressings
- Follow-up at 6 weeks with audiometry

Panendoscopy and biopsy

Description

Pandendoscopy comprises direct pharyngoscopy, direct oesophagoscopy, and direct laryngoscopy. It is performed when evidence of malignancy is found in the larynx, oesophagus, or pharynx or if there is suspicion of malignancy in a patient with enlarged cervical lymph nodes and with risk factors, e.g. smoking, excess alcohol. The relevant scopes are inserted through the mouth and the structures carefully examined visually along with manual palpation of the tongue base and tonsils. If suspicious lesions are discovered, biopsies (usually three separate samples of each lesion) are done. It is, therefore, usually a diagnostic procedure.

Mode of anaesthesia/sedation

- General anaesthesia

Intended benefits

- Diagnostic

Additional procedures that may become necessary

- None

Alternative procedures/conservative measures

- None

Serious/frequently occurring risks/complications

- *Common*: minor postoperative pain, bleeding, sore throat, temporary hoarse voice
- *Rare*: damage to teeth, oesophageal or pharyngeal perforation

Blood transfusion necessary

- Not required

Follow-up/need for further procedure

- The procedure is usually a day case and follow-up is arranged for 2–3 weeks to discuss the histology results (this may be sooner depending on the speed of your hospital's pathology lab)

Pharyngeal pouch stapling

Description

A pharyngeal pouch (or Zenker's diverticulum) develops between the two heads of the inferior constrictor muscle (see Fig. 14.4). A combination of mechanisms, including uncoordinated swallowing, spasm, and impaired relaxation of cricopharyngeus, conspire to increase pressure in the distal pharynx, causing herniation through the point of greatest potential weakness as described (which is also known as Killian's dehiscence/triangle). Thus a pouch develops through the posterior pharyngeal wall just above cricopharyngeus. This may become several centimetres in diameter.

The pouch may be asymptomatic but will more likely cause symptoms such as dysphagia, cough, and, through the build-up of swallowed food in the pouch, halitosis, and regurgitation of food boluses that may be aspirated and cause recurrent chest infections due to both aerobic and anaerobic bacteria. The pouch may be easily demonstrated with a barium swallow. Large and problematic pouches are treated by endoscopic stapling to seal the pouch after any contents are evacuated.

Mode of anaesthesia/sedation

- General anaesthesia

Intended benefits

- To close the pharyngeal pouch
- Improve dysphagia
- Prevent recurrent chest infections

Additional procedures that may become necessary

- Pharyngo-oesophageal repairs if perforation occurs

Alternative procedures/conservative measures

- *Conservative*: if the pouch is small and the symptoms minor or if the patient is a poor surgical candidate—watchful waiting is a reasonable course of action
- *Alternative*: open neck surgery to resect the diverticulum and incise cricopharyngeus thereby reducing spasm was the traditional course of treatment but has now been largely superseded by endoscopic stapling, though it remains an option for cases with poor access (e.g. a small mouth that will not permit the staple gun)

Serious/frequently occurring risks/complications

- *Common complications*: bleeding, damage to teeth, sore throat
- *Major risks*: conversion to open surgery, infection, fistula, oesophageal perforation, repeat procedure for persistent pouch, death

Blood transfusion necessary

- Not usually required
- Group and save

Follow-up/need for further procedure

- The patient should commence oral intake the next day, starting with sterile water, gradually progressing to free fluid, soft diet and normal diet over 24–48h
- Any evidence of leakage (e.g. chest pain, pyrexia) will require immediate cessation of oral feeding and investigation
- If all goes well the patient is discharged and followed up at 2–4 weeks

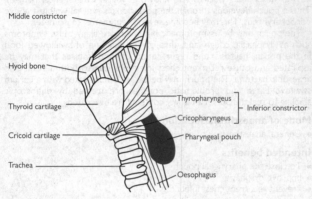

Fig. 14.4 Pharyngeal pouch.

Pinna haematoma or abscess drainage

Description

Trauma to the ear may result in a haematoma of the pinna. A pinna abscess may be the result of an infected haematoma or due to infection entering via an ear piercing or lacerating injury. Both these accumulations occur between the perichondrium and cartilage of the pinna, thus devascularizing the cartilage. If they are not evacuated subsequent fibrosis, loss of cartilage, and disfigurement ('cauliflower ear') may result in the case of haematoma; or, with an abscess, spread of infection and complete obliteration of either the local or entire pinna cartilage.

Aspiration with a large bore (16G) needle may be attempted but this will likely result in residual pus re-forming the abscess or reaccumulation of the haematoma. To ensure adequate drainage an incision should be made (usually in the shade of the helical fold; Fig. 14.5a), the haematoma or abscess aspirated, and in the case of the latter the cavity is washed out with saline. With a haematoma the incision is sutured with dental rolls as bolsters to provide fixed compression and prevent reaccumulation of blood. An abscess may be closed in the same fashion or a small, corrugated drain left *in situ* to allow any further pus to drain and for the cavity to close slowly by secondary intention.

Mode of anaesthesia/sedation
- Local (regional) or general anaesthesia

Intended benefits
- To drain the haematoma or abscess
- To prevent cartilage loss and pinna distortion

Additional procedures that may become necessary
- None

Alternative procedures/conservative measures
- As described aspiration may be attempted for pinna haematoma but the risk of reaccumulation is greater

Serious/frequently occurring risks/complications
- *Common*: Infection, pain, reaccumulation of haematoma or abscess, cauliflower ear
- *Rare*: Loss of pinna cartilage (especially if the patient presents late)

Blood transfusion necessary
- Not required

Follow-up/need for further procedure
- In both cases the patient should receive 1 week of oral broad-spectrum antibiotics (e.g. co-amoxiclav 625mg three times daily) for 1 week
- Follow up at 5–7 days for removal of dressings and inspection of pinna

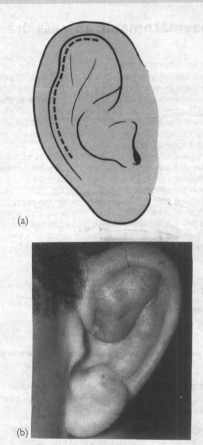

(a)

(b)

Fig. 14.5 Pinna haematoma (a) site of incision, (b) example of a typical haematoma.

Reproduced with permission from Corbridge R and Steventon N. *Oxford Handbook of ENT and Head and Neck Surgery* 2nd edition. 2010. Oxford: Oxford University Press, p.369, Figure 23.7.

Reduction of inferior turbinates

Description

The inferior turbinate mucosa hypertrophies in all forms of rhino-sinusitis but particularly in allergic rhinitis. This causes severe functional impairment through nasal obstruction, but, in addition, makes the delivery of topical medication to the nose and sinuses impossible. Several methods of reducing the turbinates are possible:

- Submucous diathermy—submucosal cautery induces shrinking of inflamed mucosa
- Surface linear cautery—at the top, middle and bottom of the turbinate to induce shrinking
- Cryotherapy—freezing the mucosa to induce shrinking
- Laser turbinate reduction
- Out fracture—pushing the turbinate laterally and out of the airway
- Submucous conchopexy—to change the turbinate shape
- Trimming or excision of the turbinate

All of these methods will improve the airway for up to 18 months but medical treatment is necessary in this period to prevent recurrence. Trimming or excision provides the best long-term result but runs the risk of potentially torrential postoperative haemorrhage.

Mode of anaesthesia/sedation

- General anaesthesia

Intended benefits

- Relieve nasal obstruction
- Allow the delivery of topical medication to the nose and sinuses

Additional procedures that may become necessary

- Nasal packing if bleeding is problematic
- Septoplasty if a deviated nasal septum continues to cause nasal obstruction

Alternative procedures/conservative measures

- Topical treatment will usually have been exhausted as an initial treatment before turbinate reduction is considered

Serious/frequently occurring risks/complications

- *Common*: bleeding, pain, infection
- *Occasional*: recurrence of nasal obstruction

Blood transfusion necessary

- Not usually required
- Group and save

Follow-up/need for further procedure

- Postoperatively the patient may need to continue steroid topical treatment in the form of a spray or drops, particularly if they have allergic rhino-sinusitis
- Follow-up at 2–3 months

Repair of pinna laceration

Description
Any kind of trauma to the external ear may result in a pinna laceration. These are common, particularly in young men. As with any laceration the wound should be cleaned thoroughly with normal saline, all debris removed, and non-viable tissue at the wound edges debrided. If necessary the wound should be scrubbed clean with dilute iodine or chlorhexidine solution. It is imperative to be meticulous in apposing the wound edges as any discrepancy may result in a poor cosmetic result in the form of a ledge deformity of the helical fold. The wound can be closed in a single layer that only comprises the skin, using small non-absorbable sutures such as 5-0/6-0 Prolene. Any head trauma should be treated as such first and the accompanying injuries dealt with subsequently. In addition, a trauma capable of lacerating the pinna should always warrant examination of the EAC and eardrum for haemotympanum.

Mode of anaesthesia/sedation
- Local (regional) or general anaesthesia

Intended benefits
- Repair laceration with good cosmetic outcome

Additional procedures that may become necessary
- None

Alternative procedures/conservative measures
- None—the wound must be cleaned and closed to prevent infection of the cartilage

Serious/frequently occurring risks/complications
- *Common*: bleeding, infection
- *Occasional*: pinna haematoma

Blood transfusion necessary
- Not required

Follow-up/need for further procedure
- As with any dirty wound, the patient's tetanus status should be checked and if necessary they should have a booster
- The patient will require broad-spectrum antibiotics (e.g. co-amoxiclav 625mg three times daily) for 1 week
- No formal follow-up is required as stitches can be removed by the patient's general practitioner or a practice nurse after 5–7 days. However, they should be advised that any worsening pain, swelling, or discharge warrants medical advice

Rhinoplasty

Description

Rhinoplasty may be performed for nasal obstruction due to an external deformity of the nose that is congenital or secondary to trauma, or for cosmetic reasons to correct an external deformity of the nose without obstruction that is congenital or secondary to trauma.

Rhinoplasty involves manipulation of the bone and cartilage that form the shape of the nose. These are the nasal bones, upper lateral and lower lateral cartilages, and alar cartilages. Any combination of these may be altered to produce the desired cosmetic effect. The septal cartilage sits in the midline and divides the nose into left and right nostrils and is also integral to the shape of the external nose, providing support as its 'backbone'. Cartilage may be harvested from the ribs, ear or nasal septum to be used as graft material. A plaster of Paris or similar splinting dressing is applied after the procedure. In altering the structure of the nose its function may be detrimentally affected so this must be a consideration for the surgeon. However, the patient's desired shape may not be one that yields satisfactory function for the surgeon.

Mode of anaesthesia/sedation

- General anaesthesia

Intended benefits

- To yield the desired cosmetic effect while maintaining function

Additional procedures that may become necessary

- Septorhinoplasty: if surgery on the external nose is combined with surgery of the nasal septum, the procedure is known as septorhinoplasty

Alternative procedures/conservative measures

- None

Serious/frequently occurring risks complications

- *Common*: bleeding, infection, swelling, bruising
- *Rare*: poor cosmesis (reoperation rate of 5–10%), poor function, nasal septal perforation, temporary numbness of the upper teeth, temporary loss of smell

Blood transfusion necessary

- Not usually required
- Group and save

Follow-up/need for further procedure

- Follow up after 1 week to remove the plaster of Paris
- Review at 4–6 weeks
- Patients are advised to avoid blowing the nose and to sne mouth open for the first postoperative week
- They are to expect crusting and blood stained watery first 2 weeks. Nasal douching can be prescribed for t

- Nasal obstruction, stiffness, and numbness are to be expected and this may last up to 3 months
- The skin of the nose will be highly sensitive to the sun and the patient should be advised to wear high factor sunscreen and a hat for at least 6 months postoperatively
- It is important for patients to be well informed preoperatively that the final result of the rhinoplasty is not evident until 9–12 months postoperatively and changes continue throughout this period

Septoplasty

Description

The nasal septum is an integral part of the external nasal skeleton. Any procedure whereby the shape of the nasal septum is altered is known as septoplasty. Congenital (e.g. during birth) or traumatic events later in life may precipitate damage, which causes cosmetic (e.g. saddle deformity) or functional (e.g. nasal obstruction) problems through deviation of the septum. Deviation at the nasal valve, a point approximately 1cm posterior to the nares and defined by the border of the upper and lower lateral cartilages superiorly, anterior origin of the inferior turbinate laterally, the floor of the nose inferiorly, and the septum medially, will result in the greatest functional impairment.

The procedure is usually performed endo-nasally via the nostrils. An incision is made in the nasal mucosa along the inferior border of the septum and above the skin of the columella in order to raise a mucoperichondrial flap. This allows for the deviated parts of the septum to be removed and the rest of the septal cartilage to be realigned in the midline. This is a tissue-sparing procedure and the dorsal aspect of the septum is maintained. The mucosa can be closed with a quilting suture to reduce the risk of haematoma. The nose may or may not be packed.

Mode of anaesthesia/sedation

- Usually performed under general anaesthesia
- Can be performed under local anaesthesia with sedation

Intended benefits

- To repair septal deviation and improve symptoms
- To allow access and treatment of tumours of the nose, sinuses, and pituitary gland
- To facilitate nasal polyp or lacrimal gland surgery
- To enable the use of continuous positive airway pressure (CPAP) in patients with OSA
- To treat refractory epistaxis caused by a septal spur that alters airflow through the nostril, causing the overlying mucosa to desiccate and increasing the chances of bleeding

Additional procedures that may become necessary

- Rhinoplasty

Alternative procedures/conservative measures

- Septoplasty should not be performed for children younger than 17 years as the nose continues to grow until this age. If septoplasty is performed too early further structural problems may arise iatrogenically. It is advisable, therefore, to delay in young children
- *Conservative*: if there is any evidence of mucosal inflammation a trial of topical steroid drops should be undertaken as this may suf[?] reduce nasal obstruction and avoid the need for surgery
- *Alternative*: submucous resection involves far more exten[?] of cartilage and bone including part of the vomer and p[?]

plate of the ethmoid. A 1cm dorsal and caudal strut is left to support the external nose structure and avoid saddle deformity

Serious/frequently occurring risks/complications
- Common: bleeding
- Rare: septal haematoma, infection with septal abscess, septal perforation, epistaxis, persisting nasal obstruction, cosmetic deformity (e.g. saddle nose), cerebrospinal fluid leak, anosmia

Blood transfusion necessary
- Not usually required
- Group and save

Follow-up/need for further procedure
- Follow-up in 4–6 weeks

Tonsillectomy

Description

The palatine tonsils are MALT, and found in the oropharynx between the anterior and posterior pillars of the fauces. They may become infected, particularly with the frequent upper respiratory tract infections of childhood, resulting in acute tonsilitis (viral or bacterial—primarily *Streptococcus* sp). Bacterial tonsillitis may be complicated by a paratonsillar abscess (quinsy). Hypertrophic tonsils may result in oropharyngeal obstruction and contribute to OSA or glue ear.

Absolute indications for tonsillectomy are:[1]

• Chronic/recurrent acute tonsillitis (disabling episodes occurring five or more times per year for at least 1 year)
• Tonsillar hypertrophy causing OSA (a cause of high morbidity and potential mortality, especially in children)
• Suspicion of tonsillar malignancy (usually SCC or lymphoma)

If the patient experiences very frequent (>8 per year) episodes of tonsillitis or has two or more episodes of quinsy within a year, it is reasonable to offer them tonsillectomy within a year of symptom onset.[1] Enlarged but asymptomatic tonsils do not require excision.

Intraoperatively, the patient is positioned supine with shoulder bolsters and a head ring. This extends the head on the body. A Boyle–Davis gag is inserted to hold the mouth open and held in position with Draffin rods. The tonsils are commonly excised using blunt dissection and/or bipolar diathermy, although other methods are also in use, e.g. Coblation® and laser.

Haemostasis is achieved using pressure, bipolar diathermy, and/or ligatures. Blood pools in the postnasal space during the procedure. This is suctioned and the postnasal space checked for clotting. The teeth, temporomandibular joints, and adequate haemostasis are also checked at the end of the procedure.

Mode of anaesthesia/sedation

• General anaesthesia

Intended benefits

• Include:
  • Prevent recurrent tonsillitis
  • Treat OSA
  • Diagnosis of tonsillar cancer

Additional procedures that may become necessary

• Often performed in conjunction with adenoidectomy and/or grommet insertion ('As, Ts, and Gs')

Alternative procedures/conservative measures

Conservative: the standard treatment of debilitating cases of acute bacterial tonsillitis is admission, intravenous fluid support, and intravenous antibiotics (e.g. benzylpenicillin 500mg four times daily; amoxicillin is avoided as it may cause a reactive rash if the patient has glandular fever), if there is evidence of airway obstruction a single dose of intravenous dexamethasone 8mg may also be given. Standard treatment of quinsy involves intraoral drainage by needle aspiration or incision in the conscious patient with subsequent antibiotic treatment (drainage often provides such relief that antibiotic treatment may be oral, otherwise intravenous therapy is required). However, if the patient meets the requirements as set out, they should be listed for tonsillectomy.

Serious/frequently occurring risks/complications

- *Common*: pain, infection, offensive breath (transient), secondary haemorrhage (>24h postoperatively—incidence 3–5%), taste disturbance (in adults)
- *Rare*: primary haemorrhage (<24h postoperatively—incidence <1%), damage to teeth

Blood transfusion necessary

- Not usually required. Group and save

Follow-up/need for further procedure

- The patient is discharged with adequate and regular analgesia (e.g. paracetamol, diclofenac ± codeine phosphate) for up to 2 weeks
- No work/school/strenuous activity for 2 weeks
- The patient is encouraged to eat normal foods immediately postoperatively as rough textures will aid removal of tissue debris from the tonsillar bed and help prevent infection
- Advise patients that pain often becomes worse 5–7 days postoperatively and they should expect this as well as halitosis
- They may expect some spotting of blood but anything greater should warrant medical advice, especially in small children
- Follow-up:
  - For recurrent tonsillitis—no formal follow-up necessary
  - For OSA—follow-up at 2–3 months
  - If suspected malignancy—10–14 days with histology

Reference

1. ENT UK. *Indications for Tonsillectomy: Position Paper, ENT UK 2009*. Available at: ℘ www.entuk. org/position_papers/documents/tonsillectomy (accessed 4 May 2011).

Tracheostomy

Description

A tracheostomy provides a secure airway for a patient who is either unable or will soon be unable to maintain their own airway or breathe spontaneously. In essence, a surgical hole is created in the trachea below the vocal cords and a rigid tube inserted via which the patient can be ventilated. The exact circumstances are varied but the indications for tracheostomy fall into four broad categories:

- Relief of upper airway obstruction (e.g. foreign body, trauma, epiglottitis, laryngeal tumour)
- To improve respiratory function (e.g. fulminant bronchopneumonia flail chest)
- Respiratory paralysis (e.g. head injury causing comatose state)
- Preoperatively in patients with a large, obstructing laryngeal tumour

Tracheostomy lessens the work of breathing by reducing anatomical dead space, and this can be useful when weaning patients from mechanical ventilation.

To perform a tracheostomy the patient is supine with shoulder bolsters to extend the neck. A transverse skin incision extending to the medial borders of the sternocleicomastoid muscles is made 1cm above the suprasternal notch in the skin crease of the neck (Fig. 14.6). This can be difficult in patients with short or stiff necks. The fascial planes are dissected and the anterior jugular veins and strap muscles retracted. The thyroid isthmus is divided and oversewn for haemostasis. A tracheostoma (opening in the trachea) is fashioned between the 3rd and 4th tracheal rings and the anterior portion of the ring is removed. This level is chosen as the trachea is narrowest just below the vocal cords, therefore, stenosis here after a tracheostomy tube would be most problematic. The endotracheal tube is retracted to the glottis and an appropriately sized tracheostomy tube (internal diameter two-thirds that of the trachea) is inserted, the cuff inflated and the tube fixed with a collar and connected to the ventilation source. The endotracheal tube can be removed.

An emergency tracheostomy is a different affair entirely and is performed only in a rapidly emergent situation when to delay would be to risk life. A longitudinal incision is made in the midline and deepened to the trachea, dividing the thyroid (rapid bleeding is expected). The scalpel is inserted between the 3rd and 4th tracheal rings, twisted vertically to hold the rings apart and the fenestration open. A cuffed tracheostomy tube is inserted into the airway, the cuff inflated, and the patient ventilated. The bleeding can then be dealt with.

A variety of tracheostomy tubes exists, supplied by numerous manufacturers, but they can essentially be any combination of the following:

- Cuffed versus non-cuffed
- Inner tube versus no inner tube
- Fenestrated versus fenestrated

Mode of anaesthesia/sedation

- General anaesthesia

Intended benefits
- To provide a secure airway

Additional procedures that may become necessary
- None

Alternative procedures/conservative measures
- Endotracheal tube: this is always the first option for a secure airway. However, if it is likely that the patient will require long-term ventilatory support, tracheostomy should be used if available. The advantages are:
  - Reduces discomfort and need for sedation
  - Improves ability to maintain oral and bronchial hygiene
  - Reduces risk of glottis trauma
  - Reduces anatomical dead space and, therefore, work of breathing, thereby augmenting weaning from ventilator support
- Percutaneous tracheostomy: this is an option for patients requiring ventilation for more than 2 weeks and is usually performed at the bedside in the ITU using a guide-wire and dilators. Complications are similar to those of the open procedure (rates 5–15%). Displaced tubes may be harder to replace

Serious/frequently occurring risks/complications
- *Immediate*: haemorrhage, trauma to oesophagus/recurrent laryngeal nerve, pneumothorax
- *Intermediate*: tracheal erosion, tube displacement, tube obstruction, subcutaneous emphysema, aspiration and pneumonia, neck scar
- *Late*: persistent trachea-cutaneous fistula, trachea-oesophageal fistula, laryngeal and/or tracheal stenosis, tracheomalacia

Blood transfusion necessary
- Not usually required
- Group and save (risk of bleeding when thyroid isthmus divided)

Follow-up/need for further procedure
- Care of the tracheostoma and the tube is essential postoperatively. The patient should be nursed in the HDU/ITU if required, otherwise on an ENT ward where the staff are trained and experienced in the care of tracheostomies
- Airway patency must be maintained. This will involve:
  - Humidified air and oxygen
  - Chest physiotherapy and encouraged coughing
  - Regular atraumatic suction
  - Mucolytic agents
  - Bronchial lavage if necessary (usually on HDU/ITU only)
- Prevention of infection and complications is paramount:
  - Prophylactic antibiotics
  - *Aseptic technique for suction and handling of tube*
  - Deflate cuff for 5min every hour
  - Avoid tube compressing posterior tracheal wall

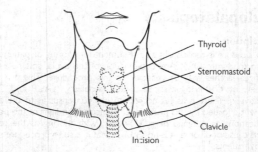

Fig. 14.5 Site of tracheostomy incision.

Reproduced with permission from McLatchie GR and Leaper DJ. *Oxford Specialist Handbook of Operative Surgery* 2nd edition. 2005. Oxford: Oxford University Press, p.641, Figure 15.1.

Uvulopalatoplasty

Description
This procedure is carried out as a treatment for snoring or patients with mild to moderate OSA. Any combination of the uvula, soft palate, and pharyngeal arches may be resected in this procedure. This can either be laser, or diathermy assisted uvulopalatoplasty (LAUP and DAUP, respectively). There is as yet no widespread consensus as to the degree of benefit afforded by this procedure, particularly in light of the possible complications as outlined here. However, with snoring as the primary medical cause of divorce, it is no surprise that it is still a procedure sought after by patients.

Mode of anaesthesia/sedation
- General anaesthesia

Intended benefits
- To reduce/stop snoring

Additional procedures that may become necessary
- Tonsillectomy and/or adenoidectomy are sometimes performed concomitantly

Alternative procedures/conservative measures
- *Conservative*: CPAP—however, some patients (or their partners!) may not tolerate this

Serious/frequently occurring risks/complications
- *Common*: very severe throat pain lasting up to 2 weeks and in rare cases longer, infection
- *Rare*: velopharyngeal insufficiency and nasopharyngeal regurgitation, long-term voice changes, persistent palatal dryness, partial loss of taste, narrowing of the airway and difficulty breathing, iatrogenic precipitation or worsening of OSA due to subsequent fibrosis of pharyngeal tissue

Blood transfusion necessary
- Not usually required

Follow-up/need for further procedure
- Follow-up at 2 months

Vocal cord medialization (medialization laryngoplasty)

Description

Unilateral palsy or paralysis of a vocal cord results in lateralization of the cord due to muscle atrophy and weakness/complete immobility. As a result the pathological cord cannot meet its partner in the midline, resulting in a weak, breathy voice, ineffectual cough, and risk of aspiration. The long course of the recurrent laryngeal nerves leave them exposed to potential pathology from the skull base to the lung hila. The pathology is idiopathic, iatrogenic, or neoplastic. Vocal cord medialization aims to bring the pathological cord to towards the midline.

A horizontal incision is made in the neck over the thyroid cartilage, on the pathological side and within a skin crease. The incision is deepened to the strap muscles, which are retracted and elevated to reveal the thyroid cartilage. A window is made in the thyroid cartilage just below the vocal cords (hence the other name for the procedure, thyroplasty) and an implant inserted (typical materials include Gortex® and Silastic®), while the extent of cord medialization is judged by watching the cords via a nasendoscope, which gives an endoluminal view of the larynx (see Fig. 14.7). The wound is then closed in layers.

Mode of anaesthesia/sedation

- General anaesthesia
- The procedure may also be performed under local anaesthesia ± sedation. The advantage of this being the effect of the implant on the voice can be assessed intraoperatively and if necessary a different-sized implant fashioned

Intended benefits

- Prevent aspiration and subsequent infection
- Improve voice

Additional procedures that may become necessary

- Arytenoid adduction: in some instances an implant alone is insufficient to fully correct the paralysis. A suture through the arytenoid, which when tightened brings the cord more medially, may also be necessary

Alternative procedures/conservative measures

- Speech therapy: in cases where the gap in the cords is small, speech therapy may be enough to strengthen the mobile cord, allowing it to compensate sufficiently to give a strong voice
- Vocal cord injection: here, the atrophied cord is bulked up by injection of an implant material. The injection may be applied via the mouth or through the skin and thyroid cartilage. In both instances the cord is visualized endoluminally with a nasendoscope/laryngoscope. Both general and local anaesthesia are options. Potential implant materials are either permanent (e.g. Bioplastique, calcium hydroxyapatite) or temporary (e.g. collagen, fat). The temporary materials are gradually absorbed into the body. Temporary injections will last 3–6 months.

The advantage of injection is that if vocal cord palsy is temporary (e.g. compression neurapraxia after surgery) and expected to recover then it may be used as a stop-gap (giving an adequate voice and preventing aspiration) until the nerve recovers

Serious/frequently occurring risks/complications

- Bleeding, infection, suboptimal result, laryngeal oedema or occlusion due to excessive injection of implant material, airway compromise ± tracheostomy, implant dislocation

Blood transfusion necessary

- Not usually required

Follow-up/need for further procedure

- The voice will usually be hoarse for the first 24–48h postoperatively but will improve after this
- Follow-up at 4–6 weeks for assessment of voice and airway safety with nasendoscopy

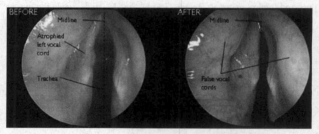

Fig. 14.7 Laryngoscopic view of vocal cord medialization. Left panel: Before injection of the implant material the atrophied left vocal cord is seen to lie in the lateral position. Right panel: After injection the left cord has sufficient bulk to allow its partner to meet it in the midline to provide adequate voice, strong cough and airway protection.

General paediatric surgery

Introduction to paediatric surgery

This section is written with the assumption that disclosure is being provided to, and consent obtained from, the parents. It goes without saying that the competent child should also be involved in the disclosure, so in this situation, the conversation should be couched in terms that enable the child to participate. Some competent children will want to provide their own consent, and are entitled to do so. However, many competent children exercise their autonomy by choosing to allow their parents to sign the consent form on their behalf.

The frequency with which a complication may occur has no bearing on whether it should be disclosed. Historically, courts have toyed with the notion that a numerical threshold for disclosure could be considered, where risks whose incidence lay below an arbitrary threshold, e.g. 1%, did not require automatic disclosure (see Box 15.1). This has been abandoned by the courts, and should equally be abandoned by surgeons. Risks should be disclosed if it is reasonably foreseeable that they could occur, and if the reasonable patient would consider them to be significant. Deaths during neuroblastoma surgery or bladder paralysis following the excision of a sacrococcygeal teratoma are rare, but they do occur. A reasonable parent would consider these complications significant. Surgeons sometimes forget, however, that the possibility of such outcomes may never occur to parents. Whether the knowledge will alter their decision to consent is quite a different matter, but it is proper that they are given the appropriate information, irrespective of the likelihood of the complication occurring. It is appropriate to put a rare risk into the context of its infrequency, but not to exclude its disclosure on this basis.

In this chapter, disclosure for quintessentially general paediatric surgical procedures is reviewed. Thus, pyloric stenosis and branchial remnants are, hopefully, fully addressed. There is also a group of diagnoses falling into both paediatric and adult practice. In examples where we have an equal interest, e.g. appendicectomy, the disclosure is provided. But in topics where the expertise is largely in adult practice, such as cholecystectomy, where the paediatric aspects of the clinical picture have no bearing on disclosure, we defer to our adult surgical colleagues, and the relevant section will thus be covered elsewhere.

The reader will note, perhaps with initial surprise, that the disclosure for children's surgery is not necessarily proportional to the complexity, difficulty, or rarity of the procedure. Experience reveals that it is the rather more prosaic operations, often day cases, which generate the most damning criticism from parents, who consider that they were inadequately informed before providing consent. Circumcision and umbilical surgery forms the lion's share of litigation over consent in routine elective children's surgery, while litigation over imperfect consent in complex (non-cardiac) neonatal surgery is almost unheard of.

Box 15.1 Should numbers be quoted?

We generally, avoid allotting specific numerical values to complication rates. In reality, the complication rates derived from any of the procedures listed in the text should not be expected to exceed 5–10%. For reasons already given, the actuarial risk of a complication should not influence its disclosure. However, if parents request an estimation of the risk of a particular complication, the local rate of occurrence of the complication should already have been identified by audit, and this is the figure that should be disclosed. It is the pertinent risk estimate for this patient's operation.

Surgery is ever changing, and it is common to find that several commonly and acceptable operations are available for the same condition. Obvious examples include the option of laparoscopic or open surgery; of percutaneous or open venous access; or of the several approaches to distal hypospadias. Where these options exist, their existence should be disclosed to the parents; and furthermore, the reasons why you have selected your proposed option should also be disclosed.

For the purposes of these descriptions, it is assumed that disclosure will reflect that all operations may result in pain, swelling, scarring, infection, and bleeding. In the clinical circumstances when one of these consequences is particularly pertinent, it will be addressed.

Groin hernias

Description

Groin hernias are commoner in males and are predominately caused by the failure of closure of the processus vaginalis. Thus, inguinal herniae arise due to persistence of the processus vaginalis, with an open deep ring large enough to allow viscera to slip down into the inguinal canal. If narrower, the ring may only allow fluid to enter (patent processus vaginalis—PPV), leading to hydrocele formation (Fig. 15.1). Femoral hernias are uncommon in children.

Alternative procedures/conservative measures

- Since many PPVs will resolve spontaneously in the first few years of life, this natural history should be disclosed if the surgery is being offered before the age of 3 years

Benefits

- *Therapeutic*: Repair hernia

Significant/frequently occurring risks[1-3]

Inguinal hernia repair
- Hernia repair can fail, and the most commonly performed repair in children (inguinal herniotomy) has its highest recurrence rate in preterm babies
- Surgery in the inguinal region carries the risk of damage to the spermatic cord; thus division of the vessels, vas, or nerve are all foreseeable
- The consequences of damage to cord structures include testicular loss, increased chances of infertility and paraesthesias
- Bleeding—sometimes causing a scrotal haematoma

PPV ligation
- Children undergoing PPV ligation face similar risks

Femoral hernia repair
- Femoral hernia repair may additionally result in damage to the femoral vein

Incarceration/ischaemia
- Since the contents of the inguinal or femoral sac may include bowel, damage to this is foreseeable, but rare
- However, the parents need to acknowledge that ischaemic damage to entrapped viscera, or due to pressure on the spermatic cord, may itself lead to visceral and or testicular damage, or loss, quite separate from the risk attributable to surgery
- This risk is proportionate to the period of ischaemic obstruction, and occurs irrespective of damage that may be caused during surgery

Type of anaesthesia/sedation

- General anaesthesia

Follow-up/need for further procedure

- Routine outpatient review

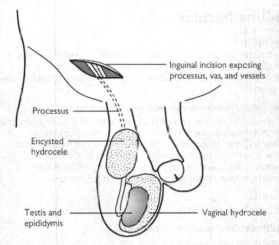

Fig. 15.1 PPV and hydrocele.

Reproduced with permission from McLatchie GR and Leaper DJ. *Oxford Specialist Handbook of Operative Surgery* 2nd edition. 2006. Oxford: Oxford University Press. p.629, Figure 14.14.

References

1. Vogels HDE, Bruijnen CJP, Beasley SW. Establishing a benchmark for the outcome of herniotomy in children. *Br J Surg* 2010;**97**:1135–9.
2. Eir SH, Njere I, Ein A. Six thousand three hundred sixty-one pediatric inguinal hernias: a 35-year review. *J Pediatr Surg* 2006;**41**:980–6.
3. Steinau G, Treutner KH, Feeken G, et al. Recurrent inguinal hernias in infants and children. *World J Surg* 1995;**19**:303–6.

Midline hernias

Description

Umbilical hernias are common and are usually caused by a delay in the formation of an umbilical cicatrix. This becomes evident at or soon after birth. Most will gradually reduce over time and close spontaneously by 3–5 years.[1]

Alternative procedures/conservative measures

- The main risk of repairing umbilical hernias is that it could prove to be an unnecessary procedure, since they are rarely symptomatic
- Many will resolve spontaneously by 3–5 years. This natural history should be disclosed to the parents. Litigation, on the basis that imperfect disclosure has led to a procedure to which the parents would not have otherwise consented, is not uncommon

Benefits

- *Therapeutic*: Repair hernia

Significant/frequently occurring risks

- Recurrence postoperatively is uncommon
- If the sac is large and associated with an elephant's 'trunk' of redundant skin, a period of many months may elapse before the bulge flattens into a normal contour. Some surgeons excise the redundant skin, but risk an inferior result than that obtained by natural healing
- For those using an incision outside the curtilage of the umbilicus, the parents need to be advised of an additional skin-crease scar
- Supraumbilical hernias may be more prone to complication, and less frequently resolve
- Epigastric hernias are notoriously easy to miss at operation, since although the swelling that they cause is easily perceived; the defect through which this emerges is often only 1 or 2mm in diameter. The sac is diaphanous, contains extraperitoneal fat, and emerges into the subcutaneous fat layer. The sac and its contents are thus difficult to identify, and unless the preoperative marking is meticulous, finding the defect can be impossible. The possibility of missing the defect must thus be disclosed
- If there is extensive subcutaneous dissection, this increases the risk of seroma formation, which should be disclosed. This difficulty is sometimes reflected in a surprisingly extensive scar, which should be anticipated during consent

Type of anaesthesia/sedation

- General anaesthesia

Follow-up/need for further procedure

- *Routine outpatient review*

Reference

1. Cilley RE. Disorders of the umbilicus. In: Grosfeld JL, O'Neill JA, Fonkalsrud EW, *et al.* (eds), *Pediatric Surgery*. Philadelphia, PA: Mosby, 2006:1143–56.

Orchidopexy

Description

Undescended testes (UDT) can be congenital or acquired. Congenital UDT has been described as being due to failure of embryological testicular descent and is present from birth. Acquired UDT, on the other hand, is described as being due to failure of spermatic cord elongation as the child grows, where the testis is initially intrascrotal and later re-ascends.[1] It has an incidence of 2–4% in term males at birth, which falls to about 1% at one year.[2] Timing of orchidopexy is controversial but current opinion ranges from 6 to 18 months.

Benefits

UDT is associated with infertility and is a risk factor for testicular cancer. Orchidopexy positions the testicle in the optimal place for spermatozoa production and research suggests that timely orchidopexy decreases the risk of testicular cancer.[3]

Additional procedures that may become necessary

- Disclosure should include the possibility that an orchidectomy may be required intraoperatively, if the quality of the testicular remnant precludes its fixation. If a 'good quality' testis lies on a spermatic cord that is of inadequate length, a staged operation may be required
- Disclosure may become complicated when at the outpatient examination, a testis cannot be found on one side
- The likely surgical plan will be an examination under anaesthesia, and routine orchidopexy if the testis can be palpated at this stage
- If not, during the same anaesthesia, a laparoscopy may then reveal an abdominal testis; which may be suitable for an orchidopexy in one or two stages
- Alternatively, laparoscopy may reveal the testicular vessels and vas entering the deep ring, after which an open groin exploration is required, to identify and in all likelihood excise a blighted (and thus impalpable) testis
- Some surgeons believe that exploration of the closed deep ring is unwarranted as no viable testicular tissue will be found
- A blighted testis may be identified lying intra-abdominally, and excised
- However, the performance of this sequence differs widely between paediatric surgical units. Given the potential for confusion during disclosure, it is prudent to be utterly sure what the operative plan will be before trying to explain it to the parents

Significant/frequently occurring risks

- The main risk of orchidopexy is testicular loss, following inadvertent damage to the testicular vessels
- Division of the vas deferens is also a well-recognized complication
- Parents need to realize that moving the undescended testis into the scrotum will not necessarily make it function normally, and the principal reason for performing the operation is to bring the testis into a subcutaneous site where it can be periodically examined by the

mature patient. Self-examination is part of prudent healthy living, akin to self-examination of the breast, and can facilitate the early diagnosis of malignancy

- The increased risk of malignancy in the originally undescended testis is also an important element of disclosure, although the numerical risk, while greater than that of the normal population, is still low
- If the spermatic cord is not adequately freed, residual tension may drag the testis back out of the scrotum postoperatively, causing recurrence. Equally, this may occur after a competent operation
- The risks of spermatic cord damage during surgery for recurrence are higher than in the primary procedure

Type of anaesthesia/sedation

- General anaesthesia

Follow-up/need for further procedure

- Routine outpatient review

References

1. Bonney T, Hutson JM, Southwell BR, et al. Congenital versus acquired undescended testes: incidence, diagnosis and management. *ANZ J Surg* 2008;**78**(11):1010–13.
2. Barthold JS, Gonzalez R. The epidemiology of congenital cryptorchidism. Testicular ascent and orchidopexy. *J Urol* 2003;**170**:2396–401.
3. Petterson A, Lorenzo R, Nordenskjold A, et al. Age at surgery for undescended testis and risk of testicular cancer. *N Engl J Med* 2007;**356**:1835–41.

Circumcision

Description
Circumcision is the removal of some or all of the foreskin from the penis (Fig. 15.2). Dual parental consent is required for cultural circumcision, originating in English common law and now reiterated by the General Medical Council.

Additional procedures that may become necessary
- Meatal dilatation in cases of severe BXO

Benefits
- Remove scarred foreskin in BXO and obtain a histological diagnosis
- Relief from recurrent balanitis
- If circumcision is performed on a healthy foreskin for cultural reasons or parental wishes, notwithstanding the lack of medical benefit to the child

Significant/frequently occurring risks
- Whatever the indication for circumcision, postoperative bleeding is a ubiquitous risk
- Meatal stenosis is more common when the circumcision is performed for BXO
- Transient urinary retention is variously reported
- The possibility of a postoperative result that does not accord with parental expectations should be addressed, particularly in those children having a cultural circumcision. In this group, a parental wish to have the glans completely and permanently exposed may not adequately be expressed preoperatively, and should be anticipated by relevant disclosure
- If too much skin is removed, a tight or bent erection may result, which again should be disclosed in consent
- The initial postoperative appearance can be alarming, with a combination of swelling and bruising. This may cause both the parents and child some distress
- Glanular hyperaesthesia should be disclosed, which may be experienced postoperatively
- A description of what the circumcised penis will look like will ensure that the parents know what to expect, and give them an opportunity to influence the final result

Type of anaesthesia/sedation
- General anaesthesia

Follow-up/need for further procedure
- Routine outpatient review only required in cases of recurrent balanitis or suspected BXO

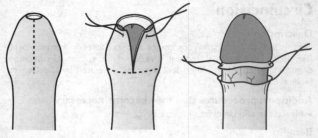

Fig. 15.2 Circumcision.

Reproduced with permission from Davenport M and Pierro A. *Oxford Specialist Handbook of Paediatric Surgery.* 2009. Oxford: Oxford University Press, p.323, Figure 7.1.

Hypospadias

Description

The name hypospadias is derived from the Greek *hypo*, 'under' and *spadon*, 'a tear'. It is a congenital abnormality of the penis in which the urethral meatus opens at varying positions in the line of the urethra on the ventral surface of the penis. It may be associated with a hooded foreskin and a penile chordee. It occurs in about 1 in 300 males.[1]

Benefits

- Cosmetic appearance
- Gives the child a normal axial urinary stream
- Straightens an otherwise bent erection

Significant/frequently occurring risks[2]

- Complications inherent in hypospadias surgery include:
  - Fistula formation
  - Meatal stenosis
  - Urethral stenosis
  - Flap failure and consequent asymmetry of the resulting skin cylinder
  - Deformity
  - Residual curvature of the erect penis
- Urethral diverticulae secondary to meatal stenosis may also be described
- To put this into some context, you may choose to quote the local unit's reoperation rate for children with a similar severity of hypospadias that corresponds with the index patient
- However, the near-inevitable postoperative swelling and bruising should be disclosed, which may alarm unsuspecting parents; and the potential difficulties associated with postoperative urinary drainage and dressings

Type of anaesthesia/sedation

- General anaesthesia

Follow-up/need for further procedure

- Depends on unit protocol
- Catheter out usually around 1 week postoperatively
- Outpatient review at 2–3 months followed by a review when patient's around 4 years old and is potty trained

References

1. Baskin LS, Ebbers MB. Hypospadias: anatomy, etiology and technique. *J Pediatr Surg* 2006;**41**:463–72.
2. Snodgrass W, Macedo A, Hoebeke P, *et al*. Hypospadias dilemmas: A round table. *J Pediatr Urol* 2011;**7**:145–57.

Branchial remnants

Description

There are four paired branchial arches in humans and these are analogous to the gills of our evolutionary ancestors. Branchial anomalies occur as a result of abnormal development of the branchial arches during embryogenesis. They may present as cysts, sinuses or less commonly fistulas.[1,2] The most common are the second branchial arch sinuses, which present as an external opening along the anterior border of the lower third of sternocleidomastoid. The internal part of these sinuses opens into the tonsillar fossa. First branchial arch anomalies are the next most common. These can present externally anywhere in the region between the external auditory meatus and the submandibular area.

Benefits

• Generally parental preference for cosmetic reasons
• Excision prevents later infection

Alternative procedures/conservative measures

• *Conservative*: With preauricular remnants, consent for excision should focus on the justification for the procedure. Preauricular pits and swellings are often asymptomatic in childhood, and it should be made clear that the reason for the removal in infancy and early childhood is almost invariably based upon parental preference rather than clinical necessity

Significant/frequently occurring risks[3]

• When excising branchial remnants or fistulas, persistent residual infection is the most obvious risk
• Scarring is also a frequently occurring risk and must be discussed during disclosure. This latter is pertinent because of the occasional necessity to make a second incision, so that the upper part of the fistulous tract, as it ascends to the pharynx, can be removed
• Potential damage to contiguous structures should be disclosed
• Risks of postoperative scarring and infection should be disclosed, together with risks to the facial nerve in appropriate cases
• Postoperative infection is relatively common; the risk of deep-seated infection in the cartilaginous structures of the external ear may be rare, but is difficult to eradicate, so should be disclosed

Type of anaesthesia/sedation

• General anaesthesia

Follow-up/need for further procedure

• Depends on unit protocol
• Outpatient review at 2 months to check for scarring or recurrence

References

1. De Cauwé D, Hayes R, McDermott M, et al. Complex branchial fistula: a variant arch anomaly. *J Pediatr Surg* 2001;**36**(7):1087–8.
2. Davenport M. ABC of general surgery in children: Lumps and swelling of the head and neck. *BMJ* 1996;**312**:368.
3. Agator-Bonilla FC, Gay-Escoda C. Diagnosis and treatment of branchial cleft cysts and fistulae. A retrospective study of 183 patients. *Int J Oral Maxillofac Surg* 1996;**25**:449–52.

External angular dermoid

Description

Dermoid cysts are painless, mobile, subcutaneous cysts that are common in children. They may become symptomatic if the cyst becomes infected. The cysts are found along the lines of embryological fusion, in this case at the lateral border of the eyebrow. Many surgeons attempt to place the skin crease incision within the region of the putative eyebrow, thus anticipating its camouflage by the growth of hair.[1] The cyst wall may be closely associated with or fused to the skull periosteum, through which a feeding vessel may emerge; and the cyst may have induced a bony depression in the outer table of the skull.

Alternative measures

- Conservative management would include a non-operative 'watch and wait' policy but these cysts gradually enlarge and treatment is by excision

Benefits

- Cosmetic
- Avoids the complication of the cyst becoming infected

Significant/frequently occurring risks[1]

- The main risks to be disclosed relate to:
  - Scarring
  - Recurrence
- A lateral or high dermoid may make scar placement within the eyebrow impractical, and a swelling is thus exchanged for a visible scar, which the parents need to be warned of
- If the cyst is closely associated with or fused to the periosteum, combined with a delicate cyst wall, it can make complete excision of the intact cyst difficult
- Bursting the cyst during excision will result in spillage of its contents, and this may lead to local inflammation of the surrounding tissues for a few days postoperatively, but has no long-term sequelae. Fragmentation of the wall, with retention of a fragment within the wound, may result in recurrence, the risk of which should be disclosed
- Dermoid cysts, less commonly, can be found in the midline on the face, or related to the medial canthus. The same risks of scarring and recurrence apply. However, the surgeon should be immediately wary, since the diagnosis may be wrong, and in reality, the lesion may originate either from the frontal or ethmoid sinuses, or deeper intracranial structures, via meningeal herniation through a skull defect
- This differential diagnosis, and the need for further investigations preoperatively, should be openly discussed with the parents, who may otherwise be perplexed that the lesion is not simply removed as a matter of routine

Type of anaesthesia/sedation
- General anaesthesia

Follow-up/need for further procedure
- Depends on unit protocol
- Outpatient review at 2 months to check for scarring

Reference
1. Cozzi DA, Mele E, d'Ambrosio G, et al. The eyelid crease approach to angular dermoid cysts in pediatric general surgery. *J Pediatr Surg* 2008;43(8):1502–6.

Thyroglossal cyst

Description

Thyroglossal cysts arise as a midline swelling, usually just inferior to the hyoid bone, and may elevate with protrusion of the tongue. They develop from epithelial remnants left as the thyroid gland descends from the foramen caecum during embryological development. Thyroglossal cysts may be hard clinically to differentiate from a midline dermoid cyst in the neck, and disclosure is thus, to an extent, conditional on confirming the diagnosis at operation. Sistrunk's operation involves removing the cyst together with the underlying track and the central part of the hyoid bone, to reduce the incidence of recurrence.[1]

Alternative measures

- Parents, initially unwilling to proceed with surgery, may elect for a trial of conservative management
- This is not unreasonable, but their decision should be tempered by disclosing that if they wait too long, the cyst may become infected, and the operation may become more difficult

Benefits

- Improved cosmetic appearance
- Prevent further infection

Significant/frequently occurring risks

- The risk of inadvertently removing all thyroid tissue by excising the thyroglossal cyst can be avoided by ensuring that in addition to the cyst, a normal thyroid gland is visible on ultrasound preoperatively
- The cyst will almost certainly recur if the body of the hyoid bone is not removed, together with any obvious superior track. Recurrence may also be more likely if there has been pre-existing infection
- The cysts are often associated with a history of infection; the possibility of postoperative infection should be disclosed
- The dissection and excision of the body of the hyoid sometimes causes a sore throat for a few days; although the surgery is usually done as a day case procedure, the possibility of an overnight stay for pain relief should be anticipated during disclosure
- Although the need for a scar is self-evident to most parents, the length of the scar may take them by surprise, since they base their own estimate on the diameter of the cyst, rather than the need to dissect the track, thus this requires discussion before consent

Type of anaesthesia/sedation

- General anaesthesia

Follow-up/need for further procedure

- *Depends on unit protocol*
- Outpatient review at 2 months to check for scarring or recurrence

Reference

1. Goldsztein H, Khan A, Pereira KD. Thyroglossal duct cyst excision—the sistrunk procedure. *Oper Tech Otolaryngol* 2009;**20**(4):256–9.

Tongue tie

Description
Disclosure needs to include the observation that the indications for surgery are still a matter of some controversy, although the current trend may favour intervention in infancy. Current NICE guidelines[1] suggest dividing tongue-ties in babies to improve breastfeeding, when symptomatic.[2,3] However, in older children, there is no evidence to suggest that division improves either speech or feeding.

Alternative procedures/conservative measures
- Tongue tied babies who are having difficulties breastfeeding will usually be able to bottle feed without difficulty
- Breastfeeding advice and counselling

Benefits
- May improve breastfeeding
- May improve nipple pain in breastfeeding mothers

Significant/frequently occurring risks
- Bleeding
- Incomplete division
- Collateral damage from diathermy (monopolar diathermy should be avoided)

Type of anaesthesia/sedation
- In some centres it is performed in the swaddled awake baby; in others, under general anaesthesia; so whatever technique is locally adopted, the alternative approach should be acknowledged
- In older children, it is performed under general anaesthesia, often using bipolar scissors

References
1. National Institute for Health and Clinical Excellence. *Division of Ankyloglossia (Tongue–Tie) for Breast Feeding*. Guideline IPG149. London: NICE, 2005. Available at: ℘ www.nice.org.uk.
2. Hogan M, Westcott C, Griffiths DM. Randomized, controlled trial of division of tongue-tie in infants with feeding problems. *J Paediatr Child Health* 2005;**41**(5–6):246–50.
3. Khoo AK, Dabbas N, Sudhakaran N, et al. Nipple pain at presentation predicts success of tongue-tie division for breast feeding problems. *Eur J Pediatr Surg* 2009;**19**(6):370–3.

Appendicectomy

Description

Appendicitis is a disease that many parents have heard of and may have experienced themselves. Such familiarity may breed a temptation to assume that disclosure may be minimized, particularly in the hastened circumstances, when the anaesthetist has called for the patient, and you are in danger of losing the emergency slot on the list.

Alternative procedures/conservative measures

- Conservative management with antibiotics and subsequent delayed appendicectomy if an appendix mass is present

Benefits

- To remove inflamed appendix and treat infection

Significant/frequently occurring risks

- The parents need to know that successful appendicectomy may still be followed by sepsis, so postoperative antibiotics over several days may be required
- It may not be possible to find a faecalith in an inflamed pelvis, making postoperative abscess formation more likely
- It also needs to be made clear that if a pelvic mass is encountered following a preliminary examination under anaesthesia, the procedure may be abandoned, and the mass treated conservatively[1]
- Damage to contiguous structures is unusual during open appendicectomy, but should be acknowledged; as should stump perforation
- Since open and laparoscopic approaches are both commonly performed, disclosure should include the rationale for why the proposed approach has been chosen
- Whether it is a 'risk' is debatable but the likelihood of finding and removing a normal appendix should be disclosed

Type of anaesthesia/sedation

- General anaesthesia

Follow-up/need for further procedure

- Outpatient review at around 2 months to check for resolution of pain and appendix histology

Reference

1. Gillick J, Velayudham M, Puri P. Conservative management of appendix mass in children. *Br J Surg* 2001;**88**:1539–42.

Excision of Meckel's diverticulum

Background

Meckel's diverticulum results from the failure of complete obliteration of the embryonic vitelline or omphalomesenteric duct. In many children presenting with rectal bleeding, Meckel's diverticulum can be included within the differential diagnosis.[1] If a positive radionuclide scan is obtained, disclosure to the parents can reasonably assert that the diverticulum is the source of the bleeding. Excision involves resection of a wedge or sleeve of ileum (Fig. 15.3) to ensure that the base of Meckel's diverticulum is resected.

Benefits

- Removal of the source of bleeding

Significant/frequently occurring risks

- The general risks of open or laparoscopic access to the abdomen, evisceration of the ileal segment bearing the diverticulum, its resection and primary anastomosis can then be disclosed, with the general risks of anastomotic leakage, infection and bleeding
- However, in many cases, the child will go to theatre without a firm diagnosis, since radionuclide scans have a high false negative rate, and both upper and lower gastrointestinal bleeding still lies within the differential
- Disclosure thus needs to be tailored to local practice. Upper and lower gastrointestinal endoscopy, which if negative can be followed by laparoscopy and/or laparotomy all have a role in the management, but it is important to be utterly sure of the operative sequence before disclosing it to the parents
- Furthermore, the possibility of finding no bleeding lesion within the gut, despite all these efforts, must be disclosed, since this is not an uncommon result

Type of anaesthesia/sedation

- General anaesthesia

Follow-up/need for further procedure

- Outpatient review at 6–8 weeks

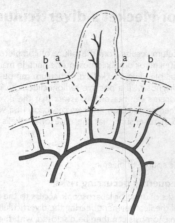

Fig. 15.3 Meckel's diverticulectomy: a = wedge excision; b = with sleeve of ileum.

Reproduced with permission from MacKay GJ, Dorrance HR, Molloy RG, *et al. Oxford Specialist Handbook of Colorectal Surgery.* 2010. Oxford: Oxford University Press, p.375, Figure 8.3.

Reference

1. Schropp KP, Garey CL. Meckel's diverticulum. In: Holcomb GW, Murphy JP, eds. *Ashcraft's Pediatric Surgery,* 5th edn. USA: Elsevier, 2010:526–31.

Pyloric stenosis

Description

Pyloric stenosis is due to hypertrophy of the pyloric muscle, leading to gastric outflow obstruction It typically occurs between the 3rd and 6th weeks of life and presents with non-bilious, projectile vomiting. The baby is often unsettled and may be dehydrated. On examination, visible peristalsis may be present, together with an olive-sized tumour in the epigastrium or right hypochondrium. A test feed may help display these signs.

If the history suggests pyloric stenosis, yet examination is equivocal, an ultrasound may help confirm the diagnosis (sensitivity ~95%). Initial treatment is rehydration and correction of electrolyte imbalance due to vomiting (hypokalaemic, hyponatraemic, metabolic alkalosis), followed by surgery in the form of pyloromyotomy (either open or laparoscopic).[1]

Benefits

- Resolution of vomiting and return to normal feeding

Significant/frequently occurring risks[1]

- The risk of a false-positive diagnosis should be acknowledged
- The risk of an inadequate pyloromyotomy, and persistence of symptoms must be acknowledged
- Equally, the risk of mucosal perforation, and the steps that will be taken if this occurs, should be discussed
- Wound infection is still common; if both right upper quadrant and peri-umbilical incisions are used in the local unit, it would be prudent to inform the parents if the wound infection rates from these alternative approaches differ markedly
- Parents also need to realize that postoperative vomiting is common for the first few days, and that an instant cessation of this sign may not occur
- For children undergoing a laparoscopic pyloromyotomy, the generic risks associated with this approach, including damage to contiguous structures, should be disclosed
- In all patients, the risk of incisional hernias could be addressed when the rationale for choosing the planned route of access, i.e. laparoscopic, peri-umbilical is presented. During the period when these commonly used alternatives are still widely employed, the reason for preferring one above the others needs to be disclosed

Type of anaesthesia/sedation

- General anaesthesia

Follow-up/need for further procedure

- Outpatient review at 6–8 weeks to assess feeding and review scar

Reference

1. Aspelund G, Langer JC. Current management of hypertrophic pyloric stenosis. *Semin Pediatr Surg* 2007;**16**:27–33.

Reduction of intussusception

Description

Intussusception is caused when one section of bowel invaginates into another section of bowel; most commonly occurring between the terminal ileum and ascending colon (Fig. 15.4). The majority of intussusceptions are reduced by air enema; the radiologist performing this will doubtless warn the parents of the risk of gut perforation, and failure to reduce. However, before the child goes to the radiology department, surgical consent will also be required, anticipating the possibility of failure of the radiological reduction.

Additional procedures that may become necessary[1]

- Surgical reduction (either open or laparoscopic) if radiological reduction by air enema fails, or if perforation occurs
- Bowel resection and anastomosis may be required and must be disclosed
- If it is local policy to perform an appendicectomy in addition to the surgical reduction, the reasoning behind this, and the related risks, should be disclosed
- The possibility of finding a lead point, and how this will be dealt with, should also be discussed

Serious/frequently occurring risks[1]

- Perforation during attempted air enema reduction
- The potential for gut resection and anastomotic leak must be disclosed
- The risk of recurrence, which is applicable to both open and closed reductions, should also be discussed
- The potential for adhesions to form and possible subsequent small bowel obstruction

Type of anaesthesia/sedation

- General anaesthesia

Follow-up/need for further procedure

- Outpatient review at 6–8 weeks to assess bowel habit

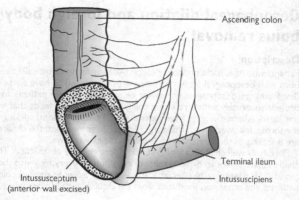

Ascending colon

Terminal ileum

Intussuscipiens

Intussusceptum
(anterior wall excised)

Fig. 15.4 Intussusception of terminal ileum.

Reproduced with permission from McLatchie GR and Leaper DJ. *Oxford Specialist Handbook of Operative Surgery* 2nd edition. 2006. Oxford Oxford University Press, p.615, Figure 14.12.

Reference

1. Davis CF, McCabe AJ, Raine PAM. The ins and outs of intussusception: History and management over the past fifty years. *J Pediatr Surg* 2003 **38**(7 Suppl 1):60–4.

Oesophageal dilation and foreign body/ bolus removal

Description

Patients who have had a previous oesophageal anastomosis, typically those born with oesophageal atresia or those with severe reflux, have a risk of developing an oesophageal narrowing or stricture.[1] These patients may present subacutely with a reducing ability to swallow any feeds that are not liquid. Alternatively, as emergencies, with a history of food sticking in the throat, followed by coughing and choking. In some cases, the children are dribbling, as they are unable to swallow their own saliva.

Previously well children are also at risk of foreign body obstruction. The child's innate desire to explore the world by putting everything into their mouths often leads to the paediatric surgeon being asked to remove coins, batteries and other non-foodstuffs from the inquisitive child's oesophagus.

Benefits

- Remove foreign body/food bolus
- Resumption of normal swallowing

Serious/frequently occurring risks[1,2]

- With any oesophageal manipulation, oesophageal perforation and its consequences represents the most serious complication, and should be disclosed, together with the steps that will be taken to treat it if it is seen to occur, or to check that it has not, once the operation is over
- Details of the consent disclosure for dilation will depend on whether it is performed with bougies or balloons, and flexible or rigid oesophagoscopy
- Equally, patients with foreign bodies or bolus obstruction may suffer perforation, although in this case, there is the additional possibility that the foreign body may pass into the stomach during the induction of anaesthesia. The parents therefore need to appreciate that the offending item may not be retrieved immediately, or even during the hospital stay

Type of anaesthesia/sedation

- General anaesthesia

Follow-up/need for further procedure

- Timing of outpatient review depending on the severity of the stricture, on average three dilations are required
- For oesophageal foreign body removal in a patient with no previous oesophageal problems, no follow-up is required

References

1. Serhal L, Gottrand F, Sfeir R, et al. Anastomotic stricture after repair of esophageal atresia: frequency, risk factors and efficacy of oesophageal bougie dilatations. *J Pediatr Surg* 2010;**45**(7):1459–62.
2. Little DC, Shah SR, St Peter SD, et al. Esophageal foreign bodies in the pediatric population: our first 500 cases. *J Pediatr Surg* 2006;**41**:914–18.

Central venous access

Description

This routine procedure may require surprising variations of consent, because of the widely different potential approaches. Catheters may be short or long term; single or multi-lumen; external or connected to a subcutaneous port. The insertion may be via a percutaneous approach to the jugular, subclavian, or more distal veins, with or without ultrasound guidance.[1,2] Alternatively, insertion may be achieved by an open operation, usually to the jugular venous system or its tributaries. As a result, disclosure may vary, although there are common elements running through all procedures.

Benefits

Delivery of chemotherapy, most commonly, other medications (e.g. antibiotics in children with cystic fibrosis), or parenteral nutrition.

Serious/frequently occurring risks[1,2]

- Haemorrhage is a prominent risk, together with damage to contiguous structures, including artery, nerves, and pleura during the percutaneous subclavian approach and the contents of the carotid sheath in open or percutaneous jugular insertions. This damage itself may lead to the need to control leaks of blood and air
- In the longer term, open venotomy may preclude reuse of the vein on a later occasion, while a long-term subclavian line may induce subclavian stenosis and render the vein equally unusable
- Equally, the presence of the catheter itself, although safely inserted, may cause complications, notably thrombosis, perforation, and infection
- Furthermore, catheters may fracture and become dislodged

Disclosing complications of such complexities may be too burdensome for parents of children who have other acute concerns, such as the very recent diagnosis of malignancy. For this reason, disclosure for central venous catheterization is a topic well suited to an information sheet, allowing parents to digest the information at a more palatable rate than can usually be achieved during oral disclosure.

Type of anaesthesia/sedation

- General anaesthesia

Follow-up/need for further procedure

- These patients are not routinely followed up in an outpatient setting as they are usually looked after by an oncology or paediatric team. Any line problems will be promptly brought to your attention
- Often long-term lines will need replacing as a result of complications such as infection and displacement
- Long-term catheters will need removing when the treatment period is over and this will require a brief general anaesthesia

References

1. Groff DB, Ahmed N. Subclavian vein catheterization in the infant. *J Pediatr Surg* 1974;**9**:171–4.
2. Arul GS, Lewis N, Bromley P, *et al.* Ultrasound guided percutaneous insertion of Hickman lines. Prospective study of 500 consecutive procedures. *J Pediatr Surg* 2009;**44**:1371–6.

Tissue and lymph node biopsy

Description

The mode of biopsy needs to be discussed, together with the reasoning behind selecting the proposed method. It is also important to emphasize that the histology results may take some time to be ready, and that depending on the rarity of disease or difficulty of histological diagnosis, this may be a matter of weeks.

Benefits

- Diagnostic[1]
- Curative[2]

Serious/frequently occurring risks

- Most parents initially fail to realize that an excisional biopsy may fail to excise a tumour. Furthermore, in some diagnoses such as soft tissue sarcoma, an incisional biopsy is often strongly preferred, and an initial excisional procedure avoided. Neither an excisional nor an incisional biopsy can guarantee a firm diagnosis. This must be carefully explained preoperatively
- The risk of bleeding and damage to contiguous anatomical structures must be acknowledged, together with the perioperative actions that may be needed to rectify the situation
- Most usually performed in the head and neck, axilla, and groin, node biopsy is notably associated with damage to contiguous structures, such as inferior branches of the facial nerve in submandibular biopsy or the accessory nerve as it courses across the posterior triangle of the neck
- Parents need to be warned that the biopsy may yield false-negative results, and that the results may take many days, sometimes weeks, to emerge from the laboratory
- They also need to realize that pathological nodal masses are often bosselated, reminiscent of a bunch of grapes. In these circumstances, only one or two nodes will be excised from the mass, which thus will not be much reduced in size. Without this warning, they may immediately be dissatisfied that the 'excision biopsy' is apparently incomplete
- It is sometimes necessary to biopsy a node which proves to be enlarged due to atypical mycobacterial infection. The biopsy may thus result in a discharging sinus, which may be persistent. In circumstances where this is foreseeable, the parents should be warned of this potential result, and the almost inevitable phase of an ugly and puckered scar

Type of anaesthesia/sedation

- General anaesthesia

Follow-up/need for further procedure

- Follow-up should be expedient and with the histology results, and may require oncology involvement
- It will include a discussion of 'where we go from here', which will depend on the histology

References

1. Knight PJ, Mulne AF, Vassy LE. When is lymph node biopsy indicated in children with enlarged peripheral nodes? *Pediatrics* 1982;**69**(4):391–6.
2. Neville HL, Andrassy RJ, Lally KP, et al. Lymphatic mapping with sentinel node biopsy in pediatric patients. *J Pediatr Surg* 2000;**35**:961–4.

Lymphatic malformation in head and neck (cystic hygroma)

Description

Cystic hygromas are congenital lymphatic malformations. They may be diagnosed antenatally and if large, some may cause airway obstruction at birth. Alternatively, they may present in early childhood as multilocular cystic swellings, most commonly in the neck or axilla, although they can occur anywhere.

Indications for surgery include disfigurement, infection, or if the malformation was causing symptoms (depending on site and size).

Alternative procedures/conservative measures[1,2]

- Disclosure should ensure that the parents appreciate that in cases where the lesion is not impinging on the airway, or impeding swallowing or vision, there may be a strong case to adopt a conservative approach, since many of these lesions resolve spontaneously
- Equally, if eradication is desired, the injection of sclerosants may present a realistic alternative (in some cases) to excisional surgery, while posing less threat of structural damage

Benefits

- May improve cosmetic appearance
- May improve function of any structures impinged upon

Serious/frequently occurring risks

- If parents wish to embark on excisional surgery, disclosure should include:
  - The risk of incomplete excision and recurrence of the lesion
  - Even if the hygroma is successfully removed, the majority of patients will acquire a postoperative transient lymphocoele, due to leakage of lymph from the transected lymphatic channels (which originally supplied the lesion), during the first month postoperatively
  - The preoperative cross-sectional imaging will give an idea of the anatomical ramification of the lesion, and can usefully be shown to the parents during disclosure, to help them appreciate the risk of damage to contiguous structures within the operative field
  - A large scar is likely

Type of anaesthesia/sedation

- General anaesthesia

Follow-up/need for further procedure

- Follow-up may be long term and include evaluation often with clinical photography

References

1. Dasgupta R, Adams D, Elluru R, et al. Noninterventional treatment of selected head and neck lymphatic malformations. *J Pediatr Surg* 2008;**43**:869–73.
2. Wheeler JS, Morreau P, Mahadevan M, et al. OK-432 and lymphatic malformations in children: the Starship Children's Hospital experience. *Aust N Z J Surg* 2004;**74**:855–8.

Neonatal surgery

Details to consider when consenting for neonatal surgery

Neonatal surgical procedures are often performed in the first few hours or days of life and this is usually a time of great parental anxiety and stress.

Many neonatal conditions are now antenatally diagnosed, and there may have been an opportunity for antenatal counselling to help prepare the parents for surgery.

Where possible, consent should be obtained face-to-face. However, sick neonates often require transportation to tertiary referral centres for a surgical opinion and parents may be unable to accompany their baby at the time. In these circumstances it may be necessary to obtain consent over the telephone. In such cases, the following things should happen:

- The parents must identify themselves and confirm their relationship to the patient and that they have parental responsibility
- They must confirm that they understand the nature of the call (they understand it is for consent for surgery)
- The patient's diagnosis, the treatment plan, the complications, risks, and alternatives should be disclosed
- There should be a specific request for consent, which is agreed to
- The call should be witnessed and agreement of consent should be repeated to the witness
- It is then acceptable for the person obtaining consent and the witness to sign the consent form on behalf of the parents

Primary repair of oesophageal atresia and tracheo-oesophageal fistula

Description

Oesophageal atresia represents a congenital failure of the oesophagus to develop in continuity with the stomach, ending as a blind pouch. Although oesophageal atresia can be an isolated anomaly it most commonly occurs with a tracheo-oesophageal fistula (TOF), an abnormal communication between the trachea and oesophagus (usually distal).

- The diagnosis is suspected on antenatal ultrasound scans when there is an absent stomach bubble and polyhydramnios
- Postnatally the infant may present with frothing and inability to swallow their own secretions or feed
- A chest X-ray will often show the nasogastric tube curled up in the upper pouch at the level of T3–T5
- Diagnosis should be confirmed following passage of a Replogle tube. Once the Replogle tube is in place continuous suction should be initiated to reduce the risk of aspiration

Parents should be counselled that there might be other abnormalities present, for example VACTERL association (Vertebral, Anorectal, Cardiac, Tracheo-Esophageal, Renal and Limb anomalies).

Surgery

Some surgeons perform preliminary bronchoscopy to identify the fistula
1. Right posterolateral muscle-sparing thoracotomy
2. Extrapleural approach
3. Ligation of the azygous vein
4. Identification, division, and over-sewing of the TOF
5. Mobilization of the upper oesophageal pouch
6. Oesophageal anastomosis if gap allows
7. Trans-anastomotic feeding tube (use will vary according to unit or surgeon preference)

Additional procedures that may become necessary

- In an unstable infant requiring respiratory support, it may be necessary to perform emergency TOF ligation alone to allow stabilization. If the baby's condition allows, subsequent anastomosis may be attempted, otherwise delayed repair will be necessary
- Babies with a 'long gap' (greater than three vertebral bodies) may require a delayed primary closure at several weeks of age. An initial gastrostomy will be required to allow the baby to feed enterally
- Formal oesophageal anastomosis after gap assessment demonstrates this to be possible
- Oesophageal replacement will be required when anastomosis is not possible. This requires an initial cervical oesophagostomy to allow drainage of saliva followed by a delayed gastric transposition or intestinal interposition

Benefits
- Restoring oesophageal continuity

Alternative procedures/conservative measures
- Untreated this condition is incompatible with life

Significant/frequently occurring risks

Early complications
- Bleeding
- Anastomotic leak occurs in around 10%[1,2]
  - Radiologic leaks are usually not clinically significant
  - Minor leaks with persistent drainage of saliva into a chest drain make up the majority of significant leaks. They heal with conservative management
  - Complete disruption of the anastomosis. These are major leaks and commonly present within the first few days of surgery, often with a tension pneumothorax. They will require re-exploration when the baby is stable
- Wound infection
- Death (coexisting cardiac anomalies and low birthweight (<1500g) increase risk of death)

Late complications
- Food bolus impaction
- Anastomotic stricture which may require rigid or balloon dilatation on more than one occasion
- Oesophageal dysmotility
- Gastro-oesophageal reflux
- Recurrent fistula (about 8%[3])
- Tracheomalacia
- Chest wall deformity and scoliosis[4]

Type of anaesthesia/sedation
- General anaesthesia

Follow-up/need for further procedure
- Long-term outcome depends on presence and severity of associated anomalies. Multidisciplinary follow-up is required in order to diagnose and manage some of the long-term complications of both the condition and the surgery

References
1. Spitz L. Lessons I have learned in a 40-year experience. *J Pediatr Surg* 2006;**41**:1635–40.
2. Chittmittrapap S, Spitz L, Brereton RJ, *et al.* Anastomotic leakage following surgery for esophageal atresia. *J Pediatr Surg* 1992;**27**:29–32.
3. Ghandour KE, Spitz L, Brereton RJ, *et al.* Recurrent tracheo-oesophageal fistula: experience with 24 patients. *J Paediatr Child Health* 1990;**26**:89–91.
4. Chetcuti P, Myers NA, Shelan PD, *et al. Chest wall deformity in patients with repaired* esophageal atresia. *J Pediatr Surg* 1989;**24**(3):244–7.

Closure of abdominal wall defects: exomphalos and gastroschisis

Description

During the 6th week of gestation rapid growth of the midgut causes a physiological herniation of the intestine through the umbilical ring. The midgut rotates as it re-enters the abdominal cavity and the intestine then migrates so that the small intestine and colon come to lie in their correct anatomical positions by the end of the 10th week of development.

- Exomphalos and gastroschisis are congenital abdominal wall defects. Exomphalos arises as a result of failure of closure of the abdominal wall following return of viscera
- In exomphalos the viscera are covered with a clear sac made of amnion, Wharton's jelly, and peritoneum, to which the umbilical chord is attached. In exomphalos minor the defect is less than 5cm in diameter and can usually be closed at one operation. Exomphalos major is greater than 5cm, may contain stomach, liver, and bowel and may require staged closure
- Exomphalos is associated with chromosome abnormalities in about 50% of cases (commonly trisomy 13, 18, or 21) and other congenital anomalies in up to 70% of cases.[1,2] Beckwith–Wiedemann syndrome (BWS) is usually associated with exomphalos minor, and includes:
  - Exomphalos
  - Macroglossia
  - Macrosomia
  - Visceromegaly
  - Hemihypertrophy
  - Hypoglycaemia
  - Various types of solid tumour
- Pentalogy of Cantrell includes:
  - Exomphalos
  - Anterior diaphragmatic hernia (Bochdalek)
  - Sternal cleft
  - Ectopia cordis
  - Intracardiac anomaly
- Giant exomphalos, with the whole liver out, is often associated with significant pulmonary hypoplasia
- Gastroschisis is thought to be due to a vascular accident involving the abdominal musculature following full closure. There is no sac covering bowel protruding through a defect, which is usually to the right of a normally sited umbilical cord. The intestine has been exposed to amniotic fluid and as a result may be foreshortened, thickened and matted together
- Unlike exomphalos, infants with gastroschisis do not have an increased risk of chromosomal abnormalities but do have an increased incidence of atresias, felt to be due to vascular compromise of the abnormal bowel or a closing defect

Exomphalos minor

The goal of surgical management is primary closure with fascial apposition and complete skin closure, without causing excessive intra-abdominal pressure.

Additional procedures that may become necessary
- Ladd's procedure after assessment of intestinal rotation

Benefits
- *Therapeutic:* Closure of abdominal defect

Alternative procedures/conservative measures
- A very small defect (hernia into the chord) may be amenable to simple ligation of the sac at the base of the cord after reduction of bowel

Significant/frequently occurring risks[2]
- Early complications:
  - Bleeding
  - Wound infection
  - Postoperative sepsis (respiratory, central venous catheter related)
- Late complications:
  - Ventral hernia
  - Adhesive bowel obstruction

Type of anaesthesia/sedation
- General anaesthesia

Follow-up/need for further procedure
- Medical follow-up depends on severity of associated congenital anomalies
- Patients with BWS have lifelong risk of solid tumours, e.g. Wilms', hepatoblastoma, and as a result must have lifelong surveillance
- Cosmetic scar revision

Major exomphalos

Again the goal of surgery is to achieve fascial and skin closure. However, with exomphalos major this may not be possible without causing excessively raised intra-abdominal pressure and the risk of abdominal compartment syndrome. If skin closure is possible, fascial repair can be achieved with a prosthetic patch. Otherwise, a staged surgical closure using a surgical silo will be necessary.

Additional procedures that may become necessary
- Ladd's procedure after assessment of intestinal rotation
- Prosthetic patch to facilitate fascial closure
- Surgical silo formation

Benefits
- *Therapeutic:* Closure of abdominal defect

Alternative procedures/conservative measures
- *Initial non-operative management:* A small unstable preterm infant or a neonate with a very large sac can be managed by application of topical agents to promote epithelialization from the skin edges

This conservative management creates a large ventral hernia, which can then be closed when the child is older. Surgery is often staged and represents a technical challenge[3]

Significant/frequently occurring risks[2]
- Early complications:
  - Significant risk of bleeding when dissecting sac from the liver
  - Skin flap haematoma
  - Wound infection and breakdown
  - Patch infection
  - Postoperative sepsis (respiratory, CVC-related)
  - Drug toxicity due to systemic absorption of active agents such as silver, iodine, or mercury has been reported
- Late complications:
  - Ventral hernia
  - Adhesive bowel obstruction
  - Gastro-oesophageal reflux

Type of anaesthesia/sedation
- General anaesthesia

Follow-up/need for further procedure
- Delayed closure where a surgical silo was required
- Long-term follow-up to observe for late complications
- Revision surgery of abdominal scar

Gastroschisis

Protection of the eviscerated bowel after birth is paramount in these babies, quickly followed by stabilization with fluid resuscitation and warming.

A variety of closure techniques are available.[4] Currently, two strategies are employed in the main: staged reduction and closure, and primary closure. If there is volvulus, necrosis, or perforation, or a closing defect noted at birth, emergency surgery is required.

Staged reduction and closure[5,6]
Staged reduction and closure involves placing the bowel inside a pre-formed Silastic silo (PFS) at the cot-side using only analgesia or sedation. This allows gradual reduction of the intestine over a period of 3–5 days. When the intestine is fully reduced the defect can be closed either as an operative procedure in theatre or using a cot-side closure technique.

PFS application
- A silo large enough to contain the volume of herniated bowel is selected
- Bowel is passed into the silo, maintaining alignment and rotation
- The ring is deformed into an elongated shape to allow insertion through the defect after ensuring there are no congenital bands between the bowel and edge of defect
- The silo is suspended vertically inside cot

Additional procedures that may become necessary
- An umbilical defect may need to be incised to make it large enough to accept a PFS at the cot-side

Benefits
- *Therapeutic:* reducing abdominal viscera and closing defect
- Allows enteral feeding

Alternative procedures/conservative measures
- Primary closure

Significant/frequently occurring risks[5,6]
- Risks of PFS:
  - Missed intestinal atresia
  - Bowel ischaemia within the silo, due to inappropriate choice of size (volume of silo must be adequate)
  - Silo detachment
  - Entrapment of viscus between silo ring and abdominal wall
  - Sepsis

Type of anaesthesia/sedation
- Analgesia or sedation

Follow-up/need for further procedure
- All patients treated with a silo will need either surgical closure or cot-side closure

Cot-side closure
- Carefully remove the silo with one person ensuring bowel stays reduced
- Clean and dry abdomen and apply tincture of benzoin compound to the skin surrounding the defect
- Lift and pull the umbilical cord to the opposite side of the defect to oppose skin edges
- Place large 12mm Steri-strips horizontally to keep skin edges together
- Vertical Steri-strips can be used to reinforce this
- Clear dressings over Steri-strips, allowing the cord to protrude, are used to cover the Steri-strips
- Leave dressing for 5–7 days

Additional procedures that may become necessary
- Surgical/primary closure may be required

Benefits
- *Therapeutic:* reducing abdominal viscera and closing defect
- No need for anaesthesia

Alternative procedures/conservative measures
- Primary closure

Significant/frequently occurring risks
- Risks of cot-side closure:
  - Skin closed only, not the fascia so increased risk of umbilical hernia
  - Dressings lifting from the skin due to serum build up beneath
  - *Raised intra-abdominal* pressure if dressings too tight
  - Failure of closure

Type of anaesthesia/sedation
- Analgesia or sedation

Follow-up/need for further procedure
- Umbilical hernia repair
- Cosmetic revision

Primary closure

Primary closure involves urgent surgery soon after birth. The intestines are carefully examined for atresias and first the muscle and then the fascia are closed. The umbilical skin is then closed and an attempt is made to re-fashion the umbilicus. The same technique is used to close the abdomen after a PFS has been used to reduce the bowel.

Additional procedures that may become necessary
- Prosthetic patch
- Bowel resection and anastomosis
- Enterostomy formation
- Silo placement if abdominal compartment is not large enough to house all the eviscerated organs

Benefits
- *Therapeutic:* reducing abdominal viscera and closing defect
- Allows enteral feeding

Alternative procedures/conservative measures
- Staged reduction with preformed silo

Significant/frequently occurring risks

Risks of surgical closure

- Early complications:
  - Bleeding
  - Wound infection or dehiscence
  - Anastomotic leak
  - Abdominal compartment syndrome
- Late complications:
  - Sepsis
  - Anastomotic stricture
  - Adhesional bowel obstruction
  - NEC
  - Gastro-oesophageal reflux
  - Abdominal wall hernias
  - Short-bowel syndrome as a result of multiple atresias or a 'closing' defect
  - Parenteral nutrition-associated liver disease (PNALD) as a result of prolonged parenteral nutrition

Type of anaesthesia/sedation
- General anaesthesia for primary closure
- Analgesia or sedation for preformed silo application

Follow-up/need for further procedure
- All children need long-term follow-up to assess feeding, growth, and bowel habit
- Cosmetic revision may be required

References

1. Lakasing L, Cicero S, Davenport M, *et al.* Current outcomes of antenatally diagnosed exomphalos: an 11-year review. *J Pediatr Surg* 2006;**41**:1403–6.
2. Rijhwana A, Davenport M, Dawrant M, *et al.* Definitive surgical management of antenatally diagnosed exomphalos. *J Pediatr Surg* 2005;**40**:516–22.
3. Nuchtern JG, Baxter R, Hatch EI. Nonoperative initial management versus silon chimney for treatment of giant omphalocele. *J Pediatr Surg* 1995;**30**:771–6.
4. Marven S, Owen A. Contemporary postnatal surgical management strategies for abdominal wall defects. *Semin Pediatr Surg* 2008;**17**(4):222–35.
5. Owen A, Marven S, Jackson L, *et al.* Experience of preformed silo staged reduction and closure for gastroschisis. *J Pediatr Surg* 2006;**41**:1830–5.
6. Lansdale N, Hill R, Gull-Zamir S, *et al.* Staged reduction of gastroschisis using preformed silos: practicalities and problems. *J Pediatr Surg* 2009;**44**:2129–9.

Congenital diaphragmatic hernia repair

Description

Congenital diaphragmatic hernia (CDH; Fig. 16.1) occurs in around 1 in 2500 live births. The defect is most commonly on the left side and results in pulmonary hypoplasia and invariably concomitant pulmonary hypertension.[1,2]

There remains a high mortality and morbidity for a 'severe' subset of patients despite recent advances in the antenatal and postnatal management of these babies including:

- high frequency oscillatory ventilation (HFOV)
- extra-corporeal membrane oxygenation (ECMO)
- fetal endoscopic tracheal occlusion (FETO)[3]

Where diagnosed antenatally, parents will have had extensive input from fetal medicine specialists and counselling.

Some of these babies are not diagnosed until after birth, often presenting with varying degrees of respiratory difficulty.

Surgery is only offered if the neonate achieves a degree of stability in terms of oxygenation and ventilation, usually after 48h. Surgery is not indicated in those patients who do not achieve this.

Surgery

1. Open, thoracoscopic, or laparoscopic
2. Return bowel to abdominal cavity
3. Excise hernial sac if present
4. Dissect a diaphragmatic rim if possible and aim for primary repair using non-absorbable sutures
5. A prosthetic or bioprosthetic patch can be used if the defect is too large for primary closure

Additional procedures that may become necessary

- Ladd's procedure after assessment of intestinal rotation
- Insertion of prosthetic patch

Benefits

- Close diaphragmatic defect and return abdominal viscera to the abdomen

Alternative procedures/conservative measures

- Untreated, this condition is not compatible with life

Significant/frequently occurring risks[1-3]

- Early complications:
  - Bleeding
  - Wound infection
  - Chylous effusion
  - Death
- Late complications:
  - Recurrence of hernia
  - Need for patch revision
  - Adhesive bowel obstruction
  - Gastro-oesophageal reflux
  - Chronic lung disease

- Hearing difficulties
- Neurocognitive deficits
- Chest asymmetry/pectus deformity
- Nutritional morbidity/growth failure
- Tracheomegaly in infants treated by FETO
- Death

Type of anaesthesia/sedation

- General anaesthesia

Follow-up/need for further procedure

- Patients will usually need to be reviewed every 3–6 months for the first 1–2 years and annually thereafter
- With increased survival a range of complications may be seen at follow up, and long-term multidisciplinary follow-up is therefore required

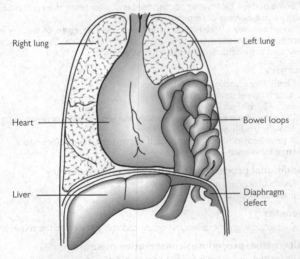

Right lung

Left lung

Heart

Bowel loops

Liver

Diaphragm defect

Fig. 16.1 Congenital diaphragmatic hernia.

Reproduced with permission from McLatchie GR and Leaper DJ. *Oxford Specialist Handbook of Operative Surgery* 2nd edition. 2006. Oxford: Oxford University Press, p.595, Figure 14.6.

References

1. de Buys Roessingh AS, Dinh-Xuan AT. Congenital diaphragmatic hernia: current status and review of the literature. *Eur J Pediatr* 2009;**168**(4):393–406.
2. Almendinger N, West SL, Wilson J. Congenital diaphragmatic hernia. In: Stringer MD, Oldham KT, Mouriquand PDE (eds) *Pediatric Surgery and Urology. Long Term Outcomes*, 2nd edn. Cambridge: Cambridge University Press, 2006:150–7.
3. Hedrick HL. Management of prenatally diagnosed congenital diaphragmatic hernia. *Semin Fetal Neonatal Med* 2010;**15**:21–7.
4. Deprest J, Nicolaides K, Done E, *et al.* Technical aspects of fetal endoscopic tracheal occlusion for congenital diaphragmatic hernia. *J Pediatr Surg* 2011;**46**:22–32.
5. McHoney M, Giacomello L, Nah SA, *et al.* Thoracoscopic repair of congenital diaphragmatic hernia: intraoperative ventilation and recurrence. *J Pediatr Surg* 2010;**45**:355–9.

Ladd's procedure for malrotation with or without volvulus

Description

Bilious vomiting in a neonate is a surgical emergency as this represents midgut malrotation and volvulus (Fig. 16.2) until proven otherwise.[1]

- Following normal intestinal development, the small bowel mesentery runs from the ligament of Treitz at the duodenojejunal flexure on the left of the second lumbar vertebra to the ileocaecal region. The caecum is then fixed in the right iliac fossa. This gives a long base to the small bowel mesentery, which provides a stable arrangement for the superior mesenteric vessels, which lie within it
- If normal rotation does not occur the caecum can lie near the duodeno-jejunal flexure with a narrow base to the small bowel mesentery, making this more susceptible to volvulus. Acute torsion can lead to obstruction of the superior mesenteric vessels and catastrophic midgut ischaemia if untreated
- Elective surgery may be performed in order to reduce the risk of volvulus once malrotation is diagnosed. In a collapsed infant emergency laparotomy is indicated
- The goal of surgery is to produce a more stable mesenteric pedicle, and in the acute situation to restore gut perfusion and preserve as much bowel length as possible

Surgery

1. Open for emergency. Laparoscopic approach is an option for malrotation without volvulus
2. Assess gut for viability
3. Untwist volvulus
4. Assess position of the duodenojejunal flexure
5. After blood supply has been restored, resect any gangrenous bowel
6. Primary anastomosis or enterostomy formation
7. Divide Ladd's bands (peritoneal bands fixing the duodenum)
8. Straighten duodenal loop and mobilize colon
9. Broaden the base of the mesentery
10. Place the large bowel in the left side of the abdomen and the small bowel on the right (Ladd's position[2])
11. Appendicectomy, inversion, or resection

Additional procedures that may become necessary

- Bowel resection (may be massive)
- Enterostomy formation
- Primary anastomosis
- If there is doubt over the viability of the bowel, a second-look laparotomy can be done in 24–48h after initial untwisting
- Further bowel resection
- Central venous access for parenteral nutrition

Benefits
- Restore blood flow to the gut
- Place bowel in a safe position so this cannot happen again

Alternative procedures/conservative measures
- 'Open and shut' laparotomy in overwhelming gut necrosis

Significant/frequently occurring risks[1]
- Early complications:
  - Bleeding
  - Wound infection
  - Anastomotic leak
  - Death
- Late complications:
  - Anastomotic stricture
  - Adhesional bowel obstruction
  - Short bowel syndrome
  - PNALD

Type of anaesthesia/sedation
- General anaesthesia

Follow-up/need for further procedure
- Early outpatient review to check the patient is thriving
- Patients with stomas may have major fluid and electrolyte losses and will require close monitoring and nutritional support
- Patients with short bowel syndrome may need long-term total parenteral nutrition and may benefit from bowel-lengthening surgery

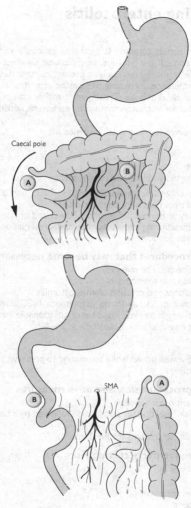

Fig. 16.2 Malrotation volvulus.

Reproduced with permission from Davenport M and Pierro A. Oxford Specialist Handbook of Paediatric Surgery. 2009. Oxford: Oxford University Press, p.142, Figure 4.6 and p.144, Figure 4.7.

References

1. Millar AJW, Rode H, Cywes S. Malrotation and volvulus in infancy and childhood. *Semin Pediatr Surg* 2003;**12**(4):229–36.
2. Ladd WE. Surgical diseases of the alimentary tract in infants. *N Engl J Med* 1936;**215** 705–8.

Necrotizing enterocolitis

Description

NEC is one of the most common surgical emergencies in neonates. It can affect small sections of the intestine, be multifocal or affect the intestine in its entirety. Seen more commonly in premature neonates,[1] symptoms include feed intolerance, increasing nasogastric aspirates, abdominal distension, and bloody diarrhoea. Treatment is mainly conservative with a long period of bowel rest, intravenous total parenteral nutrition, and antibiotics.

Surgery is reserved for those with evidence of:
• Perforation
• Obstruction
• Palpable mass
• Failure to progress with medical management

Mortality rates of 24% for medically treated NEC and 37% for NEC needing surgical treatment have been reported.[2,3]

Aim of surgery is removal of necrotic bowel and anastomosis where possible, or defunctioning enterostomies and preservation of as much intestinal length as possible.

Additional procedures that may become necessary

• Bowel resection (may be massive)
• Single resection and anastomosis
• Multiple resections and creation of enterostomies
• Limited resection or 'clip and drop' in multifocal NEC aims to salvage bowel length by retaining areas of questionable viability to be reassessed at a second look laparotomy in 24–48h[2]

Benefits

• To remove diseased bowel while attempting to preserve as much length as possible

Alternative procedures/conservative measures

• Initial treatment is conservative
• Peritoneal drain insertion for stabilization followed by a timely 'rescue' laparotomy[3]
• 'Open and shut' laparotomy for NEC totalis

Significant/frequently occurring risks

Early complications
• Bleeding
• Massive bowel resection
• Wound infection
• Anastomotic leak
• *Sepsis*
• Enterostomy complications (📖 see 'Enterostomy complications', p.505)
• Death

Late complications
- Anastomotic stricture
- Post-NEC stricture
- Abscess or fistula formation
- Adhesional bowel obstruction
- Gastro-oesophageal reflux
- Recurrence of NEC (5%)
- Short-bowel syndrome
- PNALD
- Death

Enterostomy complications
- Prolapse
- Stricture
- Retraction
- Parastomal hernia
- Fluid and electrolyte disturbance
- Inadequate weight gain
- Peristomal skin excoriation and bleeding

Type of anaesthesia/sedation
- General anaesthesia

Follow-up/need for further procedure
- Patients with a peritoneal drain will require a laparotomy
- Stoma closure
- Strictureplasty or stricture resection for post-NEC stricture
- Short-bowel syndrome babies will have a prolonged hospital stay requiring total parenteral nutrition, central venous access
- Surgery that may be required to ameliorate short-bowel syndrome includes bowel tapering, bowel lengthening, and intestinal transplantation
- Multidisciplinary follow-up is required to monitor nutrition and growth
- Patients with stomas may have major fluid and electrolyte losses and will require close monitoring and nutritional support
- These patients may also have developmental and intellectual delay

References
1. Guthrie SO, Gordon PV, Thomas V, et al. Necrotizing enterocolitis among neonates in the United States. *J Perinatol* 2003;**23**(4):278–85.
2. Ron O, Davenport M, Patel S, et al. Outcomes of the 'clip and drop' technique for multifocal necrotizing enterocolitis. *J Pediatr Surg* 2009;**44**(4):749–54.
3. Rees CM, Eaton S, Kiely EM, et al. Peritoneal drainage or laparotomy for neonatal bowel perforation? A randomized controlled trial. *Ann Surg* 2008;**248**:44–51.

Duodenal and small intestinal atresias

Description
Duodenal atresia occurs in around 1 in 5000 live births and is associated with other congenital anomalies.
- Half of these are detected on antenatal ultrasound scans
- The remainder will present in the first day of life with:
  - Vomiting (bilious or non-bilious depending on the relation of the atresia to the ampulla of Vater)
  - Abdominal distension
  - 'Double bubble' on the abdominal X-ray
- Improved operative techniques along with enhanced provision of neonatal care have improved survival rates to around 90%[1]
- Half of all patients with duodenal atresia will have chromosomal abnormalities; trisomy 21 occurs in about a third

Jejuno-ileal atresias occur due to vascular accidents usually late in the second or third trimester.
- Multiple atresias may occur if different segments are involved with viable portions of intestine surviving in between
- Most patients will be diagnosed antenatally but those who are not, typically present in the first days of life with symptoms of intestinal obstruction. They may still pass meconium
- An abdominal X-ray taken at least 24h after birth will demonstrate multiple dilated loops
- An upper gastro-intestinal contrast study can be used if there is diagnostic doubt
- A preoperative contrast enema may also be useful
- Unlike duodenal atresia, associated anomalies are uncommon

Duodenal atresia
The preferred operation for duodenal atresia is a duodeno-duodenostomy, which can be performed open or laparoscopically.[2]

Surgery
1. Mobilize duodenum
2. Duodenoduodenostomy
3. Check distal intestine for further atresias

Additional procedures that may become necessary
- Further distal anastomoses

Benefits
- Restore intestinal continuity
- Enable enteral feeding

Alternative procedures/conservative measures
- Can be performed laparoscopically or open
- Without surgical correction duodenal atresia is incompatible with life

Significant/frequently occurring risks[1]

Early complications
- Bleeding
- Wound infection
- Anastomotic leak
- Prolonged ileus
- Damage to the bile ducts has been reported

Late complications
- Anastomotic stricture
- Adhesive bowel obstruction
- Gastro-oesophageal reflux
- Duodenogastric reflux
- Gastric and duodenal ulcers
- Megaduodenum

Type of anaesthesia/sedation
- General anaesthesia

Follow-up/need for further procedure
- Late duodenal dysmotility resulting in megaduodenum may require tapering duodenoplasty
- Multidisciplinary follow-up may be required for ongoing care of associated abnormalities

Jejunal or ileal atresias
Jejunal and ileal atresias are classified into five types (Table 16.1).

Table 16.1 Classification of jejunal or ileal atresias

Type I	A complete occluding web (Fig. 16.3a)
Type II	Proximal and distal segments (Fig. 16.3b)
Type IIIa	Complete separation with a mesenteric defect (Fig. 16.3c)
Type IIIb	Proximal jejunal atresia with complete absence of the mesentery to the distal bowel—'Christmas tree' or 'apple peel' atresia
Type IV	Multiple atresias

Associated anomalies are uncommon with jejuno-ileal atresias. However, some atresias are as a result of complicated meconium ileus *in utero*. Genetic testing for cystic fibrosis should be performed.

Surgical repair involves anastomosing the proximal and distal atretic segments to restore continuity and aims to preserve intestinal length.

Surgery
1. Usually a transverse supra-umbilical incision
2. Assess length
3. Trace dilated bowel distally to the atresia
4. Resect proximal dilated bowel in case of major size discrepancy if sufficient length allows

5. Perform tapering or imbrication enteroplasty of proximal bowel if necessary to preserve bowel length
6. Perform enterostomy if baby is unstable
7. Examine for further atresias by flushing distal loop

Additional procedures that may become necessary

- Bowel resection
- Anastomosis
- Formation of enterostomy

Benefits

- Restore intestinal continuity
- Enable enteral feeding

Alternative procedures/conservative measures

- Without surgical correction intestinal atresias are incompatible with life

Significant/frequently occurring risks[3]

Early complications

- Bleeding
- Wound infection
- Anastomotic leak

Late complications

- Anastomotic stricture
- Adhesive bowel obstruction
- Gastro-oesophageal reflux
- Short bowel syndrome
- PNALD
- Sepsis
- Death

Type of anaesthesia/sedation

- General anaesthesia

Follow-up/need for further procedure

- Bowel length influences the long-term outcome in these patients: 5–10% of children may develop short-bowel syndrome and need long-term parenteral nutrition or even a liver or small bowel transplant
- Motility problems may occur many years after surgical repair. Dilatation of the proximal bowel with anastomotic narrowing may require anastomotic revision, tapering, or plication

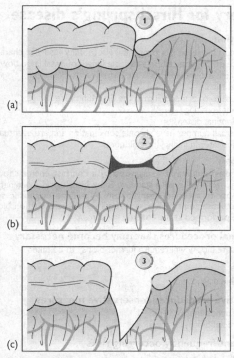

Fig. 16.3 Bland–Sutton classification of intestinal atresia: (a) complete occluding web, mural continuity; (b) cord joining proximal and distal segments; and (c) complete separation with mesenteric defect.

Reproduced with permission from Davenport M and Pierro A. *Oxford Specialist Handbook of Paediatric Surgery*. 2009. Oxford: Oxford University Press. p.146, Figure 4.8.

References

1. Escobar MA, Ladd AP, Grosfeld JL, *et al.* Duodenal atresia and stenosis: Long-term follow-up over 30 years. *J Pediatr Surg* 2004;**39**(6):867–71.
2. Kimura K, Mukohara N, Nishijima E, *et al.* Diamond shaped anastomosis for duodenal atresia: an experience with 44 patients over 15 years. *J Pediatr Surg* 1990;**25**:977–9.
3. Dalla Vekkia LK, Grosfeld JL, West KW, *et al.* Intestinal atresia and stenosis: a 25 year experience with 277 cases. *Arch Surg* 1998;**133**:490–6.

Surgery for Hirschsprung's disease

Description

Hirschsprung's disease is a congenital gut motility disorder characterized by absence of ganglion cells in a variable length of distal large bowel.

- Incidence is around 1 in 5000 live births[1]
- Classical triad:
  - Failure to pass meconium in the first 48h of life
  - Bilious vomiting
  - Abdominal distension
- A very small number have chronic constipation and are eventually diagnosed later in infancy or childhood

Rectal biopsy

Although diagnosis may be suggested by a contrast enema showing the 'transitional zone', the gold standard is by histological examination of a rectal biopsy to ascertain aganglionosis. A suitable diagnostic specimen of rectal mucosa and submucosa is required. A rectal suction biopsy can usually be performed at the cot-side in infants.

Additional procedures that may become necessary

- Inadequate biopsy will require further biopsy to be taken

Benefits

- To enable diagnosis

Alternative procedures/conservative measures

- Rectal suction biopsy
- Open rectal biopsy

Significant/frequently occurring risks

- Bleeding
- Inadequate biopsy
- Infection

Type of anaesthesia/sedation

- Anaesthesia is not required for rectal suction biopsy in infants as biopsy is taken from above the dentate line
- General anaesthesia—for larger children having open biopsy

Follow-up/need for further procedure

- If Hirschsprung's disease is confirmed, a daily rectal washout regimen will need to be initiated. Parents can be taught to perform rectal washout and definitive surgery discussed. This is commonly performed as a single procedure primary pull-through
- If adequate bowel decompression cannot be achieved by washouts, defunctioning enterostomy will be required

Duhamel's retro-rectal pull-through and Soave's endorectal pull-through[2,3]

The aim of surgery is to resect aganglionic bowel and to re-anastomose the remaining ganglionic bowel to the anal canal. Both of these operations aim to preserve the innervation of the pelvic organs by minimizing the pelvic dissection.

- In the Duhamel procedure (Fig. 16.4c) the distal rectum is left *in situ* and the normal bowel is brought down in a retro-rectal tunnel. An end-to-side anastomosis is performed before stapling the common septum to create a rectal pouch
- In the Soave operation (Fig. 16.4a) the seromuscular layer is separated from the mucosal layer of the rectum, which is then removed leaving a sheath of muscle. The normal bowel is then pulled through this muscle and anastomosed to the anus

Both techniques are suitable for laparoscopic assisted repair.

Additional procedures that may become necessary

- A colostomy may be fashioned to protect the pelvic anastomosis
- Closure of stoma

Benefits

- Remove aganglionic colon
- Enable patients to pass stool

Alternative procedures/conservative measures

- Can be performed laparoscopically or open
- Can be done as a one-stage or a two-stage procedure with a covering stoma in the newborn
- A levelling colostomy can be performed followed by definitive pull through at a later stage for those patients who present late and have significant colonic distension
- Can be performed via a abdominal and transanal approach or totally via the transanal approach

Significant/frequently occurring risks

Early complications
- Bleeding
- Wound infection
- Perianal excoriation
- Rectal prolapse
- Anastomotic leak
- Pelvic sepsis

Late complications
- Anastomotic stricture
- Rectocolonic spur formation (Duhamel)
- Adhesional bowel obstruction
- Constipation (~30%)
- Enterocolitis (15–30%)
- Incontinence
- Death

Type of anaesthesia/sedation
- General anaesthesia

Follow-up/need for further procedure[4-6]
- Urinary incontinence and sexual dysfunction may affect a small number of adult and adolescent patients
- Patients who have had a Duhamel may develop constipation due to a recurrent rectocolonic spur which may need re-division
- Constipation can be a problem following both procedures
- Frequent bowel movements can also be a problem but should usually subside within 6–12 months; 80% of patients should have fewer than three to four bowel motions per day 2–3 years after a pull-through procedure

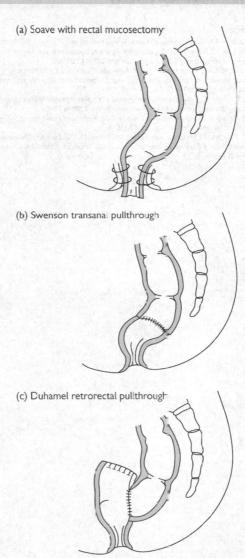

(a) Soave with rectal mucosectomy

(b) Swenson transanal pullthrough

(c) Duhamel retrorectal pullthrough

Fig. 16.4 (a) Soave, (b) Swenson, and (c) Duhamel procedures for Hirschsprung's disease.

Reproduced with permission from MacKay GJ, Dorrance HR, Molloy RG, et al. Oxford Specialist Handbook of Colorectal Surgery. 2010. Oxford: Oxford University Press, p.235, Figure 5.11.

References

1. Spouge D, Baird PA. Hirschsprung's disease in a large birth cohort. *Teratology* 1985;**32**:171–7.
2. Keckler SJ, Yang JC, Fraser JD, *et al*. Contemporary practice patterns in the surgical management of Hirschsprung's disease. *J Pediatr Surg* 2009;**44**:1257–60.
3. Teitelbaum DH, Cilley RE, Sherman NJ, *et al*. A decade of experience with the primary pull-through for Hirschsprung's Disease in the newborn period: A multicenter analysis of outcomes. *Ann Surg* 2000;**232**:372–80.
4. Dasgupta R, Langer JC. Evaluation and management of persistent problems after surgery for Hirschsprung disease in a child. *J Pediatr Gastroenterol Nutr* 2008;**46**:13–19.
5. Rintala RJ, Pakarinen MP. Outcome of anorectal malformations and Hirschsprung's disease beyond childhood. *Semin Pediatr Surg* 2010;**19**:160–7.
6. Rintala RJ, Pakarinen M. Hirschsprung's disease. In: Stringer MD, Oldham KT, Mouriquand PDE (eds) *Pediatric Surgery and Urology. Long-term Outcomes*. Cambridge: Cambridge University Press, 2006:385–400.

Neurosurgery

Introduction to neurosurgery

The fundamental aim of neurosurgical intervention is the improvement of neurological symptoms by relieving structures of the nervous system from the pathological effects of pressure. However modest this aim might be, it nevertheless entails a significant amount of risk, largely due to the inherent complexity of the nervous system and its associated disorders. The brain and spine are notoriously challenging operative territories with very little tolerance to surgical insult. The difference between gain and catastrophic loss in neurosurgery can quite easily be a matter of millimetres. Consequently, obtaining informed consent requires that the consenting surgeon possesses a clear understanding of neuroanatomical structure and function. Moreover, there must also be a firm understanding of what is realistically achievable within the context of the presenting problem.

Presented in this chapter are consent templates for a number of basic neurosurgical procedures that junior surgical trainees should be familiar with. The general indications and benefits are listed, along with what the authors feel to be the significant associated risks and complications. It is by no means an exhaustive selection of procedures, as the number of approaches to the three-dimensional space of the nervous system are far too numerous to be covered within a single chapter. There is deliberate omission of consent templates for deep brain and skull base surgery, as well as approaches to the complex spine. This has been done with the belief that consent in such circumstances should ideally be done in light of presenting symptoms and individual anatomy. Nevertheless, a few principles regarding the general complications of intracranial and spinal procedures, as well as regional neurological syndromes, are provided for reference.

General risks and complications

Intracranial procedures

The full range of risks and complications cannot be generalized across all intracranial procedures. The nature of the underlying surgical lesion (e.g. bleed vs. tumour vs. aneurysm), as well as the location of the lesion influences the type and degree of risk. However, a few significant complications, with a collective complication rate in the region of 5–10%, are shared by the vast majority of intracranial procedures:

- Risk of general anaesthesia
- Wound infection (<5%)[1–3]
- Bleeding (~1%)[4,5]
- Leak of cerebrospinal fluid (requiring repair) (<5%)[2,3]
- Meningitis (<2%)[6]
- Injury to surrounding neural/vascular structures
- Deterioration of neurology
- Chest infection
- DVT (8%)[7,8]
- Pulmonary embolism (~0.1%)[7]
- Seizure (15–25%)[9–11]
- Stroke
- Coma
- Death

Spinal procedures

As with cranial procedures, the specific risks for spinal procedures are dependent on the level of the pathology and operation. In general, however, there are few notable common complications:

- Risk of general anaesthesia
- Superficial infection (<5%)[12]
- Deep infection (discitis, epidural abscess) (<1%)[13,14]
- Dural tear (0.3–13%)[15]
- Cerebrospinal fluid leak, pseudomeningocoele, cerebrospinal fluid fistula, meningitis (<2%)[13,15]
- Failure to relieve symptoms
- Increased pain, numbness
- Increased motor deficit: quadriplegia/paraplegia ± double incontinence (according to level)
- Recurrent herniated disc (4%)[16]
- Chest infection
- DVT (<2%)[7,8]
- Pulmonary embolus (0.1%)[7]
- Death

References

1. Lietard C, Thebaud V, Besson G, *et al.* Risk factors for neurosurgical site infections: an 18-month prospective survey. *J Neurosurg* 2008;**109**(4):729–34.
2. Korinek AM. Risk factors for neurosurgical site infections after craniotomy: a prospective multicenter study of 2944 patients. *Neurosurgery* 1997;**41**(5):1073–9.
3. Blomstedt GC. Craniotomy infections. *Neurosurg Clin Am* 1992;**3**(2):375–85.
4. Kalfas IH, Little JR. Postoperative hemorrhage: A survey of 4992 intracranial procedures. *Neurosurgery* 1988;**23**(3):343–7.
5. Palmer JD, Sparrow OC, Iannotti FI. Postoperative hematoma: A 5 year survey and identification of avoidable risk factors. *Neurosurgery* 1994;**35**(6):1061–5.
6. Van de Beek D, Drake DM, Tunkel AR. Nosocomial bacterial meningitis. *N Engl J Med* 2010;**362**:146–54.
7. Epstein NE. A review of the risks and benefits of differing prophylaxis regimens for the treatment of deep venous thrombosis and pulmonary embolism in neurosurgery. *Surg Neurol* 2005;**64**(4):295–301.
8. Flinn WR, Sandager GP, Silva MB, *et al.* Prospective surveillance for perioperative venous thrombosis. Experience in 2643 patients. *Arch Surg* 1997;**132**(2):212–13.
9. Rabinstein AA, Chung SY, Rudzinski LA, *et al.* Seizures after evacuation of subdural hematomas : incidence, risk factors, and functional impact. *J Neurosurg* 2010;**112**(2):455–80.
10. Sabo RA, Hanigan WC, Aldag JC. Chronic subdural haematomas and seizures: the role of prophylactic anticonvulsant medication. *Surg Neurol* 1995;**43**(6):579–82.
11. Shaw MD, Foy PM. Epilepsy after craniotomy and the place of prophylactic anticonvulsant drugs: discussion paper. *J R Soc Med* 1991;**84**(4):221–3.
12. Shektman A, Granick MS, Solomon MP, *et al.* Management of infected laminectomy wounds. *Neurosurgery* 1994;**35**(2):307–9.
13. Spiegelmann R, Findler G, Faibel M. Postoperative spinal epidural empyema: Clinical and computed tomography features. *Spine* 1991;**16**(1):1146–9.
14. Rawlings CE, Wilkins RH, Gallis HA. Postoperative intervertebral disc space infection. *Neurosurgery* 1983;**13**(4):371–6.
15. Goodkin R, Laksa LL. Unintended 'incidental' durotomy during surgery of the lumbar spine: medicolegal implications. *Surg Neurol* 1995;**43**(1):4–14.
16. Davis RA. A long-term outcome analysis of 984 surgically treated herniated lumbar discs. *J Neurosurg* 1994;**80**(3):415–21.

Regional neurological syndromes

Applied anatomy and lesion localization is crucial to understanding the risks associated with operating in and around specific structures within the brain. The regional brain syndromes that occur following insult to portions of the functional lobes of the brain may produce characteristic patterns of deficit that should be noted preoperatively, and potentially highlighted during consent.

Frontal
- Hemiparesis, apathy, personality change, impairment of gaze (with posterior frontal lesions)

Parietal
- *Dominant side*: aphasias, bilateral astereognosis, dyscalculia
- *Non-dominant side*: apraxia, geographical disorientation
- *Either side*: cortical sensory syndrome, sensory extinction, contralateral homonymous hemianopia, contralateral neglect

Occipital
- Homonymous hemianopia

Temporal
- Aphasias, memory impairment, emotional lability

Pituitary
- Visual field loss, endocrine disturbance

Brainstem
- Cardiorespiratory compromise, mixture of cranial nerve deficits and long tract signs

Cerebellum
- *Hemispheric*: ipsilateral limb ataxia
- *Vermian*: truncal ataxia

The identification and documentation of preoperative deficit is crucial to the neurosurgical consent process. The motor and sensory cortices, and the deep brain nuclei and long tracts, can be affected by a wide variety of pathology, as well as during surgery. Typically, great care is taken to avoid these structures, but where symptoms already exist, or where the possibility of loss may occur, it should be highlighted in the consent process that weakness, sensory loss, or worsening of existing deficit may occur either transiently or permanently.

Craniotomy and evacuation of acute subdural haematoma

Description

This procedure involves evacuation of the acute subdural haematoma (which is usually but not always the result of a severe brain injury, and often performed as an emergency). A suitable area of the scalp is shaved, and an appropriately sited scalp incision ± raising of a scalp flap is performed. A bone flap is created and the dura is opened to access the subdural space. Using a combination of generous irrigation and suction, the visible clot is removed, and any obvious bleeding points controlled. Unless there is significant brain swelling, the dura, bone, and skin flaps are closed, usually with a temporary subdural drain left *in situ* for 24–48h. This drain is generally removed on the ward.

Additional procedures that may become necessary

- Insertion of an arterial line
- Insertion of CVP line
- Insertion of urinary catheter

Benefits

- To evacuate the compressive clot
- To ameliorate the secondary effects of cerebral compression, and hopefully save life
- To prevent further neurological deterioration, and achieve best possible survival

Alternative procedures/conservative measures

- Observation to allow maturation/absorption of clot

Serious/frequently occurring risk

- Wound infection
- Bleeding and recollection of clot
- Repeat operation
- Cerebral swelling, leak of cerebrospinal fluid
- Meningitis
- Tension pneumocephalus
- Electrolyte disturbance
- Injury to local neural/vascular structures
- Neurological deterioration
- Seizure, stroke, coma
- Thromboembolic disease
- Chest infection
- Death

Blood transfusion necessary

- Cross-match 2 units

Type of anaesthesia/sedation
- General anaesthesia

Follow-up/need for further procedure
- Recollection requiring further procedure

Craniotomy and evacuation of acute extradural haematoma

Description

This procedure involves evacuation of the acute extradural haematoma (which classically follows skull fracture with rupture of the underlying meningeal artery). A suitable area of the scalp is shaved, and an appropriately sited (usually temporo-frontal) scalp incision is performed ± raising of a skin/temporalis muscle flap. A bone flap is created to access the extradural space. Using a combination of generous irrigation and suction, the visible clot is removed, and any obvious source of bleeding (e.g. middle meningeal artery) controlled. Unless there is significant brain swelling, the bone and skin flaps are closed, usually with a temporary extradural drain left *in situ* for 24–48h. This drain is generally removed on the ward.

Additional procedures that may become necessary

- Insertion of an arterial line
- Insertion of CVP line
- Insertion of urinary catheter

Benefits

- To evacuate the compressive clot
- To alleviate intracranial pressure and limit secondary cerebral damage
- To prevent further neurological deterioration and improve neurological outcome

Alternative procedures/conservative measures

- Observation to allow maturation/absorption of clot

Serious/frequently occurring risk

- Wound infection
- Bleeding and recollection of clot
- Repeat operation
- Leak of cerebrospinal fluid
- Meningitis
- Neurological deterioration
- Seizure
- Stroke
- Coma
- Thromboembolic disease
- Chest infection
- Death

Blood transfusion necessary

- Cross-match 2 units

Type of anaesthesia/sedation

- General anaesthesia

Follow-up/need for further procedure

- Recollection requiring further procedure

Burrhole evacuation of chronic subdural haematoma

Description

This procedure involves evacuation of the chronic subdural haematoma (usually as the result of trivial or unforgotten trauma without underlying brain injury). A 3–4cm scalp incision is appropriately sited to the location and dimensions of the subdural collection, followed by the drilling of a 1.5cm burrhole through the cranium. A small opening is made in the dura to access the subdural space and relieve symptomatic pressure. Using generous irrigation, liquid clot is evacuated, and any obvious bleeding points controlled. The skin is closed over the burrhole(s), usually with a temporary subdural drain left *in situ* for 24–48h. This is generally removed on the ward.

Additional procedures that may become necessary

- Insertion of an arterial line
- Insertion of CVP line
- Insertion of urinary catheter

Benefits

- To evacuate the liquid collection and improve neurological symptoms/ headache
- To prevent further neurological deterioration and hasten natural recovery

Alternative procedures/conservative measures

- Observation with natural absorption of clot
- Intravenous/oral steroids

Serious/frequently occurring risk

- Wound infection
- Bleeding and recollection of clot (10% with drain vs. 19% without)[1]
- Leak of cerebrospinal fluid, meningitis
- Tension pneumocephalus
- Injury to local neural/vascular structures
- Neurological deterioration
- Seizure, stroke, coma
- Thromboembolic disease
- Chest infection
- Death

Blood transfusion necessary

- Group and save

Type of anaesthesia/sedation

- General anaesthesia

Follow-up/need for further procedure

- Recollection requiring further procedure

Reference

1. Lind CR, Lind CJ, Mee EW. Reduction in the number of repeated operations for the treatment of subacute and chronic subdural hematomas by placement of subdural drains. *J Neurosurg* 2003;**99**(1):44–6.

Ventricular catheterization (insertion of an external ventricular drain)

Description

Indicated in the presence of acute hydrocephalus requiring emergency cerebrospinal fluid diversion, this procedure involves insertion of a ventricular catheter into the frontal horn of the lateral ventricle of the non-dominant (usually right) hemisphere. A small sagittal scalp incision is made 1–2cm anterior to the coronal suture in the mid-pupillary line (Kocher's point). A single burrhole is made, followed by a small durotomy and cortical puncture to allow passage of the ventricular catheter. The catheter is inserted perpendicular to the surface of the brain to a depth of approximately 5–7cm, with the expectation of ventricular penetration and cerebrospinal fluid drainage prior to that depth. The distal end of the catheter is tunnelled underneath the scalp to exit at a separate site at least 5cm from the initial incision. The scalp is closed over the frontal burrhole site, and the ventricular catheter is fixed in place with non-absorbable sutures/clips and connected to an appropriate drain/manometer.

Additional procedures that may become necessary

- Insertion of an arterial line
- Insertion of CVP line
- Insertion of urinary catheter

Benefits

- To reduce intracranial pressure by decompressing the ventricles
- To prevent further neurological deterioration

Alternative procedures/conservative measures

- Serial lumbar puncture (In the absence of contraindications)
- Serious/frequently occurring risk
- Wound infection
- Bleeding
- Haematoma requiring evacuation (0.5–2.5%)[1]
- Drain misplacement
- Leak of cerebrospinal fluid; meningitis/ventriculitis (1–27%)[2]
- Injury to local neural/vascular structures
- Neurological deterioration
- Seizure, stroke, coma
- Thromboembolic disease
- Chest infection
- Death

Blood transfusion necessary

- Rarely required
- Group and save

Type of anaesthesia/sedation

- General anaesthesia

References

1. Maniker AH, Vaynman AY, Karimi RJ. Hemorrhagic complications of external ventricular drainage. *Neurosurgery.* 2006;**59**(4 Suppl 2):419–24.
2. Lovzier AP, Sciacca RR, Romanoli M. Ventriculostomy-related infection: A critical review of the literature. *Neurosurgery* 2002;**51**(1):170–82.

Ventriculoperitoneal shunt

Description

Indicated in the presence of hydrocephalus requiring long-term cerebrospinal fluid diversion. This procedure involves insertion of a ventricular catheter into the lateral ventricle to drain cerebrospinal fluid in a controlled fashion via a valve and longer catheter, which is tunnelled inferiorly under the skin and subcutaneous tissues to drain in the peritoneal cavity. There are therefore two scars: one cranial, one on the ipsilateral abdomen.

A small patch of hair is shaved behind the ear, and a small horseshoe-shaped incision is made to site an burrhole on either the parietal eminence (roughly 3cm above and 3cm behind the tip of the ear), lambdoid suture or at the precoronal position (both 3cm from midline). Deep to the burrhole, a small durotomy and corticotomy is made to allow passage of the ventricular catheter. The catheter is inserted perpendicular to the surface of the brain to a depth of approximately 4–5cm, with the expectation of intraventricular access and cerebrospinal fluid drainage. The catheter is attached to a reservoir that typically sits flush to the surface of the skull, and which may be palpated post-operatively to confirm shunt functioning.

At the abdomen, a transverse subcostal incision lateral and superior to the umbilicus is one of several sites used to access the peritoneal cavity. Skin, anterior abdominal musculature, and pre-peritoneal fat is encountered en route to the peritoneal cavity. A subcutaneous trochar is passed between the two incisions taking care to avoid injuring the subclavian structures cranially, or inadvertently entering the thoracic/abdominal cavities. The peritoneal catheter is threaded through the trochar and implanted in the free peritoneum.

Additional procedures that may become necessary

- Insertion of an arterial line
- Insertion of CVP line
- Insertion of urinary catheter

Benefits

- To reduce intracranial pressure by decompressing the ventricles
- To prevent further neurological deterioration and hopefully to improve neurological symptoms/headache

Alternative procedures/conservative measures

- Observation to allow maturation/absorption of clot

Serious/frequently occurring risk

- Wound infection
- Shunt misplacement
- Shunt infection (<5%)[1]
- Shunt blockage (12–34%)[2]
- Reoperation
- Cerebrospinal fluid leak, meningitis/ventriculitis
- Injury to local neural/vascular structures

- Bowel injury
- Peritonitis
- Neurological deterioration
- Seizure (5.5%),[3] stroke, coma
- Thromboembolic disease
- Chest infection
- Death

Blood transfusion necessary

- Cross-match 2 units

Type of anaesthesia/sedation

- General anaesthesia

References

1. Yogev R. Cerebrospinal fluid shunt infections: A personal view. *Pediatr Infect Dis* 1985;**4**(2): 113–18.
2. Cozzens JW, Chandler JP. Increased risk of distal ventriculoperitoneal shunt obstruction associated with slit valves or distal slits in the peritoneal catheter. *J Neurosurg* 1997;**87**(5):682–6.
3. Dan NG, Wade MJ. The incidence of epilepsy after ventricular shunting procedures. *J Neurosurg* 1986;**65**(1):19–21.

Insertion of an intracranial bolt/pressure monitor

Description

This is indicated where intracranial pressure monitoring is required for diagnostic purposes, or to aid in the critical care management of head-injured or otherwise unconscious patients. This procedure involves insertion of a fine pressure sensor wire into the substance of the frontal lobe of the non-dominant (usually right) hemisphere (Fig. 17.1). A small sagittal scalp incision is made 1–2cm anterior to the coronal suture in the mid-pupillary line (Kocher's Point). A single 3–5mm hole is drilled through the cranium, followed by a dural puncture to allow passage of the pressure monitor. A securing bolt is inserted into the hole, through which the intracranial pressure line is inserted perpendicular to the surface of the brain with adequate length to ensure that 2–3cm of it lie within the brain substance. Both the line and the securing bolt will be removed when no longer required.

Additional procedures that may become necessary

- Insertion of an arterial line (for head-injured patients)
- Insertion of CVP line (for head-injured patients)
- Insertion of urinary catheter (for head-injured patients)

Benefits

- To aid in the diagnosis of raised intracranial pressure states
- To provide a means of dynamic intracranial pressure monitoring

Alternative procedures/conservative measures

- Burr hole or open craniotomy and insertion of intracranial pressure line in the subdural, parenchymal, or ventricular space

Serious/frequently occurring risk

(In addition to those associated with the underlying pathology)
- Wound/intracranial pressure line infection
- Bleeding
- Formation of haematoma requiring evacuation (0.5–2.5%)[1]
- Leak of cerebrospinal fluid
- Meningitis
- Seizure
- Coma
- Death

Blood transfusion necessary

- Rarely required

Type of anaesthesia/sedation

- General anaesthesia

Microsensor options

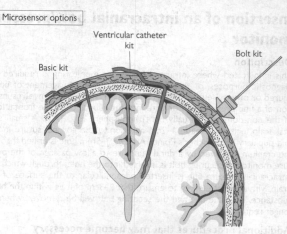

Ventricular catheter
kit

Bolt kit

Basic kit

Fig. 17.1 Intracranial pressure monitor.

Reproduced with permission from O'Connor IF and Urdang M. *Oxford Handbook of Surgical Cross-Cover.* 2008. Oxford: Oxford University Press, p.266, Figure 6.17.

Reference

1. Maniker AH, Vaynman AY, Karimi RJ. Hemorrhagic complications of external ventricular drainage. *Neurosurgery* 2006;**59**(4 Suppl 2):419–24.

Lumbar laminectomy/discectomy

Description

Indicated for cauda equina syndrome, progressive neurological deficit, radicular pain refractory to non-surgical management. This procedure involves positioning the patient in a face-down position in theatre. The lumbar vertebrae/discs are approached via an appropriately sited longitudinal midline lower back incision. The fascia is opened and the paralumbar muscles are retracted to expose the appropriate spinal segment. The interlaminar ligamentum is opened/removed and the surrounding bone ± disc material carefully removed to achieve decompression of the affected lumbar nerve roots.

Additional procedures that may become necessary

- Insertion of an arterial line
- Insertion of CVP line
- Insertion of urinary catheter

Benefits

- To improve pain
- To prevent further neurological deterioration

Alternative procedures/conservative measures

- Conservative physiotherapy
- Caudal/nerve root/facet injections
- Analgesic management

Serious/frequently occurring risk

- Failure to relieve symptoms
- Wound infection
- Dural tear
- Leak of cerebrospinal fluid
- Meningocele/cerebrospinal fluid fistula
- Meningitis
- Discitis
- Recurrent disc protrusion
- Reoperation
- Injury to local neural/vascular structures
- Neurological deterioration—increased pain numbness and weakness
- Quadriplegia/paraplegia ± double incontinence (according to level)
- Thromboembolic disease
- Chest infection
- Death

Blood transfusion necessary

- Cross-match 2 units

Type of anaesthesia/sedation

- General anaesthesia

Cardiac surgery

Consent in cardiac surgery

Individual surgeons' mortality data have been in the public domain for several years and most patients now expect a detailed discussion on the likely outcome from surgery. The Parliamentary Ombudsman's report[1] on consent in cardiac surgery recommends that during the consent process patients should be told about:

• Potential benefits
• Potential side effects
• Potential complications (differentiating between side effects and complications)
• The outcomes for high-volume operations, e.g. how many people have had complications in the unit during the year (on an institutional basis and where appropriate on a surgeon-specific basis)
• Chances of success, i.e. will the operation deliver what it is designed to achieve
• Unit infection rates

It is also necessary to have some discussion on alternative treatments (i.e. medical and interventional therapy).

Signing of the consent form records only one stage in an ongoing process. Many NHS trusts operate a two-stage consent process. In the first stage the consultant in charge of a patient's care should discuss the proposed surgery with the patient. Alternatively, consent may be obtained either by a surgeon who is capable of performing the procedure independently and who understands the risks and benefits, or a professional who has been specifically trained to do so. For elective cardiac surgery the first stage of consent should occur in the outpatient setting some time prior to admission to hospital. In the second stage, consent is confirmed prior to surgery.

An accurate prediction of the risk of death or morbidity is essential to a process of informed consent. Taking just one commonly predictive factor, age, between 2004 and 2008 the mortality from isolated carotid artery bypass graft (CABG) in the UK ranged from 0.7% in those aged <61 to 8.7% in those aged >85. Several risk-scoring systems have been developed in cardiac surgery, predominately the Parsonnet, additive Euroscore, and Logistic Euroscore. All of these have now been shown to underestimate survival, due to a combination of improving survival and increasingly high-risk patients. A better risk estimate *may* be obtained by multiplying the logistic Euroscore by a value of 0.5.[2]

In addition it is clear that specific operations carry their own particular operative risk, and it is no longer enough to classify procedures as 'CABG' or 'non-CABG' (as per the Euroscore). The United States Society of Thoracic Surgeons has developed new models that incorporate patient specific data for several procedures (ℰ www.sts.org/riskmodels). These models have yet to be validated against UK data but it is likely that they will represent an improvement on existing methods, and they have been accepted for the assessment of surgical risk in the current European guidelines on myocardial revascularization.[3] These models predict not only survival and overall risk of major morbidity but also specific risks such as prolonged ventilation, stroke and new or significantly worsened renal failure. At the time of writing new UK-specific models are being developed by the Society for Cardiothoracic Surgery,[4] based on the wealth of information collected in the National Adult Cardiac Surgical Database. Data collection is also underway for a new version of Euroscore. In time these models will allow more accurate risk prediction utilizing UK and Europe-specific data.

As well as getting the statistics right, it is also essential in cardiac surgery (as in all specialties) that information is presented in the way that patients are most likely to understand. Written information should be provided to patients in their primary language, and diagrams will also be helpful. No risk scoring system can predict complications accurately for the individual patient—only for a statistical population of similar patients- this can be challenging to convey, as few people truly understand risk. Patients have discouraged the use of metaphors. It is preferable to use survival data rather than mortality, and avoid percentages, instead using 'If I were to operate on 100 people like you, then I would expect 98 of them to survive and leave hospital.'[5] Cardiac surgery is performed on diverse patient populations for whom different complications may be given different weight. A worker with dependents may prioritize an early return to work while an elderly patient may pragmatically prioritize complications resulting in loss of independence or quality of life over mortality risk. It is not possible for the clinician to predict a patient's priorities, and good communication is essential.[6]

In most centres, on-table transoesophageal echocardiography (TOE) will be performed when valve surgery is under consideration. Where the operative process of valve repair versus replacement may partly depend upon intraoperative findings this must be made clear to patients when consent is obtained, for example 'mitral valve repair/replacement'. Consent should be obtained for foreseeable outcomes. It may be appropriate to include in the consent process information about any expected ITU or overnight intensive recovery unit stay, and the predicted duration of hospital stay.

The anaesthetist bears responsibility for obtaining consent for general anaesthesia, and this process can begin when the patient is first referred for surgery. Patient information booklets should contain information about the anaesthetic aspects of care.

References

1. The Health Service Ombudsman. *Consent in Cardiac Surgery: A Good Practice Guide to Agreeing and Recording Consent*. London: The Health Service Ombudsman, 2005.
2. Choong CK, Sergeant P, Nashef SA, *et al*. The EuroSCORE risk stratification system in the current era: how accurate is it and what should be done if it is inaccurate? *Eur J Cardiothorac Surg* 2009;**35**(1):59–61.
3. Guidelines on Myocardial Revascularization. The task force on myocardial revascularsation of the European Society of Cardiology (ESC) and the European Association for Cardio-Thoracic Surgery (EACTS). *Eur Heart J* 2010;PMID 20802243.
4. The Society for Cardiothoracic Surgery in Great Britain & Ireland. *Sixth National Adult Cardiac Surgical Database Report*. The Society for Cardiothoracic Surgery in Great Britain & Ireland. Dendrite Clinical Systems Ltd. 2009.
5. Kurbaan AS, Rickards AF, Ilsley CD, *et al*. Consent in cardiac practice. *Heart* 2001;**86** 593–4.
6. Bridgewater B, Keogh B. Surgical 'league tables'. *Heart* 2008;**94**:936–42.

Coronary artery bypass grafting

Major indications

Interpretation of the results of randomized controlled trials in cardiac surgery is complicated by several factors, predominantly the ongoing improvements in surgical (technique, choice of graft, choice of cardioprotection) and medical therapy (Fig. 18.1). A major new European guideline was published in 2010 by the European Society of Cardiology (ESC) and the European Association for Cardio-Thoracic Surgery (EACTS);[1] these guidelines provide a comprehensive source of evidence on which the multi-disciplinary 'heart team' can base decisions and it should be read in full. CABG is performed to improve the patient's life expectancy or symptoms. For asymptomatic or in well-controlled patients, clearly only a prognostic benefit is of value.[2,3] It is important to be clear what the intended benefits of the procedure are when obtaining consent. The major indications (largely supported by multiple randomized controlled trials or meta-analyses) are summarized as follows.[4]

Major indications in stable disease

- For life expectancy:
  - Left main stenosis >50%
  - Proximal left anterior descending (LAD) stenosis >50%
  - Two- or three-vessel disease with impaired left ventricular (LV) function
  - A proven area of ischaemia (>10% myocardium)
- For symptoms:
  - >50% stenosis with angina (or equivalent) that is unresponsive to optimal medical therapy
  - Possibly for dyspnoea/congestive heart failure and >10% area of ischaemia, supplied by an artery with >50% stenosis

Indications in non-ST-segment elevation myocardial infarction (STEMI)

- One or two-vessel disease involving proximal LAD
- Three-vessel disease (preference over percutaneous coronary intervention (PCI) is even stronger for complex lesions, when incomplete revascularization is achievable and with a SYNTAX score >22)
- Left main stem stenosis (regardless of the ostium/shaft/bifurcation location of the stenosis) with one-, two-, or three-vessel disease. Preference over PCI is even stronger with two-/three-vessel disease and SYNTAX score ≥33

Indications in STEMI

- PCI is the primary treatment. CABG may be indicated when:
  - PCI has failed or when the anatomy is unfavourable for PCI, and
  - The area of ischaemic myocardium is very large, and
  - *CABG can be carried out within 3–4h*

There appears to be an inverse relationship between time delay after STEMI and CABG mortality; delay for several days may be beneficial when ongoing symptoms are absent.

CABG with valve surgery

When there is an indication for aortic/mitral valve surgery CABG is *recommended* when the coronary stenosis is ≥70% and should be *considered* when it is 50–70%.

Risks

Evidence-based mortality and major morbidity rates should be estimated on an individual patient basis where possible, using the best available data (📖 see 'Consent in cardiac surgery', p.534) Morbidity rates (the first five factors listed after death) may currently be estimated using the Society of Thoracic Surgeons' models. These risks vary widely with operative and patient factors and general estimates are listed here. Much of this detail would be described in the preoperative information booklet, as this represents more information than is likely to be retained from a single consultation.

- Death
- Permanent stroke
- New renal impairment (including dialysis)
- Reoperation for any reason, e.g. infection, bleeding, rewiring
- Prolonged ventilation
- Deep sternal wound infection
- Bleeding requiring reoperation (~3.5%)
- Postoperative atrial fibrillation (~30%)
- Perioperative myocardial infarction (~1%)
- Graft failure and angina recurrence: 16–30% of saphenous vein grafts (SVGs) fail within 1 year, ~50% fail within 10 years. This is likely to be responsible for the recurrence rate of angina—4–9% per year
- Depression, 'post-op blues' (up to 18%)
- Pneumonia (up to 20% in active smokers)
- Other neurological dysfunction
  - Type 1: transient or permanent motor, speech, or sensory deficit. (~1–3%)
  - Type 2: intellectual impairment (~3%)

Screening for significant carotid stenosis prior to coronary surgery

In the current joint ESC/EACTS guidelines, preoperative duplex assessment of the carotid arteries is recommended for all patients with a prior transient ischaemic attack (TIA)/CVA or a bruit on auscultation. Duplex assessment should be considered in those aged ≥75, or with left main stem disease, or severe peripheral arterial disease.

CABG may be performed with or without (off-pump, OPCABG) cardiopulmonary bypass. OPCABG may have benefits in experienced hands, but a recent trial randomized 2203 patients to either on-pump or off-pump CABG and found no significant difference in mortality, and a higher graft failure rate with OPCABG.[5] This study has been criticized as participants were relatively lower risk, operations were mostly carried out by supervised trainees and there was a 12% intraoperative cross-over (to on-pump). At the time of writing NICE guidance[6] is being updated. OPCABG may be of greater benefit in high-risk patients (under investigation in the CRISP trial).

Information to help explain the procedure
- Veins or arteries taken from elsewhere in the body are used to bypass the blocked arteries supplying the heart with blood. One artery is usually taken from within the chest; additional arteries and veins are usually required. It is not always possible to know in advance how many bypasses will be performed
- *Having Heart Surgery*—💾 www.bhf.org.uk/publications.aspx
- British Cardiac Patients Association—💾 www.bcpa.co.uk
- Heart UK—💾 www.heartuk.org.uk/

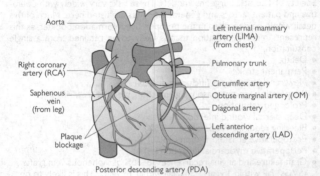

Aorta

Left internal mammary artery (LIMA) (from chest)

Right coronary artery (RCA)

Pulmonary trunk

Saphenous vein (from leg)

Circumflex artery

Obtuse marginal artery (OM)

Diagonal artery

Left anterior descending artery (LAD)

Plaque blockage

Posterior descending artery (PDA)

Fig. 18.1 Anatomy and vasculature: coronary artery bypass grafting (CABG).

Reproduced with permission from O'Connor IF and Urdang M. *Oxford Handbook of Surgical Cross-Cover*. 2008. Oxford: Oxford University Press p.163, Figure 5.2.

References

1. Guidelines on Myocardial Revascularization. The task force on myocardial revascularsation of the European Society of Cardiology (ESC) and the European Association for Cardio-Thoracic Surgery (EACTS). *Eur Heart J* 2010;**31**(20):2501–55.
2. The Society for Cardiothoracic Surgery in Great Britain & Ireland. *Sixth National Adult Cardiac Surgical Database Report*. The Society for Cardiothoracic Surgery in Great Britain & Ireland, 2008.
3. Eagle KA, Guyton RA, Davidoff R, *et al*. The ACC/AHA 2004 guideline update for coronary artery bypass graft surgery. *Circulation* 2004;**110**;e340–e437.
4. ACC/AHA Pocket Guideline. *Coronary Artery Bypass Graft Surgery*. American College of Cardiology/American Heart Association Task Force on Practice Guidelines, 2005.
5. Shroyer AL, Grover FL, Hattler B, *et al*. On-pump versus off-pump coronary-artery bypass surgery. *N Engl J Med* 2009;**361**:1827–37.
6. National Institute for Clinical Excellence. *Off-pump Coronary Artery Bypass (OPCAB): Guidance*. IPG 35. London: National Institute for Clinical Excellence, 2004 (Currently undergoing revision).

Internal mammary artery harvest for CABG

Indications

Approximately 50% of vein grafts are blocked after 10 years. Use of the internal mammary artery (IMA) in revascularization (ideally of the LAD artery) not only provides a long-term survival benefit but also improves immediate operative mortality. Bilateral IMAs may be grafted and this further increases long-term survival but may increase wound infection and sternal dehiscence rates. In those with 'reasonable life expectancy' arterial grafting to LAD and also non-LAD systems is a class 1 recommendation in the current ESC/EACTS guidelines.

Risks

- Wound infection/mediastinitis
- Bleeding

Other procedures that should also be consented for

- The harvested IMA (Fig. 18.2) may be damaged, exhibit poor flow, or be too small to use as a conduit. Other sources of conduit may be required
- Information about sources of graft may be included in an information booklet

Information to help explain the procedure to the patient

- The IMA is harvested from within the chest during the CABG procedure, thereby avoiding an additional incision

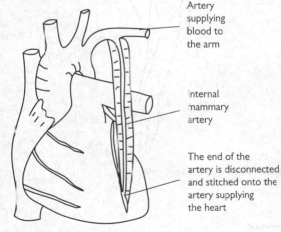

Artery supplying blood to the arm

Internal mammary artery

The end of the artery is disconnected and stitched onto the artery supplying the heart

Fig. 18.2 IMA harvest.

Reference

1. Buxton.B, Tatoulis J, Fuller J. Arterial conduits update. *Heart Lung Circ* 2005;**14S**:S14–S17.

Radial artery harvest for CABG

Indications
- While the left IMA graft is preferred for the LAD, the radial artery, right IMA or SVG are commonly used for other target sites. Radial artery harvest requires an additional lengthy incision (Fig. 18.3) unless endoscopic harvest techniques are used[1]

Risks
- Sensory abnormalities (mostly numbness, 3–15%)
- Forearm haematoma (0.5%)
- Fingertip ischaemia (~0.1%)
- (The incidence of forearm/hand ischaemia is virtually nil)

Information to help explain the procedure to the patient
- *Having Heart Surgery*—✍ www.bhf.org.uk/publications.aspx

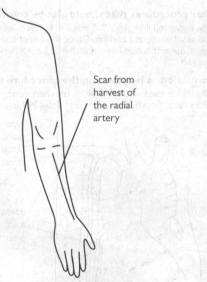

Scar from harvest of the radial artery

Fig. 18.3 Scar following radial artery harvest.

Reference
1. Tatoulis J, et al. Total arterial coronary revascularization: techniques and results in 3220 patients. *Heart Lung Circ* 2005;**14S**:S14–S17.

Long saphenous vein harvest for CABG

Indications

The long saphenous vein (LSV) remains the most commonly used conduit for CABG. Harvest is traditionally via an open technique, but newer minimally invasive endoscopic techniques are available.[1] Open harvest obviously requires a longer incision and attracts a higher incidence of wound infection[2] but there are little data supporting the long-term patency of veins harvested via minimally invasive techniques. Recent data have suggested that endoscopic harvest may result in higher rates of vein graft failure and increased mortality.[3] Haematoma and vein injury rates, harvest time and pain scores are similar, but endoscopic harvest is associated with early mobilization and reduced rates of infection and postoperative stay. NICE currently recommends that the endoscopic harvesting 'should be used only with special arrangements for clinical governance, consent and audit or research'.[4] ►► Scars (Fig. 18.4) may be bilateral, and may be from ankle to groin (typically much shorter).

Risks

- Numbness related to skin incision and saphenous nerve injury (some anaesthesia—90%)
- Leg oedema (7–30%)
- Haematoma formation (8–15%)
- Wound infection (3–13%)
- Seroma (1–14%)
- Skin necrosis (1–8%)
- Wound dehiscence (1–10%)
- Carbon dioxide embolization (moderate to massive ~1–3%, where endoscopic techniques are used)

Information to help explain the procedure to the patient

- *Having Heart Surgery*—℅ www.bhf.org.uk/publications.aspx
- *Keyhole Saphenous Vein Harvesting for CABG*—℅ www.nice.org.uk/nicemedia/live/11361/48781/48781.pdf

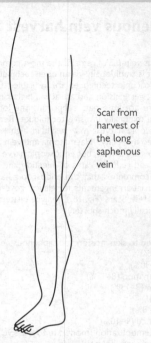

Scar from
harvest of
the long
saphenous
vein

Fig. 18.4 Scar following long saphenous vein harvest.

References

1. Lopes RD, Hafley GE, Allen KB, et al. Endoscopic versus open vein-graft harvesting in coronary-artery bypass surgery. *N Engl J Med* 2009;**361**(3):235–44.
2. Athanasiou T, Aziz O, Skapinakis P, et al. Leg wound infection after coronary artery bypass grafting: a meta-analysis comparing minimally invasive versus conventional vein harvesting. *Ann Thorac Surg* 2003;**76**:2141–6.
3. Markar SR, Kutty R, Edmonds L, et al. A meta-analysis of minimally invasive versus traditional open vein harvest technique for coronary artery bypass graft surgery. *Interact Cardiovasc Thorac Surg* 2010;**10**:266–70.
4. National Institute for Health and Clinical Excellence. *Endoscopic Saphenous Vein Harvest for Coronary Artery Bypass Grafting*. London: National Institute for Health and Clinical Excellence, 2010.

Cardiac valve surgery—repair/replacement

The commonest isolated valve procedures are aortic followed by mitral. Tricuspid and pulmonary procedures are *relatively* uncommon. For multivalve procedures the commonest are combined aortic valve replacement (AVR; Fig. 18.5) and mitral valve replacement (MVR) while other multivalve operations are performed in small numbers.[1] In the UK the mitral valve is now repaired (rather than replaced) in ~65–70% of cases affected by degenerative disease.[2]

These operations are frequently performed in association with CABG, particularly AVR + CABG. Mortality from a combined operation is significantly higher. ESC/EACTS guidelines *recommend* CABG when coronary artery diameter stenosis is ≥70%. CABG should be *considered* for 50–70% stenoses.[3]

The most common approach used is a median sternotomy, but various 'less invasive' approaches are used, which are beyond the scope of this chapter.

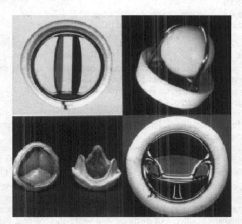

Fig. 18.5 Common types of prosthetic heart valve. From top left clockwise: St Jude's medical bileaflet, Star–Edwards ball and cage, Bjork–Shiley tilting disc, and stented porcine prosthesis.

Reproduced from Blomfield P (2002). *Heart* **87**:583–9, with permission from BMJ Publishing.

References

1. National Institute of Health and Clinical Excellence. *Guidance Both for Patients Their Carers and Health Professionals*. London: National Institute of Health and Clinical Excellence. Available at: ℞ http://guidance.nice.org.uk/ (accessed 17 May 2011).
2. Bonow RO, Carabello BA, Chatterjee K, et al. 2008 focused update incorporated into the ACC/AHA 2006 guidelines for the management of patients with valvular heart disease. *J Am Coll Cardiol* 2008;**52**(13):e1–142.
3. The Task Force on Myocardial Revascularisation of the European Society of Cardiology (ESC) and the European Association for Cardio-Thoracic Surgery (EACTS). Guidelines on Myocardial Revascularization. *Eur Heart J* 2010;**31**(20):2501–55.

Aortic valve replacement

(📖 *Oxford Handbook of Cardiothoracic Surgery*, p.370)

Indications

Aortic stenosis (AS)

- Symptomatic severe AS (with a valve area <1.0cm^2 or peak gradient >50mmHg across the valve)
- Moderate AS undergoing other cardiac surgery
- Asymptomatic patients with severe AS and LV systolic dysfunction, abnormal response to exercise for example hypotension, severe LV hypertrophy (>15mm), valve area <0.60cm^2

Aortic regurgitation (AR)

- Acute severe AR
- Severe AR and New York Heart Association (NYHA) class III symptoms, Canadian Heart Association (CHA) class II symptoms, left ventricular end-systolic diameter (LVESD) >5.5cm or ejection fraction (EF) <55%
- Severe AR undergoing other cardiac surgery
- Native or prosthetic valve endocarditis
- Failure of a previously inserted bioprosthetic valve[1]

Specific risks

- As for other cardiac surgical procedures, patient-specific data should be given where possible, using the best available data[2]
- Requirement for a permanent pacemaker (1–2%)
- Prosthetic endocarditis (1–2%)
- Prosthesis failure (reflected in reoperation rate)
- Need for reoperation (📖 see 'Mechanical versus bioprosthetic aortic valve replacement', p.545)
- The risk of reoperation for bleeding is increased after AVR: overall rate of 5.5% for isolated AVR and 7% for combined AVR and CABG (6th National Adult Cardiac Surgical Database Report (NACSDR)[3])

Aortic bioprostheses are thought to have improved since randomized controlled trials of mechanical versus bioprosthetic valves were carried out. In the 6th NACSDR, survival in patients aged <61 years was better with a mechanical valve, but in those >70 years survival was better for those having biological valves. In those between 61 and 70 years, there was no difference.

Alternatives

- Balloon valvuloplasty for AS is recommended by NICE only in those unfit for surgery, as the recurrence rate is high[4]
- Trans-catheter valve insertion (e.g. via the LV apex, ascending aorta, peripheral arteries). To date only performed in patients at increased *risk from open surgery, and associated with a significant risk of* stroke and other major complications. There is no evidence supporting long-term outcomes, although short-term efficacy has been demonstrated. NICE recommend these procedures should only be performed in high-risk patients, and after assessment by a multidisciplinary team

Information for patients

- See comparison of bioprosthetic and mechanical valves in Table 18.1
  - ℘ www.patient.co.uk/health/Aortic-Regurgitation.htm
  - ℘ www.patient.co.uk/health/Aortic-stenosis.htm
  - ℘ http://guidance.nice.org.uk/Topic/SurgicalProcedures/HeartArteriesVein

Mechanical versus bioprosthetic aortic valve replacement

Table 18.1 Comparison of bioprosthetic and mechanical valves

	Bioprosthetic	Mechanical
Anticoagulation	May require 3 months warfarin.	Required, usually with warfarin. Valve thrombosis 0.2–5.7% per patient year.
Haemodynamics and valve duration.	Better haemodynamics, but affected by activity of patient: valve failure at 10 years in >40% in those 0–39 years-old, Vs 10% aged >70 years.	Abnormal haemodynamics, especially in small sizes. Durable beyond patient's lifetime but re-operation is rarely required, e.g. for tissue ingrowth or recurrent bleeding on warfarin.
Noise	Silent	Mechanical 'click' (rarely a problem)
Endocarditis prophylaxis	Antibiotic prophylaxis/chlorhexidine mouthwash before dental procedures not recommended by NICE since 2008 (for biological or mechanical valves)[5]	
Source of valve material	Either bovine pericardium, or porcine valve, or cadaveric homograft.	Entirely prosthetic
Typical patient groups	Patients aged >60–65 years Patients aged <60 years who wish to avoid warfarin, or accept need for re-operation Patients in whom warfarin is contra-indicated. Women who may wish to become pregnant and therefore avoid warfarin (teratogenic). Patients unable to access regular INR checks.	Patients <60 years who accept anti-coagulation and wish to reduce the need for re-operation. Any patient with a mechanical valve at another position or taking warfarin for another reason.

References

1. Bonow RO, Carabello BA, Chatterjee K, et al. Focused update incorporated into the ACC/AHA 2006 guidelines for the management of patients with valvular heart disease. *Circulation* 2008;**118**(15):e523–661.

2. British Heart Foundation. *Factfile—Prosthetic Heart Valves.* London: British Heart Foundation, 2009.

3. Bridgewater B, Keogh B, Kinsman R, Walton KH. *Sixth National Adult Cardiac Surgical Database Report 2008: Demonstrating Quality.* Dendrite Clinical Systems.

4. National Institute for Clinical Excellence. *Balloon Valvuloplasty for Aortic Valve Stenosis in Adults and Children.* London: National Institute for Clinical Excellence, 2004.

5. National Institute for Health and Clinical Excellence. *Prophylaxis Against Infective Endocarditis: Antimicrobial Prophylaxis Against Infective Endocarditis in Adults and Children Undergoing Interventional Procedures.* London: National Institute for Health and Clinical Excellence, 2008.

The Ross procedure

(📖 *Oxford Handbook of Cardiotroracic Surgery*, pp.375, 388)

This is transfer of the pulmonary valve to the aortic position, with replacement of the pulmonary valve (now usually with a cadaveric human pulmonary valve). This is a highly specialized procedure.[1]

Indications

The benefits of the Ross procedure include potential for growth, excellent flow characteristics, and freedom from complications of anticoagulation. However, age <30 years, associated mitral valve disease, and rheumatic valve disease may independently predict autograft failure. Compared with other biological valves, the rate of structural degeneration with the pulmonary autograft is very low.[2] The autograft will grow with a child. As long as pulmonary artery pressure is low, pulmonary homograft insufficiency can be well tolerated for many years. There is, however, a significant need for reoperation at both the aortic and pulmonary positions.[3]

Specific risks

- 'Single valve' disease is converted into 'double valve' disease
- Mortality: ~2.3%; ~95% survival reported at 10 years, 80% at 20 years
- Reoperation: at the pulmonary position in ~5% at 10 years, ~7% at the aortic position
- Some have demonstrated a 0–1.2% risk of thromboembolism per year, with similarly low incidence of endocarditis

Information to explain the procedure to patients

- 📖 See 'Mechanical versus bioprosthetic aortic valve replacement', p.545
- 🖱 www.patient.co.uk/doctor/Aortic-Valve-Operations.htm

References

1. Ross D. Replacement of aortic and mitral valves with a pulmonary autograft. *Lancet* 1967;**2**(7523):956–8.
2. Ross D. The pulmonary autograft—a permanent aortic valve. *Eur J Cardiothorac Surg* 1992;**6**:113–17.
3. Yacoub MH, Klieverik LM, Melina G, et al. An evaluation of the Ross operation in adults. *J Heart Valve Dis* 2006;**15**(4):531–9.

Mitral valve repair/replacement

(📖 *Oxford Handbook of Cardiothoracic Surgery*, p.402)

It should be made clear whether the surgeon's intention is to attempt to repair the valve but replace it if repair is not possible, or to proceed directly to replacement. Replacement is often with a mechanical valve. Thoracoscopic approaches are possible; this is a highly specialized procedure and specific unit risks should be consented for.[1]

Indications

Mitral regurgitation (MR)

- Acute symptomatic MR
- Severe MR, NYHA II symptoms, and normal LV
- Severe MR and LVESD >4.5cm, or EF <50%
- Severe MR and pulmonary artery pressure (PAP) >50mmHg systolic at rest or AF

Stenosis

- MV area <1.5cm^2 and NYHA III symptoms or thromboembolic risk
- MV area <1cm^2 and PAP >60mmHg and NYHA class I symptoms

Specific risks

In the 6th NACSDR, the overall mortality for isolated mitral valve *repair* was around 2% while the mortality from mitral valve *replacement* was 6.1%. In those aged >80 years, mortality was 5.5% and 15.6%, respectively. ▶▶Average UK mortality from MVR + CABG is ~10–13% (6th NACSDR[2]).

- Endocarditis
- Need for reoperation
- Valve failure, although where the valve is replaced this is most commonly with a mechanical valve

Patient-specific risks should be estimated using models (📖 see 'Consent in cardiac surgery', p.534). Warfarin is commonly prescribed for 3 months following mitral valve repair.

Alternatives

- Non-operative management
- Percutaneous repair—'clipping' for MR. NICE currently recommends that this procedure is carried out only in those 'unfit' for surgery, and within a research programme

Information to help explain the procedure to the patient

- ℘ www.bhf.org.uk/publications.aspx (several patient-oriented publications covering heart valve disease, valve surgery, and warfarin)
- ℘ www.patient.co.uk/health/Mitral-Regurgitation.htm
- ℘ www.patient.co.uk/health/Mitral-Stenosis.htm

References

1. National Institute for Health and Clinical Excellence. *Percutaneous Mitral Valve Leaflet Repair for Mitral Regurgitation*. London: National Institute for Health and Clinical Excellence, 2009.
2. Bridgewater B, Keogh B, Kinsman R, Walton KH. *Sixth National Adult Cardiac Surgical Database Report 2008: Demonstrating Quality*. Dendrite Clinical Systems.

Tricuspid valve replacement

(📖 *Oxford Handbook of Cardiothoracic Surgery* p416)

While tricuspid regurgitation (TR) may be secondary to MR, the TR does not reliably resolve after surgery to correct the MR, and some authors have advocated a more aggressive approach to TR in order to avoid the mortality associated with reoperation to correct persistent or worsening TR.

Indications

Regurgitation

- Severe TR during surgery for multivalvular disease (usually respond well to annuloplasty[1])
- Tricuspid annuloplasty for mild TR in patients undergoing MV surgery (2° pulmonary hypertension and annular dilatation[2])

Stenosis

- Tricuspid stenosis (usually rheumatic)

Risks

- Mortality is as high as 10% at 30 days; 10-year survival: ~47% after tricuspid valve (TV) repair, ~37% after TV replacement (most as part of multi-valve surgery). Mortality should be estimated on a patient-specific basis. (📖 www.euroscore.org/calc.html)
- Recurrence of regurgitation: ~18% at 15 years following ring annuloplasty
- There are no data clearly showing the advantage of one type of tricuspid prosthesis over another[3]

Information to help explain the procedure to the patient

- 📖 www.bhf.org.uk/publications.aspx (several patient-oriented publications covering heart valve disease, valve surgery, and warfarin)

References

1. Tang GH, David TE, Singh SK, *et al.* Tricuspid valve repair with an annuloplasty ring results in improved long-term outcome. *Circulation* 2006;**114**:I577–81.
2. Rogers JH, Bolling SF. The tricuspid valve: current perspective and evolving management of tricuspid regurgitation. *Circulation* 2009;**119**:2718–25.
3. Guenther T, Noebauer C, Mazzitelli D, *et al.* Tricuspid valve surgery: a thirty-year assessment of early and late outcome. *Eur J Cardiothorac Surg* 2008;**34**(2):402–9.

Procedures for atrial fibrillation

(📖 *Oxford Handbook of Cardiothoracic Surgery*, p604)

Indications for the Maze procedure

Without anticoagulation, atrial fibrillation (AF) carries a 4–5% risk per stroke per year. AF ablation carries a much greater chance of restoration of sinus rhythm than mitral valve surgery alone.

- After failed catheter ablation
- Those with symptomatic AF undergoing other cardiac surgery
- Possibly those with asymptomatic AF undergoing cardiac surgery (when ablation can be performed with minimal risk)[1–3]

Specific risks

- Risks vary depending on exact procedure performed (cut and sew, radiofrequency ablation, etc.)
- Recurrence of AF in ~8–40%
- Oedema (variable, 2° to ↓ atrial natriuretic peptide)
- Need for permanent pacemaker in up to 3–7%
- Death ~1%
- Oesophageal injury
- Heart block
- Perforation of the heart
- Coronary artery damage

Information for patients

- NICE: *Radiofrequency Ablation for Atrial Fibrillation in Association With Other Cardiac Surgery (For patients/carers).* 🔗 http://guidance.nice.org.uk/IPG121[4]
- 🔗 www.atrialfibrillation.org.uk—multiple patient information leaflets available
- 🔗 www.sts.org/doc/4511—the Maze procedure

References

1. Lee R, Kruse J, McCarthy PM. Surgery for atrial fibrillation. *Nat Rev Cardiol* 2009;**6**:505–13.
2. Dewire J, Calkins H. State-of-the-art and emerging technologies for atrial fibrillation ablation. *Nat Rev Cardiol* 2010;**7**:129–38.
3. Albrecht A, Kalil RA, Schuch L, et al. Randomized study of surgical isolation of the pulmonary veins for correction of permanent atrial fibrillation associated with mitral valve disease. *J Thorac Cardiovasc Surg* 2009;**138**:454–9.
4. National Institute for Health and Clinical Excellence. *Radiofrequency Ablation for Atrial Fibrillation in Association With Other Cardiac Surgery.* London: National Institute for Health and Clinical Excellence, 2005. Available at: 🔗 www.nice.org.uk/nicemedia/live/11144/31268/31268.pdf (accessed 17 May 2011).

Pericardectomy and pericardial window

(📖 Oxford Handbook of Cardiothoracic Surgery, pp.608–10)

Indications

In constrictive pericarditis (which may or may not be accompanied by an effusion) the upper limit of the cardiac volume is constrained by the inelastic pericardium. This occurs in mid to late diastole when the cardiac volume approximates that of the pericardium.

Surgery (pericardectomy, including visceral pericardium) is indicated in patients with chronic constrictive pericarditis who have persistent and prominent symptoms.[1]

Pericardectomy may also be required for relief of tamponade from a pericardial collection, often ~6 weeks after cardiac surgery (or s = secondary to malignancy). Some form of pericardial window is also recommended in the event of recurrent large effusion after pericardiocentesis.[2]

Techniques

- Subxiphoid pericardial window, video-assisted thoracoscopic (VATS) pericardial window (usually anterior to the phrenic nerve), open pericardiectomy. The approach is largely dependent on underlying cause of tamponade[2]

Specific risks

- Operative mortality ~5%, but up to 8% for postoperative constrictive pericarditis and 20% for postradiation constrictive pericarditis
- A long stay in ITU may be inevitable
- 7-year survival 27–88% dependent on aetiology and other patient factors
- Recurrence (variable)
- General complications specific to approach (sternal, subxiphoid, VATS)[3]

Other procedures that should also be consented for

- Conversion of a non-median sternal approach to a median sternotomy

Information to help explain the procedure to the patient

- 🖱 www.patient.co.uk/doctor/Chronic-Pericarditis.htm
- 🖱 www.patient.co.uk/showdoc/27000359/
- 🖱 www.bhf.org.uk/publications/view-publication.aspx?ps=1000729

References

1. Imazio, M. Brucato A. Trinchero R, et al. Diagnosis and management of pericardial diseases. *Nat Rev Cardiol* 2009;**6**:743–51.
2. Maisch B, Seferovic PM, Ristic AD, et al. Guidelines on the diagnosis and management of pericardial diseases executive summary: the task force on the diagnosis and management of pericardial diseases of the European Society of Cardiology *Eur Heart J* 2004;**25**:587–610.
3. Bertog SC, Thambidorai SK, Parakh K, et al. Constrictive pericarditis: etiology and cause-specific survival after pericardiectomy. *J Am Coll Cardiol* 2004;**43**(8):1445–52.

Surgery for Stanford type A aortic dissection

(📖 *Oxford Handbook of Cardiothoracic Surgery*, pp.428–45)

Indications

- Surgery is currently indicated in all cases of type A (Debakey I and II) dissection, except when the patient is not a candidate for surgery (for example due to advanced age/dementia/malignancy) to reduce the risk of death from aortic rupture, acute AR, cardiac tamponade, or myocardial ischaemia[1,2]
- Untreated mortality is as high as 1–1.4% per hour. Treated medically early mortality is ~53%, reduced to ~25% with operative intervention

Techniques

Various techniques of surgical repair are practised, and are beyond the scope of this chapter. Typically the ascending aorta is replaced with an interposition tube graft. The aortic valve and arch may or may not be replaced.[3]

Risks

- Death ~25%. In the UK in 2004–08, early mortality for non-elective surgery for aortic dissection was 21% with interposition tube graft and 33% with a composite valve-graft. Mortality ~50% in those aged >85
- Paraplegia
- Stroke
- Renal failure
- Wound infection
- Pneumonia
- Need for further surgery/intervention to deal with distal dissection

Information to help explain the procedure to the patient

- 🖉 www.patient.co.uk/doctor/Aortic-Dissection.htm
- 🖉 www.bhf.org.uk/publications/view-publication.aspx?ps=1001122

References

1. Tsai TT, Neinaber CA, Eagle KA. Acute aortic syndromes. *Circulation* 2005;**112**:3802–13.
2. Karthikesalingam A, Holt PJE, Hinchliffe RJ, *et al.* The diagnosis and management of aortic dissection. *Vasc Endovascular Surg* 2010;**44**(3):165–9.
3. Erbel R, Alfonso F, Boileau C, *et al.* Diagnosis and management of aortic dissection. Recommendations of the Task Force on Aortic Dissection, European Society of Cardiology. *Eur Heart J* 2001;**22**:1642–81.

Aortic surgery

Aortic procedures are highly variable, with many permutations of common techniques for the management of pathology involving the various aortic segments. Composite aortic root replacement, interposition grafts and valve replacement plus interposition graft (depending on involvement of the aortic valve and coronary arteries) make up the bulk of the UK cardiothoracic surgical workload.[1,2]

Indications
- Aneurysmal dilatation
- Dissection
  - Type A—📖 see 'Surgery for Stanford type A aortic dissection', p.552
  - Type B—usually performed by a vascular surgeon (uncomplicated cases are usually managed medically)
- Transection
- Coarctation

Specific risks
- Death—highly dependent on the urgency of surgery. For interposition tube graft UK average mortality varies from 9.3% (elective) to 42% (salvage). For non-elective dissection repair, average mortality is 22.8%, rising to 32.5% for those requiring a composite root replacement
- Stroke
- Renal failure
- Paraplegia[3]

Alternatives

Type B dissection, and aneurysms involving the descending thoracic aorta are now most commonly managed by insertion of an endovascular stent-graft, in order to cover the primary entry tear. Aneurysms involving the distal arch can also be treated with a stent graft after a carotid-subclavian or carotid-carotid-subclavian cross-over procedure has been performed to create a proximal landing zone. In addition the brachiocephalic artery origin may also be moved more proximally to the aortic valve.

Information to help explain the procedure
- ℘ www.patient.co.uk/showdoc/40000540/
- ℘ www.bhf.org.uk/publications/view-publication.aspx?ps=1001122

References
1. Trimarchi S, Nienaber CA, Rampoldi V, et al. Contemporary results of surgery in acute type A aortic dissection: the international registry of acute aortic dissection experience. *J Thorac Cardiovasc Surg* 2005;**129**(1):112–22.
2. Feldman M, Shah M, Elefteriades J. Medical management of acute type A aortic dissection. *Ann Thorac Cardiovasc Surg* 2009;**15**(5):286–93.
3. National Institute for Health and Clinical Excellence. *Endovascular Stent–Graft Placement in Thoracic Aortic Aneurysms and Dissections.* London: National Institute for Health and Clinical Excellence, 2005.

Thoracic surgery

Consent in thoracic surgery

Risk stratification

As in many other surgical specialties, the main source of information regarding surgical risk assessment is via self-reported morbidity and mortality figures. In Great Britain and Ireland this is collected and published by the Society for Cardiothoracic Surgery (SCTS).

Mortality figures, such as those reported annually by the SCTS, reflect population risk and also serve as a tool for clinical governance. This, however, poorly translates into predicting the individual risk a patient undergoing a surgical procedure would face.

Several tools have been suggested to stratify an individual's risk when deciding whether to proceed with surgery, and the tool most widely anticipated to fill this need in the field of thoracic surgery is the Thoracoscore.

Thoracoscore

The Thoracoscore is a clinical tool used for predicting a the risk of death for patients admitted for first-time thoracic surgery. It was developed using a multivariate regression analysis of 15 183 patients evaluated at 59 French hospitals. The following factors were identified to predict an increased risk:

- Increasing age
- Male sex
- Higher ASA score
- Higher Performance status classification
- Pneumonectomy
- Procedures for malignant disease
- Higher co-morbidity score

Current opinion is that the risk model used to calculate the Thoracoscore is a good predictor of the mortality risk, however at the time of publication it has not been externally validated in the UK population.[1]

It can be easily calculated using online tools such as the one provided at ℘ www.sfar.org/scores2/thoracoscore2.php.

Reference

1. Falcoz PE, Conti M, Brouchet L, *et al.* The thoracic surgery scoring system (Thoracoscore): Risk model for in-hospital death in 15,183 patients requiring thoracic surgery. *J Thorac Cardiovasc Surg* 2007;**133**:325–32.

Bronchoscopy

Background

Bronchoscopy provides a means to inspect the airway and bronchial tree (Fig. 19.1), and has both diagnostic and therapeutic applications. It can be performed using either a flexible or rigid bronchoscope. Flexible bronchoscopy is usually performed under sedation and gives access to the entire bronchial tree from the larynx to the sub-lobar bronchial orifices. Rigid bronchoscopy requires general anaesthesia and access to the distal airways is more limited. However, rigid bronchoscopy can provide larger biopsies and may be a better option for therapeutic procedures.

Indications

- Diagnostic (assessment and/or investigation of bronchiectasis, inhalation injury, stridor, vocal cord paralysis, trauma)
- Biopsy of airways tumours
- Biopsy of structures outside but adjacent to the airway using techniques such as endobronchial ultrasound, transbronchial needle aspiration)
- Obtaining bronchial lavage cytology
- Evaluation of known tumours to determine position and extent of required resection
- Removal of inhaled foreign objects
- Disobliteration of the airway using manual techniques, electrocautery, cryotherapy or laser
- Evaluation and treatment of haemoptysis
- Bronchial and tracheal stent insertion/removal
- As an aid in tracheostomy

Complications

- Haemoptysis and bleeding (more common after biopsy)
- Damage to teeth, caps, and crowns (rigid bronchoscopy)
- Laryngospasm, bronchospasm
- Cardiac arrhythmia
- Pneumothorax
- Tracheal perforation
- Airway obstruction
- Death: Respiratory and cardiac arrest
  - SCTS mortality rate for diagnostic bronchoscopy: 0.2%
  - Therapeutic bronchoscopy: 1.2%
- Tracheo-oesophageal stenosis or fistula (rare, late complications)[1]

Patient resources

- 🖰 www.patient.co.uk/health/Bronchoscopy.htm

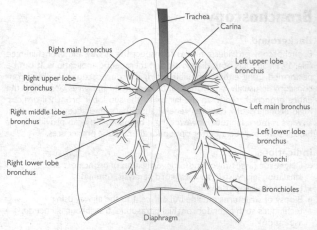

Fig. 19.1 Anatomy of the trachea and bronchial tree.

Reference

1. Jin F, Mu D, Chu D, *et al.* Severe complications of bronchoscopy. *Respiration* 2008;**76**(4):429–33.

Anatomical lung resections

Background

Anatomical lung resection is defined as the resection of one or more bronchopulmonary segments. The term can include either resection of a single segment (segmentectomy), a single lobe (lobectomy), two adjacent lobes (bilobectomy) or the entire lung (pneumonectomy).

Anatomical lung resection combined with mediastinal lymph node resection is considered the gold standard surgical treatment for early stage primary lung cancer. There is an increased risk of local recurrence when less than lobectomy (sublobar resection) is performed for primary lung cancer, but this may be necessary in patients with borderline lung function.

Alternatively resection and reconstruction of the airway or pulmonary vasculature may enable a surgeon to limit the amount of lung parenchyma resected (bronchoplastic/sleeve resection).

Long-term survival following surgery for primary lung cancer depends on final pathological staging, histological diagnosis, and achieving a complete resection.

It is important when obtaining consent for an anatomical lung resection to differentiate between operative mortality and long-term survival. Table 19.1 shows the difference in survival for various stages of non-small cell lung cancer (NSCLC), while Table 19.2 presents the SCTS operative mortality rates for different anatomical lung resections.

Table 19.1 International Association for the Study of Lung Cancer (IASLC) 5-year survival rates according to clinical and pathological staging[1]

Stage	Clinical (%)	Pathological (%)
IA	50	73
IB	43	58
IIA	36	46
IIB	25	36
IIIA	19	24
IIIB	7	9
IV	2	13

Table 19.2 SCTS operative mortality rates according to type of resection performed for period 2002–08

Procedure	Resection for primary lung cancer (%)	Resection for other than primary lung cancer (%)
Pneumonectomy	6.6	5.7
Lobectomy, bilobectomy	2.3	2.4
Sleeve lobectomy	2.7	0.8
Segmentectomy, wedge resection	1.6	0.8
Any resection which includes chest wall or diaphragmatic resection, etc.	4.2	3.4
Exploratory thoracotomy	2.4	–

Anatomical lung resection can also be undertaken to treat:
• Lung abscess
• Chronic infections
• Bronchiectasis
• Pulmonary metastases

Preoperative assessment

Careful preoperative assessment is essential to select those patients who would benefit from pulmonary resection. The British Thoracic Society (BTS) has published guidelines to aid the distinction between high- and low-risk individuals (see ℘ www.brit-thoracic.org.uk/Clinical-Information/Lung-Cancer/Lung-Cancer-Guidelines.aspx).

Although risk stratification and assessment is less well-defined in thoracic surgery compared with cardiac surgery, preoperative lung function and the amount of intended lung resection are important determinants of perioperative morbidity and mortality.

The incidence of adverse respiratory complications and death increases proportionally with the degree of preoperative respiratory compromise (as indicated by lung function and cardiopulmonary function testing) and the extent of resection intended. The influence of other factors such as age, current smoking status, and the presence of cardiovascular and renal comorbidities are less well-defined.

A postoperative forced expiratory volume in 1s (ppFEV$_1$) and/or transfer factor (carbon monoxide diffusion capacity (DLCO)) of <40% predicted implies that an individual would be at increased risk for complications after a lung resection. The predicted postoperative FEV$_1$ or DLCO can be calculated using the formula:

$$ppFEV_1 = FEV_1 \left[(a - b)/a \right]$$

• a = total number of functioning bronchopulmonary segments (which equates to 19 minus the number of non-functional segments removed)
• b = number of functional segments to be removed

Segments are divided as shown in Table 19.3 and Fig. 19.2.

Table 19.3 The lobes of the lungs

Right lung		Left lung	
Upper lobe	3	Upper lobe	3
Middle lobe	2	Lingula	2
Lower lobe	5	Lower lobe	4

Approaches that may be used for anatomical lung resection
- Posterolateral thoracotomy (>90% of open resections)
- VATS
- Anterolateral thoracotomy
- Axillary thoracotomy
- Median sternotomy
- Sternothoracotomy (clamshell or hemi-clamshell thoracotomy)
- Anterior and posterior approaches to superior sulcus tumours
  (Pancoast tumour)
- Resections that may be performed:
  - Wedge resection, segmentectomy (sublobar)
  - Lobectomy, bilobectomy
  - Bronchoplastic/angioplastic lobectomy (sleeve lobectomy)
  - Pneumonectomy
- Special considerations with lung resection
  - Consider consenting for a more extensive resection when operating
    for centrally placed tumours, or tumours abutting the pulmonary
    fissures
  - When a mass involves or abuts the mediastinum, one should warn
    about the possibility of an exploratory thoracotomy alone, as the
    tumour may be deemed irresectable at the time of surgery (2–8%)
  - Increased risk of respiratory complications including long-term
    oxygen dependence and prolonged intubation—difficult to predict,
    but more likely if postoperative predicted DLCO and/or FEV_1 is less
    than 40%
  - Death (refer to Table 19.2 for specific rates)

Risks
- General thoracic surgery complications
  - Atelectasis, retention of pulmonary secretions, chest infection,
    pneumonia, respiratory failure requiring ventilatory support
  - Arrhythmias—AF develops in up to 15% of all pulmonary resections
    and is more common with left-sided surgery and when pericardial
    surgery is performed
  - Venous thromboembolism (15–40% without prophylaxis)—more
    common in patients undergoing surgery for malignant conditions
  - Ischaemic cardiac events—lung cancer patients also at risk for
    ischaemic heart disease through shared risk factors and withdrawal
    of antiplatelet drugs and anticoagulation in the perioperative period

- Thoracotomy
  - The thoracotomy approach is associated with significant postoperative pain. Regional anaesthesia (epidural, spinal, paravertebral blockade) may be employed. One or more intercostals drains are likely to be inserted at the time of surgery
  - Thoracotomy pain syndrome is well described. It is reported in 25–60% in patients who have had a thoracotomy[2]
  - Damage to intercostal nerve leading to numbness
  - Wound infection
  - Empyema (infection in the pleural cavity)
- Median sternotomy
  - Sternal wound infection, empyema, mediastinitis (0.2–0.4%)[3]
  - Injury to major blood vessels and heart (with haemorrhage)
- Anterior and posterior approach for superior sulcus tumours
  - Brachial plexus injury
  - Thoracic outlet obstruction
- Segmentectomy, lobectomy, wedge resection
  - Prolonged parenchymal air leak may necessitate prolonged intercostal drainage of the pleural cavity
- Sleeve lobectomy
  - Prolonged air leak
  - Anastomotic air leak, stricture, bronchopleural fistula
  - Increased risk of haemorrhage with vascular sleeve procedures

Pneumonectomy

- Pneumonectomy (removal of whole lung) is associated with an increased risk of complications and higher morbidity and mortality rates
- Risk of blood loss requiring transfusion is increased
- Pulmonary oedema and acute respiratory distress syndrome (ARDS; due to relative doubling of the blood flow through the remaining lung)
- Long term oxygen dependence, prolonged intubation and ventilation (increasing risk as preoperative lung function decreases)
- Bronchopleural fistula (breakdown of bronchial stump)
- Pneumonectomy space infection
- Incidence of recurrent laryngeal nerve palsy increased after left pneumonectomy
- Post-pneumonectomy syndrome (late)(<1%—obstruction of contralateral bronchus due to mediastinal shift)

Other procedures that should also be consented for

Synchronous chest wall resection
- Peripherally placed tumours may invade chest wall structures such as the ribs (staged as T3) or the vertebral column (T4). In selected cases en-bloc resection of the tumour and chest wall structures may be appropriate
- It is only necessary in about 5% of all resections performed for lung cancer

- Large defects need to be closed to prevent herniation of the lung. A chest wall reconstruction using prosthetic material and/or musculocutaneous flaps may be required
- Prosthesis can form a nidus for chronic infection
- Chest wall resection is associated with an increased incidence of chronic pain syndromes

Patient resources

- ℘ www.patient.co.uk/health/Cancer-of-the-Lung.htm
- ℘ www.cancerhelp.org.uk/type/lung-cancer/index.htm

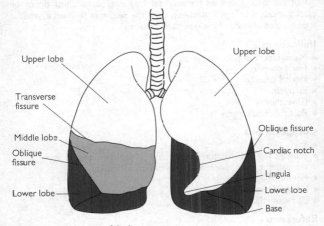

Fig. 19.2 Lobar divisions of the lungs.

References

1. Goldstraw P, Crowley J, Chansky K, et al. International association for the study of lung cancer international staging committee; Participating institutions the IASLC lung cancer staging project: proposals for the revision of the TNM stage groupings in the forthcoming (seventh) edition of the TNM classification of malignant tumours. *J Thorac Oncol* 2007;**2**:706–14.
2. Wildgaard K, Ravn J, Kehlet H. Chronic post-thoracotomy pain: a critical review of pathogenic mechanisms and strategies for prevention. *Eur J Cardiothorac Surg* 2009;**36**(1):170–80.
3. Salehi Omran A, Karimi A, Ahmadi SH, et al. Superficial and deep sternal wound infection after more than 9000 coronary artery bypass graft (CABG): incidence, risk factors and mortality. *BMC Infect Dis* 2007;**7**:112.

Chest tube insertion

Background

Percutaneous intercostal tube thoracostomy is a procedure performed for a variety of thoracic conditions. Its main use is for the evacuation of air and fluid (blood, effusion, pus, chyle) from the pleural cavity and restoration of the negative intrapleural pressure.

It can be performed in various settings including in emergency units and on wards under local anaesthesia. Chest tubes are also routinely placed in theatre for most surgical procedures involving the thorax.

Current BTS guidelines recommend that intercostal chest drains be placed under radiological guidance, using the Seldinger technique, when it is performed outside of the operating theatre.

Indications

- Management of pneumothorax
- Haemothorax
- Pleural effusion
- Empyema
- Chylothorax
- Post thoracic surgery

Complications

- Pain
- Damage to local structures (lung, heart, diaphragm, oesophagus, sympathetic chain, intercostal neurovascular bundle)
- Haemorrhage
- Misplacement of tube
- Empyema thoracis[1]

Reference

1. Bailey RC. Complications of tube thoracostomy in trauma. *J Accid Emerg Med* 2000;**17**:111–14.

Metastasectomy

Background

Pulmonary metastases often indicate advanced disease, but there is mounting evidence that in highly selected individuals, surgical resection of lung metastases may provide enhanced survival.

Removal can be achieved through open or thoracoscopic procedures. Thoracoscopic techniques are prone to missing smaller nodules, as palpation of the entire lung is not possible through small portholes. The most common practice in Europe is wedge resection of peripheral nodules by open thoracotomy.

Indications

Metastasectomy is reserved for a very select group of patients where:
- The primary malignancy site is controlled or controllable
- The patient is fit enough for the intended resection based on preoperative lung function testing
- Complete clearance is potentially achievable by surgical resection
- No extra-thoracic spread (excluding liver metastases) is present[1]

Some centres will further specify a minimum disease-free interval from the time of diagnosis and limit the amount of nodules that they would consider removing. There is little evidence-based information for a survival advantage following pulmonary metastasectomy, but registry data suggest that in a highly selected group of patients the 5-year survival rate can be improved, provided that complete resection is obtained. Five-year survival rates are dependent on various factors, including the type of malignancy, type of resection (☐ see 'Anatomical lung resections', p.559), and performance status[2]

Complications

- General thoracic surgery complications
- Disease recurrence
- DVT and pulmonary embolism

Special considerations

- It has been shown that in patients who perform well, redo procedures are possible for disease recurrence, provided the same conditions previously mentioned are met

References

1. Erhunmwunsee L, D'Amico TA. Surgical management of pulmonary metastases. *Ann Thorac Surg* 2009;**88**:2052–60.
2. Pastorino U, Buyse M, Friedel G, et al. Long-term results of lung metastasectomy: prognostic analyses based on 5206 cases. *J Thorac Cardiovasc Surg* 1997;**113**:37–49.

Cervical mediastinoscopy

Background

Cervical mediastinoscopy is a minimally invasive procedure that provides access to the superior mediastinum. It is used to obtain biopsies of mediastinal lymph nodes (stations 1, 2, 4, 7, 10R) and superior mediastinal tumours.

A transverse cervical incision is made and the surgeon then dissects down to the pretracheal fascia. A mediastinoscope is introduced into this plane, into the superior mediastinum.

Complications

Complications are rare but serious (<2%).

- Major haemorrhage from large mediastinal blood vessels—requiring sternotomy, thoracotomy
- Recurrent nerve palsy
- Mediastinitis
- Pneumothorax
- Oesophageal injury
- Death (0.4%)

Special considerations

- Patients should be consented for a median sternotomy or thoracotomy as an additional procedure in case significant bleeding occurs
- Video mediastinoscopy has been shown to be superior to traditional techniques, with fewer complications and higher yield biopsies
- Video-assisted mediastinal lymphadenectomy and transcervical extended mediastinal lymphadenectomy—these are new techniques of mediastinal lymphadenectomy, performed through the same approach as a mediastinoscopy, with similar complication rates, however, their effect on long-term survival is still uncertain[1]

Patient resources

- ℘ www.patient.co.uk/health/Mediastinoscopy.htm

Reference

1. Lerut T, De Leyn P, Coosemans W, et al. Cervical videomediastinoscopy. *Thorac Surg Clin* 2010;**20**(2):195–206.

Mediastinotomy (Chamberlain procedure)

Background

Left and/or right anterior (parasternal) mediastinotomy are procedures performed to biopsy lesions in the anterior mediastinum. Hilar lymph nodes and mediastinal lymph node stations 5 and 6 are also accessible via this approach.

A transverse, parasternal incision (3–4cm) is made in an appropriate intercostal space (usually second or third) and biopsies are performed. It may be necessary to resect the costal cartilage for access.

Complications

- Pneumothorax
- Wound infection (3.4%)
- Postoperative bronchopneumonia (2.6%)
- Pleural effusion (2.6%)
- Wound haematoma (1.7%)
- Wound pain (severe) (0.9%)
- Chest wall asymmetry if costal cartilage is resected
- Death (0.4%)[1]

Reference

1. Evans DS, Hall JH, Harrison GK. Anterior mediastinotomy. *Thorax* 1973;**28**:444–7.

Surgery for mediastinal mass

Background

The most common tumours of the superior mediastinum include thymoma, germ cell tumours, retrosternal goitre, and lymphoma. Benign masses found in the mediastinum include thymic, pericardial, dermoid, oesophageal, and bronchogenic cysts.

Surgery is reserved mainly for removal of thymic tumours and benign masses causing local compression. The preferred surgical access for these tumours is median sternotomy or mediastinotomy. Mediastinoscopy/mediastinotromy or VATS approaches can be used for some select tumours.

Thymic tumours

Thymoma and thymic carcinoma represent a spectrum of thymic epithelial and neuroendocrine neoplasms that vary in their behaviour from slow, indolent growing tumours (some thymomas) to very aggressive, invasive, and metastasizing tumours (thymic carcinomas).

Thymoma is associated with a range of paraneoplastic syndromes, which may resolve when the tumour is removed. These include:

- Myasthenia gravis (35% of thymomas, and thymic tumours are found in up to 15% of patients diagnosed with myasthenia gravis)
- Haematological abnormalities, e.g. pure red cell aplasia, thrombocytopaenia
- Hypogammaglobulinaemia (Good's syndrome)
- Pemphigus foliaceus (rare)
- Giant cell myocarditis (rare)

Complications

- Recurrence (thymoma and thymic carcinoma—dependent on the Masaoka stage: stage I: <5%, stage II: 5–20%, stage III: 15–30%; and stage IV: 25–55%
- Phrenic nerve damage
- Failure of resolution of paraneoplastic syndromes
- Wound site seeding
- Death (0.6%)

Chest wall resection

Background

Chest wall resection can be performed as part of the resection of a primary lung cancer, or to treat a primary chest wall tumour. Primary chest wall tumours are rare, but approximately 50% will be malignant.

Resection of primary chest wall tumours requires large, disease-free margins. Chest wall resection may involve removing soft tissue, one or more consecutive ribs, vertebral bodies, and may include resecting lung, pericardium, and diaphragm.

Reconstruction of the chest wall will be necessary in most cases, but it is dependent on the location of the tumour and the extent of the resection. Reconstruction may involve placement of prosthetic mesh, methyl methacrylate sheets and the use of tissue flaps (latissimus dorsi, pectoralis major, rectus abdominis, omentum).[1]

Complications

- Prolonged postoperative pain, chronic pain syndromes
- Prosthesis infection
- Lung herniation (if defects created are not closed)
- Skin flap failure
- Death 4–6%

Reference

1. Stoelben E, Ludwig C. Chest wall resection for lung cancer: indications and techniques. *Eur J Cardiothorac Surg* 2009;35(3):450–6.

Pectus surgery

Pectus excavatum 'funnel chest' and pectus carinatum 'pigeon chest' are congenital developmental anomalies of the anterior chest wall. Surgical correction is usually undertaken for cosmetic reasons, but in severe excavatum deformities, there is some evidence that cardiac and respiratory function is improved following surgery.

Various procedures have been described but the most common procedures performed are as follows.

Nuss bar insertion

Background

- A C-shaped bar is inserted behind the sternum and fixed to the lateral ribs. The bar exerts anterograde pressure on the sternum and corrects the anomaly. It is preferred in younger patients as the chest wall is more malleable.
- It has the following advantages:
  - Relative quick procedure
  - Performed using small peripheral incisions

Risks

- Pain
- Reoperation (planned as bar will eventually need to be removed, and also unplanned because of bar migration or persistent deformity)
- Pneumothorax, haemothorax
- Damage to heart—rare -isolated case reports only
- In older patients chronic pain syndrome attributed to the bar has been described
- Infection (rare)

Modified Ravitch procedure

Background

The modified Ravich procedure involves surgical excision of bilateral costal cartilages over the extent of the deformity, and correction of any sternal angular deformity. A prosthesis (pectus bar or mesh) is placed retrosternally to stabilize the sternum in cases of pectus excavatum.

The procedure necessitates an open repair, either through a transverse incision at the midpoint of the deformity or through a vertical midline incision over the sternum. Both approaches necessitate mobilization of the pectoralis muscle off the sternum.

The Ravich procedure is preferred in post-pubertal patients.[1]

Advantages

- Associated with less recurrence, pneumothorax, and haemothorax than Nuss procedure
- Allows correction of pectus carinatum anomaly

Risks

- Larger scar on chest wall, increased incidence of hypertrophic and keloid scar formation
- Longer procedure
- Recurrence of anomaly

- Infection
- Bleeding
- Haemothorax, pneumothorax

Special considerations

- In both procedures patient satisfaction is similar but the patient should be warned that their expected correction may not be achieved
- Contact sports should be avoided after the procedure for at least 3 months
- The presence of a pectus bar renders cardiac compressions during cardiopulmonary resuscitation ineffective

Patient resource

- www.pectus.org/index.htm

Reference

1. Nasr A, Fecteau A, Wales PW. Comparison of the Nuss and the Ravitch procedure for pectus excavatum repair: a meta-analysis. *J Pediatr Surg* 2010;45(5):880–6.

Pleural decortication

Background

In situations where a thick cortex has formed around the lung, a decortication can be performed to aid in re-expansion. The cortex may develop as a result of infection (empyema), long-standing pleural effusion, haemothorax, or pleural malignancy and is often seen in associated with rib crowding and loss of lung volume.

Decortication involves removing the visceral and/or parietal pleura. This potentially allows the ribs to separate and the lung to re-expand and once again fill the pleural cavity. Decortication is a major procedure with significant associated morbidity and mortality, which reflects both the extent and duration of surgery and the poor performance status of patients requiring this intervention. It is, however, the only definitive way to re-expand the lung once a cortex has developed, will often improve symptoms of dyspnoea, and assist eradication of chronic pleural sepsis.

Complications

- Bleeding—both parietal and visceral pleura surfaces are highly vascular, particularly in the presence of active infection and may be exacerbated by underlying sepsis-related coagulopathy
- Prolonged parenchymal air leak—often two to three chest drains are placed to help the lung expand
- Pain—due to large thoracotomy, stripping of parietal pleura
- Failure of lung to re-expand—in chronic diseased pleura it may be difficult to perform the procedure without damaging the lung and major blood vessels
- Recurrence of empyema
- Systemic inflammatory response syndrome (SIRS), ARDS, multiple organ dysfunction syndrome (MODS)—exacerbation of a localized septic focus as a result of surgery
- Damage to lung and mediastinal structures (heart, phrenic nerve, thoracic aorta, oesophagus, sympathetic trunk, thoracic duct)
- Death (3%)

Video-assisted thoracoscopic surgery

Background

VATS is minimal access surgery of the chest. It can potentially provide access to the pleural cavity and mediastinum, and is usually undertaken through one or more 2–5cm incisions that are sited according to the target organ. A thoracoscope and instruments are then introduced to perform the surgery.

VATS techniques are potentially applicable to most open thoracic operations and have been described for:

- Pleural disease (pleural biopsy, pleurectomy, pleurodesis)
- Pneumothorax surgery (bullectomy, pleurectomy, pleural abrasion)
- Mediastinal procedures (removal of mediastinal masses, pericardial window formation, thymectomy, lymphadenectomy)
- Drainage of pleural effusion and empyema
- Thoracic sympathectomy
- Sublobar wedge resections of lung
- Anatomical lung resections

General considerations

- Benefits include smaller scars, reduced pain, quicker recovery and fewer complications than open procedures
- When consenting for VATS always consent for converting to open surgery, via thoracotomy or median sternotomy. It is more common to convert in more complicated procedures with VATS biopsy rates quoted up to 2.4% and VATS lobectomies up to 12%
- Table 19.4 lists the operative mortality for various VATS procedures

Table 19.4 Operative mortality for VATS procedures

Procedure	Mortality (%)
Lung resection (primary malignant)	
Wedge resection	1.0
Lobectomy	1.7
Pneumonectomy	6.7
Lung resection (other)	
Wedge resection	0.8
Lobectomy	0.0
Pneumonectomy	0.0
Pleural procedures	
Closure of air leak	0.8
Any other pleural procedure	1.8
Mediastinal procedures	0.5

VATS pleural biopsy

Background

A pleural biopsy is one of the commonest procedures performed via VATS, followed by pleural symphysis (pleurodesis) and placement of indwelling pleural catheters.

The procedure is used in both obtaining a diagnosis in exudative pleural effusions when alternative diagnostic modalities have failed, and in managing chronic or recurrent pleural effusions.

Talc insufflation is used most commonly to cause the pleurodesis, but various other substances (including autologous blood) can be used. Severe talc reactions are uncommon but can be life-threatening. Pleural symphysis is most commonly performed as a palliative procedure in advanced metastatic malignancy. It does not cure the underlying cause and can make future thoracic surgery technically difficult.

Indications

- Obtaining histology in recurrent or persistent pleural effusions
- Pleural symphysis in known recurrent malignant pleural effusions, when medical talc infusion failed

Complications

- Bleeding and haemothorax, especially when the cause of effusion is metastatic tumours, known to be highly vascular (renal cell carcinoma)
- Failure of pleurodesis
- Talc reactions (anaphylaxis, lung damage, ARDS, SIRS, renal failure)
- Empyema thoracis

Indwelling pleural catheter insertion (PleurX®)

- Indwelling pleural catheters provide an alternative way to manage chronic pleural effusions when a pleurodesis has failed or the lung is chronically trapped by tumour or infection. Because the catheter is tunnelled, the risk for introducing infection into the pleural cavity is lower
- The catheters are placed when an encorticated lung is discovered during a VATS pleural biopsy. Because the lung is unable to expand, talc pleurodesis is not likely to be successful in this setting

Surgery for pneumothorax

Background

Pneumothorax can be divided into:

- Primary pneumothorax—pneumothorax developing in seeming healthy individuals with no underlying lung disease. Often the result of apical blebs
- Secondary pneumothorax—pneumothorax caused by underlying lung disease such as bullous emphysema, cystic fibrosis, infection, and tumours

Surgery is reserved for cases of recurrent pneumothorax and persistent air leaks (>7days). Surgical procedures that may be performed include:

- Tube thoracostomy/pleural aspiration
- Resection of blebs, bullae, lesions causing the pneumothorax
- Pleurectomy
- Pleural abrasion
- Chemical pleurodesis (talc)

These procedures can be performed via open thoracotomy or via minimal access surgery such as VATS. Surgery is most successful in primary spontaneous pneumothorax.

Complications

- Similar to complications according to access used (thoracotomy, VATS) and extent of resection (wedge resections)
- Recurrence—depends on the procedure performed (Table 19.5)
- In primary spontaneous pneumothorax, 10% of patients will develop a contralateral pneumothorax
- Bleeding—especially after pleurectomy and pleural abrasion
- Talc reaction (SIRS, ARDS)
- Empyema
- Open procedures are associated with significant more postoperative pain
- Death—0.8%(VATS)—1.8% (open procedures)

Table 19.5 Rates of recurrence after surgery for pneumothorax

Tube thoracostomy/aspiration	20% after 1st episode
	50% after 2nd episode
Open pleurectomy, blebbectomy	<2%
VATS pleurectomy/pleural abrasion, blebbectomy	5%
Chemical pleurocesis	5–10%

Surgery for bullous lung disease

Background

It has long been established that bullous lung disease can be alleviated by resecting the affected area. This allows the remaining lung tissue to expand and eliminates dead space ventilation. It may take the form of giant bullectomy or lung volume reduction surgery.

Giant bullectomy

- Giant bullae are most commonly found in the apical part of the upper and lower lobes
- Surgical resection may be performed via open or VATS approach

Lung volume reduction surgery

- 20–30% of the upper lobe is resected following the contour of the lung
- Severely diseased areas are also resected
- Most commonly performed via thoracotomy—bilateral staged approach, but may also be performed by single stage median sternotomy, or transverse sternothoracotomy
- Patients with predominantly upper lobe disease and that are symptomatic at the time of the procedure, will benefit the most
- It is a palliative procedure in emphysematous lung disease, and does not improve long-term survival
- Although it offers symptomatic improvement, after 3–5 years most patients' functional status will revert to levels similar to those experienced before the surgery[1]

Complications

- Prolonged air leak
- Recurrence of symptoms
- Empyema thoracis
- Long term oxygen requirement
- Death (1.8%)

Patient resources

- ℘ www.lunguk.org/you-and-your-lungs/diagnosis-and-treatment/lung-volume-reduction-surgery

Reference

1. National Emphysema Treatment Trial Research Group. A randomized trial comparing lung-volume–reduction surgery with medical therapy for severe emphysema. *N Engl J Med* 2003;**348**:2059–73.

Thoracic sympathectomy

Background

Interruption of the thoracic sympathetic chain is performed mainly to treat hyperhidrosis. Depending on the desired outcome the chain is interrupted at different levels (referring to the sympathetic ganglia):

- Facial hyperhidrosis and rubor (flushing)—T2
- Palmar hyperhidrosis—T3
- Axillary hyperhidrosis—T3 & T4

The procedure is usually performed using single-stage, bilateral VATS approach. The lung on one side is collapsed the procedure performed, and the lung re-expanded. After closure of the wounds, the surgeon then proceeds to perform the same procedure on the contralateral side.

Techniques described include:

- Resection of the chain
- Electrocautery
- Laser ablation
- Compression with clips

Similar outcomes are reported, regardless of the technique used.[1]

Complications

- Pneumothorax (8%)
- Postoperative pain (60%)
- Neurologic (Horner's syndrome, radial paralysis, dysaesthesia of the arm) (3%)
- Failure of procedure (2% in palmar, up to 35% in axillary hyperhidrosis)
- Compensatory sweating (87%)—compensatory hyperhidrosis over chest, back, abdomen, which is usually well tolerated (>90%)

Alternatives available

- Subcutaneous botulinum toxin (axillary hyperhidrosis)
- Medical treatment (doxazosin, aluminium salts, anticholinergics)—results vary widely

Patient resources

- 🔊 www.hyperhidrosisuk.org

Reference

1. Baumgartner FJ. Surgical approaches and techniques in the management of severe hyperhidrosis. *Thorac Surg Clin* 2008;**18**(2):167–81.

Empyema thoracis

Background

Infection of the pleural cavity is known as empyema thoracis. A collection of pus, bounded by the visceral and parietal pleura is found. It is often the consequence of pneumonia and para-pneumonic effusions.

In patients with loculated pleural effusions and empyema thoracis, surgical evacuation of the pleural cavity may be necessary to control the infection and re-expand the lung. The surgical procedure of choice will depend on the extent of the disease and the physiological status of the patient.

Empyema thoracis can be represented as three overlapping consecutive stages:

- Stage I: exudative stage—drainage alone with tube thoracostomy is often successful, however, if the lung does not fully expand, treatment is as in stage II
- Stage II: fibrinopurulent stage—VATS debridement, evacuation, and irrigation of pleural cavity, removing all loculations is the preferred procedure. If the lung does not fully expand the treatment is the same as in Stage III
- Stage III: organization stage—a pleural cortex forms around the lung and pleural decortication becomes necessary, however, this is often delayed to optimize the patient and allow for the development of a mature cortex[1]

Special considerations

- Thoracoplasty is an alternative to decortication, where the space is obliterated by collapsing the chest wall. It results in resolution of the infection, but with an alteration in the appearance of the chest wall. It is not commonly performed
- In debilitated patients where thoracoplasty is not a viable alternative, and if tube thoracostomy ± VATS cannot control the disease an open window thoracostomy with rib resection can be performed

Complications

- SIRS, ARDS, MODS
- Recurrence of empyema
- Prolonged air leak
- Postoperative pain

Reference

1. Molnar TF. Current surgical treatment of thoracic empyema in adults. *Eur J Cardiothorac Surg* 2007;**32**:422–30.

Maxillofacial surgery

Open reduction and internal fixation of fractured mandible

Description

The mandible is one of the most frequently fractured bones of the face (Fig. 20.1). Fractures of the mandible are most common in young males and are frequently the result of interpersonal violence. Sporting accidents and motor vehicle accidents are other common causes.

Fractures of the mandible may also be the result of underling bony pathology of the mandible such as large jaw cysts or tumours that weaken the bone structure thereby predisposing to fracture. These are referred to as 'pathological' fractures.

The mandible can be likened to a ring structure (much like the pelvis) and therefore more than one fracture is commonly present.

Treatment consists of open reduction and internal fixation of fractures with titanium mini-plates usually via an intraoral approach. A small incision (<1cm) through the cheek may be required to facilitate this. Occasionally in the case of comminuted fractures, or pathological fractures, an extraoral approach with subsequent reconstruction achieved using larger and stronger plates may be required.

The procedure involves the placement of screws, buttons, or archbars so that the patient's occlusion (bite) may be restored using inter-maxillary wiring. The fracture sites are then exposed and the fractures reduced and fixed with bone plates. The incisions are closed using absorbable sutures.

Postoperatively the patient will need to maintain immaculate oral hygiene, keep to a very soft diet and refrain from smoking. Postoperative radiographs are usually required to ascertain the adequacy of the reduction and position of the plates.[1]

Additional procedures that may become necessary

- Extraction of teeth in fracture line
- Need for rigid intermaxillary fixation

Benefits

- Restore occlusion, reduction of fractures
- Promote favourable union, prevent infection
- Reduction of pain

Alternative procedures/conservative measures

- For isolated undisplaced fractures, conservative management may be indicated; close observation will be required

Serious/frequently occurring risks[2]

- *Common*: bleeding, pain, infection, temporary numbness or altered sensation in the distribution of the mandibular branch of the trigeminal nerve (i.e. lower lip and chin)
- *Occasional*: prolonged or permanent altered sensation of lower lip and chin, need to have plates removed at a later date
- *Rare*: malunion, non-union

Blood transfusion necessary
- None/group and save

Type of anaesthesia/sedation
- General anaesthesia (fibreoptic intubation may be required)

Follow-up/need for further procedure
- Regular review in outpatient clinic for up to 6 weeks
- In the case of a malunion or non-union, further procedures including bone grafting may be required

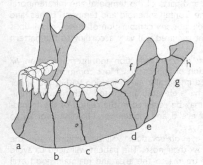

a - Symphysis
b - Parasymphysis
c - Body
d - Angle
e - Ramus
f - Coronoid process
g - Low condylar
h - High condylar

Fig. 20.1 Sites of mandibular fracture.
Reproduced with permission from O'Connor IF and Urdang M. *Oxford Handbook of Surgical Cross-Cover.* 2008. Oxford: Oxford University Press, p.367, Figure 9.7.

References
1. Stacey DH, Doyle JF, Mount DL, Snyder MC, Gutowski KA. Management of mandible fractures. *Plast Reconstr Surg* 2006;**117**:48e–60e.
2. Lamphier J, Ziccardi V, Ruvo A, et al. Complications of mandibular fractures in urban teaching centre. *J Oral Maxillofac Surg* 2006;**61**:745.

Open reduction and internal fixation of fractured zygoma

Description

The zygoma is the most commonly fractured facial bone, usually as a result of interpersonal violence. Sporting accidents and motor vehicle accidents are also common causes. The left side is more commonly fractured than the right.

The zygoma forms the prominence of the cheek, part of the lateral wall, and floor of the orbit and parts of the temporal and infratemporal fossae. It articulates with the frontal, sphenoid and temporal bones, and the maxilla. Fractures may disrupt any combination of these articulations (Fig. 20.2) and the treatment required will vary according to the pattern of fracture.

Treatment usually consists of open reduction and internal fixation via either a single or combination of approaches. Most commonly the fractured zygoma is approached intraorally via an incision within the upper buccal sulcus and the zygoma is elevated and plated with titanium miniplates. However, incisions may be required in the region of the frontozygomatic suture, the lower eyelid, and the temporal hairline in order to fully reduce and fix the fractures.[1]

Postoperatively, regular eye observations will be required and the patient is advised not to blow their nose. The patient will need to avoid contact sports and further trauma to the area and maintain good oral hygiene. Postoperative radiographs are usually required to establish the adequacy of the reduction. Skin sutures will need to be removed at follow-up.

Additional procedures that may become necessary

- Nil

Benefits

- Restore cheek prominence, reduction of fracture
- Restore function, if ocular signs are present or there is restriction of mandibular movement

Alternative procedures/conservative measures

- If the patient is unwilling to undergo operative intervention, the fracture may be treated conservatively but the patient must understand that there is a relatively small time window for operative intervention and any facial deformity will be permanent

Serious/frequently occurring risks

- *Common*: bleeding, pain, infection, temporary numbness or altered sensation in the distribution of the maxillary branch of the trigeminal nerve (i.e. upper lip and cheek), facial scar from surgical incision
- *Occasional*: prolonged or permanent altered sensation of upper lip, cheek and teeth. Ectropion from lower eyelid incision
- *Rare*: blindness in the ipsilateral eye as a result of retrobulbar haemorrhage (this is a rare but catastrophic complication whereby

bleeding behind the globe leads to an increase in orbital tissue pressures compromising the blood supply to the eye; if untreated blindness results)[2] malunion, non-union

Blood transfusion necessary

- None/group and save

Type of anaesthesia/sedation

- General anaesthesia

Follow-up/need for further procedure

- Regular review in outpatient clinic for up to 6 weeks with radiographs

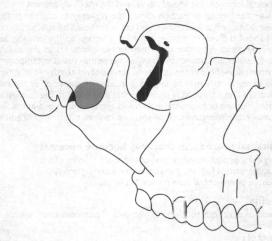

Fig. 20.2 Zygomatic fracture.
Reproduced with permission from Kerawala C and Newlands C. *Oxford Specialist Handbook of Oral and Maxillofacial Surgery.* 2010. Oxford: Oxford University Press, p.46, Figure 1.15.

References

1. Zingg M, Laedrach K, Chen J, et al. Classification and treatment of zygomatic fractures: A review of 1,025 cases. *J Oral Maxillofac Surg* 1992; **50**:778–90.
2. Ord RA. Post-operative retrobulbar haemorrhage and blindness complicating trauma surgery. *Br J Oral Surg* 1981; **19**:202–7.

Extraction of teeth

Description

Teeth may need to be extracted for a number of reasons. The most common causes are dental caries (decay) and periodontal (gum) disease. Lower third molars or wisdom teeth are frequently impacted and may become symptomatic necessitating extraction.

Each group of teeth requires its own technique for extraction and the risks of the procedure depend on the position of the tooth, the tooth morphology and the position of adjacent structures. Structures to be aware of include adjacent teeth, the mandibular branch of the trigeminal nerve (inferior dental nerve), including where it exits the mandible through the mental foramen, the lingual nerve, and the maxillary antrum.[1]

Lower third molar extraction carries the highest risk of damage to the inferior dental and lingual nerves, and patients should be specifically counselled about the risk of damage to them. Damage to the inferior dental nerve may result in temporary or permanent numbness to the ipsilateral lower lip and chin; damage to the lingual nerve may result in temporary or permanent numbness of the ipsilateral anterior two-thirds of the tongue.[2]

The upper molars may be intimately related to the floor of the maxillary antrum and occasionally their removal may result in the formation of a communication between the mouth and antrum, i.e. an oro-antral fistula This may close spontaneously, if small or require a formal procedure to close.

Additional procedures that may become necessary

- Surgical approach to extraction of the tooth (raising of a mucoperiosteal flap and removal of surrounding bone)
- Closure of oro-antral communication/fistula

Benefits

- Removal of carious tooth/teeth, removal of potential/actual source of infection
- Relief of pain

Alternative procedures/conservative measures

- If the tooth is not too badly broken down, there is the option of restoring the tooth
- Root canal treatment is nearly always required with a symptomatic tooth

Serious/frequently occurring risks

- *Common*: pain, bleeding, infection
- *Occasional*: damage to adjacent teeth, damage to the mandibular branch of the trigeminal nerve, creation of an oro-antral communication
- *Rare: damage to the lingual nerve, fracture of the mandible*[2]

Blood transfusion necessary

- None/group and save

Type of anaesthesia/sedation

- Commonly performed under local anaesthesia, but may require either intravenous sedation or general anaesthesia for complex cases or for the anxious patient

Follow-up/need for further procedure

- Routine follow-up not usually required

References

1. Robinson P. *Tooth extraction a practical guide*. 2000. Oxford Butterworth–Heinemann, 100–27.
2. Rerton T, McGurk M. Evaluation of factors predictive of lingual nerve injury in third molar surgery. *Br J Oral Maxillofac Surg* 2001; **39**:432–8.

Orbital floor reconstruction

Description

Direct blows to the globe may result in fractures to the delicate bones of the walls or floor of the orbit as the force is dissipated. This may lead to an increased orbital volume.

Clinical features of such injuries include enophthalmos and restriction of eye movements with associated diplopia, as the orbital contents herniate through the fracture and may become trapped. Hypoaesthesia in the distribution of the infraorbital nerve may also result if the fracture involves the infraorbital canal, thereby damaging the infraorbital nerve. Formal ophthalmological and orthoptic assessment are required prior to surgery.

The orbital floor may be accessed through a subciliary or blepharoplasty incision in the lower eyelid or via a transconjunctival approach. The orbital contents are retrieved from the fracture and the orbital floor reconstructed using either autologous (bone) or alloplastic (titanium mesh) materials.[1]

Postoperatively the patient will require regular eye observations, as for a fractured zygoma and is advised to refrain from nose blowing. It may take some weeks for the oedema to settle and for ocular function to return to normal.

Additional procedures that may become necessary
• None

Benefits
• Restoration of orbital volume and retrieval of orbital contents
• Restore eye movements and correct diplopia
• Correction of hypoglobus

Alternative procedures/conservative measures
• In the presence of significant ocular signs, there is no other effective way of managing such fractures

Serious/frequently occurring risks
• *Common*: pain, swelling
• *Occasional*: infection, persistent hypoaesthesia of ipsilateral upper lip, cheek and teeth
• *Rare*: retrobulbar haemorrhage, persistent diplopia, blindness[2]

Blood transfusion necessary
• None/group and save

Type of anaesthesia/sedation
• General anaesthesia

Follow-up/need for further procedure
• *Regular follow-up in clinic to ensure resolution of symptoms*
• Further orthoptic assessment may be required

Reference
1. Burnstine, M. Clinical recommendations for repair of orbital facial fractures. *Current Opinion Ophthalm* 2003; **14**(5): 236–40.

Elevation of fractured zygomatic arch

Description

The zygomatic arch consists of the zygomatic process of the temporal bone and the temporal process of the zygomatic bone. It may be fractured in isolation by a direct blow. There is characteristically a dimple evident in the region when the swelling subsides. There may also be associated limitation of mouth opening due to the depressed arch impinging on the coronoid process of the mandible.

The temporalis fascia attaches to the upper border of the arch whereas the temporalis muscle itself attaches to the coronoid process of the mandible. It is this anatomical arrangement that facilitates the surgical elevation of a fractured arch. Surgical elevation is achieved through a temporal hairline incision and dissection made down to the temporalis fascia. This fascia is then incised and an elevator inserted down between the fascia (Fig. 20.3) and the muscle extending beneath the zygomatic arch. The fracture can then be elevated and reduced.[1]

Postoperative radiographs are usually required to ascertain the adequacy of the reduction. The patient should be advised to sleep on the contralateral side and to avoid contact sports for 6 weeks.

Additional procedures that may become necessary

- Nil

Benefits

- Restoration of facial contour; restoration of function, in the case of limitation of mouth opening

Alternative procedures/conservative measures

- Conservative management may be indicated if there is no functional impairment and the patient is happy with their appearance

Serious/frequently occurring risks

- *Common*: pain, swelling, bleeding
- *Rare*: residual deformity, need for further procedure

Blood transfusion necessary

- None/group and save

Type of anaesthesia/sedation

- General anaesthesia

Follow-up/need for further procedure

- Generally one follow-up visit to ensure adequate healing and aesthetics

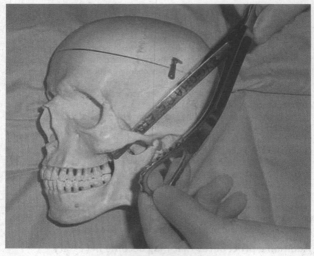

Fig. 20.3 Gillie's approach to zygomatic arch fracture.
Reproduced with permission from Kerawala C and Newlands C. *Oxford Specialist Handbook of Oral and Maxillofacial Surgery*. 2010. Oxford: Oxford University Press, p.48, Figure 1.18.

Reference

1. Werner J, Frenkler JE, Lippert B, *et al.* Isolated zygomatic arch fracture: report on a modified surgical technique. *Plastic Recon Surg* 2002; **109**(3): 1085–9.

Bilateral sagittal split osteotomy

Description

The bilateral sagittal split mandibular osteotomy may be used to correct mandibular prognathism, retrognathism, or asymmetry. It may be a single jaw procedure or as part of a bimaxillary procedure in conjunction with a Le Fort 1 osteotomy. The patient will usually undergo a course of orthodontic treatment prior to surgery to facilitate maximum accuracy of the procedure and optimization of their occlusion (bite).

The procedure is undertaken through an intraoral approach. Mucoperiosteal flaps are raised and a series of bone cuts made in the sagittal plane. The mandible is then split on either side. The free distal portion is repositioned into an appropriate occlusion using a prefabricated splint, the jaws wired together, and the osteotomized fracture sites fixed with titanium mini-plates or screws. Small incisions (<1cm) may be required on either cheek to facilitate this. Closure is with resorbable sutures.

Postoperative radiographs are taken and the patient may need to wear intermaxillary elastic bands. A further period of orthodontics is usually required.

An alternative approach may be considered for patients with isolated mandibular prognathism. The *vertical subsigmoid mandibular osteotomy* involves bone cuts made vertically to section the ramus of the mandible from the sigmoid notch down to its inferior border. The body of the mandible is then repositioned posteriorly with the fragments now overlapping. A major disadvantage of this procedure is that a 4–6-week period of rigid intermaxillary fixation is required.

Additional procedures that may become necessary

- Removal of mandibular third molars (wisdom teeth)
- Placement of drains
- Rigid intermaxillary fixation
- Bone grafting (frequently taken from the iliac crest)

Benefits

- Improve facial profile, improve dental occlusion

Alternative procedures/conservative measures

- A bimaxillary approach may be more appropriate for those with severe skeletal discrepancies
- For patients with relatively minor skeletal discrepancies, a course of orthodontic treatment to 'camouflage' the problem may be considered

Serious/frequently occurring risks[1]

- *Common*: pain, swelling, bleeding, temporary numbness of lower lip and chin
- *Occasional*: infection, permanent altered sensation of lower lip and chin, need for removal of plates at a later date[2]
- *Rare*: need for further procedure, malunion, non-union

Blood transfusion necessary

- None/group and save

Type of anaesthesia/sedation

- General anaesthesia

Follow-up/need for further procedure

- Careful prolonged follow-up in joint maxillofacial/orthodontic clinics

References

1. Teltzrow T, Kramer F, Schulze A, et al. Perioperative complications following sagittal split osteotomy of the mandible. *J Cranio-Maxillofac Surg* 2005; **33**(5): 307–13.
2. Westermark A, Bystedt H, von Konow L. Inferior alveolar nerve function after mandibular osteotomies. *Br J Oral Maxillofac Surg* 1998; **36**(6): 425–8.

Le Fort 1 maxillary osteotomy

Description

The Le Fort 1 maxillary osteotomy is a procedure whereby the maxilla is separated from the skull base so that it may be repositioned in order to correct an underlying skeletal deformity. It may be a single-jaw procedure or as part of a bimaxillary procedure in conjunction with a mandibular osteotomy. The patient will usually undergo a course of orthodontic treatment prior to surgery to facilitate maximum accuracy of the procedure and optimization of their occlusion (bite).

The procedure is undertaken through an intraoral approach. An incision is made in the upper buccal sulcus and cuts made through the lateral, medial, and posterior maxillary walls. The maxilla is then dis-impacted (Fig. 20.4) and repositioned into an appropriate position using a prefabricated splint, the jaws are wired together, and the fracture sites fixed with titanium mini-plates. Closure is with absorbable sutures.

Postoperatively, radiographs are taken, and the patient may need to wear intermaxillary elastic bands. A further period of orthodontic treatment is usually required.

Additional procedures that may become necessary

- Bone grafting from the iliac crest—where the vertical height of the maxilla is being increased

Benefits

- Improve facial profile, improve dental occlusion

Alternative procedures/conservative measures

- A bimaxillary approach may be more appropriate for those with more severe skeletal discrepancies
- For patients with relatively minor skeletal discrepancies, a course of orthodontic treatment to 'camouflage' the problem may be considered

Serious/frequently occurring risks[1,2]

- *Common*: pain, swelling, bleeding, temporary numbness of upper lip, cheek and teeth
- *Occasional*: infection, permanent altered sensation of upper lip, cheek and teeth, need for removal of plates at a later date
- *Rare*: need for further procedure

Blood transfusion necessary

- None/group and save

Type of anaesthesia/sedation

- General anaesthesia

Follow-up/need for further procedure

- Careful prolonged follow-up in joint maxillofacial/orthodontic clinics

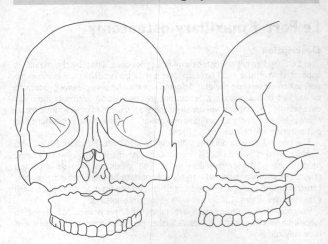

Fig. 20.4 Le Fort 1 fracture.

Reproduced with permission from Kerawala C and Newlands C. *Oxford Specialist Handbook of Oral and Maxillofacial Surgery*. 2010. Oxford: Oxford University Press, p.42, Figure 1.12.

References

1. Kramer FJ, Baethge C, Swennen G, et al. Intra- and perioperative complications of the Le Fort 1 osteotomy: A prospective evaluation of 1000 patients. *J Craniofac Surg* 2004; **15**(6): 971–7.
2. Bendor-Samuel R, Chen YR, Chen PK. Unusual complications of the Le Fort 1 osteotomy: a case report. *Int J Oral Maxillofac Surg* 2004; **33**(1): 101–4.

Enucleation of jaw cysts

Description

A cyst is a pathological cavity, usually lined by epithelium and filled with fluid, semifluid, or gaseous material. They can vary in size from the very small to involving the majority of one or both jaw bones. They may be developmental or inflammatory, odontogenic or non-odontogenic in origin. Patients may be asymptomatic and the cyst found incidentally on routine radiographs or they may occasionally present with swelling of the jaw, with pain and discharge if the cyst has become infected.[1]

The treatment required depends on the histological subtype. The majority of cysts respond well to simple enucleation. A mucoperiosteal flap is raised intraorally, and the cyst accessed through the bone and removed in its entirety. The specimen is then sent for histological analysis. Large cysts may significantly weaken the bone and fracture of the mandible, either at the time of surgery or during the recovery period is a recognized complication. Large mandibular cysts may also envelop the inferior dental nerve as it passes through the mandible and therefore the patient must be counselled about the possibility of damage to the nerve at time of surgery.[2]

Additional procedures that may become necessary

- Removal of associated teeth
- Apicectomy and retrograde root filling of associated teeth
- Open reduction and internal fixation of fractured mandible
- Insertion of drainage tube

Benefits

- Removal of cyst, diagnosis

Alternative procedures/conservative measures

- Marsupialization of cyst (not suitable for all cysts and results in slower healing)

Serious/frequently occurring risks

- *Common*: pain, swelling, bleeding, temporary hypoaesthesia of lower lip and chin (mandibular cysts)
- *Occasional*: need for further procedure, permanent hypoaesthesia of the lower lip and chin (mandibular cysts)
- *Rare*: fractured mandible

Blood transfusion necessary

- None/group and save

Type of anaesthesia/sedation

- General anaesthesia/local anaesthesia (for smaller cysts)

Follow-up/need for further procedure

- Routine follow-up with radiographs to ensure satisfactory resolution

References

1. Pogrel M. Treatment of Keratocysts: the case for decompression and marsupialization. *J Oral Maxillofac Surg.* 2005; **63**:1667–73.
2. Keise G. Odontogenic cysts and tumors of the maxilla: controversies in surgical management. *Operative Techniques in Otolaryngol Head Neck Surg.* 1999; **10**(2): 140–7.

Incision and drainage of orofacial abscesses

Description

Dental decay can allow ingress of bacteria into the pulp of a tooth and from there into the surrounding alveolar bone, resulting in a localized infection. This infection can spread, usually along the path of least resistance into the surrounding tissues. This path of spread is influenced by the position of the tooth and the position of surrounding structures, for example muscle attachments. In simple cases, resolution may be achieved by commencing root canal therapy or extracting the affected tooth. However, if left untreated such infections can progress to become very serious and in some cases life-threatening.

The procedure undertaken depends on the tissue spaces involved, whether there is a collection of pus that can be drained and the severity of the infection. For maxillary teeth, extraction of the culprit tooth, with or without intraoral incision and drainage is usually sufficient. Infections associated with mandibular teeth commonly spread into the submandibular space (i.e. beneath the attachment of mylohyoid) and will therefore require incision and drainage via an extraoral submandibular incision. This approach will leave a scar on the neck and the patient should be warned about potential damage to the marginal mandibular branch of the facial nerve.[1]

A plastic corrugated drain is usually left *in situ* for 24–48h postoperatively.

Additional procedures that may become necessary

- Examination under anaesthesia
- Removal of teeth as necessary
- Placement of drains (intraoral/extraoral)
- Tracheostomy

Benefits

- Remove source of infection, drain collection of pus

Alternative procedures/conservative measures

- Occasionally the affected tooth may be considered to be restorable and this needs to be considered before condemning it to extraction

Serious/frequently occurring risks

- *Common*: pain, swelling, bleeding, temporary weakness to the ipsilateral corner of mouth
- *Occasional*: permanent weakness to the ipsilateral corner of mouth
- *Rare*: tracheostomy
- If a mandibular third molar is to be extracted, the patient must be counselled about the further risks of this procedure

Blood transfusion necessary

- None/group and save

Type of anaesthesia/sedation

- General anaesthesia (awake fibreoptic intubation may be required)

Follow-up/need for further procedure

- Occasionally a repeat procedure is required if the patient fails to improve
- Most patients can be discharged without formal follow-up arrangements

Reference

1. Osborn T, Assael L, Bell R. Deep space neck infection: principles of surgical management. *Oral and Maxillofac Surg Clinics North Am*. 2008; **20**(3): 353–65.

Excision of submandibular gland

Description

The submandibular gland is most often removed due to recurrent infections or sialadenitis. This is usually due to obstruction of the submandibular duct by a stone or stricture. The greater the number of episodes, the more damage is done to the gland and surrounding tissues. Patients may report repeated episodes of pain and swelling from the gland. In some cases of obstruction, the gland may swell every time the patient eats as the saliva produced is unable to pass down the duct into the mouth—this is known as 'mealtime syndrome'.[1]

Neoplasms may also develop in any of the salivary glands; they may be benign or malignant. Malignancies are more common than benign lesions in the submandibular glands.

The gland is accessed by an incision in the neck below the border of the mandible, care being taken to protect the marginal mandibular branch of the facial nerve. The lingual nerve is identified and protected and the gland dissected out from the surrounding structures (Fig. 20.5). The submandibular duct is tied off and the gland excised and sent for histopathological examination.

A drain is placed to prevent haematoma formation and the wound closed in layers, usually with absorbable sutures. The drain can usually be removed the following day and the patient discharged.

Additional procedures that may become necessary

- Examination under anaesthesia
- Placement of drains

Benefits (depends on underlying pathology)

- Resolve symptoms
- Removal of mass, provide tissue for diagnosis

Alternative procedures/conservative measures

If a stone in the submandibular duct is responsible for the obstruction, then in some cases it may be amenable to removal, either endoscopically or surgically through an intraoral incision into the duct. This may provide resolution of the symptoms but often removal of the gland at a later date is required.

Serious/frequently occurring risks[2]

- *Common*: pain, swelling, bleeding, temporary weakness to the ipsilateral corner of mouth, scar
- *Occasional*: permanent weakness to the ipsilateral corner of mouth, numbness to the ipsilateral side of tongue
- *Rare*: damage to hypoglossal nerve

Blood transfusion necessary

- None/group and save

Type of anaesthesia/sedation

- General anaesthetic

Follow-up/need for further procedure
- Neck dissection, radiotherapy
- Patients may need to attend for removal of sutures; follow-up depends on the underlying pathology

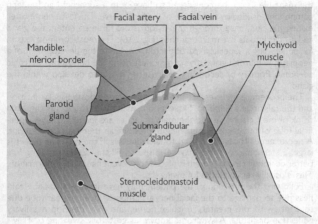

Fig. 20.5 Relations of the submandibular gland at the angle of the mandible.
Reproduced with permission from Warner G, Burgess AS, Patel S, et al. *Oxford Specialist Handbook of Otolaryngology and Head and Neck Surgery.* 2009. Oxford: Oxford University Press, p.123, Figure 7.4.

References
1. McGurk M, Makdissi J, Brown J. Intra-oral removal of stones from the hilum of the submandibular gland. *Int J Oral Maxillofac Surg.* 2004; **33**(7): 583–6.
2. Smith W, Peters W, Markus A. Submandibular gland surgery: an audit of clinical findings, pathology and postoperative morbidity. *Annals Royal College of Surgeons of England.* 1993; **75**:164–7.

Superficial parotidectomy

Description

The parotid glands lie anterior and inferior to the ear over the ramus of the mandible. It can be considered to have both a superficial and a deep component, divided by the course of the facial nerve. The facial nerve, after exiting the skull base through the stylomastoid foramen enters the gland and divides into its five main branches (Fig. 20.6). The most common reason for undergoing a superficial parotidectomy is due to the development of a neoplasm within the gland, the commonest being the benign pleomorphic adenoma. Primary or secondary malignancies may also develop within the gland.

The procedure involves making a preauricular or postauricular incision and the raising of a skin flap. Dissection is then made to identify the main trunk of the facial nerve and the main branches are identified. The superficial lobe of the parotid containing the lesion can then be dissected out. A nerve stimulator is often used to facilitate this. If the resulting defect is large, a sternomastoid flap may be raised to fill the defect resulting in a better cosmetic result. A drain is placed to prevent haematoma formation. This is usually removed the following day.

Following the procedure, the patient may have ipsilateral facial weakness due to damage to the facial nerve, numbness over the ear lobe due to damage to the greater auricular nerve, and may develop a salivary collection or fistula. A syndrome known as gustatory sweating or Frey's syndrome may develop, where the patient's skin overlying the parotid sweats excessively at mealtimes. This is due to inappropriate regeneration of parasympathetic nerve fibres that, instead of innervating salivary tissue, now innervate the sweat glands of the skin.[1]

Additional procedures that may become necessary

- Placement of drains
- Sternomastoid flap
- Neck dissection

Benefits (depends on underlying pathology)

- Resolve symptoms
- Removal of mass, provide tissue for diagnosis

Alternative procedures/conservative measures

- If a benign tumour is identified, a period of watchful waiting could be considered if the patient refuses surgical intervention
- Extracapsular dissection of lesion

Serious/frequently occurring risks[2]

- *Common*: pain, swelling, bleeding, temporary ipsilateral facial weakness, numbness of ear lobe, scar
- *Occasional*: permanent ipsilateral facial weakness, Frey's syndrome, facial asymmetry, recurrence of tumour

Blood transfusion necessary

- None/group and save

Type of anaesthesia/sedation

• General anaesthesia

Follow-up/need for further procedure

• Neck dissection
• Radiotherapy—for malignancies
• Patients may need to attend for removal of sutures; follow-up depends on the underlying pathology

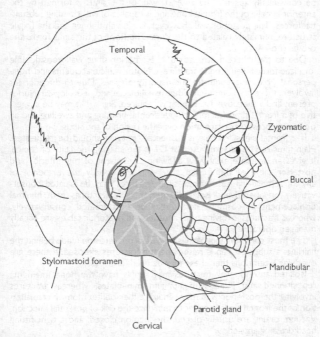

Fig. 20.6 Anatomical relations of the parotid gland and the facial nerve.

Reproduced with permission from Warner G, Burgess AS, Patel S, et al. *Oxford Specialist Handbook of Otolaryngology and Head and Neck Surgery*. 2009. Oxford: Oxford University Press, p.113, Figure 7.1.

References

1. Marchese-Ragona R, De Filippis C, Marioni G, et al. Treatment of complications of parotid gland surgery. *Acta Otorhinolartygol Ital.* 2005; **25**(3):174–8.
2. Langdon J. Complications of parotid gland surgery. *J Maxillofac Surg.* 1984; **12**:225–9.

Open reduction and internal fixation of frontal bone fractures

Description

The frontal sinuses lie within the frontal bone, varying considerably in size. Pneumatization progresses throughout childhood with the sinuses becoming fully developed in young adults. Occasionally one or both may be congenitally absent. The anterior wall of the sinus is formed by the anterior lamella of the frontal bone and is capable of withstanding substantial forces. The posterior wall, however, is a much thinner and the fragile structure intimately related to the dura. The floor of the sinus forms the orbital roof.

Due to the inherent strength of the anterior sinus wall considerable localized force is required to fracture it. Motor vehicle accidents and interpersonal violence account for the majority of cases. Due to the energies involved, there are commonly other maxillofacial and neurological injuries present and a thorough assessment is required. Signs that may be suggestive of a frontal sinus fracture include frontal bruising and swelling and an obvious depression or laceration over the region of the sinus.

If a frontal sinus fracture is suspected, imaging should be requested. Plain films can be of some use but CT is the imaging modality of choice. It gives an accurate axial view allowing assessment of the anterior and posterior table of the frontal sinus and additionally the presence of any intracranial injuries. Frontal sinus fractures may be treated conservatively or operatively. Isolated anterior table fractures with minimal displacement or cosmetic defect may be best treated conservatively, whereas fractures involving both anterior and posterior tables are usually managed operatively.[1]

The most common approach is via a bicoronal incision made behind the hairline; a subgaleal flap is raised and the fractures exposed. If there are overlying lacerations then these may be used for access.

Isolated anterior wall fractures may simply have the bone fragments repositioned and fixed with titanium mini-plates, whereas fractures involving the posterior wall may require either obliteration or cranialization of the frontal sinus in order to minimize the risk of potential infection. Vacuum drains are usually placed, the incision closed, and a tight fitting head dressing applied.[2]

Additional procedures that may become necessary

- Harvesting of bone for sinus obliteration
- Dural repair

Benefits

- Reduce fracture
- Improve cosmesis
- Prevention of infection—meningitis, sinusitis
- Dural repair—prevent cerebrospinal fluid leak

Alternative procedures/conservative measures
- Fractures may be treated expectantly, especially isolated anterior wall fractures, however, the patient must be fully informed of the risks
- An endoscopic assisted approach to anterior table fractures may be taken which avoids the need for the conventional bicoronal incision

Serious/frequently occurring risks
- *Common*: pain, swelling, scar, bleeding
- *Occasional*: infection, sinusitis, meningitis, cerebrospinal fluid leak, mucocele, alopecia in the region of the scar, paraesthesia
- *Rare*: death

Blood transfusion necessary
- None/group and save

Type of anaesthesia/sedation
- General anaesthesia

Follow-up/need for further procedure
- Routine follow-up is required

References
1. Yavuzer R, Sari A, Kelly C, et al. Management of frontal sinus fractures. *Plastic Recon Surg*. 2005; **115**(6): 79e–93e.
2. Kalavrezos N. Current trends in the management of frontal sinus fractures. *Injury*. 2004; **35**(4): 340–6.

Cranioplasty

Description

Cranioplasty is the surgical repair of a skull defect or deformity that often results from previous neurosurgery such as decompressive craniectomy or from trauma to the cranium. There is usually a significant time period between the initial surgery and cranioplasty repair. Many materials can be used for cranioplasty including bone and polymethyl-methacrylate. Custom-made titanium implants are widely used in the UK.

A CT scan of the defect is performed and a life size model produced using a computer-controlled mill. This allows for the fabrication of the implant prior to surgery. The placement of the implant is relatively straightforward. A scalp flap is raised, often using the scar from previous surgery, the defect fully exposed and the implant positioned appropriately. The implant is then secured with titanium bone screws. A vacuum drain is placed and the flap replaced. A tight fitting head bandage is placed to prevent the development of a seroma.

The cranioplasty restores the contour of the skull and provides physical protection to the intracranial structures. There is evidence emerging that the placement of a cranioplasty may also lead to an improvement in neurological function, perhaps by reducing atmospheric pressure on the brain and increasing cerebral blood flow in the area. There is, however, no way of predicting which patients will show an improvement in neurological function following surgery.[1]

Additional procedures that may become necessary
• Nil

Benefits
• Restore contour of cranium
• Physical protection of brain
• Potentially improve neurological function

Alternative procedures/conservative measures
• Nil

Serious/frequently occurring risks[1,2]
• *Common*: scarring
• *Occasional*: infection, development of seroma, bleeding necessitating return to theatre, alopecia in region of scar
• *Rare*: stroke, death

Blood transfusion necessary
• None/group and save

Type of anaesthesia/sedation
• *General anaesthesia—an HDU bed postoperatively is essential*

Follow-up/need for further procedure
• Removal of head bandage at 10 days postoperatively
• Routine follow-up is required

References

1. Kuo J-R, Wang C-C, Chio C-C, et al. Neurological improvement after cranioplasty—analysis by transcranial Doppler ultrasonography. *J Clin Neurosci*. 2004; 11(5): 486–9.
2. Wen Y-D, Yoo D-S, Kim K-T, et al. Cranioplasty effect on the cerebral hemodynamics and cardiac function. *Acta Neurochirurgica Suppl*. 2009; 1(1): 13–20.

Temporomandibular joint arthroscopy

Description

The temporomandibular joint forms the articulation between the condyle of the mandible and the glenoid fossa of the temporal bone of the skull. It is a synovial joint with a fibrocartilaginous articular disc dividing the joint into two compartments. The joint is capable of two types of movement. Initial mouth opening is a rotational movement of the condylar head against the articular disc, within the inferior joint compartment. Further opening leads to a translatory movement of the articular cartilage and condylar head around the glenoid fossa.

The temporomandibular joint can be affected by many different pathologies, the most common of which is temporomandibular joint dysfunction. This has a wide range of symptoms and presentations but generally involves one or more parts of the temporomandibular joint apparatus. Patients may complain of pain in or around the joint, reduced or painful mouth opening and a clicking or grinding sensation on mandibular movement. These symptoms may be constant or intermittent and are typically worse at certain times of day, typically in the morning.

The aetiology of such dysfunction is complex and many hypotheses have been suggested. There is often an associated psychological component. Due its multifactorial aetiology, a multidisciplinary team approach to temporomandibular joint dysfunction should be employed. The majority of patients can be managed non-operatively.

The least invasive of surgical temporomandibular joint procedures is arthroscopy. A small arthroscope can be introduced into the joint space allowing the joint to be visualized and any pathology such as adhesions, disc displacement, or perforation to be identified. In some cases, therapeutic procedures can be performed such as the lysis of adhesions and meniscopexy. This can remove the need to have open exploratory temporomandibular joint surgery with its associated risks.

Additional procedures that may become necessary

- Temporomandibular joint arthrocentesis

Benefits

- Diagnosis of underlying pathology
- Reduce symptoms (therapeutic arthroscopy)

Alternative procedures/conservative measures

- *Conservative*: this approach to temporomandibular joint dysfunction, such as soft diet, physiotherapy, jaw splints, jaw exercises, and anti-inflammatory medication should be tried initially

Serious/frequently occurring risks

- *Common*: pain, bleeding
- *Occasional*: infection
- *Rare*: damage to facial nerve

Blood transfusion necessary

- None/group and save

Type of anaesthesia/sedation
- Local anaesthesia/general anaesthesia

Follow-up/need for further procedure
- Dependent on arthroscopy findings
- Open temporomandibular joint surgery/arthroplasty may be required

Temporomandibular joint arthroplasty

Description

Temporomandibular joint arthroplasty describes any open procedure of the temporomandibular joint. There are a variety of procedures that can be performed. They include disc reposition, discectomy, recontouring of the articular eminence, and total joint replacement.

The temporomandibular joint is accessed via a preauricular incision, a skin flap is raised and dissection continued down to the joint capsule. The capsule is opened to expose the joint itself allowing further assessment of the joint and full surgical access to it.

If the articular disc has been displaced it may be relocated into its appropriate position and sutured in place. If it has been too badly damaged it is sometimes necessary to remove it—discectomy. Synthetic or autologous materials can be used to re-create the disc or the space left empty for scar tissue to fill.

If the temporomandibular joint is not suitable for such procedures or they have been unsuccessfully attempted in the past, then a partial or total joint replacement may be indicated. Replacement temporomandibular joints consist of two components, a fossa component that reproduces the glenoid fossa and a mandibular component that replaces the mandibular condyle. Two incisions are required, one preauricular and one retromandibular, to gain sufficient access. The condylar head is excised and the glenoid fossa prepared. The patient is then put into rigid inter-maxillary fixation before the implants are placed and secured. A drain is rarely used due to the risk of introducing infection and the wounds are closed.

Open temporomandibular joint procedures are not without risk and should not be undertaken lightly. They are often a last resort for intractable joint pathology.

Specific risks include damage to the facial nerve, especially the temporal and zygomatic branches. The middle ear can also be damaged with associated loss of hearing. While such procedures are undertaken with the intention of improving the patient's symptoms, the patient must be specifically warned about failure of the procedure and that such procedures may cause a worsening of their symptoms.

Additional procedures that may become necessary

- None

Benefits

- Improve temporomandibular joint function
- Reduce pain

Alternative procedures/conservative measures

- A conservative approach may be taken to temporomandibular joint dysfunction as previously mentioned

Serious/frequently occurring risks

- *Common*: scarring, swelling, pain

- *Occasional*: facial nerve dysfunction, infection—localized or systemic, failure to improve symptoms, dislocation, malocclusion
- *Rare*: neuroma formation, ear problems, loosening of implant/failure of implant

Blood transfusion necessary

- Group and save

Type of anaesthesia/sedation

- General anaesthesia

Follow-up/need for further procedure

- Routine follow-up is required

Ophthalmic surgery

Conjunctival laceration repair

Description
The conjunctiva of the eye is a thin, but important layer (see Fig. 21.1). It helps lubricate the eye, protects the eye from infection, and provides mucus for the corneal tear film.

Laceration size can affect whether surgical repair may be required or not. The larger the gap, the less chance that the conjunctiva will heal, or it will just take longer to heal. There is also a chance of scarring.

Indications
• Restore normal conjunctival anatomy

Alternatives
• Leave to heal by secondary intention (laissez-faire)

Benefits
• Faster recovery
• Prevent abnormal healing

Procedure
• Carried out under local anaesthesia ± sedation or general anaesthesia
• The edges of the conjunctiva are apposed and sutured/glued together
• The operation takes 10–15min

Complications
Common
• Bleeding

Uncommon
• Infection
• Scarring
• Suture granuloma
• Need for additional surgery

Corneal transplants/grafts

Description

The cornea is the clear window of the eye. It has an approximate thickness of 0.5mm and a diameter of 12mm. It is separated from the iris by the aqueous filled anterior chamber. It has five layers from superficial to deep: epithelium, Bowman's membrane, stroma, Descemet's membrane, and endothelium (see Fig. 21.4). Any or all of these layers can become affected by pathology, perforation, or damage to the cells from inflammation or injury. Any distortion or opacity will result in blurring of vision. A corneal graft will replace the damaged layers and restore clearer vision, particularly when there is no damage within the eye itself.

There are 2 main types of corneal grafts:
- Full thickness or penetrating grafts
- Partial thickness or lamellar grafts
  - Lamellar grafts may be anterior or posterior

Anterior lamellar graft
- Deep anterior lamellar keratoplasty (DALK)

Posterior lamellar grafts
- Deep lamellar endothelial keratoplasty (DLEK—superseded by DSEK)
- Descemet's stripping endothelial keratoplasty (DSEK)
- Descemet's stripping automated endothelial keratoplasty (DSAEK)

Posterior lamellar grafts have the advantage of being smaller operations through a small incision requiring a few stitches. The integrity of the eyeball is much stronger compared with a full-thickness graft.

Deep anterior lamellar keratoplasty

Description
Generally performed when the cornea has a normal endothelium and pathology is limited to the stroma. Compared to full thickness grafts, in the presence of ocular surface disease it is safer, but more difficult to perform and may take longer. The recipient cornea is prepared first in case the surgeon has to convert to a full-thickness graft.

Indications
- Corneal scars
- Stromal dystrophies
- Corneal perforations/thinning
- Congenital lesions (e.g. dermoid cysts)

Alternatives
- Penetrating keratoplasty

Benefits
- To improve vision
- To restore/preserve corneal integrity
- To correct abnormal corneal contour

Procedure
- Commonly performed under general anaesthesia
- Patient's cornea (only the anterior lamella) is removed, and donor cornea (only the anterior lamella) is prepared using either microkeratome or femto-second laser
- Donor cornea is inserted and sutured into position
- The procedure takes 60–90min

Complications
Common
- Penetration into anterior chamber, requiring conversion to penetrating keratoplasty
- High astigmatism/change in refractive status
- Excessive post op inflammation
- Persistent corneal defect
- Microbial keratitis
- Corneal graft infection
- Opacification and vascularization of the graft–host interface
- Need for additional surgery

Uncommon
- Cataract
- Wound leaks

Rare
- Cystoid macula oedema
- Epithelial downgrowth
- Intraocular bleeding
- Cataract
- Iris trauma
- Endophthalmitis (severe infection in the eye)
- Wound leaks

Descemet's stripping endothelial keratoplasty

Description
This is commonly performed in patients with endothelial disease only.

Indications
- Endothelial dystrophies
- Fuch's endothelial dystrophy
- Pseudophakic bullous keratopathy

Alternatives
- Penetrating keratoplasty

Benefits
- Restore corneal endothelial function

Procedure
- Usually performed under general anaesthesia
- Host cornea prepared for donor tissue insertion
- Donor tissue prepared and inserted onto host stroma
- Air tamponade used to assist graft–host interface adhesion
- No sutures required
- The procedure can take 60–90min

Complications
Common
- Intraocular bleeding during surgery
- Cataract
- Iris trauma
- Corneal oedema (water-logging of cornea)
- Dislocation of donor transplant (10–20% of patients in the first 24h)
- Excessive post op inflammation
- Corneal scarring
- Need for additional surgery

Uncommon
- Endophthalmitis (severe infection in the eye)
- Glaucoma
- Persistent epithelial defect

Rare
- Wound leaks
- Graft infection
- Graft rejection

- Epithelial downgrowth

Cyclodestructive procedures

Description

The ciliary body contains the ciliary processes that are responsible for aqueous humour production (see Fig. 21.3). Destroying the ciliary processes will ultimately reduce aqueous production and lower intraocular pressure. These procedures are associated with unwanted complications and are unpredictable in their pressure lowering effects. They are usually indicated as a last resort particularly in eyes with very limited visual potential.

Indications

- Glaucoma refractory to medical/surgical treatment
- End-stage open angle glaucoma
- Rubeotic, malignant, or congenital glaucoma
- Blind, painful (phthisical) eye
- Glaucoma secondary to penetrating keratoplasty, advanced angle closure, trauma, or silicone oil

Alternatives

- Filtration surgery with antimetabolites
- Drainage tube shunts

Benefits

- Reduce intraocular pressure
- Control pain
- Avoid enucleation (removal of eyeball)

Procedure

- Carried out under local anaesthesia ± secation or general anaesthesia
- Destruction of the ciliary processes resulting in reduced aqueous production
- Carried out by several techniques including cyclodide laser, cyclocryotherapy, and endoscopic cyclophotocoagulation (ECP)
- The procedure can take 10–30min depending on the technique

Complications

Common

- Chronic hypotony (low intraocular pressure soft eyeball)
- Severe postoperative uveitis
- Corneal oedema (water-logging of cornea)
- Bleeding (hyphaema and vitreous haemorrhage)
- Phthisis (shrinkage of eye)
- Loss of vision
- Need for additional treatment

Uncommon
- Anterior segment necrosis/ischemia
- Scleral thinning
- Retinal detachment
- Failure to control/improve pain
- Traumatic cataract (ECP only)

Rare
- Sympathetic ophthalmitis
- Endophthalmitis (severe infection in the eye)

Sympathetic ophthalmitis (also known as sympathetic ophthalmia/uveitis) is a rare, autoimmune (delayed-type hypersensitivity reaction) granulomatous uveitis (towards melanin-containing structures in the eye) that occurs following penetrating trauma (from surgery or injury) to an eye. This can result in inflammation appearing in the contralateral eye, and can lead to loss of vision in both eyes.

Dacryocystorhinostomy ± bypass tube insertion

Description

Tears are produced by the lacrimal glands and drain continuously through the nasolacrimal ducts. The nasolacrimal ducts are situated in the medial corners of the eye (see Fig. 21.8). They connect the small lower eyelid puncta to the middle meatus of the nose. The drainage channel becomes narrower with age and can become blocked. This can cause troublesome watery eyes (epiphora) which may require surgery to re-create a new drainage channel.

Silicone tubes may be inserted via the eyelid puncta into the nose for 2–3 months. They are removed in clinic although in children short general anaesthesia may be required. Permanent bypass tubes (e.g. Lester–Jones tube) are sometimes needed if there is significant canalicular damage.

Indications

- Epiphora caused by nasolacrimal duct obstruction (requiring dacryocystorhinostomy (DCR))
- Epiphora caused by canalicular system obstruction (requiring bypass tube)

Alternatives

- None (obstructions will generally not resolve spontaneously)

Benefits

- Create an alternative drainage pathway for tears into the nasal cavity, thereby reducing/stopping epiphora and associated symptoms

Procedure

- Carried out under general anaesthesia but can also be done under local anaesthesia with sedation
- This is commonly done by one of two approaches—external or endonasal (which is now not usually performed with laser)
- If done externally, a skin incision in the nasal crease is required, which will leave a scar
- Regardless of the approach used, a temporary silicone tube will be inserted
- The operation takes 40–60min
- Success rates for external DCR range from 65% to 100%, for non-laser endonasal DCR from 84% to 94%, and for laser endonasal DCR from 47% to 100%[1]

Complications

Common
- Bleeding
- Scar formation
- Early dislodging of silicone tubes
- Shifting/subluxation of bypass tube

Uncommon
- Pyogenic granuloma
- Diplopia
- Failure to improve epiphora

Rare
- Infection
- Blockage due to scarring
- Need for additional surgery (insertion of a small tube, or a bypass tube which remains permanently)
- Loss of vision
- Nerve injury
- Nasal cavity adhesions
- Cerebrospinal fluid rhinorrhoea

Reference

1. Leong SC, Macewen CJ, White PS. A systematic review of outcomes after dacryocystorhinostomy in adults. *Am J Rhinol Allergy* 2010;**24**(1):81–90.

Eyelid laceration repair ± canalicular system repair

Description

The eyelids (see Figs. 21.6 and 21.7) play an important role in protecting the eye, and in keeping it lubricated through blinking. Lacerations away from the margin and not involving deep structures can be repaired simply in the emergency department if needed. Deeper lacerations may require exploration in theatre if contaminated, or if there is a concern that damage to deeper structures (such as the LPS, which raises the upper lid) has occurred.

Lacerations involving the lid margins should ideally be taken to theatre to ensure proper repair, as incorrect healing can cause subsequent complications (e.g. irregular lid margins, lid notching, and exposure keratopathy if lids do not close properly). The margin must be aligned antero-posteriorly (using a suture through the grey line to help ensure this), in order to ensure that tissue structures are in the correct place. Until this is satisfactory, the repair should not progress any further. The tarsal plate is next repaired, with muscles and subcutaneous tissue following. The skin is repaired last.

Lacerations of the medial canthus are important as the canalicular apparati can be torn, affecting tear drainage. These must always be taken to theatre for repair, as the nasolacrimal system will likely need to be probed from both the punctual (canalicular punctum) and nasal (nasolacrimal duct) ends, in order to identify if the nasolacrimal system has been affected, and if it has, an attempt can be made to repair the damage. This is usually performed by stenting the nasolacrimal system and repairing the lid laceration, in the hope that healing will allow the nasolacrimal system to heal around the stent, so that when it is removed in the future, the system will work once more.

Sometimes it is not possible to repair the damage to the canalicular system, or the canaliculus scars up after the stent is removed. In these cases, additional surgery may be required to provide an alternative route for tear drainage. It is also important to repair the medial or lateral canthal tendons that provide support to the eyelids.

Indications
- Eyelid laceration(s)

Alternatives
- Healing by secondary intention (laissez-faire)—this may not be recommended for lacerations involving the eyelid margin

Benefits
- Restore normal eyelid anatomy
- Protect cornea from exposure

Procedure

- Carried out under local anaesthesia ± sedation or general anaesthesia
- The eyelid is closed in anatomical layers using sutures and/or tissue glue
- The operation takes 30–60min

Special considerations (canalicular injuries)

- Suspected canalicular involvement requires detailed assessment of the nasolacrimal system to ensure adequate repair
- Temporary silicone tubes may be inserted to maintain patency

Complications

Common
- Bleeding
- Infection

Uncommon
- Scarring
- Suture granuloma
- Lid margin notching
- Eyelid asymmetry
- Epiphora
- Early dislodging of silicone tubing
- Need for additional surgery

Eyelid lesion biopsy ± excision

Description

The eyelid skin with its appendages can develop various benign and malignant lesions. Many eyelid lesions can be identified by their appearance and location and do not require histological confirmation.

However, some with suspicious features will require excision and histological confirmation with the possibility of wider excisions suggested. These larger defects usually require grafts or flaps to repair.

Indications

- Remove lesions in/around the eyelid that require histological identification, or that are interfering with eyelid function and/or vision

Alternatives

- None

Benefits

- Remove lesion
- Histological diagnosis
- Improve vision and/or eyelid function

Procedure

- Carried out under local anaesthesia ± sedation or general anaesthesia
- The lesion is partially or fully excised and sent to histology for analysis
- In cases where neoplasia is suspected, further excision may be required, based on histology results
- Wound closure may require a graft
- The procedure takes 15–20min unless a graft or flap is required

Complications

Common

- Bleeding
- Infection
- Scarring
- Eyelid asymmetry
- Need for further surgery (further excision, skin grafting)

Uncommon

- Suture granuloma
- Pyogenic granuloma
- Reoccurrence
- Graft failure (if used)

Rare

- Loss of vision

Fluorescein/indocyanine green angiography

Description

Fluorescence is the emission of light of one wavelength by a substance after it has been stimulated by light of a different wavelength. The stimulating wavelength is normally shorter (closer to the ultraviolet end of the electromagnetic spectrum) than the wavelength emitted (which would be closer to the infrared end of the electromagnetic spectrum). Fluorescein is a water-soluble dye that absorbs light at a wavelength of 465–490nm (blue), and emits light at a wavelength of 520–530nm (yellow-green). Indocyanine green is a water soluble dye (that binds tightly to plasma proteins) that absorbs light at a wavelength of 805nm (infrared) and emits light at a wavelength of 835nm (infrared).

When the retinal or choroidal circulation in the eye has been damaged/affected (or if there is suspicion of damage) following an event in the eye, it needs to be assessed to determine the extent of the injury, and the subsequent potential effect on retinal function. This is done by injecting a water-soluble dye (such as fluorescein or indocyanine green) through a peripheral vein. As the dye passes through the retinal and choroidal circulation, it is exposed to light filtered (excitation filter) to only allow wavelengths designed to cause fluorescence through. A camera takes pictures using a lens filter (barrier filter) that is designed to block out all light entering except light at the wavelengths the dye fluoresces at. Areas with high/low circulation, leakage, or obstruction can then be seen.

Fluorescein angiography is used to assess the retinal circulation, whereas indocyanine green is used to assess the choroidal circulation. This is because indocyanine green binds tightly to plasma proteins and therefore remains in the choroidal circulation, and because the retinal pigment epithelium does not absorb infrared wavelengths, allowing stimulating light and fluoresced light to pass unimpeded.

Indications

- Confirmation/identification of diagnosis
- Assessment of disease progression

Alternatives

- None

Benefits

- Obtain more information regarding the retinal and/or choroidal circulation

Procedure

- The pupils are dilated
- *Fluorescein/Indocyanine dye is injected intravenously*
- Rapid sequential photographs are taken of the fundus as the dye passes through the retinal/choroidal vasculature
- The procedure takes 10–30min

Complications

Common
- Temporary discoloration of the skin for up to 48h
- Temporary discoloration of the urine for up to 48h
- Mild (nausea, vomiting)

Uncommon
- Moderate (urticaria, syncope) (0.016%)[1]

Rare
- Severe (anaphylaxis, or other respiratory, cardiac, and/or neurological manifestations) (0.0001%)[1]
- Death (0.0000045%)[1]

The quoted rates are for fluorescein angiography specifically. However, indocyanine green has been shown to have a similar level of complications and the same rates could be quoted.[2]

References
1. Yanuzzi LA, Rohrer KT, Tindel LJ, et al. Fluorescein angiography complication survey. Ophthalmology 1986; **93**: 611–17.
2. Obana A, Miki T, Hayashi K, et al. Survey of complications of indocyanine green angiography in Japan. Am J Ophthalmol 1994;**118**(6):749–53.

Focal/macula grid laser

Description

The macula is the area of the retina responsible for best vision (see Fig. 21.5). Disturbance of the normal anatomy of the macula will generally result in functional visual symptoms, such as blurred vision, or metamorphopsia (distortion of vision, such as straight lines looking wavy). One of the most common problems to affect the macula is the development of oedema (fluid swelling) within the retina (macula oedema—not to be confused with subretinal fluid). This commonly occurs as a result of a breakdown in the blood–retinal barrier in this area through microvascular damage, allowing plasma constituents to cross into the retina (which is normally not allowed to occur). The commonest conditions that can cause macular oedema are venous occlusions, and diabetes mellitus.

Argon laser photocoagulation can be used in some of these cases to try to treat such oedema. Depending on the type of oedema, different methods of laser exist. For areas of oedema that appear to be caused by a few points of leakage (such as a microaneurysm), focal laser can be used. For diffuse (spread out) oedema, grid laser is used.

In focal laser, using a relatively weak powered beam (compared with argon laser pan-retinal photocoagulation), a mild thermal coagulative effect is placed on the macula vessels caught in the beam, which is believed to help seal microvascular leaks that may exist. For this to work, the wavelength used for the laser beam should be absorbed by the blood cells inside the blood vessels. Green and yellow wavelengths work well, red works poorly. Blue is avoided as it is taken up very easily by the xanthophyll pigment present in the macula, and raises the chance that macular function could be damaged in treatment.

In grid laser, a beam (similar in strength to that used for focal laser) is fired at the macula in an ordered set of rows with regular gaps in between. There are a number of theories as to how grid laser works. One theory suggests that the underlying vascular endothelium or retinal pigment epithelial cells are stimulated to improve integrity or absorb more fluid, respectively. Another suggests that the laser removes unhealthy/poorly functioning retinal pigment epithelial cells, allowing new healthy cells to take their place. A third theory suggests retinal photoreceptors are destroyed by the laser, reducing oxygen demand locally, causing reduced blood flow in leaking vessels (and theoretically, thus reducing leakage). In reality, it may be a combination of some or all of these theories that occur (or even possibly something completely different!).

Indications

- Diabetic maculopathy
- Cystoid macula oedema associated with venous occlusions
- Closure of intraretinal microvascular abnormalities
- Focal treatment of pigment epithelium abnormalities

Alternatives
- Intravitreal triamcinolone
- Intravitreal bevacizumab (Avastin®)
- Intravitreal ranibizumab (Lucentis®)

Benefits
- To stabilize vision

Procedure
- Commonly carried out under local anaesthesia
- A contact lens is placed on the eye, after the eye is dilated
- Repeated laser burns are applied to the retina
- The number of burns depends on the indication
- Multiple laser treatment sessions may be required
- The procedure takes 10–20min

Complications
Common
- Bleeding
- Need for additional laser

Uncommon
- Abnormal colour vision
- Abnormal night vision
- Abnormal visual field

Rare
- Cataract
- Diplopia
- Corneal burns
- Choroidal neovascular membrane
- Optic neuritis
- Retinal tears/detachment
- Choroidal detachment
- Loss of driving licence
- Loss of vision (including foveal burns)

Glaucoma drainage tubes

Description

Also known as:
- Aqueous shunts
- Tube implants
- Glaucoma drainage devices
- Glaucoma tube shunts

They are used to drain aqueous from within the eye into a small bleb created beneath the upper eyelid. By draining the aqueous they reduce intraocular pressure and control glaucoma (see Figs. 21.9 and 21.10).

There are many types of devices including (but not limited to):
- Ahmed valve (valved)
- Baerveldt implant (non-valved)
- Molteno tube (non-valved)

Both valved and non-valved devices have their advantages and disadvantages. Valved devices must be blocked with a stitch at the time of surgery to prevent excessive drainage of aqueous in the first few weeks postsurgery. Draining fluid is slowly reabsorbed into the blood vessels on the conjunctival surface.

Indications
- Glaucoma refractory to trabeculectomy or where trabeculectomy has a high likelihood of failure

Alternatives
- None

Benefits
- To improve intraocular pressure control
- To stabilize vision (by preventing further visual field loss)

Procedure
- Carried out under local anaesthesia ± sedation or general anaesthesia
- The tube is connected to a plate that is placed between the conjunctiva and the sclera
- Tubes allow communication between the anterior chamber and sub-Tenon's space allowing aqueous fluid to drain
- An anti-scarring agent (mitomycin C) may be applied to the surface of the eye to reduce failure of the bleb formation
- A donor patch of sclera is used to keep the aqueous shunt in place
- The procedure takes 60–90min

Complications
Common
- *Bleeding*
- Scarring
- Hypotony
- Choroidal effusion
- Suprachoroidal haemorrhage

- Drainage failure
- Bleb encapsulation
- Failure to control intraocular pressure adequately
- Need for additional surgery
- Cataract

Uncommon
- Corneal oedema (water-logging of cornea)/decompensation
- Choroidal detachment
- Tube erosion/blockage
- Endophthalmitis (severe infection in the eye)
- Scarring
- Diplopia

Rare
- Aqueous misdirection
- Loss of vision

Globe rupture repair

Description

A globe rupture is one of the greatest significant injuries an eye can receive (see Fig. 21.3). Damage can vary, depending on the size and location of the rupture, as well as the mechanism of injury. It is important that all trauma injuries to the eye are described appropriately, so appropriate planning of management can occur.

The most common terms you should therefore be aware of are:[1]

- *Closed injury*—the corneoscleral wall of the globe is intact but intraocular damage may be present
- *Open injury*—full thickness wound of the corneoscleral wall
- *Contusion*—closed injury resulting from blunt trauma. Damage may occur at the site of impact or at a distant site
- *Rupture*—full thickness wound caused by blunt trauma. The globe gives way at its weakest point, which may not be at the site of impact
- *Laceration*—full thickness wound caused by a sharp object at the site of impact
- *Lamellar laceration*—partial thickness wound caused by a sharp object
- *Penetration*—single full thickness wound, usually caused by a sharp object, without an exit wound. Such a wound may be associated with intraocular retention of a foreign body
- *Perforation*—two full-thickness wounds, one entry and one exit, usually caused by a missile

Globe rupture injuries are therefore caused by blunt trauma, penetrating, or perforating injuries. The most common causes of these are assault, domestic, and sporting injuries.

The aim of primary repair is to close up the eye and try to replace displaced tissues back to their appropriate plan (i.e. retinal/choroidal prolapse should be replaced, and vitreous should be cleared from the wound). The injured area should be exposed clearly enough to see adequately, and the repair should be methodical, working either anterior to posterior, or vice versa. Antibiotics should be used to prevent infection, as open globe injuries have a high chance of developing endophthalmitis (severe infection in the eye) or panophthalmitis.

Once primary repair is complete, secondary repair will be required to assess and repair damaged retina, or other intraocular structures. Eyes which have no visual potential or which are damaged too severely to repair adequately should be considered for enucleation within 10 days of injury in order to prevent/reduce the chance of sympathetic ophthalmitis.

Indications

- Penetrating eye injury
- *Perforating eye injury*

Alternatives

- Enucleation within 10 days in severely damaged eyes to prevent sympathetic ophthalmitis

Benefits

- To restore globe integrity

Procedure

- Usually performed under general anaesthesia
- Corneoscleral injuries are repaired first (primary repair). The exact method of repair will depend on the nature/extent of the injuries
- Additional repair to intraocular structures (secondary repair) may be required later
- Further assessment by the vitreo-retinal team may also be required
- Secondary enucleation may be considered following primary repair if the eye is deemed to be severely and irreversibly damaged within 10 days of the initial injury
- The procedure can take up to 120min

Complications

Common

- Bleeding
- Infection
- Scarring
- Need for additional surgery

Uncommon

- Chronic uveitis
- Chronic hypotony
- Phthisis
- Loss of vision
- Endophthalmitis (severe infection in the eye) (0.70%)[2]
- Sympathetic ophthalmitis (0.37%)[2,3]

Sympathetic ophthalmitis (also known as sympathetic ophthalmia/uveitis) is a rare, autoimmune (delayed-type hypersensitivity reaction) granulomatous uveitis (towards melanin-containing structures in the eye) that occurs when penetrating trauma (from surgery or injury) occurs to an eye. This can result in inflammation appearing in the contralateral eye, and can lead to loss of vision in both eyes.

References

1. Kanski JJ. Trauma. In: Kanski JJ, Bowling B, eds. *Clinical Ophthalmology: A Systematic Approach*, 6th edn. London: Butterworth-Heinemann, 2007:852.
2. Zhang Y, Zhang MN, Jiang CH, et al. Development of sympathetic ophthalmia following globe injury. *Chin Med J (Engl)* 2009;**122**(24):2961–6.
3. Savar A, Andreoli MT, Kloek CE, et al. Enucleation for open globe injury. *Am J Ophthalmol* 2009;**147**(4):595–600.e1.

Incision and curettage of chalazion

Description
The meibomian glands in the eyelids (see Figs. 21.6 and 21.7) can become blocked. The blockage may be due to blepharitis, which is inflammation along the lid margin associated with irritation, crusting, and build-up of secretions/meibom, which is normally produced by the meibomian glands. There is development of chronic inflammation with associated formation of a lump within the tarsal plate. This lump is called a chalazion.

It can occur in both upper and lower eyelids. Some do resolve spontaneously after a few months but if they are symptomatic then they require incision and curettage.

Chalazia can sometimes become infected and lead to preseptal cellulitis. Oral/topical antibiotics can treat this overlying infection, but will do nothing to treat the underlying chalazion.

Incision and curettage should only be carried out once acute inflammation has settled. Non-surgical options are usually recommended in most cases as first-line treatment, with evidence suggesting around 50% of cases might settle with regular conservative management within 3 weeks.[1] However, there is no strong evidence for or against the effectiveness of conservative management strategies.[2]

Indications
- Chalazion refractory to hot compresses ± massage
- Astigmatism caused by chalazion
- Mechanical ptosis caused by chalazion

Alternatives
- Continue warm compresses ± massage

Benefits
- Remove chalazion
- Reverse astigmatism caused by chalazion
- Reverse mechanical ptosis caused by chalazion

Procedure
- Carried out under local anaesthesia ± sedation or general anaesthesia
- Following application of a clamp to the eyelid, the eyelid is incised and the chalazion curetted
- No sutures are required
- The procedure takes 5–15min

Complications
Common
- Bleeding
- *Infection (preseptal cellulitis)*
- Scarring
- Reoccurrence

Uncommon
- Need for additional surgery
- Pyogenic granuloma

Rare
- Misdiagnosis

Beware the recurrent chalazion, as the diagnosis may need to be re-considered. Eyelid malignancy needs to be considered in these situations.

References

1. Goawalla A, Lee V. A prospective randomized treatment study comparing three treatment options for chalazia: triamcinolone acetonide injections, incision and curettage and treatment with hot compresses. *Clin Experiment Ophthalmol* 2007;**35**(8):706–12.
2. Lindsley K, Nichols JJ, Dickersin K. Interventions for acute internal hordeolum. *Cochrane Database Syst Rev* 2010;**9**:CD007742.

Intravitreal injections

Description
Due to the presence of the blood–ocular and blood–retinal barriers, it can be difficult to develop significant concentrations of a drug inside the eye in order to treat certain conditions, as most drugs have poor ocular penetration. In situations where it is imperative to get the requisite treatment to sites inside the eye, intravitreal injection of the drug in question is the solution. This allows the drug to sit in the vitreous cavity (see Fig. 21.3), where it can get to work directly.

Indications
- Neovascularization
- Macular oedema
- Intraocular inflammation/infection
- Endophthalmitis (severe infection in the eye)

Alternatives
- None

Benefits
- To stabilize/improve vision

Procedure
- Carried out under local anaesthesia ± sedation or general anaesthesia
- The eye is prepared using antibiotic drops ± 5% povidone-iodine drops prior to the procedure
- The pupils are dilated, and injections are via the pars plana (approximately 3.5–4.0mm posterior to the limbus, depending on whether the patient is phakic or pseudophakic)
- The conjunctiva is frequently displaced prior to needle entry, so that when it settles back after needle retraction, there is no gap in the conjunctiva above the point of scleral entry
- Common agents injected are steroids, anti-VEGFs, and anti-infectives (including antibiotics, antifungals, and antivirals)
- The procedure takes about 5–10min

Complications
Common
- Bleeding
- Pain
- Scarring
- Floaters
- Raised intraocular pressure (can lead to central retinal artery occlusion and subsequent visual loss)
- *Need for additional injections/surgery*

Uncommon
- Infection
- Cataract
- Retinal detachment/breaks

Rare
- Endophthalmitis (severe infection in the eye)
- Loss of vision

Lacrimal syringing and probing

Description

Obstruction or delayed canalization of the nasolacrimal duct occurs in about 5% of newborns. A remnant of a small valve at the lower end of the nasolacrimal duct is the usual cause. This can cause persistent watering (epiphora) and sticky eyes in infants, and can sometimes lead to recurrent infections. Probing is required in a minority of children. This involves dilating the canalicular punctum and then attempting to irrigate the nasolacrimal duct. A probe is usually inserted and as it slides through the duct, distal obstruction is overcome.

A dacryocystogram (X-ray of the nasolacrimal system following injection of radiopaque dye through the canalicular punctum) or a scintillogram (using radiosensitive material to demonstrate nasolacrimal duct anatomy) can be a helpful investigation to determine the cause of epiphora. These are also helpful before DCR (📖 see 'Dacryocystorhinostomy ± bypass tube insertion', p.617).

Indications

• Nasolacrimal system assessment
• 60–90% of children with epiphora will spontaneously resolve within the first year of life, so this procedure is generally not advised until at least 10–12 months of age[1]

Additional procedures

• Dacryocystogram (x-rays of the nasolacrimal system following injection of radio-opaque dye through the canalicular punctum)

Benefits

• Reduce epiphora
• Identify nasolacrimal system obstruction

Procedure

• Carried out under local anaesthesia ± sedation or general anaesthesia
• Punctal dilators used to assist punctum visualization
• Nasolacrimal system syringing performed through both upper and lower eyelid puncta
• If successful, the patient will taste salty water at the back of their throat. If unsuccessful, regurgitation may occur
• Subjective improvement in adults with epiphora has been quoted between 52%[2] and 82%,[3] with only 35% reporting complete resolution of symptoms[2]
• Success (complete resolution of symptoms) in children has been shown to decrease with age. Within the first 2 years of life, success is around 85%[4] to 90%.[5] By the age of 4, this can drop to around 64%[4]
• *The procedure can take 10–15min*

Complications

Common
- Bleeding
- Infection
- Scarring

Uncommon
- Need for additional surgery

References

1. Royal College of Ophthalmologists. *Management of Epiphora. Focus.* London: Royal College of Ophthalmologists, 2000. Available at: www.mrcophth.com/focus1/Management%20of%20Epiphora.htm (accessed 30 May 2010).
2. Guinot-Saera A, Koay P. Efficacy of probing as treatment of epiphora in adults with blocked nasolacrimal ducts. *Br J Ophthalmol* 1998;**82**(4):389–91.
3. Bell TA. An investigation into the efficacy of probing the nasolacrimal duct as a treatment for epiphora in adults. *Trans Ophthalmol Soc U K* 1986;**105**(Pt 4):494–7.
4. Kashkouli MB, Kassaee A, Tabatabaee Z. Initial nasolacrimal duct probing in children under age 5: cure rate and factors affecting success. *J AAPOS* 2002;**6**(6):360–3.
5. Limbu B, Akin M, Saiju R. Age-based comparison of successful probing in Nepalese children with nasolacrimal duct obstruction. *Orbit* 2010;**29**(1):16–20.

Lower eyelid ectropion repair

Description

The eyelid is the thinnest external structure of the body. It is divided into skin, subcutaneous tissue, orbicularis muscle, tarsal plate, and conjunctiva (see Figs. 21.1, 21.6, and 21.7).

In the lower eyelid, there are retractors which help to maintain normal lower lid position. The retractors are the capsulopalpebral fascia and the inferior tarsal muscle.

Ectropion is an outward turning (eversion) of the eyelid away from the globe primarily due to horizontal lid laxity.

The main types of ectropion are:
- Involutional
- Congenital
- Mechanical
- Paralytic
- Cicatricial

Most cases are due to involutional ectropion, which occurs with age. This can cause corneal exposure and recurrent infections.

Indications
- Ectropion

Alternatives
- None (but this will result in corneal exposure and recurrent infections over time)

Benefits
- Restore lid anatomy

Procedure
- Carried out under local anaesthesia ± sedation or general anaesthesia
- This generally involves the use of either inverting sutures, reattachment of eyelid retractors to the tarsal plate, or both
- A lid-tightening procedure (such as a lateral tarsal strip procedure) is the most commonly performed procedure for lower lid ectropion. This will correct the lid laxity
- Scarred eyelids (cicatrisation) may require mucous membrane, tarsal plate, or skin grafts depending on the amount of scarring of the skin and tarsal plate
- The operation takes 45–90min

Complications

Common
- Bleeding
- Infection (preseptal cellulitis)
- Over-correction
- Under-correction
- Eyelid asymmetry
- Reoccurrence

Uncommon
- Skin graft failure (if used)
- Graft donor site complications
- Need for additional surgery

Rare
- Loss of vision (from a retrobulbar bleed)

Lower lid entropion repair

Description
The eyelid is the thinnest skin of the body. It is divided into skin, subcutaneous tissue, orbicularis muscle, tarsal plate and conjunctiva. In the lower eyelid, there are retractors which help to maintain normal lower lid position (see Fig. 21.6). The retractors are the capsulopalpebral fascia and the inferior tarsal muscle.

Entropion is an inward turning (inversion) of the eyelid towards the globe, due to horizontal lid laxity and disinsertion of the lower eyelid retractors.

In cicatricial cases, scarring of the conjunctiva and tarsal plate has to be corrected with a mucous membrane graft (e.g. from the inner lip).

The main types of entropion are:
- Involutional
- Congenital
- Acute spastic
- Cicatricial

Most cases are due to involutional entropion, which occurs with age. This can cause corneal irritation, infection, and scarring due to inwardly turning eyelashes rubbing on the cornea.

Eyelash irritation from entropion should be differentiated from:
- Trichiasis (misdirection of lashes towards the globe with normal eyelid position)
- Distichiasis (abnormal eyelash growth from meibomian gland orifices)

Indications
- Entropion

Alternatives
- Lid taping
- Bandage contact lens
- Botulinum toxin injections to lower eyelid

Benefits
- Restore lid anatomy
- Protect cornea from eyelash irritation

Procedure
- Carried out under local anaesthesia ± sedation or general anaesthesia
- This generally involves the use of either everting sutures, reattachment of eyelid retractors to the tarsal plate, or both
- A lateral tarsal strip procedure (shortening and tightening of the eyelid) may be required if there is horizontal lid laxity present
- The operation takes 45–90min

Complications

Common
- Bleeding
- Infection
- Over-correction (causing ectropion)
- Eyelid asymmetry
- Reoccurrence

Uncommon
- Graft failure (if used)
- Graft donor site complications
- Need for additional surgery

Rare
- Loss of vision

Macula hole/epiretinal membrane (ERM) surgery

Description

An epiretinal membrane is a proliferation of glial cells at the vitreo-retinal interface. The glial cells are from the retina, and normally arrive at the retinal surface through breaks in the internal limiting membrane. While epiretinal membranes can occur idiopathically, other causes include previous retinal surgery/procedures, trauma, intraocular inflammation, and retinal vascular conditions.

If left unchecked, epiretinal membranes can cause traction on the macula (where it commonly forms). This is commonly noted symptomatically through metamorphopsia and reduced vision. On examination, an irregular light reflex can be seen at the macula, with obvious surface distortion visible at more advanced stages.

Macular holes can occur when there has been an abnormal vitreo-macular (or more specifically a vitreo-foveolar) attachment, resulting in combined anteroposterior and horizontal traction. This results in displacement of photoreceptors at the fovea. Unless the tractional forces are relieved, displacement can continue to occur, and the hole can continue to develop into a full thickness macular hole. Holes can be differentiated from pseudoholes (other conditions which have the gross appearance of a macular hole) using the Watzke-Allen test. (Shine a thin bright beam of light that passes through the hole. Patients with a macular hole will see a break in the light where it passes through the hole, whereas those with a pseudohole will see an unbroken line.)

In both of the conditions mentioned, treatment consists of relieving the traction being applied to the macula by detaching remaining vitreous attachments that might still be having an effect, and 'peeling' away any membrane that has formed. These steps give the macula a chance to settle back anatomically within days/weeks. However, it takes longer (months) to determine final functional outcome.

Indications

- Full thickness macula hole (Gass stage 2 and above)[1]
- Reducing visual acuity
- Distortion

Alternatives

- Observe (conditions may deteriorate)

Benefits

- To improve vision and prevent further visual loss
- To reduce distortion

Procedure

- Carried out under local anaesthesia ± sedation or general anaesthesia
- Para plana vitrectomy (PPV) is performed, and the internal limiting (ILM)/epiretinal membranes (ERM) are removed
- Gas tamponade is applied

- Posturing may be required postoperatively for a variable period
- Anatomical hole closure has been seen in between 82% and 100% of patients, depending on the case series
- The procedure takes 60–90min

Complications

Common

- Bleeding
- Infection
- Scarring
- Cataract
- Raised intraocular pressure

Uncommon

- Failure to close macular hole
- Need for additional surgery
- Retinal detachment/tears

Rare

- Choroidal haemorrhage
- Endophthalmitis (severe infection in the eye
- Loss of vision

Reference

1. Johnson RN, Gass JD. Idiopathic macular holes. Observations, stages of formation, and implications for surgical intervention. *Ophthalmology* 1988;**95**(7):917–24.

Nasolacrimal duct intubation

Description
Failure, narrowed, or delayed canalization of the nasolacrimal duct can occur in babies/children (see Fig. 21.8). Adults can develop nasolacrimal duct stenosis (or have had it all their life and have just never been treated for it). Silicone tube intubation is usually recommended after multiple probing and syringing have failed. Ideally the tubes are left in place for 3–6 months before being removed. If they have not been successful in canalizing the nasolacrimal duct then a DCR will be required.

Indications
• Nasolacrimal duct stenosis

Alternatives
• Leave (symptoms may persist)

Benefits
• Allow increased drainage of tears through the nasolacrimal system, thereby reducing/stopping epiphora and other symptoms

Procedure
• Carried out under local anaesthesia ± sedation or general anaesthesia
• Tube insertion can be either mono-canalicular (inferior canaliculus only) or bi-canalicular (both superior and inferior canaliculi)
• Once inserted, tubes are fixed at either the proximal (punctal), or distal (nasal) end, or both
• In children aged between 6 and 44 months, success (defined as the absence of epiphora, mucous discharge, and increased tear lake at the outcome visit, 1 month after tube removal) has been shown to be around 90%[1]
• In adults, success (defined as complete disappearance of symptoms) has been shown to be 62% for mono-canalicular intubations, and 59% for bi-canalicular intubation[2]
• The procedure takes 30min

Complications
Common
• Bleeding
• Infection (including preseptal cellulitis)
• Scarring
• Corneal abrasion
• Movement/premature removal of tubing
• Punctal stretching

Uncommon
• Need for additional surgery

References

1. Pediatric Eye Disease Investigator Group, Repka MX, Melia BM, *et al.* Primary treatment of nasolacrimal duct obstruction with nasolacrimal duct intubation in children younger than 4 years of age. *J AAPOS* 2008;**12**(5):445–50.

2. Kashkouli MB, Kempster RC, Galloway GD, *et al.* Monocanalicular versus bicanalicular silicone intubation for nasolacrimal duct stenosis in adults. *Ophthal Plast Reconstr Surg* 2005;**21**(2):142–7.

Panretinal laser photocoagulation (PRP)

Description

There are a number of conditions (such as venous occlusion or diabetes mellitus) that can cause retinal damage through bleeding. Significant damage causes ischaemia (lack of oxygen), and results in the promotion and release of growth factors (including vascular endothelial growth factor, or VEGF) that cause new blood vessel growth to occur (neovascularization), in an attempt to fix the oxygen deficit. However, these new vessels have a tendency to break and bleed, resulting in further damage to the retina, and additional neovascularization.

In order to preserve the remaining vision in the eye (and in particular the macula, as it is responsible for best vision), this ischaemic 'demand' for oxygen needs to be dealt with, as the vascular 'supply' can no longer cope. This is achieved by applying an argon laser beam to the peripheral retina at strength sufficient to destroy the retina permanently. Such destroyed areas no longer require oxygen, and as a result, the ischaemic drive is reduced. This results in reduced VEGF release and reversal of neovascularization as the vascular 'supply' can now keep up with the oxygen 'demand' of the remaining 'live' retina.

Indications

- Retinal/iridal neovascularization secondary to ischaemia (commonly proliferative diabetic retinopathy, or post-retinal vein occlusion)

Alternatives

- None (ischaemic drive will continue)

Benefits

- To stabilize vision
- To reduce ischaemic drive, and therefore secondary sequelae

Procedure

- Carried out under local anaesthesia ± sedation or general anaesthesia
- A contact lens is placed on the eye, after the eye is dilated
- Repeated laser burns are applied to the retina
- The number of burns depends on the indication and patient comfort (the procedure can still be uncomfortable with only topical anaesthesia)
- Multiple laser treatment sessions may be required
- The procedure takes 20–30min

Complications

Common

- Bleeding
- Need for additional laser
- Abnormal colour vision
- Abnormal night vision
- Abnormal visual field
- Potential loss of driving licence

Uncommon
- Cystoid macula oedema
- Retinal tears/detachment
- Choroidal neovascular membrane
- Cataract
- Diplopia
- Corneal burns

Rare
- Optic neuritis
- Choroidal detachment
- Loss of vision (including foveal burns)

Pars plana vitrectomy

Description

In order for any surgical procedure to be performed effectively in the posterior segment of the eye, there needs to be a clear space to work in. For this reason, and to reduce the potential future risk of retinal breaks/detachments through remaining tractional attachments of vitreous, vitrectomy is performed prior to any other work being carried out.

Indications

- Retinal detachment
- Macular epiretinal membranes
- Vitreo-macular traction syndrome
- Idiopathic macula hole[1]
- High-risk proliferative diabetic retinopathy
- Submacular haemorrhage
- Postoperative endophthalmitis (severe infection in the eye)[2]
- Suprachoroidal haemorrhage
- Dropped nucleus
- Posterior dislocation of intraocular lenses

Alternatives

- None

Benefits

- Stabilize vision
- Improve vision
- Reduce distortion
- Diagnosis and treatment (endophthalmitis (severe infection in the eye))

Procedure

- Carried out under local anaesthesia ± sedation or general anaesthesia
- PPV is performed
- Vitreous samples are obtained and sent for sampling if required
- The ILM and ERM are removed if required
- Tamponade (gas or silicone oil) is applied if required
- Posturing may be required
- The procedure may take 45–90min

Complications

Common

- Bleeding
- Infection
- Scarring
- Raised intraocular pressure

Uncommon

- Need for additional surgery
- Epiretinal membrane
- Cataract
- Proliferative vitreo-retinopathy
- Hypotony
- Retinal detachment/tears
- Band keratopathy

Rare

- Endophthalmitis (severe infection in the eye)
- Choroidal haemorrhage
- Sympathetic ophthalmitis
- Loss of vision

References

1. Johnson RN, Gass JD. Idiopathic macular holes. Observations, stages of formation, and implications for surgical intervention. *Ophthalmology* 1988;**5**(7):917–24.
2. Results of the Endophthalmitis (severe infection in the eye) Vitrectomy Study. A randomized trial of immediate vitrectomy and of intravenous antibiotic for the treatment of postoperative bacterial endophthalmitis (severe infection in the eye). Endophthalmitis (severe infection in the eye) Vitrectomy Study Group. *Arch Ophthalmol* 1995;**113**(12):1479–96.

Penetrating keratoplasty

Description

This is a full thickness corneal graft that replaces all the layers of the cornea. It is performed when corneal pathology involves both the stroma and endothelium. Damaged cornea is replaced by donor tissue.

They are the most widely used type of corneal graft. One major disadvantage compared with partial thickness grafts is rejection. This is the commonest complication of full thickness grafts.

There is also a long period of aftercare with frequent clinic visits. The corneal sutures usually remain *in situ* for about 12 months during which time the vision may not be optimal. There may be suture-related problems, which will require removal and/or replacement during the long period of wound healing and stability. However, final visual outcome is usually better with a partial thickness graft.

Indications

- Keratoconus and other corneal ectasia
- Bullous keratopathy
- Corneal dystrophies
- Corneal degeneration
- Corneal scarring
- Stromal thinning
- Descemetocoeles
- Corneal oedema (water-logging of cornea)
- Trauma
- Congenital opacities
- Chemical injuries
- Previous graft failure

Alternatives

- DALK
- DSEK

Benefits

- Improve vision
- Restore/preserve corneal integrity
- Correct abnormal corneal contour
- Improve cosmetic appearance of the eye

Procedure

- Usually performed under general anaesthesia
- Donor cornea is prepared for transplant
- Host cornea is prepared for graft insertion
- Donor button sutured onto host tissue using non-absorbable sutures.
- Overall graft survival at 5 years is 66% (keratoconus 98%, viral keratitis 86%, Fuchs' dystrophy 85%, pseudophakic bullous keratopathy 84%, re-grafts 55%, and other diagnoses 57%)[1]
- The procedure can take up to 120min

Complications

Common

- Bleeding (including choroidal expulsive haemorrhage)
- Iris trauma
- Glaucoma
- Corneal graft infection often related to sutures and herpes infections
- Corneal graft rejection (20% of low-risk grafts and 80% of high-risk grafts)
- High astigmatism
- Corneal scarring
- Suture-related problems
- Need for further surgery

Uncommon

- Cataract
- Endophthalmitis
- Graft failure
- Wound leaks
- Severe postoperative inflammation
- Persistent epithelial defect
- Epithelial downgrowth
- Fixed dilated pupil (Urrets–Zavalia syndrome)

Rare

- Cystoid macula oedema (more common when corneal graft is combined with cataract surgery)
- Sympathetic ophthalmitis

Choroidal expulsive haemorrhage usually results in severe loss of vision or loss of the eye. The risk is higher than for cataract surgery. Risk factors are old age, coughing, hypertension, glaucoma, or straining during surgery if carried out under local anaesthesia.

Sympathetic ophthalmitis (also known as sympathetic ophthalmia/ uveitis) is a rare, autoimmune (delayed-type hypersensitivity reaction) granulomatous uveitis (towards melanin-containing structures in the eye), which occurs following penetrating trauma (from surgery or injury) to an eye. This can result in inflammation appearing in the contralateral eye, and can lead to loss of vision in both eyes.

Reference

1. Beckingsale P, Mavrikakis I, Al-Yousuf N, et al. Penetrating keratoplasty: outcomes from a corneal unit compared to national data. Br J Ophthalmol 2005;90(6):728–31.

Phacoemulsification ± intraocular lens (IOL) insertion

Description

The natural lens of the eye sits behind the iris (see Fig. 21.3), and provides approximately a third of the refractive (focusing) power of the eye. The lens is encased in a transparent capsule (capsular bag), and is normally suspended along the visual axis of the eye by zonules (fibrous strings), which come from the ciliary body. Contraction/relaxation of the ciliary body muscles causes changes in the tension of these zonular attachments, which is transmitted to the lens capsule and causes the lens to change shape and thus alter its refractive power (accommodation).

The width of the lens increases with age, as new lens fibres are laid down on top of existing fibres. Eventually, the lens may become large enough to touch the posterior aspect of the iris at the pupillary border (Fig. 21.2), and potentially block transmission of aqueous fluid from the posterior chamber (where it is produced by the ciliary body) to the anterior chamber (where it drains out of the trabecular meshwork at the 'angle') via the pupil. This may result in acute angle closure glaucoma developing where intraocular pressure rises extremely quickly (minutes to hours), resulting in damage to the optic nerve, and thus to the vision in the eye (see Figs. 21.9 and 21.10). If the lens only occasionally blocks passage of aqueous fluid via the pupil, the patient can develop chronic angle closure glaucoma instead (weeks to years). When the lens is responsible for causing glaucoma through its size obstructing aqueous fluid drainage, it is called phacomorphic glaucoma.

The natural lens of the eye can develop opacities and become cloudy. This is an acquired cataract. If this occurs, the only way to improve the vision is to remove the cataract and replace the natural lens with an artificial one.

Common causes for acquired cataract include (but are not limited to):
- Increasing age
- Previous eye surgery for other conditions
- Diabetes
- Chronic steroid use
- Trauma

While advanced classification systems exist, cataracts are routinely described in clinical practice by location:
- Anterior cortical
- Anterior polar
- Anterior subcapsular (shortened to 'ASCLO')
- Nuclear (shortened to 'NS')
- Posterior cortical
- Posterior polar (these are associated with a higher chance of posterior capsule rupture during surgery)
- Posterior subcapsular (shortened to 'PSCLO')

Indications
- Cataract
- Phacomorphic glaucoma

Alternatives
- Leave (vision will deteriorate further)

Benefits
- Improve vision
- Definitive treatment for phacomorphic glaucoma
- Improve refractive error

Procedure
- Carried out under local anaesthesia ± sedation or general anaesthesia
- Incisions are made in the cornea to gain access to interior of the eye
- A hole (central curvilinear capsulorrhexis) is carefully torn in the anterior aspect of the capsular bag to gain access to the cataract
- The cataract is broken up using ultrasound waves (phacoemulsification), and then aspirated via a probe
- A replacement artificial lens is inserted back into the capsular bag
- The procedure generally takes 20–30min

Special considerations
- Clear lens extraction
  - Same operation, but in an eye that does not have a cataract. This is usually done to correct refractive errors or presbyopia (loss of accommodation with advancing age), e.g. with multi-focal lens implantation
- Phacoemulsification only
  - No artificial lens is inserted, deliberately leaving the patient aphakic. The lens capsule may also be removed in some cases
- Alternative lens position
  - When the artificial lens cannot be placed in the capsular bag for any reason, alternative positions for artificial lens placement are either in the ciliary sulcus (posterior to the iris, but anterior to the capsular bag—if there is enough capsular bag remaining to support it), or in the anterior chamber (generally attached to the iris/sclera by clips or sutures)

Complications
- 95.4% of patients have no intraoperative complications[1]
- 85.6% of patients have no postoperative complications[1]

Common
- Postoperative corneal oedema (water-logging of cornea) (5.18%)[1]
- Postoperative uveitis (3.29%)[1]
- Postoperative raised intraocular pressure (2.57%)[1]

Uncommon
- Posterior capsule rupture with/without vitreous loss (1.92%)[1]
- Postoperative cystoid macular oedema (1.62%)[1]
- Postoperative posterior capsular opacification (1.22%)[1]

Rare
- Retained lens fragments (dropped nucleus) (0.18%)[1]
- Postoperative endophthalmitis (severe infection in the eye) (0.10%)[2]
- Retinal detachment/tear (0.10%)[2]
- Suprachoroidal haemorrhage (0.07%)[1]

While rare, these complications are considered to have a potential outcome of complete permanent loss of vision (1 in 1000) or eye (1 in 10 000).[3] This must be made clear to the patient when consenting. The complications mentioned here do not represent the full list of statistics. These can be obtained from the listed references.[1,2]

References

1. Jaycock P, Johnston RL, Taylor H, *et al*. UK EPR user group. The Cataract National Dataset electronic multi-centre audit of 55 567 operations: updating benchmark standards of care in the United Kingdom and internationally. *Eye (Lond)* 2009;**23**(1):38–49.
2. Desai P, Minassian DC, Reidy A. National cataract surgery survey 1997-8: a report of the results of the clinical outcomes. *Br J Ophthalmol* 1999;**83**(12):1336–40.

Photodynamic therapy (PDT)

Description

Photodynamic therapy is a treatment used for benign or malignant conditions through the use of a targeted photochemical reaction. The aim is to treat an affected area of tissue while sparing the surrounding unaffected area.

Three components are required:

- A photosensitizer (a chemical compound that is stimulated by light of a certain wavelength and excited into a high energy state)
- Oxygen (normally present in cells of tissues) to participate in energy transfer from stimulated molecules of the photosensitizer used, resulting in the creation of highly damaging oxygen-free radicals
- Light (of a specific wavelength, in order to stimulate and excite the photosensitive compound in use)

The photosensitizer is injected via a peripheral vein, and given time to enter the retinal circulation. The required wavelength laser light is then shone into the eye onto the area of retina that requires treating for a short time.

Indications

- Age-related macular degeneration
- Central serous chorioretinopathy
- Ocular tumours

Alternatives

- Intravitreal bevacizumab (Avastin®)
- Intravitreal ranibizumab (Lucentis®)

Benefits

- To stabilize vision

Procedure

- Verteporfin (for photosensitization) is injected intravenously
- Laser is then applied to the retina to activate the injected verteporfin as it traverses the retinal vasculature
- The procedure can take up to 90min

Complications

Common

- Photosensitivity
- Pain (specifically back and chest)

Rare

- Loss of vision

Pterygium excision

Description

Pterygium is a fleshy growth of fibrous tissue and elastotic degeneration of collagen from the conjunctiva that can encroach beyond the limbus. It can cause irritation initially and subsequent growth across the cornea can interfere with vision. It is common in people who live/have lived in hot, dusty climates and is usually benign. It has been associated with ultraviolet (UV) light exposure.

Indications

- Painful and/or vision-threatening pterygium

Alternatives

- Leave (visual obscuration may increase if corneal involvement progresses)
- Subconjunctival antimetabolites (may need multiple treatments)
- β-irradiation (risk of necrotizing scleritis)

Benefits

- Improve vision
- Prevent further visual obscuration
- Improve pain

Procedure

- Carried out under local anaesthesia ± sedation or general anaesthesia
- The pterygium is excised from the cornea and the conjunctival portion is excised down to bare sclera
- The bare sclera is either left bare (with or without antimetabolites applied), or covered with an amniotic membrane graft or conjunctival autograft
- The procedure takes 45–60min

Complications

Common

- Reoccurrence (rates depend on method of excision used)[1]
- Bleeding, scarring
- Graft dehiscence, corneal scarring
- Refractive astigmatic change

Uncommon

- Uveitis, corneal perforation
- Infection (including microbial keratitis and endophthalmitis (severe infection in the eye))
- Corneal endothelial cell density reduction (associated with mitomycin C use)
- Scleritis (including necrotizing scleritis)

Rare

- Scleral thinning/perforation
- Loss of vision

Reference

1. Fernandes M, Sangwan VS, Bansal AK. *et al.* Outcome of pterygium surgery: analysis over 14 years. *Eye* 2005;**19**(11):1182–90.

Ptosis repair

Description

Ptosis commonly refers to drooping of the upper eyelid, although it can apply to the lower eyelid as well.

Ptosis can be classified into six main types:

- Neurogenic (examples include IIIrd nerve palsy, and Horner's syndrome)
- Myogenic (examples include myasthenia gravis, and myotonic dystrophy)
- Aponeurotic (commonly involutional, but can be postoperative)
- Mechanical (secondary to eyelid masses or oedema)
- Neurotoxic (secondary to envenomation). This is rare
- Congenital (idiopathic, with dystrophic muscle tissue)

Pseudoptosis must be excluded. This can be due to hypotropia (squint where eyeball deviates downwards), lack of eyelid support (from atrophy of orbital fat), or lid retraction on the contralateral side.

If ptosis affects vision by obstructing the visual axis, surgery can be carried out. However, in conditions where deterioration could potentially occur again (such as myasthenia gravis) depending on disease control, this should be made clear to the patient.

Children under 6 years of age are a special consideration as there is a risk of amblyopia (lazy eye) or an abnormal head posture.

The common methods (there are others) by which repair can be carried out include:

- Levator aponeurosis repair
- Levator palpebrae superioris (LPS) resection
- Frontalis suspension with synthetic material or autogenous material (such as fascia lata)
- Müller's muscle resection

Indications

- Significant ptosis (droopy eyelid) causing peripheral sight loss

Important contraindications to be aware of

- Poor Bell's phenomenon
- Poor blink reflex
- Poor corneal sensitivity
- Poor orbicularis function
- Dry eye

Alternatives

- Leave (i.e. no surgery), but visual obscuration will persist, and may increase
- Ptosis props (special props mounted to glasses to lift upper eyelid)

Benefits

- Improve vision/field of vision
- Improve eyelid position

Procedure

- Carried out under local anaesthesia ± sedation or general anaesthesia
- The method of repair is related to the aetiology of the ptosis, and LPS function
- Common repair techniques involve reattaching LPS (aponeurosis repair) to the tarsal plate from where it has dehisced (commonly using sutures), or resecting LPS if it has become stretched/weak
- Alternatives include resection of Müller's muscle or elevating the lid via the brow through frontalis suspension
- The procedure can take 60–90min

Complications

Common

- Under-correction
- Over-correction
- Bleeding
- Infection
- Eyelid asymmetry
- Corneal abrasion
- Poor/improper upper eyelid skin crease
- Peaking of the eyelid

Uncommon

- Scarring
- Suture granuloma
- Exposure keratopathy
- Lagophthalmos
- Diplopia
- Need for additional surgery

▶▶Although not a true complication, lowering of the contralateral upper eyelid can occur due to a reduction of muscle tone to the contralateral levator.

Punctal plug insertion

Description
Patients with dry eyes have two main options. Either lubrication is increased (lubricating drops), or lubrication already present is made to remain longer. In the case of the latter, this can be achieved by preventing tear drainage through the canalicular puncta. While punctual cautery can be used, it is destructive and permanent. Punctal plugs can be used permanently without destroying/damaging the surrounding anatomy. For a more permanent solution, cauterizing the punctum with heat is possible.

Indications
- Dry eyes

Alternatives
- Topical lubricants/ciclosporin
- Punctal cautery

Benefits
- Improve vision
- Improve ocular surface lubrication

Procedure
- Carried out under local anaesthesia ± sedation or general anaesthesia
- Plug composition varies depending on whether they are temporary (collagen) or permanent (silicone)
- Plugs can be inserted or injected into the lacrimal punctum
- The procedure can take up to 5min

Complications
Common
- Irritation
- Epiphora

Uncommon
- Infection[1]
- Corneal ulceration[2]

References
1. SmartPlug Study Group. Management of complications after insertion of the SmartPlug punctal plug: a study of 28 patients. *Ophthalmology* 2006;**113**(10):1859.e1–6.
2. Toufeeq A, Mohammad-Ali FH. Peripheral corneal ulceration as a complication of silicon punctal plug: a case report. *Eye* 2007;**21**:1437–8.

Punctoplasty

Description

Patients with watery eyes who are found to have patent nasolacrimal systems (following syringe ± probe) commonly have issues with drainage of tears through small/closed canalicular puncta, rather than over-production of tears. While puncta can be dilated temporarily with punctual dilators, they tend to close up again with time. The more definitive method requires the punctal opening to be enlarged. This is done by punctoplasty.

Indications

- Punctal stenosis

Alternatives

- Punctal dilation (temporary)

Benefits

- Reduce epiphora

Procedure

- Carried out under local anaesthesia ± sedation or general anaesthesia
- Punctal dilators used to assist punctum visualization
- The punctum is widened using one of a variety of 'snip' methods
- Nasolacrimal system syringing is commonly performed at the end of the procedure
- Punctoplasty success rates have been quoted between 64% and 92%[1,2]
- The procedure can take 10–15min

Complications

Common

- Bleeding
- Infection
- Scarring

Uncommon

- Need for additional surgery

References

1. Shahid H, Sandhu A, Keenan T, et al. Factors affecting outcome of punctoplasty surgery: a review of 205 cases. *Br J Ophthalmol* 2008 **92**(12):1689–92.
2. Caesar RH, McNab AA. A brief history of punctoplasty: the -snip revisited. *Eye (Lond)* 2005;**19**(1):16–18.

Scleral buckling

Description

In patients with retinal detachment, repair is either internal (via PPV and tamponade), or externally (by buckling). In external situations, a silicone band (explant) is sutured onto the sclera in order to cause internal indentation (buckle). This causes closure of breaks through apposition of the retinal pigment epithelium to the detached neurosensory retina.

In order to be successful, the piece of silicone must be larger than the break to be buckled. It should also involve the retina anterior to the break (and the vitreous base in that region), to ensure it does not cause additional traction and pull open the break again. In some cases, subretinal fluid may need to be drained first to bring the retina close to the internal wall of the eye for the explant to work when attached.

Indications
• Retinal detachment/tears

Alternatives
• PPV

Benefits
• To stabilize the vision
• To reattach the retina

Procedure
• Carried out under local anaesthesia ± sedation or general anaesthesia
• Cryotherapy or laser treatment may be employed first
• Subretinal fluid may require drainage
• The silicone buckle is then sutured onto the sclera in the required position to act as an indent
• Additional tamponade may be required
• The procedure can take 45–60min

Complications
Common
• Bleeding
• Infection
• Scarring
• Re-detachment
• Cataract
• Raised intraocular pressure
• Altered refractive status/astigmatism
• Diplopia

Uncommon
- Retinal incarceration (at drainage site)
- Need for additional surgery
- Buckle erosion

Rare
- Ptosis
- Orbital cellulitis
- Anterior segment ischaemia
- Sympathetic ophthalmitis

Squint (strabismus) surgery

Description

Strabismus describes misalignment of the eyes.

The six extraocular ocular muscles are:

- Horizontal (medial and lateral recti)
- Vertical muscles (superior and inferior recti)
- Oblique (superior and inferior obliques)

These muscles insert into the eyeball at various locations and are responsible for eye movements through cranial nerve control. Under normal conditions our eyes work together to give us a single three-dimensional image (binocular single vision). Misalignment of the eyes results in abnormalities in binocular vision, which can result in double vision (diplopia). Such abnormalities can be due to refractive error (common in children), abnormal placement of extraocular muscle insertions (causing muscle actions to be altered), or neuromuscular control of the ocular muscles (common in adults). Diplopia is generally difficult to determine in preverbal children.

Deviations of the eyes may be horizontal or vertical depending on the affected muscles:

- Deviation nasally is known as an esodeviation (convergent squint)
- Deviation temporally is known as an exodeviation (divergent squint)
- Deviation upwards is known as a hyperdeviation
- Deviation downwards is known as a hypodeviation

It is also possible to have a combination of horizontal and vertical deviations.

When suffering from diplopia, children can learn to ignore (suppress) one of the images from one of the eyes in an attempt to relieve their symptoms. If this is not treated as early as possible, the visual function of that eye may never fully develop, which would result in amblyopia (lazy eye). As amblyopia is irreversible once visual development stops occurring, it is imperative that strabismus is treated as early as possible to sufficiently reduce/eliminate eye misalignment (and any potential diplopia), in order to allow proper development of the visual pathways to occur.

In some cases, strabismus can be treated using glasses, patching of an eye, or a combination of both. In some cases, realignment of the eyes requires surgery on the extraocular muscles. This may involve shortening muscles, or adjusting muscle insertions into the sclera. The overall aim is to strengthen/weaken certain muscle actions to reduce misalignments as much as possible.

Indications

- Diplopia
- Poor binocular single vision
- Abnormal cosmetic appearance, head posture, or ocular misalignment

Alternatives

- Botulinum toxin injections
- Do nothing (in adults, as amblyopia is now irreversible)

Benefits

- Improve diplopia
- Correct ocular misalignment and improve cosmetic appearance
- Restore/enhance binocular single vision
- Reduce abnormal head posture

Procedure

- Performed under general anaesthesia
- Muscles are repositioned and/or shortened depending on the required outcome
- Adjustable sutures are sometimes used to optimize results post-operatively
- The procedure can take 60–90min

Complications

Common

- Bleeding (including retrobulbar haemorrhage)
- Over-correction
- Under-correction
- Need for additional surgery
- Failure to improve diplopia, or new-onset diplopia
- Slipped muscle

Uncommon

- Infection (including orbital cellulitis)
- Scarring
- Anterior segment ischaemia
- Globe perforation (which can lead to retinal detachment)
- Suture granuloma

Rare

- Loss of vision

Tarsorrhaphy

Description

Patients with an inability to close their eyelids (either partially or completely) are at risk of exposure keratopathy. This is either through the loss of the blink reflex (which is normally used to spread the lubricating tear film over the eye), or from constant exposure of the cornea/conjunctiva to the air, resulting in tear film evaporation and subsequent drying out and damage of the surface epithelium. This predisposes the damaged areas to infection.

Management involves artificially protecting the eye from exposure and subsequent damage and infection. There are many methods available to do this. However, if trouble with eyelid closure is chronic, and the exposure risk is significant, it may be prudent to consider a more definitive procedure, such as tarsorrhaphy.

Tarsorrhaphy involves suturing part or all of the upper and lower lid edges together. The amount sutured depends on the reason for tarsorrhaphy, and the amount of protection required. Tarsorrhaphy can be permanent if the eye is deemed to be at permanent risk without it. Otherwise, it can be done temporarily if recovery of lid closure is expected.

Indications

- Ocular surface protection
- Lagophthalmos

Alternatives

- Taping eyelid shut
- Bandage contact lens
- Topical lubrication
- Gold weights
- Botulinum toxin

Benefits

- Protect ocular surface

Procedure

- Carried out under local anaesthesia ± sedation or general anaesthesia
- The tarsorrhaphy can be temporary or permanent
- Sutures are passed from one eyelid to the other to obtain closure
- The anterior and posterior lamellae of the eyelids can be split and sutured together separately
- The amount of closure required will be based on the amount of ocular surface protection required
- The procedure can take 30–45min

Complications

Common
- Bleeding
- Infection
- Scarring

Uncommon
- Suture dehiscence
- Trichiasis
- Adhesions between upper and lower eyelids
- Need for additional surgery

Rare
- Pyogenic granuloma

Temporal artery biopsy

Description
This is the definitive procedure used for histological confirmation of a diagnosis of temporal (giant cell) arteritis. It is typically carried out within 2 weeks of starting corticosteroid therapy (which should be started without delay in patients who are diagnosed with temporal arteritis based on clinical findings ± blood results).

Indications
- Giant cell (temporal) arteritis

Alternatives
- None

Benefits
- Histological confirmation of diagnosis

Procedure
- Carried out under local anaesthesia ± sedation or general anaesthesia
- Doppler ultrasound can be used to identify the path of the superficial temporal artery
- Hair in the region of the temple is shaved to allow a clear view of the operating site
- The skin is incised and the subcutaneous tissues dissected until the artery is identified
- At least 3cm of the artery is removed and sent to histology, and the wound closed
- The rate of a positive contralateral biopsy after an ipsilateral negative biopsy is approximately 1%[1]
- The procedure takes 30–60min

Complications
Common
- Bleeding
- Infection
- Scarring

Uncommon
- Foreign body reaction
- Need for additional surgery

Rare
- Incisional alopecia
- Scalp necrosis
- Nerve damage
- *Cerebrovascular event causing* contralateral hemiparesis

Reference
1. Ball J, Malhotra R. Efficacy of unilateral versus bilateral temporal artery biopsies for the diagnosis of giant cell arteritis. *Am J Ophthalmol* 2000;**129**(4):559–60.

Trabeculectomy

Description

This is a procedure that is most commonly used to lower intraocular pressure in glaucoma patients. It is usually indicated after failure of medical treatment or in cases of worsening of glaucoma despite adequate medical treatment.

It involves creating a channel between the drainage angle of the eye and a bleb created beneath the upper eyelid. This allows drainage of aqueous humour from within the eye into the bleb, which reduces the intraocular pressure. In order to improve drainage, antimetabolites such as 5-fluororacil or mitomycin-C can be used.

Indications

- Glaucoma refractory to topical and/or laser treatment

Alternatives

- Deep sclerectomy
- Visco-canulostomy (not widely performed by many glaucoma specialists)

Benefits

- Stabilize intraocular pressure
- Prevent further visual loss

Procedure

- Carried out under local anaesthesia ± sedation or general anaesthesia
- A drainage canal is created between the anterior chamber and sub-conjunctival bleb
- The bleb is created under the upper eyelid
- Antimetabolites can be used to prevent scarring
- Releasable sutures may be used
- The procedure takes 45–60min

Complications

Common

- Bleeding
- Hypotony
- Wound leak
- Raised intraocular pressure
- Scarring
- Bleb encapsulation
- Cataract
- Need for additional surgery (bleb needling and injection of antiscarring agents)

Uncommon
- Suprachoroidal haemorrhage
- Chronic inflammation
- Cystoid macular oedema

Rare
- Loss of vision
- Aqueous misdirection
- Endophthalmitis (severe infection in the eye)

Upper eyelid blepharoplasty

Description
Overhanging/excess eyelid skin/fat/muscle (dermatochalasis) can interfere with vision (see Figs. 21.6 and 21.7). This can be demonstrated by performing a visual field test which will show superior visual field restriction. This constitutes an important indication for surgical correction.

Indications
• Dermatochalasis

Alternatives
• None (dermatochalasis will not resolve spontaneously)

Benefits
• To improve dermatochalasis while ensuring that eyelid position remains optimal

Procedure
• Carried out under local anaesthesia ± sedation or general anaesthesia
• Through a skin incision, excess skin, fat, and/or muscle are removed
• The wound is then closed with sutures/tissue glue
• The operation takes 30–90min per eyelid

Complications
Common
• Bleeding
• Infection (preseptal cellulitis)
• Under-correction
• Over-correction
• Eyelid asymmetry
• Reoccurrence of loose eyelid skin

Uncommon
• Scarring
• Dry eye
• Ptosis
• Need for additional surgery

Rare
• Retrobulbar haemorrhage (0.055%)[1]
• Loss of vision (secondary to retrobulbar haemorrhage) (0.0045%)[1]

Reference
1. Hass AN, Penne RB, Stefanyszyn MA, et al. Incidence of postblepharoplasty orbital hemorrhage and associated visual loss. *Ophthal Plast Reconstr Surg* 2004;**20**(6):426–32.

Nd: YAG laser posterior capsulotomy

Description

Following uncomplicated phacoemulsification with intraocular lens insertion, the posterior aspect of the capsular bag can become fibrous and opacified (posterior capsular opacification). Patients can feel as if they are developing another cataract, as this opacification blurs the vision and can block out light. Vision can be improved again by making a hole in the posterior aspect of the capsular bag, so that light may pass through unimpeded again. If untreated, posterior capsular opacification will not spontaneously resolve, and will progress with time.

Indications

- Posterior capsular opacification

Alternatives

- Surgical posterior capsulotomy

Benefits

- Improve vision
- Reduce glare

Procedure

- Commonly under local (generally topical) anaesthesia
- The pupil is dilated, and a contact lens is placed on the eye
- Using the laser, a hole is made in the posterior capsular bag (thermal coagulation)
- The procedure takes 5–10min

Complications

Common

- Floaters
- Intraocular lens pitting
- Failure to improve vision (generally due to other retinal pathology being present)
- Raised intraocular pressure (5.7%)[1]
- Cystoid macular oedema (2.3%)[1]

Uncommon

- Need for repeat Nd: YAG laser (for incomplete/small capsulotomies)

Rare

- Retinal detachment/breaks (0.4%)[1]
- Intra-ocular lens dislocation
- Vitreous prolapse[2]
- Acute angle closure glaucoma (secondary to vitreous prolapse)[1]
- Malignant glaucoma[3]

References

1. Keates RH, Steinert RF, Puliafito CA, *et al.* Long-term follow-up of Nd: YAG laser posterior capsulotomy. *J Am Intraocul Implant Soc* 1984;**10**(2) 16–8.
2. Mihora LD, Bowers PJ Jr, Blank NM Acute angle-closure glaucoma caused by vitreous prolapse after neodymium: YAG posterior capsulotomy. *J Cataract Refract Surg* 2004;**30**(11):2445–7.
3. Arya SK, Kochhar S, Kumar S, *et al.* Malignant glaucoma as a complication of Nd: YAG laser posterior capsulotomy. *Ophthalmic Surg Lasers Imaging* 2004;**35**(3):248–50.

Nd: YAG peripheral iridotomy

Description

The drainage angle of the eye is the space between where the inside of the cornea and anterior iris meet (see Fig. 21.8). Angle structures and openness can be estimated by using a gonioscopy lens placed on the eyeball. There are various methods of grading the angle width from closed to wide open.

Important structures include:
- Schwalbe's line
- Trabecular meshwork
- Scleral spur
- Ciliary body

The drainage angle of the eye can become occluded by mechanical obstruction by the peripheral iris of the outflow through the trabecular meshwork. This could be acute, subacute, or chronic. It is usually caused by relative pupil block in anatomically predisposed (usually hypermetropic) eyes, and eyes with plateau iris.

Peripheral laser iridotomy is performed in order to create an alternative drainage pathway for the build up of aqueous fluid behind the iris when aqueous fluid cannot pass through the pupil.

Indications
- Narrow angle glaucoma
- Acute angle closure event
- Narrow angles on gonioscopy

Alternatives
- Surgical iridectomy
- Phacoemulsification + intra-ocular lens insertion

Benefits
- Prevent/treat acute angle closure event
- Open drainage angle (gonioscopic confirmation)

Procedure
- Carried out under local anaesthesia
- A contact lens is placed on the eye
- A laser hole is created in the iris at between 10 and 1 o'clock preferably as far peripherally as possible, which allows the upper eyelid to cover the laser hole and not cause visual problems
- Intraocular pressure is checked 1h after laser
- Anti-inflammatory drops are given for a short time
- The procedure takes 10–20min

Complications

Common
- Bleeding (commonly hyphaema from iris vessels hit during the procedure)
- Inflammation
- Raised intraocular pressure

Uncommon
- Failure to prevent angle closure event
- Cataract
- Lens capsule damage
- Diplopia
- Corneal damage
- Retinal damage
- Anterior synechiae
- Need for additional laser/surgery

Rare
- Retinal detachment/breaks
- Cystoid macular oedema
- Loss of vision

Diagrams of the eye

Figures 21.1 to 21.10 can be used to help explain procedures and eye anatomy to patients in order to aid the consent process.

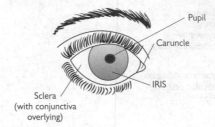

Fig. 21.1 Outside of the eye with eyelids.

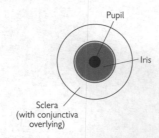

Fig. 21.2 The outside of the eye without eyelids.

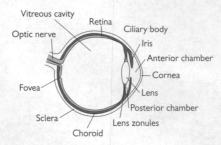

Fig. **21.3** The globe.

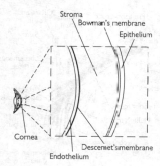

Fig. 21.4 The cornea.

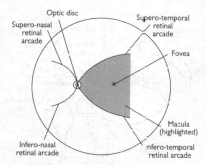

Fig. 21.5 The fundus.

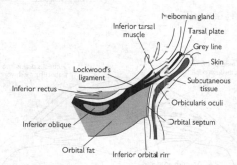

Fig. 21.6 The lower eyelid.

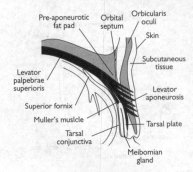

Pre-aponeurotic fat pad

Orbital septum

Orbicularis oculi

Skin

Subcutaneous tissue

Levator palpebrae superioris

Levator aponeurosis

Superior fornix

Muller's muslcle

Tarsal plate

Tarsal conjunctiva

Meibomian gland

Fig. 21.7 The upper eyelid.

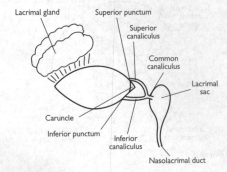

Lacrimal gland

Superior punctum

Superior canaliculus

Common canaliculus

Lacrimal sac

Caruncle

Inferior punctum

Inferior canaliculus

Nasolacrimal duct

Fig. 21.8 The lacrimal system.

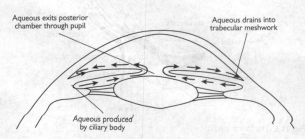

Aqueous exits posterior chamber through pupil

Aqueous drains into trabecular meshwork

Aqueous produced by ciliary body

Fig. 21.9 Normal drainage of aqueous fluid.

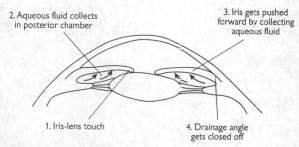

2. Aqueous fluid collects in posterior chamber

3. Iris gets pushed forward by collecting aqueous fluid

1. Iris-lens touch

4. Drainage angle gets closed off

Fig. 21.10 Acute angle closure glaucoma.

Obstetrics and gynaecological surgery

Amniocentesis and chorionic villus sampling

Description

Amniocentesis is a procedure in which a sample of amniotic fluid is obtained by passing a needle through the maternal abdomen into the amniotic sac. Fluid can then be analysed, usually to provide information about the karyotype of the fetus. It is performed from 15 weeks' gestation onwards.

Chorionic villus sampling (CVS) is performed from 11 to 14 weeks, and differs from amniocentesis in that a sample of placental tissue is obtained, either using a transabdominal or transcervical approach. Should the decision be to terminate the pregnancy, after receipt of the results, the timeframe in which CVS is performed is likely to allow surgical termination of the pregnancy (as opposed to medical termination of pregnancy which is recommended after 15 weeks). However, CVS is associated with a higher rate of miscarriage.

The procedures will usually be recommended in the event of abnormal screening results, or where there is a high risk of genetically carried disease (e.g. where there is a family history of cystic fibrosis or thalassaemia).

Additional procedures that may become necessary

- A second passage of the needle—in the event of a dry tap

Benefits

- Provides information regarding the karyotype (genes) of the fetus
- Occasionally biochemical or metabolic information is gained

Alternative procedures/conservative measures

- *Conservative*: no diagnostic testing. *Disadvantage*: no definite diagnosis on which to base decision to terminate pregnancy, or prepare for the additional needs of the child during and after delivery

Serious/frequently occurring risks[1,2]

- *Common*: mild discomfort at needle insertion site, failure to obtain sample (6%), miscarriage (risk above background rate quoted as 1% for amniocentesis, 2% for CVS): risk actually felt likely to be lower than this (but limited trial evidence); half of these will occur within the first 2 weeks after the procedure
- *Occasional*: amniotic fluid leakage
- *Rare*: fetal injury, maternal bowel injury, failure of cell culture (no results even after sample obtained), chorioamnionitis causing maternal sepsis

Blood transfusion necessary

- *None*

Type of anaesthesia/sedation
- Local anaesthesia often used for CVS, occasionally used for amniocentesis

Follow-up/need for further procedure
- Follow-up with results from laboratory tests
- Anti-D immunoglobulin for all rhesus-negative women
- Advised to seek help in the event of any fluid loss, bleeding, contractions or fever (chorioamnionitis usually occurs in the first 24–72h)

References
1. Royal College of Obstetricians and Gynaecologists. *Consent Advice 6: Amniocentesis*. London: RCOG, 2006.
2. Royal College of Obstetricians and Gynaecologist. *Greentop Guideline No 8: Amniocentesis and Chorionic Villus Sampling*. London: RCOG, 2010.

External cephalic version

Description

External cephalic version (ECV) describes the turning of the fetus, through the maternal abdomen, to a cephalic presentation, thereby reducing the risk of vaginal breech. It may be performed after 36 weeks' gestation.

A tocolytic (such as terbutaline or atosiban) may be given prior to the procedure.

Additional procedures that may become necessary

- Emergency caesarean section in the event of fetal distress

Benefits

- Reduces risks associated with vaginal breech delivery

Alternative procedures/conservative measures

- *Conservative*: resulting in either (a) vaginal breech delivery– *disadvantages*: higher fetal morbidity and mortality compared to caesarean section and cephalic vaginal delivery, or (b) spontaneous version to cephalic presentation (occurs in 8% after 36 weeks)
- *Surgical*: elective caesarean section. *Disadvantages*: higher maternal morbidity

Serious/frequently occurring risks[1,2]

- *Common*: failure (60% in nullips, 40% in multips), reversion to breech after version (<5%), pain (which may cause procedure to be abandoned)
- *Occasional*: emergency caesarean section due to bradycardia with cord entrapment (0.5%)
- *Rare*: placental abruption, uterine rupture, fetomaternal haemorrhage

Blood transfusion necessary

- Group and save required prior to procedure

Type of anaesthesia/sedation

- *None*: currently the procedure is stopped if discomfort is intolerable for mother
- Studies are underway to assess the usefulness of regional anaesthesia, though there are concerns about its safety

Follow-up/need for further procedure

- Presentation must be confirmed in labour, as spontaneous reversion to breech can occur
- All rhesus-negative women requite prophylactic anti-D

References

1. *Royal College of Obstetricians and Gynaecologists. Guideline No 20a: External Cephalic Version and Reducing the Incidence of Breech Presentation.* London: RCOG, 2006.
2. Royal College of Obstetricians and Gynaecologists. *Guideline No 20b: The Management of Breech Presentation.* London: RCOG, 2006.

Instrumental delivery

Description

Instrumental delivery is the use of either forceps or ventouse to aid delivery of the fetus (Fig. 22.1). It accounts for 10–15% of all vaginal deliveries.

Indications for instrumental delivery include prolonged second stage of labour, or presumed fetal or maternal compromise. An instrumental delivery should only be considered if the cervix is fully dilated, the fetal head is ≤1/5 palpable abdominally, the membranes are ruptured, and the patient has adequate analgesia. The clinician should choose the appropriate instrument based on the clinical situation.

Additional procedures that may become necessary

- Episiotomy + repair
- Repair of third/fourth degree perineal tears
- Caesarean section if unsuccessful

Benefits

- To expedite delivery of baby
- Avoidance of emergency caesarean section if successful

Alternative procedures/conservative measures

- *Conservative*: observe. *Disadvantage*: potentially poor fetal and maternal outcome
- *Medical*: oxytocin infusion can help aid delivery if there is poor uterine contractility, malposition, and in the absence of fetal compromise
- *Surgical*: caesarean section. *Disadvantages*: invasive, higher maternal morbidity

Serious/frequently occurring risks

- *Common*: bleeding, pain, vaginal wall laceration, perineal damage (other than episiotomy)—with associated complications. More likely with forceps delivery
- *Occasional*: infection (endometrial/systemic) cephalohaematoma to baby (collection of blood under the periosteum due to suction), urinary stress incontinence, urogenital prolapse
- *Rare*: fetal scalp injuries, serious fetal injury/death, fetal nerve palsy, uterine rupture, thromboembolic disease

Blood transfusion necessary

- Depends on overall blood loss during delivery

Type of anaesthesia/sedation

- Spinal/epidural anaesthesia
- Local anaesthesia, e.g. pudendal block can be used but regional anaesthesia is more appropriate in cases where there is a significant likelihood of proceeding to caesarean

Follow-up/need for further procedure

- If delivery is not imminent after three pulls of a correctly applied instrument, instrumental delivery should be abandoned and a caesarean section considered
- Paired cord samples should be analysed following all instrumental deliveries
- The mother should be debriefed regarding indication for instrumental delivery
- Attention paid to bladder care

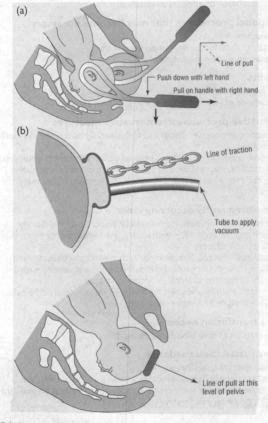

Fig. 22.1 Assisted delivery techniques (a) forceps (b) ventouse.

Reproduced from Chamberlain, G et al. ABC of labour care: operative delivery. BMJ 1999; **318**:1260–4, with permission. © BMJ Publishing Group Ltd 1999.

Caesarean section

Description

Caesarean section is the delivery of the fetus through a direct incision in the abdominal wall and uterus. It may be performed where the anticipated risks to the mother and/or baby of an alternative mode of delivery outweigh those of a caesarean section.

Indications for caesarean may be immediate (grade I, e.g. for uterine rupture, fetal scalp pH 7.2), urgent (grade I, e.g. for failure to progress with an abnormal cardiotocograph (CTG)), scheduled (grade III, e.g. for intrauterine growth retardation) or elective (grade IV, e.g. for breech, multiple previous caesarean sections, placenta previa).

Additional procedures that may become necessary

- Repair of damage to bowel, bladder or blood vessels
- Hysterectomy

Benefits

- To secure the safest and/or quickest route of delivery

Alternative procedures/conservative measures

- *Conservative*: vaginal delivery (with or without instruments).
  Disadvantages: increased risk of fetal and maternal morbidity and mortality (depending on indication)
- *Medical*: augmentation or induction of labour may occasionally be an appropriate alternative, depending on the indication

Serious/frequently occurring risks[1]

- ▶▶Risks are higher in crash caesarean section, and in women who are obese, have pre-existing significant medical conditions, or who have had previous surgery
- *Common*: bleeding, infection, wound and abdominal discomfort (often lasting a few weeks), risk in future pregnancy (placenta previa/accreta, uterine rupture, increased risk of further caesarean section)
- *Occasional*: fetal lacerations, adhesions, small bowel obstruction (late complication)
- *Rare*: hysterectomy (more common with placenta previa), thromboembolic disease, bowel or bladder injury, ureteric injury, maternal death

Blood transfusion necessary

- Usually group and save only: cross-match may be indicated if previous haemorrhage, placenta previa, or fibroids in lower segment

Type of anaesthesia/sedation

- Usually regional anaesthesia
- General anaesthesia in case of crash caesarean section if deemed faster, platelets <80, or difficulty with regional techniques

Follow-up/need for further procedure

- Future pregnancies are usually followed up in a doctor-led clinic

Reference

1. Royal College of Obstetrics and Gynaecology. *Consent Advice No 7: Caesarean Section*. London: RCOG, 2009.

Third and fourth degree perineal tear repair

Description

Obstetric anal sphincter injury complicates 1% of all vaginal deliveries and encompasses third and fourth degree perineal tears.[1] A third degree perineal tear involves a partial or complete disruption of the anal sphincter muscles whereas a fourth degree perineal tear involves disruption of the anal sphincter muscles plus a breach of the rectal mucosa.

Additional procedures that may become necessary

- Referral to tertiary centre or colorectal surgeon for secondary repair

Benefits

- To restore anorectal and perineal anatomy
- Facilitate wound healing
- Reduced risk of faecal incontinence

Alternative procedures/conservative measures

- *Conservative*: not recommended

Serious/frequently occurring risks

- *Common*: bleeding, infection (wound/urinary tract/systemic), dyspareunia, faecal urgency, perineal pain
- *Occasional*: incontinence of faeces/flatus, knot migration to the perineal surface
- *Rare*: failure of repair, haematoma, rectovaginal fistula, thromboembolic disease

Blood transfusion necessary

- Dependent on overall blood loss during delivery

Type of anaesthesia/sedation

- Epidural/spinal anaesthesia

Follow-up/need for further procedure

- Physiotherapy referral required
- Commenced on laxatives and antibiotics post-procedure
- Outpatient clinic at 6/52 to assess for faecal continence and dyspareunia, and for discussion regarding mode of delivery in future pregnancies

Reference

1. Royal College of Obstetricians and Gynaecologists. *Consent Advice No. 9: Repair of Third- and Fourth- Degree Tears Following Childbirth*. London: RCOG, 2004.

Manual removal of placenta

Description

The incidence of retained placenta after vaginal delivery is approximately 0.6–2%. It is more common after physiological management of the 3rd stage, in women who have previously had retained placenta or who have had uterine surgery, after preterm deliveries and with young maternal age. There is a high risk of postpartum haemorrhage and infection if the tissue is not removed.

It can be caused by failed separation (especially in placenta accreta), an accessory lobe (which does not separate with the rest of the placenta), trapping of the placenta behind a closed cervix or cord detachment (often related to excess cord traction).

The procedure involves placing a gloved hand inside the uterus and manually separating the placenta in its entirety. The removed tissue is examined to ensure that the placenta and membranes are intact; if they are not, further exploration will be performed. After the procedure, IV oxytocin is given to promote contraction of the uterus. IV antibiotic cover is generally used, though there are no data as yet confirming its efficacy to prevent infection.[1]

Additional procedures that may become necessary

- Hysterectomy in the event of uncontrollable bleeding or irreparable damage to the uterus

Benefits

- Removal of retained placenta, which, if left, can cause ongoing bleeding and infection

Alternative procedures/conservative measures

- *Conservative*: conservative management is sometimes needed in case of morbidly adherent placenta
- *Medical*: oxytocin injection into umbilical vein.[2] *Advantages*: reduces need for manual removal by 20%
- *Surgical*: none

Serious/frequently occurring risks

- *Common*: bleeding, infection,[1] incomplete removal necessitating further procedure
- *Rare*: inversion of uterus, broad ligament haematoma, perforation resulting in trauma to pelvic organs

Blood transfusion necessary

- Up to 10% of women requiring manual removal may require blood transfusion

Type of anaesthesia/sedation

- Usually regional anaesthesia; general anaesthesia less commonly

Follow-up/need for further procedure

- Given increased risk of recurrence, should be made note of in any future pregnancies

References

1. Chongsomchai C, Lumbiganon P, Laopaiboon M. Prophylactic antibiotics for manual removal of retained placenta in vaginal birth. *Cochrane Database Syst Rev* 2006;**2**:CD004904.
2. Carroli G, Bergel E. Umbilical vein injection for management of retained placenta. *Cochrane Library* 2004;**3**:CD001337.

Long-acting reversible contraception

Description

Methods of long-acting reversible contraception (LARC) are: intrauterine system (IUS, Mirena Coil®), intrauterine device (IUD, the 'copper coil'), injectable contraceptives and implants (Implanon®).

They are all more cost-effective at 1 year of use than the combined oral contraceptive pill, and reduce the number of unwanted pregnancies.

The intrauterine device mechanically prevents fertilization and implantation, and lasts 5–10 years depending on the manufacturer. The intrauterine system delivers local progestagens, which inhibit implantation, and possibly fertilization, and offer protection for 5 years.

The implant is a single rod containing 68mg of etonogestrel, which is released at 6–70micrograms/day. It is inserted subdermally by trained practitioners in the non-dominant arm, in the biceps/triceps groove 8–10cm above the medial epicondyle. It acts by preventing ovulation and lasts for 3 years from the time of insertion.

Progesterone-only injectable contraceptives (POICs) also act by preventing ovulation. Injections are required every 8–12 weeks depending on the progesterone. There is therefore more potential for user error if appointments for repeat injections are missed or delayed.

Additional procedures that may become necessary

- Triple swabs to exclude infection are usually taken before, or at the time of, IUD or IUS insertion

Benefits

- Prevention of unwanted pregnancy
- IUD can be used as emergency postcoital contraception

Alternative procedures/conservative measures

- *Oral contraceptives* (combined and progesterone only). *Disadvantages*: higher rates of unwanted pregnancy, subject to user error, hormonal side effects, combined pill contraindicated in certain groups (e.g. sufferers of migraine with aura)
- *Barrier contraceptives*: condoms, female diaphragm. *Disadvantages*: higher rates of unwanted pregnancy
- *Surgical*: laparoscopic tubal sterilization/vasectomy. *Disadvantages*: irreversible

Serious/frequently occurring risks[1]

- *Common*:
  - *IUS/IUD*: discomfort during and after insertion of IUS and IUD: patients warned to expect cramping lower abdominal pain and spotting after procedure, failure of insertion, expulsion (<1 in 20, usually in first 3 months and during menstruation), changes in bleeding pattern (IUS: irregular bleeding/spotting common during first 6 months, oligomenorrhoea/amenorrhoea likely by end of 1st year. IUD: heavier bleeding, dysmenorrhoea)
  - *Implant*: discomfort during, and bruising after, insertion, changes in bleeding pattern (frequent, infrequent or prolonged)

- *POIC*: delay in return of fertility by <1year, weight gain, changes in bleeding pattern (persistent bleeding or amenorrhoea common)
- *Occasional*:
  - Pregnancy
  - IUD 20 in 1000 over 5 years
  - IUS <10 in 1000 over 5 years
  - ►►If pregnancy occurs while the IUS/IUD is in situ, there is an increased risk of ectopic pregnancy <1 in 20 (overall risk of ectopic pregnancy <1 in 1000, i.e. less than if no contraception used)
  - Implant <1 in 1000 over 3 years
  - POIC 4 in 1000 over 5 years if given at correct time interval
- *Rare*:
  - Uterine perforation at time of insertion of IUS/IUD <1 in 1000
  - Deep/impalpable implants in 1 in 1000

Blood transfusion necessary

- None

Type of anaesthesia/sedation

- Local anaesthesia only for implant

Follow-up/need for further procedure

- IUS/IUD follow-up in 3–6 weeks to exclude infection/perforation/expulsion
- Every 8 or 12 weeks for repeat POIC

Reference

1. National Institute of Health and Clinical Excellence. *Long-acting Reversible Contraception; the Effective and Appropriate use of LARC.* London: NICE, 2005.

Laparoscopic sterilization

Description

Laparoscopic sterilization is intended to permanently prevent pregnancy. Two port sites are generally used to place Filshie clips or rings over both fallopian tubes (Fig. 22.2).

It is essential during any conversation regarding this procedure that reversible alternatives are discussed. These must include vasectomy of the partner, Mirena® IUS, and Implanon®. Increased regret rate is recognized in women under age of 30, and those immediately following a pregnancy.[1]

It is imperative that the procedure is considered permanent. Reversal procedures, *in vitro* fertilization (IVF), and intracytoplasmic sperm injection (ICSI) are not available on the NHS, and are associated with significantly reduced success rate.

Effective contraception must be used up to the day of the surgery and until her next menstrual period. If there is a chance of pregnancy then the operation must be delayed until the follicular phase of the next cycle.

Additional procedures that may become necessary

- Repair of damage to blood vessels, bladder or bowel, which may necessitate laparotomy

Benefits

- Intended to permanently prevent pregnancy

Alternative procedures/conservative measures

- *Conservative*: rhythm or withdrawal method. *Disadvantage*: high failure rate
- *Medical*: short-acting contraception (including barrier methods and daily pills) *Disadvantages*: user dependent, increased risk of pregnancy mainly due to user error, hormonal side effects
- LARC (implant, progesterone injection, IUD or IUS). *Disadvantages*: hormonal side effects (see 📖 'Long-acting reversible contraception', p.690 for more details)
- *Surgical*: male vasectomy. *Advantage*: lower failure rate and less procedure related risks

Serious/frequently occurring risks[1]

- *Common*: bruising, pain, including post-operative shoulder pain
- *Occasional*: failure (lifetime pregnancy rate 1 in 200, ectopic more likely if pregnancy occurs), wound infection, damage to the bladder, bowel, uterus or major blood vessels, development of port-site hernia
- *Very rare*: death as a result of major complications of laparoscopy

Blood transfusion necessary

- Rarely, in the event of damage to surrounding structures

Type of anaesthesia/sedation
- General anaesthesia

Follow-up/need for further procedure
- None required

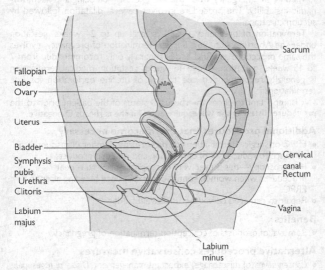

Fig. 22.2 Sagittal view of the female pelvis showing fallopian tube, uterus, and ovary.
Reproduced with permission from Pocock G and Richards CD. *Human Physiology: the basis of medicine* 3rd edition. 2006. Oxford: Oxford University Press, p.437, Figure 20.7.

Reference

1. Royal College of Obstetricians and Gynaecologists *Consent Advice No 2: Diagnostic Laparoscopy*. London: RCOG, 2009.

ERPC and termination of pregnancy

Description

Evacuation of retained products of conception (ERPC) is the surgical procedure performed for an incomplete or missed miscarriage. It is performed as an emergency when there is excessive bleeding and haemodynamic instability. The procedure involves cervical dilatation followed by suction curettage.

Termination of pregnancy (TOP) is legal up to 24 weeks' gestation under the Abortion Act 1967. Surgical termination of pregnancy involves the same procedure as ERPC and is generally only recommended from 7 to 15 weeks' gestation. Above 15 weeks' gestation, medical termination is generally recommended due to risk of uterine perforation for late terminations.[1]

It is important to check the rhesus D status of the patient prior to the procedures listed as she will require anti-D if she is rhesus D negative.

Additional procedures that may become necessary

- ERPC or surgical termination can be performed under ultrasound guidance to reduce risk of perforation and retained products
- Hysteroscopy—this is used very occasionally prior to repeat procedures when women continue to experience bleeding after an ERPC
- Repair to damaged cervix/uterus/bowel/bladder

Benefits

- Removal of products of conception/termination of pregnancy

Alternative procedures/conservative measures

- *Conservative*: (of miscarriage) expectant management. *Disadvantages*: pain and heavy bleeding, may be less effective in gestations above 12 weeks (ERPC may be required at a later date), unacceptable to patient, not recommended in cases of suspected gestational trophoblastic disease
- *Medical*: mifepristone followed by misoprostol. *Disadvantages*: pain and heavy bleeding, wide variation in efficacy depending on gestation, more effective for TOP below 8 weeks' gestation

Serious/frequently occurring risks[1]

- *Common*: bleeding, pain
- *Occasional*: infection (endometrial/systemic), damage/perforation to uterus, failure to dilate the cervix, cervical trauma
- *Rare*: damage to bowel/bladder, retained products, haemorrhage leading to disseminated intravascular coagulation, thromboembolism

Blood transfusion necessary

- Occasionally group and save and rhesus D status required

Type of anaesthesia/sedation

- Mainly general anaesthesia, but some units are beginning to offer under local anaesthesia for gestations less than 8 weeks

Follow-up/need for further procedure

- No follow-up required unless histology indicates a molar pregnancy. In the UK such patients should be referred for follow-up to one of the three tertiary referral centres in the country
- If women have not been screened for sexually transmitted diseases prior to procedure, prophylaxis may be offered
- Per vaginal (PV) bleeding is normal for 7 days
- Anti-D needed if rhesus D negative

Reference

1. Royal College of Obstetricians and Gynaecologists. *Consent Advice No. 10: Surgical Evacuation of the Uterus for Early Pregnancy Loss.* London: RCOG, 2010.

Laparoscopic management of tubal ectopic pregnancy

Description

Ectopic pregnancy is a significant cause of maternal mortality. It occurs when the embryo implants outside of the uterine cavity. The most common location of ectopic pregnancy is within the fallopian tube, known as a tubal ectopic. An ectopic pregnancy can be asymptomatic, or it may present with abdominal pain, vaginal bleeding or, in extremis, with maternal collapse. It is diagnosed by ultrasound scan in which an adnexal mass is visualized. There may be free fluid visible if the ectopic pregnancy has ruptured. A suboptimal rise in serum β-human chorionic gonadotrophin (hCG) may raise clinical suspicion.

The surgical management of a tubal ectopic pregnancy is usually performed laparoscopically,[1] but laparotomy may be indicated in cases of haemodynamic compromise, or if extensive bleeding is obscuring laparoscopic views.[2] A salpingectomy, which is removal of the fallopian tube, is the preferred surgical option unless there is disease or absence of the contralateral fallopian tube. In this case, a salpingotomy is performed: an incision is made in the fallopian tube through which the pregnancy is removed.

Rhesus D status must be determined preoperatively and anti-D is given if the patient is rhesus D negative.

Additional procedures that may become necessary

- Conversion to laparotomy if difficulties encountered at laparoscopy
- Repair of damaged bowel/bladder/ureters

Benefits

- To remove ectopic pregnancy that can be life-threatening

Alternative procedures/conservative measures

- *Conservative*: expectant management—only acceptable in women who are asymptomatic, with no blood in the pouch of Douglas and with a decreasing HCG level, usually less than 1000iu/L initially. *Disadvantages*: risk of tubal rupture, risk of failure, requirement for follow-up
- *Medical*: methotrexate—only acceptable in women with minimal symptoms and hCG <3000iu. *Disadvantages*: risk of tubal rupture, risk of failure, requirement for follow-up, abdominal pain, other side effects including conjunctivitis, stomatitis, and gastrointestinal upset
- *Surgical*: as previous bullet

Serious/frequently occurring risks[1,2]

- *Common*: infection (wound/systemic), scar, pain (including shoulder-tip pain secondary to pneumoperitoneum), persistent trophoblastic tissue (4–8%) when salpingotomy performed
- *Occasional*: bleeding, port-site hernias
- *Rare*: damage to bladder/bowel/uterus/ureters/blood vessels, thromboembolic disease, gas embolism, conversion to laparotomy

Blood transfusion necessary
- Likely if ruptured (ensure group and save performed for patients with suspected ectopic)

Type of anaesthesia/sedation
- General anaesthesia

Follow-up/need for further procedure
- Anti D immunoglobulin should be given to all rhesus negative women post-procedure
- As per unit guidelines: consider outpatient clinic at 6 weeks to assess wound healing and review histology
- Increased risk of further ectopic pregnancy in the future
- All patients should be advised to arrange for an ultrasound scan at 6 weeks gestation in future pregnancies to exclude an ectopic

References
1. Royal College of Obstetricians and Gynaecologists. *Consent Advice No. 8: Laparoscopic Management of Tubal Ectopic Pregnancy.* London: RCOG, 2010.
2. Royal College of Obstetricians and Gynaecologists. *Green-top Guidelines No. 21: The Management of Tubal Pregnancy.* London: RCOG, 2004.

Diagnostic laparoscopy

Description

A diagnostic laparoscopy allows the surgeon direct visualization of the patient's abdominal and pelvic organs. It may be performed to diagnose the cause of abdominal and pelvic pain where no diagnosis has been made with non-invasive investigations. When pathology is found such as endometriosis, adhesions, or ovarian cysts, further surgery can then be carried out if consent has been sought beforehand.

The most common approach is first to insert a Veress' needle through the umbilicus to inflate the peritoneal cavity. A trochar is then inserted through the umbilicus. Further ports may be inserted as necessary under direct vision.

A dye test is often performed during diagnostic laparoscopy to assess tubal patency, specifically in cases of subfertility. Saline dyed with methylene blue is syringed through the cervical canal, and dye spillage from both fallopian tubes is monitored.

Additional procedures that may become necessary

- Conversion to laparotomy
- Repair of bowel/uterus/bladder/ureters
- Dependent on findings: adhesiolysis or treatment to endometriosis may be indicated
- Definitive treatment
- Dye test to assess for tubal patency in cases of subfertility

Benefits

- *Diagnosis*: to find the cause of the symptoms
- *Treatment*: as appropriate, e.g. ovarian cyst aspiration/cystectomy

Alternative procedures/conservative measures in case of normal imaging and chronic pelvic pain

- *Conservative*: observation
- *Medical*:
  - Analgesia: *Disadvantage*: non-diagnostic
  - Imaging: *Disadvantages*: reduced sensitivity and specificity, non-therapeutic

Serious/frequently occurring risks[1]

- *Common*: pain—wound/shoulder-tip, bruising, infection (wound/systemic)
- *Occasional*: bleeding
- *Rare*: damage to bladder/bowel/ureters/uterus/major blood vessels, failure to gain entry into abdominal cavity, port site hernias, thromboembolic disease

Blood transfusion necessary

- *Rarely (group and save required preoperatively)*

Type of anaesthesia/sedation

• General anaesthesia

Follow-up/need for further procedure

• Outpatient clinic appointment in 6/52 may need to be arranged if pathology found during laparoscopy

Reference

1. Royal College of Obstetricians and Gynaecologists. *Consent Advice 2: Diagnostic Laparoscopy.* London: RCOG, 2008.

Laparoscopy and treatment of endometriosis

Description

Laparoscopy is considered the gold standard diagnostic test for endometriosis. Usually surgical treatment of endometriosis will be undertaken at the time of diagnosis, provided disease is not so severe as to require extensive resection, which may involve the bladder or bowel. This would usually be performed in a tertiary centre by a surgeon with the necessary laparoscopic expertise. Consent for such resections is not covered here.

The aim of surgical resection is to excise or ablate areas of ectopic endometrium in order to improve symptoms, and/or increase the chance of pregnancy. Techniques include diathermy, laser ablation or excision, ovarian cystectomy, nerve ablation, and helium plasma coagulation.

Additional procedures that may become necessary

- Repair of damage to blood vessels, bladder or bowel, which may necessitate laparotomy
- Resection of deposits on the bladder or bowel (usually not consented for at first laparoscopy)

Benefits[1]

- Diagnosis
- Reduced pain (in 30–40% of women)
- Improved fertility (though role remains uncertain)

Alternative procedures/conservative measures[2]

- *Conservative*: observation. *Disadvantages*: lack of definite diagnosis, continuing pain
- *Medical*: hormonal treatment (combined oral contraceptive pill, progesterone, intrauterine system) *Disadvantages*: recurrence, interfere with ovulation (and therefore inappropriate for patients seeking treatment of infertility)
- Gonadotropin-releasing hormone (GnRH) agonists. *Disadvantages*: recurrence, iatrogenic menopause, loss of bone mineral density (thereby limiting treatment duration), interfere with ovulation

Serious/frequently occurring risks[2,3]

- *Common*: bruising, pain, including postoperative shoulder pain, wound infection, relapse of symptoms (50% require analgesia or hormonal treatment at 1 year, <50% reoperation rate[1])
- *Occasional*: wound infection, damage to the bladder, bowel or major blood vessels
- *Rare*: port site hernias, thromboembolic disease
- *Very rare*: 3–4 women in every 100 000 die as a result of complications of laparoscopy

Blood transfusion necessary

- Rarely, in the event of damage to surrounding structures
- Group and save should be performed

Type of anaesthesia/sedation

- General anaesthesia

Follow-up/need for further procedure

- Review in outpatient clinic in 3 months with menstrual diary

References

1. Vercellini P, Crosignani PG, Abbiati A, et al. The effect of surgery for symptomatic endometriosis: the other side of the story. *Hum Reprod Update* 2009;**15**(2):177–83.
2. Royal College of Obstetricians and Gynaecologists. *The Investigation and Management of Endometriosis.* London: RCOG, 2006.
3. Royal College of Obstetricians and Gynaecologists. *Consent Advice No 2: Diagnostic Laparoscopy.* London: RCOG, 2009.

Cervical cone biopsy

Description

A cervical cone biopsy is the excision of a cone of cervical tissue containing the transformation zone (the area of squamous metaplasia due to the influence of low vaginal pH on cervical columnar epithelium).

Women requiring cone biopsy are generally picked up asymptomatically through the cervical screening programme, which recommends that all women between the ages of 25 and 64 are invited for cervical smear on a regular basis.[1,2] If moderate or severe cytological abnormalities are detected on a smear test, or in cases of persistent mild or borderline dyskaryosis or mild dyskaryosis associated with high-risk HPV infection (depending on unit guidelines), women are referred for colposcopy. During colposcopy, biopsies of any suspicious areas are taken. Histology is graded CIN (cervical intraepithelial neoplasia) I, II, or III depending on the depth of abnormal cells within the epithelium.

Women with CIN II or III are usually recommended to have a cone biopsy or large loop excision of the transformation zone (LLETZ) procedure. These procedures may also be considered for CIN I (especially if persistent). Cone biopsy is also usually the treatment of choice for Stage 1a1 cervical cancer (microscopic invasive carcinoma where there is stromal invasion of less than 3mm depth and less than 7mm diameter), and for 1a2 cervical cancer (stromal invasion 3–5mm, less than 7mm diameter) in women wishing to retain fertility.

Additional procedures that may become necessary

- Repair of damage to uterus/cervix

Benefits

- Removal of precancerous cervical cells
- Removal of early cervical cancers

Alternative procedures/conservative measures

- None recommended

Serious/frequently occurring risks

- *Common*: bleeding (which may continue for up to 4 weeks), pain
- *Occasional*: infection leading to late bleeding (within 2 weeks of procedure)
- *Rare*: cervical incompetence—leading to increased risk of miscarriage, cervical stenosis/distortion, hysterectomy with uncontrollable bleeding

Blood transfusion necessary

- Rarely

Type of anaesthesia/sedation

- *Dependent on unit and on patient preference; can be performed under local or general anaesthetic*

Follow-up/need for further procedure

- Most units will have a system to write to the patient with the histology results after the procedure
- Routine follow-up of cone biopsies for CIN is a colposcopy and smear test after 6 months

References

1. National Institute of Health and Clinical Excellence. *Liquid-based Cytology for Cervical Screening*. London: NICE, 2005.
2. Mohan S, Ind T. Cervical screening in England and Wales: an update. *Curr Opin Obstet Gynecol* 2004;**16**(6):491–6.

Marsupialization of Bartholin's cyst

Description

Bartholin's glands are situated bilaterally at the posterior vaginal entrance (Fig. 22.3), and secrete lubricant that enters the vagina via a duct.

Blockage of a duct leads to development of Bartholin's cyst, a hard and usually painless lump. If the blockage continues the cyst may become infected, leading to formation of a painful abscess. Cysts which do not respond to conservative measures, and those with infection, will require definitive management, usually by surgically creating a permanent tract though which fluid can drain.

Marsupialization is the most commonly performed surgical procedure for the treatment of Bartholin's abscess. The edges of the cyst wall are everted and sutured to the vulval skin with absorbable sutures, thus creating a pouch (hence 'marsupialization').

Other methods may be chosen based on local expertise and facilities.[1] The use of a balloon catheter,[2] which is inserted into the cyst cavity, expanded, and left for a period of 2–6 weeks to allow epithelialization around the balloon, is gaining popularity. The use of silver nitrate to ablate the gland has also been found to be associated with less scar formation and similar recurrence rates.

Additional procedures that may become necessary
- Excision of gland

Benefits
- Reduction in swelling and/or pain
- Treatment of infection

Alternative procedures/conservative measures[1]
- *Conservative*: warm baths/warm compresses. *Disadvantages*: unlikely to resolve infection, recurrence
- *Medical*: oral antibiotics. *Disadvantages*: large, painful abscess unlikely to completely respond, recurrence
- *Surgical*: balloon catheter insertion, silver nitrate ablation and carbon dioxide laser. All have similar efficacy: choice depends on local facilities

Serious/frequently occurring risks
- *Common*: pain (including dyspareunia), recurrence, bleeding, haematoma formation

Blood transfusion necessary
- None

Type of anaesthesia/sedation
- Usually performed under general anaesthesia

Follow-up/need for further procedure
- None usually required. Biopsies should be taken in any women above the age of 40 presenting with a suspected Bartholin's mass to exclude malignancy

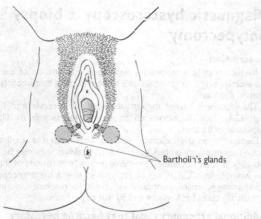

Bartholin's glands

Fig. 22.3 Location of Bartholin's glands.
Reproduced with permission from O Connor IF and Urdang M. *Oxford Handbook of Surgical Cross-Cover*. 2008. Oxford: Oxford University Press, p.504, Figure 13.4.

References

1. Wechter ME, Wu JM, Marzano D, et al. Management of Bartholin duct cyst and abscess: a systematic review. *Obstet Gynecol Surv* 2009;**64**(6):395–40⁵
2. National Institute of Health and Clinical Excellence. *Balloon Catheter Insertion for Bartholin's Cyst or Abscess*. London: NICE, 2009.

Diagnostic hysteroscopy ± biopsy ± polypectomy

Description

A hysteroscopy is a procedure that allows examination of the inside of the womb using a narrow tube-like camera called a hysteroscope (usually 5mm in diameter).

The camera is passed through the vagina and cervix into the womb (Fig. 22.4). Fluid is introduced to distend the womb to allow close inspection of its cavity.

Depending on the indication, and on what is seen, a small sample of tissue may be taken for histology. Endometrial washings may be taken for cytology. It is also possible to remove polyps (protrusions of the lining of the womb). An IUD/IUS can be introduced after a hysteroscopy (📖 see 'Long-acting reversible contraception', p.690 for relevant consent advice).

It usually takes between 10 and 30 min to perform.

Additional procedures that may become necessary

- Laparoscopy or laparotomy, and repair of damage, in the event of a uterine perforation

Benefits

- *Diagnostic*: to exclude endometrial pathology responsible for symptoms such as heavy periods or postmenopausal bleeding
- *Therapeutic*: remove polyps. A hysteroscopic approach can also be used for resection of submucous fibroids, endometrial ablation, and adhesiolysis

Alternative procedures/conservative measures

- *Conservative*: ultrasound diagnosis. *Disadvantages*: less sensitive, not therapeutic
- *Surgical*: endometrial aspiration[1] (Pipelle® biopsy) *Advantage*: can be performed in clinic without anaesthesia. *Disadvantages*: may miss pathology due to small sample area, no therapeutic options

Serious/frequently occurring risks[2,3]

- *Common*: cramping pelvic pain, bleeding, infection
- *Occasional*: perforation of the uterus, failure to gain entry to the womb, failure to attain representative sample requiring repeat procedure
- *Rare*: damage to the bladder, bowel, or major blood vessels

Blood transfusion necessary

- Rarely, in the case of damage to surrounding structures

Type of anaesthesia/sedation

- *Local/general anaesthesia*

Follow-up/need for further procedure

- Results from histology/cytology need to be followed up

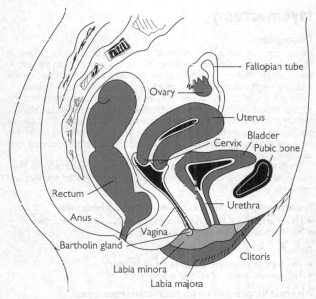

Fig. 22.4 Saggital view of the female pelvis, its contents and relationships.
Reproduced with permission from Pattman R, Sankar KN, Elawad B, et al. Oxford Handbook of Genitourinary Medicine, HIV, and Sexual Health 2nd edition. 2010. Oxford: Oxford University Press, p.55, Figure 3.1.

References

1. Bedner R, Rzepka-Górska I. Hysteroscopy with directed biopsy versus dilatation and curettage for the diagnosis of endometrial hyperplasia in perimenopausal women. Eur J Gynecol Oncol 2007;**28**(5):400–2.
2. Royal College of Obstetricians and Gynaecologists. Consent Advice 1: Diagnostic Hysteroscopy Under General Anaesthesia. London: RCOG, 2008.
3. Jansen FW; Vredevoogd CB; van Ulzen K, et al. Complications of hysteroscopy: a prospective, multicenter study. Obstet Gynaecol 2000;**96**(2):266–70.

Myomectomy

Description

Myomectomy is the surgical removal of uterine fibroids, also known as uterine leiomyomas. Fibroids are benign tumours originating from the uterine myometrium. Fibroids only need to be removed if they are causing pain, pressure symptoms, menorrhagia, or if they interfere with reproduction.

For subserosal and intramural fibroids the procedure involves location of the fibroid once inside the peritoneal cavity and then incision of the uterine muscle and subsequent removal of the fibroid. This can be performed by laparotomy or laparoscopy, although it may be preferable to use the open approach for larger fibroids. Postoperative recovery for an open procedure may take up to 6 weeks.

Submucosal fibroids are generally visualized via a hysteroscope. Myomectomy is then performed with a resectoscope (so-called transcervical resection of fibroids or TCRF).

Additional procedures that may become necessary

- Hysterectomy—if excessive bleeding which cannot be controlled
- Repair to damaged bowel/bladder/ureters

Benefits

- To improve symptoms associated with fibroids
- To improve chance of successful pregnancy

Alternative procedures/conservative measures[1]

- *Conservative*: observation
- *Medical*:
  - Analgesia, antifibrinolytics, e.g. tranexamic acid. *Disadvantages*: symptomatic relief only, compliance
  - GnRH analogues. *Disadvantages*: short-term treatment, iatrogenic menopause, reduced bone mineral density
  - Oral contraceptive pill. *Disadvantages*: symptomatic relief for menorrhagia only, compliance
- *Surgical*:
  - Intrauterine system. *Disadvantages*: symptomatic relief for menorrhagia only, uterine cavity often distorted by fibroids and therefore unsuitable
  - Uterine artery embolization. *Disadvantages*: small risk of ovarian failure leading to subfertility, limited response (especially if fibroids are large)
  - Hysterectomy. *Advantage*: definitive solution. *Disadvantages*: permanent infertility

Serious/frequently occurring risks[1]

- *Common*: bleeding, pain, scar, infection (wound/systemic), recurrence
- *Occasional*: damage to bladder/ureters ± long-term bladder dysfunction
- *Rare*: damage to bowel, adhesions, conversion to hysterectomy, thromboembolic disease

Blood transfusion necessary
- Group and save. In cases of large/multiple fibroids, or low pre-operative haemoglobin, cross match of 2–4 units may be indicated

Type of anaesthesia/sedation
- General anaesthesia

Follow-up/need for further procedure
- Outpatient clinic in 6/52 for histology results and to assess wound healing
- If the cavity is breeched during an open or laparoscopic myomectomy a caesarean section is advised for future pregnancies to avoid the risk of uterine rupture

Hysterectomy ± bilateral salpingo-oophorectomy

Description

Hysterectomy is the surgical removal of the uterus. Indications include benign conditions such as menorrhagia, fibroids, and uterine prolapse, and malignant conditions including endometrial, cervical, and ovarian carcinoma.

Three different types of hysterectomy are performed:

- Total hysterectomy—removal of the uterus and cervix, with or without bilateral salpingo-oophorectomy
- Subtotal hysterectomy—removal of the uterus with conservation of the cervix, with or without bilateral salpingo-oophorectomy
- Radical hysterectomy—removal of uterus, cervix, both fallopian tubes, ovaries, part of the vagina, parametrium, and surrounding lymph nodes

The procedure is performed under general anaesthesia and the three different surgical approaches are: open abdominal hysterectomy, vaginal hysterectomy and laparoscopic-assisted vaginal hysterectomy (LAVH). The approach is dependent on surgical preference and also on indication, for example the open technique would be preferred for the removal of a large fibroid uterus or in the case of an ovarian tumour.

In the general, regardless of the approach, the procedure consists of removing the uterus from its supporting ligaments and ligating the uterine vessels. The uterus is either removed from the abdominal cavity or from the vagina. After the operation the woman will be infertile and if the ovaries are removed concurrently this will produce a surgical menopause. This needs to be discussed, along with the pros and cons of hormone replacement therapy, prior to the procedure.

Additional procedures that may become necessary

- Conversion of laparoscopic/vaginal approach to open abdominal approach
- Repair of damage to bowel/bladder/ureters/blood vessels

Benefits

- Removal of cancer
- Abolishes menstruation (thereby offering a definitive solution to menorrhagia and dysmenorrhoea)
- Relief of symptoms from uterine prolapse
- Relief of pressure symptoms from fibroids

Alternative procedures/conservative measures

- *Conservative*: uterine prolapse—pelvic floor exercises, weight loss, ring/shelf pessary. *Disadvantages*: less effective, non-curative
- *Medical*:
  - Menorrhagia—IUS (Mirena®), antifibrinolytics, e.g. tranexamic acid. *Disadvantages*: limited efficacy. IUS may be unsuitable in cases where uterine cavity is large or distorted by fibroids, non-curative
- *Surgical*:
  - Menorrhagia—endometrial ablation. *Disadvantages*: higher dissatisfaction rates compared to hysterectomy
  - Uterine fibroids—open/laparoscopic/hysteroscopic myomectomy, uterine artery embolization. *Disadvantages*: fibroids recur

Serious/frequently occurring risks

- *Common*: bleeding, pain, scarring, wound infection, surgical menopause
- *Occasional*: damage to ureters, bladder and bowel, thromboembolic disease
- *Rare*: future vault prolapse, adhesions leading to bowel obstruction

Blood transfusion necessary

- Group and save only, unless high blood loss suspected

Type of anaesthesia/sedation

- General anaesthesia

Follow-up/need for further procedure

- Outpatient clinic in 6/52 for histology results and to assess wound healing
- Routine cervical screening is no longer required except in cases of subtotal hysterectomy

Reference

1. Royal College of Obstetricians and Gynaecologists. *Consent Advice 4: Abdominal Hysterectomy for Benign Conditions.* London: RCOG, 2009.

Prolapse and incontinence surgery

Description

Urogenital prolapse is a condition in which the bladder, uterus, vaginal vault, and/or bowel protrudes into the vaginal canal. This can cause symptoms including a sensation of a lump within the vagina, constipation, stress incontinence, and dyspareunia.

If the anterior aspect of the vaginal wall weakens the bladder can protrude producing a cystocele. This is often managed with an anterior wall repair procedure (anterior colporrhaphy). Weakness of the posterior aspect of the vaginal wall leads to protrusion of the rectum forming a rectocoele, which can be treated with a posterior wall repair (posterior colporrhaphy). Uterine prolapse can be surgically managed with hysterectomy (usually performed vaginally), or with various suspension procedures. Vaginal vault prolapse can occur after hysterectomy and can be also be managed by suspension techniques.

Stress incontinence is a condition in which there is impaired urethral support from pelvic floor muscle weakness. As a result, there is leakage of urine with increases in abdominal pressure, for example with coughing or sneezing. Various surgical techniques, using an ever-evolving range of surgical materials, aim to lift the bladder neck to its original position and thereby achieve continence.

Procedures for prolapse and stress incontinence are often combined.

Additional procedures that may become necessary

- Conversion to laparotomy
- Repair of damaged bowel/bladder/ureters/urethra

Benefits

- To improve the symptoms of prolapse/stress incontinence

Alternative procedures/conservative measures

- *Conservative*:
  - Pelvic floor muscle exercises. *Disadvantages*: of unproven efficacy
  - Weight loss. *Disadvantages*: difficult to maintain
- *Medical*:
  - Vaginal pessary. *Disadvantages*: uncomfortable, risk of ulceration, implications for sexual intercourse, usually requires changing 6 monthly

Serious/frequently occurring risks

- *Common*: bleeding, pain, dyspareunia, infection (wound/urinary tract/ systemic, or of mesh requiring surgical removal), damage to bladder
- *Occasional*: urinary frequency, failure to control prolapse, recurrence of prolapse, new or continuing bladder dysfunction, need for long-term catheterization, risk of mesh erosion
- *Rare*: damage to ureters/bowel, thromboembolic disease

Blood transfusion necessary
- Occasionally/group and save

Type of anaesthesia/sedation
- Usually general anaesthesia

Follow-up/need for further procedure
- Outpatient clinic at 6–8 weeks to assess success of surgery

Reference

1. Royal College of Obstetricians and Gynaecologists. *Green-top Guideline No 35: Surgical Treatment of Urodynamic Stress Incontinence*. London: RCOG, 2003.

Example consent form for patients able to consent for themselves

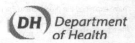

(DH) Department of Health

[NHS organisation name] consent form 1

Patient agreement to investigation or treatment

Patient details (or pre-printed label)

Patient's surname/family name.................................

Patient's first names ....

Date of birth ....

Responsible health professional.................................

Job title ....

NHS number (or other identifier).................................

☐ Male   ☐ Female

Special requirements ....
(eg other language/other communication method)

To be retained in patient's notes

Patient identifier/label

Name of proposed procedure or course of treatment (include brief

explanation if medical term not clear) ....

....

....

Statement of health professional (to be filled in by health professional with

appropriate knowledge of proposed procedure, as specified in consent policy)

I have explained the procedure to the patient. In particular, I have explained:

The intended benefits ....

....

....

Serious or frequently occurring risks ....

....

....

Any extra procedures which may become necessary during the procedure

☐ blood transfusion..

☐ other procedure (please specify) ....

....

I have also discussed what the procedure is likely to involve, the benefits and risks of any
available alternative treatments (including no treatment) and any particular concerns of this
patient.

☐ The following leaflet/tape has been provided ....

This procedure will involve:

☐ general and/or regional anaesthesia   ☐ local anaesthesia   ☐ sedation

Signed:................................   Date ....

Name (PRINT) ....   Job title ....

Contact details (if patient wishes to discuss options later) ....

Statement of interpreter (where appropriate)

I have interpreted the information above to the patient to the best of my ability and in a way
in which I believe s/he can understand.

Signed ....   Date ....

Name (PRINT) ....

Top copy accepted by patient: yes/no (please ring)

Statement of patient

Patient identifier/label

Please read this form carefully. If your treatment has been planned in advance, you should already have your own copy of page 2 which describes the benefits and risks of the proposed treatment. If not, you will be offered a copy now. If you have any further questions, do ask – we are here to help you. You have the right to change your mind at any time, including after you have signed this form.

I agree to the procedure or course of treatment described on this form.

I understand that you cannot give me a guarantee that a particular person will perform the procedure. The person will, however, have appropriate experience.

I understand that I will have the opportunity to discuss the details of anaesthesia with an anaesthetist before the procedure, unless the urgency of my situation prevents this. (This only applies to patients having general or regional anaesthesia.)

I understand that any procedure in addition to those described on this form will only be carried out if it is necessary to save my life or to prevent serious harm to my health.

I have been told about additional procedures which may become necessary during my treatment. I have listed below any procedures **which I do not wish to be carried out** without further discussion. ....
....
....
....

Patient's signature .... Date................................
Name (PRINT) ... .

A witness should sign below if the patient is unable to sign but has indicated his or her consent. Young people/children may also like a parent to sign here (see notes).

Signature .... Date ....
Name (PRINT) ....

Confirmation of consent (to be completed by a health professional when the patient is admitted for the procedure, if the patient has signed the form in advance)

On behalf of the team treating the patient, I have confirmed with the patient that s/he has no further questions and wishes the procedure to go ahead.

Signed:.. Date ....
Name (PRINT) .... Job title ....

Important notes: (tick if applicable)

☐ See also advance directive/living will (eg Jehovah's Witness form)

☐ Patient has withdrawn consent (ask patient to sign /date here) ....

Guidance to health professionals (to be read in conjunction with consent policy)

What a consent form is for

This form documents the patient's agreement to go ahead with the investigation or treatment you have proposed. It is not a legal waiver – if patients, for example, do not receive enough information on which to base their decision, then the consent may not be valid, even though the form has been signed. Patients are also entitled to change their mind after signing the form, if they retain capacity to do so. The form should act as an *aide-memoire* to health professionals and patients, by providing a check-list of the kind of information patients should be offered, and by enabling the patient to have a written record of the main points discussed. In no way, however, should the written information provided for the patient be regarded as a substitute for face-to-face discussions with the patient.

The law on consent

See the Department of Health's *Reference guide to consent for examination or treatment* for a comprehensive summary of the law on consent (also available at www.doh.gov.uk/consent).

Who can give consent

Everyone aged 16 or more is presumed to be competent to give consent for themselves, unless the opposite is demonstrated. If a child under the age of 16 has "sufficient understanding and intelligence to enable him or her to understand fully what is proposed", then he or she will be competent to give consent for himself or herself. Young people aged 16 and 17, and legally 'competent' younger children, may therefore sign this form for themselves, but may like a parent to countersign as well. If the child is not able to give consent for himself or herself, some-one with parental responsibility may do so on their behalf and a separate form is available for this purpose. Even where a child is able to give consent for himself or herself, you should always involve those with parental responsibility in the child's care, unless the child specifically asks you not to do so. If a patient is mentally competent to give consent but is physically unable to sign a form, you should complete this form as usual, and ask an independent witness to confirm that the patient has given consent orally or non-verbally.

When NOT to use this form

If the patient is 18 or over and is not legally competent to give consent, you should use form 4 (form for adults who are unable to consent to investigation or treatment) instead of this form. A patient will not be legally competent to give consent if:
*   they are unable to comprehend and retain information material to the decision and/or
*   they are unable to weigh and use this information in coming to a decision.
You should always take all reasonable steps (for example involving more specialist colleagues) to support a patient in making their own decision, before concluding that they are unable to do so. Relatives **cannot** be asked to sign this form on behalf of an adult who is not legally competent to consent for himself or herself.

Information

Information about what the treatment will involve, its benefits and risks (including side-effects and complications) and the alternatives to the particular procedure proposed, is crucial for patients when making up their minds. The courts have stated that patients should be told about 'significant risks which would affect the judgement of a reasonable patient'. 'Significant' has not been legally defined, but the GMC requires doctors to tell patients about 'serious or frequently occurring' risks. In addition if patients make clear they have particular concerns about certain kinds of risk, you should make sure they are informed about these risks, even if they are very small or rare. You should always answer questions honestly. Sometimes, patients may make it clear that they do not want to have any information about the options, but want you to decide on their behalf. In such circumstances, you should do your best to ensure that the patient receives at least very basic information about what is proposed. Where information is refused, you should document this on page 2 of the form or in the patient's notes.

Example consent form for those with parental responsibility consenting on behalf of a child

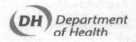

(DH) Department of Health

[NHS organisation name]
consent form 2

Parental agreement to investigation or treatment for a child or young person

Patient details (or pre-printed label)
Patient's surname/family name....................................
Patient's first names ....
Date of birth ....
Age ....
Responsible health professional....................................
Job title ....
NHS number (or other identifier)....................................
☐ Male ☐ Female
Special requirements .... (eg other language/other communication method)

To be retained in patient's notes

Patient identifier/label

Name of proposed procedure or course of treatment (include brief explanation if medical term not clear) ....
....
....

Statement of health professional (to be filled in by health professional with appropriate knowledge of proposed procedure, as specified in consent policy)

I have explained the procedure to the child and his or her parent(s). In particular, I have explained:

The intended benefits ....
....
Serious or frequently occurring risks ....
....
....

Any extra procedures which may become necessary during the procedure

☐ blood transfusion..

☐ other procedure (please specify) ....
....

I have also discussed what the procedure is likely to involve, the benefits and risks of any available alternative treatments (including no treatment) and any particular concerns of this patient and his or her parents.

☐ The following leaflet/tape has been provided ....

This procedure will involve:

☐ general and/or regional anaesthesia   ☐ local anaesthesia   ☐ sedation

Signed:..   Date ....
Name (PRINT) ....   Job title ....

Contact details (if child/parent wish to discuss options later) ....

Statement of interpreter (where appropriate)

I have interpreted the information above to the child and his or her parents to the best of my ability and in a way in which I believe they can understand.

Signed ....   Date ....
Name (PRINT) ....

Top copy accepted by patient: yes/no (please ring)

Statement of parent

Patient identifier/label

Please read this form carefully. If the procedure has been planned in advance, you should already have your own copy of page 2 which describes the benefits and risks of the proposed treatment. If not, you will be offered a copy now. If you have any further questions, do ask – we are here to help you and your child. You have the right to change your mind at any time, including after you have signed this form.

I agree to the procedure or course of treatment described on this form and **I confirm** that I have 'parental responsibility' for this child.

I understand that you cannot give me a guarantee that a particular person will perform the procedure. The person will, however, have appropriate experience.

I understand that my child and I will have the opportunity to discuss the details of anaesthesia with an anaesthetist before the procedure, unless the urgency of the situation prevents this. (This only applies to children having general or regional anaesthesia.)

I understand that any procedure in addition to those described on this form will only be carried out if it is necessary to save the life of my child or to prevent serious harm to his or her health.

I have been told about additional procedures which may become necessary during my child's treatment. I have listed below any **procedures which I do not wish to be carried out** without further discussion. ....
....
....
....

Signature .... Date.............................
Name (PRINT) ....Relationship to child..............................

Child's agreement to treatment (if child wishes to sign)

I agree to have the treatment I have been told about.

Name .... Signature ....
Date ....

Confirmation of consent (to be completed by a health professional when the child is admitted for the procedure, if the parent/child have signed the form in advance)

On behalf of the team treating the patient, I have confirmed with the child and his or her parent(s) that they have no further questions and wish the procedure to go ahead.

Signed:............ .... Date ....
Name (PRINT) .... Job title ....

Important notes: (tick if applicable)

☐ See also advance directive/living will (eg Jehovah's Witness form)

☐ Parent has withdrawn consent (ask parent to sign /date here) ....

Guidance to health professionals (to be read in conjunction with consent policy)

This form

This form should be used to document consent to a child's treatment, where that consent is being given by a person with parental responsibility for the child. The term 'parent' has been used in this form as a shorthand for 'person with parental responsibility'. Where children are legally competent to consent for themselves (see below), they may sign the standard 'adult' consent form (form 1). There is space on that form for a parent to countersign if a competent child wishes them to do so.

Who can give consent

Everyone aged 16 or more is presumed to be competent to give consent for themselves, unless the opposite is demonstrated. The courts have stated that if a child under the age of 16 has "sufficient understanding and intelligence to enable him or her to understand fully what is proposed", then he or she will be competent to give consent for himself or herself. If children are not able to give consent for themselves, some-one with parental responsibility may do so on their behalf.

Although children acquire rights to give consent for themselves as they grow older, people with 'parental responsibility' for a child retain the right to give consent on the child's behalf until the child reaches the age of 18. Therefore, for a number of years, both the child and a person with parental responsibility have the right to give consent to the child's treatment. In law, health professionals only need the consent of one appropriate person before providing treatment. This means that in theory it is lawful to provide treatment to a child under 18 which a person with parental responsibility has authorised, even if the child refuses. As a matter of good practice, however, you should always seek a competent child's consent before providing treatment unless any delay involved in doing so would put the child's life or health at risk. Younger children should also be as involved as possible in decisions about their healthcare. Further advice is given in the Department's guidance *Seeking consent: working with children*. Any differences of opinion between the child and their parents, or between parents, should be clearly documented in the patient's notes.

Parental responsibility

The person(s) with parental responsibility will usually, but not invariably, be the child's birth parents. People with parental responsibility for a child include: the child's mother; the child's father if married to the mother at the child's conception, birth or later; a legally appointed guardian; the local authority if the child is on a care order; or a person named in a residence order in respect of the child. Fathers who have never been married to the child's mother will only have parental responsibility if they have acquired it through a court order or parental responsibility agreement (although this may change in the future).

Information

Information about what the treatment will involve, its benefits and risks (including side-effects and complications) and the alternatives to the particular procedure proposed, is crucial for children and their parents when making up their minds about treatment. The courts have stated that patients should be told about 'significant risks which would affect the judgement of a reasonable patient'. 'Significant' has not been legally defined, but the GMC requires doctors to tell patients about 'serious or frequently occurring' risks. In addition if patients make clear they have particular concerns about certain kinds of risk, you should make sure they are informed about these risks, even if they are very small or rare. You should always answer questions honestly.

Guidance on the law on consent

See the Department of Health publications *Reference guide to consent for examination or treatment* and *Seeking consent: working with children* for a comprehensive summary of the law on consent (also available at www.doh.gov.uk/consent).

Example consent form for procedures performed with no impairment of consciousness

[NHS organisation name] consent form 3

Patient identifier/label

Patient/parental agreement to investigation or treatment

(procedures where consciousness not impaired)

Name of procedure (include brief explanation if medical term not clear)

....

....

Statement of health professional (to be filled in by health professional with appropriate knowledge of proposed procedure, as specified in consent policy)

I have explained the procedure to the patient/parent. In particular, I have explained:
The intended benefits ....

....

....

Serious or frequently occurring risks:...

....

....

I have also discussed what the procedure is likely to involve, the benefits and risks of any available alternative treatments (including no treatment) and any particular concerns of those involved.

☐ The following leaflet/tape has been provided ....

Signed: .... Date ....
Name (PRINT) .... Job title ....

Statement of interpreter (where appropriate)
I have interpreted the information above to the patient/parent to the best of my ability and in a way in which I believe s/he/they can understand.

Signed ....Date....................Name (PRINT).............................

Statement of patient/person with parental responsibility for patient
I agree to the procedure described above.

I understand that you cannot give me a guarantee that a particular person will perform the procedure. The person will, however, have appropriate experience.

I understand that the procedure will/will not involve local anaesthesia.

Signature .... Date ....
Name (PRINT) .... Relationship to patient ....

Confirmation of consent (to be completed by a health professional when the patient is admitted for the procedure, if the patient/parent has signed the form in advance)

I have confirmed that the patient/parent has no further questions and wishes the procedure to go ahead.

Signed: .... Date ....
Name (PRINT) .... Job title ....

Top copy accepted by patient: yes/no (please ring)

Guidance to health professionals (to be read in conjunction with consent policy)

This form
This form documents the patient's agreement (or that of a person with parental responsibility for the patient) to go ahead with the investigation or treatment you have proposed. **It is only designed for procedures where the patient is expected to remain alert throughout and where an anaesthetist is not involved in their care: for example for drug therapy where written consent is deemed appropriate.** In other circumstances you should use either form 1 (for adults/competent children) or form 2 (parental consent for children/young people) as appropriate.

Consent forms are not legal waivers – if patients, for example, do not receive enough information on which to base their decision, then the consent may not be valid, even though the form has been signed. Patients also have every right to change their mind after signing the form.

Who can give consent
Everyone aged 16 or more is presumed to be competent to give consent for themselves, unless the opposite is demonstrated. If a child under the age of 16 has "sufficient understanding and intelligence to enable him or her to understand fully what is proposed", then he or she will be competent to give consent for himself or herself. Young people aged 16 and 17, and legally 'competent' younger children, may therefore sign this form for themselves, if they wish. If the child is not able to give consent for himself or herself, some-one with parental responsibility may do so on their behalf. Even where a child is able to give consent for himself or herself, you should always involve those with parental responsibility in the child's care, unless the child specifically asks you not to do so. If a patient is mentally competent to give consent but is physically unable to sign a form, you should complete this form as usual, and ask an independent witness to confirm that the patient has given consent orally or non-verbally.

When NOT to use this form (see also 'This form' above)
If the patient is 18 or over and is not legally competent to give consent, you should use form 4 (form for adults who are unable to consent to investigation or treatment) instead of this form. A patient will not be legally competent to give consent if:
• they are unable to comprehend and retain information material to the decision and/or
• they are unable to weigh and use this information in coming to a decision.
You should always take all reasonable steps (for example involving more specialist colleagues) to support a patient in making their own decision, before concluding that they are unable to do so. Relatives **cannot** be asked to sign this form on behalf of an adult who is not legally competent to consent for himself or herself.

Information
Information about what the treatment will involve, its benefits and risks (including side-effects and complications) and the alternatives to the particular procedure proposed, is crucial for patients when making up their minds about treatment. The courts have stated that patients should be told about 'significant risks which would affect the judgement of a reasonable patient'. 'Significant' has not been legally defined, but the GMC requires doctors to tell patients about 'serious or frequently occurring' risks. In addition if patients make clear they have particular concerns about certain kinds of risk, you should make sure they are informed about these risks, even if they are very small or rare. You should always answer questions honestly. Sometimes, patients may make it clear that they do not want to have any information about the options, but want you to decide on their behalf. In such circumstances, you should do your best to ensure that the patient receives at least very basic information about what is proposed. Where information is refused, you should document this overleaf or in the patient's notes.

The law on consent
See the Department of Health's *Reference guide to consent for examination or treatment* for a comprehensive summary of the law on consent (also available at www.doh.gov.uk/consent).

Example consent form for adults without capacity to consent for themselves

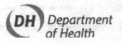

(DH) *Department of Health*

**[NHS organisation name]
consent form 4**

Form for adults who are unable to consent to investigation or treatment

---

Patient details (or pre-printed label)

Patient's surname/family name.................................

Patient's first names ....

Date of birth ....

Responsible health professional..............................

Job title ....

NHS number (or other identifier)............................

☐ Male   ☐ Female

Special requirements ....
(eg other language/other communication method)

To be retained in patient's notes

Patient identifier/label

All sections to be completed by health professional proposing the procedure

A Details of procedure or course of treatment proposed

(NB see guidance to health professionals overleaf for details of situations where court approval must first be sought)

B Assessment of patient's capacity

I confirm that the patient lacks capacity to give or withhold consent to this procedure or course of treatment because:

the patient is unable to comprehend and retain information material to the decision; and/or

the patient is unable to use and weigh this information in the decision-making process; or

the patient is unconscious

Further details (excluding where patient unconscious): for example how above judgements reached; which colleagues consulted; what attempts made to assist the patient make his or her own decision and why these were not successful.

C Assessment of patient's best interests

To the best of my knowledge, the patient has not refused this procedure in a valid advance directive. Where possible and appropriate, I have consulted with colleagues and those close to the patient, and I believe the procedure to be in the patient's best interests because:

(Where incapacity is likely to be temporary, for example if patient unconscious, or where patient has fluctuating capacity)

The treatment cannot wait until the patient recovers capacity because:

D Involvement of the patient's family and others close to the patient

The final responsibility for determining whether a procedure is in an incapacitated patient's best interests lies with the health professional performing the procedure. However, it is good practice to consult with those close to the patient (eg spouse/partner, family and friends, carer, supporter or advocate) unless you have good reason to believe that the patient would not have wished particular individuals to be consulted, or unless the urgency of their situation prevents this. "Best interests" go far wider than "best medical interests", and include factors such as the patient's wishes and beliefs when competent, their current wishes, their general well-being and their spiritual and religious welfare.

(to be signed by a person or persons close to the patient, if they wish)

I/We have been involved in a discussion with the relevant health professionals over the treatment of ....(patient's name). I/We understand that he/she is unable to give his/her own consent, based on the criteria set out in this form. I/We also understand that treatment can lawfully be provided if it is in his/her best interests to receive it.

Any other comments (including any concerns about decision)

Name ....Relationship to patient................................. ....
Address (if not the same as patient.. ....
....
....

Signature .... Date........................ ....

If a person close to the patient was not available in person, has this matter been discussed in any other way (eg over the telephone)?

☐ Yes   ☐ No

Details:

Signature of health professional proposing treatment

The above procedure is, in my clinical judgement, in the best interests of the patient, who lacks capacity to consent for himself or herself. Where possible and appropriate I have discussed the patient's condition with those close to him or her, and taken their knowledge of the patient's views and beliefs into account in determining his or her best interests.

I have/have not sought a second opinion.

Signature:........... .... Date .. ..
Name (PRINT) .... Job title ....

Where second opinion sought, s/he should sign below to confirm agreement:

Signature:.. Date .. ..
Name (PRINT) .... Job title ....

Guidance to health professionals (to be read in conjunction with consent policy)

This form should only be used where it would be usual to seek written consent but an adult patient (18 or over) lacks capacity to give or withhold consent to treatment. If an adult **has** capacity to accept or refuse treatment, you should use the standard consent form and respect any refusal. Where treatment is very urgent (for example if the patient is critically ill), it may not be feasible to fill in a form at the time, but you should document your clinical decisions appropriately afterwards. If treatment is being provided under the authority of Part IV of the *Mental Health Act 1983*, different legal provisions apply and you are required to fill in more specialised forms (although in some circumstances you may find it helpful to use this form as well). If the adult now lacks capacity, but has clearly refused particular treatment in advance of their loss of capacity (for example in an advance directive or 'living will'), then you must abide by that refusal if it was validly made and is applicable to the circumstances. For further information on the law on consent, see the Department of Health's *Reference guide to consent for examination or treatment* (www.doh.gov.uk/consent).

When treatment can be given to a patient who is unable to consent

For treatment to be given to a patient who is unable to consent, the following **must** apply:
- the patient must lack the capacity ('competence') to give or withhold consent to this procedure AND
- the procedure must be in the patient's best interests.

Capacity

A patient will lack capacity to consent to a particular intervention if he or she is:
- unable to comprehend and retain information material to the decision, especially as to the consequences of having, or not having, the intervention in question; and/or
- unable to use and weigh this information in the decision-making process.

Before making a judgement that a patient lacks capacity you must take all steps reasonable in the circumstances to assist the patient in taking their own decisions (this will clearly not apply if the patient is unconscious). This may involve explaining what is involved in very simple language, using pictures and communication and decision-aids as appropriate. People close to the patient (spouse/partner, family, friends and carers) may often be able to help, as may specialist colleagues such as speech and language therapists or learning disability teams, and independent advocates or supporters.

Capacity is 'decision-specific': a patient may lack capacity to take a particular complex decision, but be quite able to take other more straight-forward decisions or parts of decisions.

Best interests

A patient's best interests are not limited to their best medical interests. Other factors which form part of the best interests decision include:
- the wishes and beliefs of the patient when competent
- their current wishes
- their general well-being
- their spiritual and religious welfare

Two incapacitated patients, whose *physical* condition is identical, may therefore have different best interests.

Unless the patient has clearly indicated that particular individuals should not be involved in their care, or unless the urgency of their situation prevents it, you should attempt to involve people close to the patient (spouse/partner, family and friends, carer, supporter or advocate) in the decision-making process. Those close to the patient cannot require you to provide particular treatment which you do not believe to be clinically appropriate. However they will know the patient much better than you do, and therefore are likely to be able to provide valuable information about the patient's wishes and values.

Second opinions and court involvement

Where treatment is complex and/or people close to the patient express doubts about the proposed treatment, a second opinion should be sought, unless the urgency of the patient's condition prevents this. Donation of regenerative tissue such as bone marrow, sterilisation for contraceptive purposes and withdrawal of artificial nutrition or hydration from a patient in PVS must never be undertaken without prior High Court approval. High Court approval can also be sought where there are doubts about the patient's capacity or best interests.

Index